Falls in Older People

Falls in Older People

Risk Factors, Strategies for Prevention and Implications for Practice

Third Edition

Edited by

Stephen R. Lord
Neuroscience Research Australia and University of New South Wales

Catherine Sherrington
Sydney Local Health District and University of Sydney

Vasi Naganathan
Concord Hospital and University of Sydney

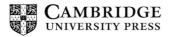
CAMBRIDGE
UNIVERSITY PRESS

CAMBRIDGE
UNIVERSITY PRESS

University Printing House, Cambridge CB2 8BS, United Kingdom

One Liberty Plaza, 20th Floor, New York, NY 10006, USA

477 Williamstown Road, Port Melbourne, VIC 3207, Australia

314–321, 3rd Floor, Plot 3, Splendor Forum, Jasola District Centre,
New Delhi – 110025, India

103 Penang Road, #05–06/07, Visioncrest Commercial, Singapore 238467

Cambridge University Press is part of the University of Cambridge.

It furthers the University's mission by disseminating knowledge in the pursuit of
education, learning, and research at the highest international levels of excellence.

www.cambridge.org
Information on this title: www.cambridge.org/9781108706087
DOI: 10.1017/9781108594455

First published 2001

Second Edition 2007

Third Edition 2021

Printed in the United Kingdom by TJ Books Limited, Padstow Cornwall

A catalogue record for this publication is available from the British Library.

ISBN 978-1-108-70608-7 Paperback

Cambridge University Press has no responsibility for the persistence or accuracy of
URLs for external or third-party internet websites referred to in this publication
and does not guarantee that any content on such websites is, or will remain,
accurate or appropriate.

Every effort has been made in preparing this book to provide accurate and up-to-date information
that is in accord with accepted standards and practice at the time of publication. Although case
histories are drawn from actual cases, every effort has been made to disguise the identities of the
individuals involved. Nevertheless, the authors, editors, and publishers can make no warranties that
the information contained herein is totally free from error, not least because clinical standards are
constantly changing through research and regulation. The authors, editors, and publishers therefore
disclaim all liability for direct or consequential damages resulting from the use of material contained
in this book. Readers are strongly advised to pay careful attention to information provided by the
manufacturer of any drugs or equipment that they plan to use.

Contents

Preface

In the preface to the second edition of our book published in 2005, we remarked on the large amount of work on risk factors for falls in older people and fall prevention strategies published in the preceding 25 years. Since then, a further 15,000 articles and reviews have been published on this topic in the international literature (see Figure 0.1) and there have been many substantial gains in the evidence base that have increased our understanding of fall risk factors, prevention strategies, and how to translate this research into practice. The aim of this third edition of our book is to review and incorporate this new material to provide researchers, students, and health care workers with a means for gaining access to current thinking and best clinical practice. Listed below are some highlights of progress and encouraging findings.

- Studies aimed at understanding balance have used paradigms such as tripping, slipping, and stepping to more accurately reflect situations in which people fall.
- A large body of neuropsychological research has shown that balance activities that were generally considered to be reflex or automatic require attention, and that impaired executive functioning is an important risk factor for falls.
- New wearable sensor technologies have allowed mobility and fall risk to be remotely assessed, paving the way for unobtrusive at-home monitoring.
- Several cognitive-motor interventions comprising exergames have been evaluated in randomized controlled trials, where they have been shown to improve balance. These may be an enjoyable way to facilitate adherence.
- Cognitive behaviour therapy in association with exercise can substantially reduce fear of falling.
- Systematic reviews have synthesized the findings of randomized controlled trials that have examined the effects of a range of exercise interventions in preventing falls in community dwellers. From this large body of evidence, it is now possible to conclude that effective exercise programs must comprise challenging, weight-bearing balance exercises.

- It is less clear how to prevent falls in residential care, but a recent well-designed randomized controlled trial has shown that an exercise intervention can prevent falls in nursing home residents.
- Several fall prevention interventions have now also been demonstrated to be cost-effective, again particularly exercise interventions in community dwellers.

Two areas of investigation have been less encouraging and will require further research and consideration.

- Intervention studies aimed at preventing falls in frail older people including those with dementia and stroke, have generally not been successful, despite well planned and executed studies.
- A further large trial of risk-factor-based assessment and intervention in the hospitals setting has failed to prevent falls. The most promising interventions to date have involved communication with patients and carers so future research could focus on this area.

The growing literature is evidenced by the change in the title to include implications for practice and the increase in chapters, from 18 to 31, with the new chapters addressing exciting new research and implementation areas developed over the last decade. This edition also differs from the previous two in that the editors have enlisted the assistance of multiple authors who are expert in the book chapter fields.

As suggested by the title, the book has three major themes: fall risk factors, fall prevention strategies, and implications for practice. Part 1 includes an initial chapter on the epidemiology of falls and fall-related injuries in older people. Chapters 2 to 12 present critical appraisals of fall risk factors addressed under the headings of postural stability, gait, sensory and neuromuscular, biomechanics, feet and footwear, brain function, cognition, depression and fear of falling, medical, medication, and environmental risk factors. Chapter 13 reviews research from the emerging field of fall detection with new technologies and Chapter 14 presents findings in fall risk screening and assessment. The final chapter weighs the importance of the risk factors described in the above chapters as weak, moderate, or strong, using a simple evidence-based metric.

Part 2 commences with an overview of fall prevention strategies that address the multitude of fall risk factors. Chapters 16 to 23 summarize the published findings on 'single' strategies for addressing fall risk: exercise, step training, exergames, cognitive behaviour therapy, medical management, vision correction, use of safe footwear, aids and appliances, and environmental modifications. Chapter 24 addresses strategies for minimizing fall injury, Chapter 25 summarizes the evidence for multi-factorial interventions to prevent falls, and the final two chapters (Chapters 26 and 27) discuss suggested strategies for preventing falls in hospitals and residential aged care.

Part 3 synthesizes the information on successful fall prevention strategies in a format that can be used to facilitate the translation of research findings into clinical practice. It contains chapters on behaviour change, research translation, health economics of fall prevention strategies, and optimal interventions for specific sub-groups of older people. The final chapter reviews the research and clinical practice issues that still need to be addressed in this field.

In each chapter we have attempted to be analytical in nature. Thus, we have not simply presented lists of the many and varied factors that have been suggested as possible (but unproven) risk factors for falls and the suggested (but untested) fall prevention strategies. Instead, we have attempted to evaluate the evidence for each factor implicated with falls to determine whether they constitute important areas for consideration and intervention. For example, we present arguments that challenge some traditional approaches to the management of older persons at risk of falls. We question the utility of fall risk assessment based solely on diagnoses of disease processes and the value of standard clinical tests of vision, sensation, strength, and balance. We also discuss the role of particular medications in predisposing older people to falls and why factors such as alcohol use, vestibular disorders, and postural hypotension have not often been shown to be

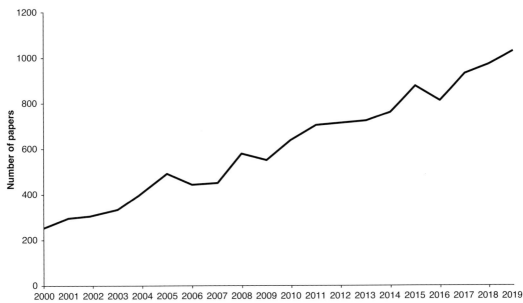

Figure 0.1   Research publications pertaining to falls in people between 2000 and 2019 (source: PubMed).

significant risk factors for falls in well-planned epidemiological studies. With regard to interventions, we examine the effectiveness of suggested strategies for preventing falls and attempt to unravel why many fall prevention interventions have not been effective.

We hope our book will be of interest to medical practitioners, nurses, physiotherapists, occupational therapists, podiatrists, research workers in the fields of gerontology and geriatrics, health service managers, medical and allied health care undergraduate and postgraduate students, scientists, and health care workers in the disciplines of public health, injury, and occupational health. We feel that this book is of relevance to those working in community, hospital, and residential aged care settings.

Contributors

Clemens Becker, Department of Clinical Gerontology, Robert-Bosch-Hospital, Auerbachstr. 110, 70376 Stuttgart, Germany

Matthew A. Brodie, Falls, Balance and Injury Research Centre, Neuroscience Research Australia, Sydney, NSW, Australia and Graduate School of Biomedical Engineering, Faculty of Engineering, UNSW Sydney, Sydney, NSW, Australia

Michele Callisaya, Menzies Institute for Medical Research, University of Tasmania, Hobart, Tasmania, Australia and Peninsula Clinical School, Central Clinical School, Monash University, Melbourne, Victoria, Australia

Ian Cameron, John Walsh Centre for Rehabilitation Research, Kolling Institute of Medical Research, The University of Sydney, Sydney, NSW, Australia

Lindy Clemson, Faculty of Health Sciences, The University of Sydney, Sydney, NSW, Australia

Carly Chaplin, Falls, Balance and Injury Research Centre, Neuroscience Research Australia, Sydney, NSW, Australia

Jennifer C. Davis, Centre for Hip Health and Mobility, Vancouver Coastal Health Research Institute, The University of British Columbia, Vancouver, Canada and Faculty of Management, The University of British Columbia-Okanagan, Kelowna, Canada

Kim Delbaere, Falls, Balance and Injury Research Centre, Neuroscience Research Australia, UNSW Sydney, NSW, Australia and School of Public Health and Community Medicine, UNSW Sydney, Sydney, NSW, Australia

Nicola Fairhall, Institute for Musculoskeletal Health, School of Public Health, Sydney Medical School, The University of Sydney, Sydney, NSW, Australia

Thomas Hadjistavropoulos, Department of Psychology and Centre on Aging and Health, University of Regina, Regina, Saskatchewan, Canada

Leanne Hassett, Institute for Musculoskeletal Health, School of Public Health, Sydney Medical School, The University of Sydney, Sydney, NSW, Australia

Cameron Hicks, Falls, Balance and Injury Research Centre, Neuroscience Research Australia, Sydney, NSW, Australia

Anne-Marie Hill, School of Physiotherapy and Exercise Science, Faculty of Health Sciences, Curtin University, Perth, Western Australia, Australia

Chun-Liang Hsu, Aging, Mobility and Cognitive Neuroscience Lab, Department of Physical Therapy, The University of British Columbia, Vancouver, Canada

Oshadi Jayakody, Menzies Research Institute, University of Tasmania, Hobart, Australia

Alexandra M.B. Korall, Simon Fraser University, Burnaby, British Columbia, Canada and Centre for Hip Health and Mobility, Vancouver, British Columbia, Canada

Susan Kurrle, Cognitive Decline Partnership Centre, Faculty of Medicine and Health, The University of Sydney, Sydney, NSW, Australia

Sarah E. Lamb Mireille Gillings Professor of Health Innovation, University of Exeter, Institute of Health Research, College of Medicine and Health, St Luke's Campus, Heavitree Road, Exeter, UK

Mark D. Latt, Sydney Medical School, The University of Sydney, Sydney, NSW, Australia, and Geriatrician, Royal Prince Alfred Hospital, Sydney, NSW, Australia

Teresa Liu-Ambrose, Aging, Mobility, and Cognitive Neuroscience Lab, Department of Physical Therapy, The University of British Columbia, Vancouver, British Columbia, Canada

Hopin Lee, Centre for Statistics in Medicine, Rehabilitation Research in Oxford, Nuffield Department of Orthopaedics Rheumatology and Musculoskeletal Sciences (NDORMS), University of Oxford, Oxford, UK and School of Medicine and Public Health, University of Newcastle, Newcastle, NSW, Australia

Stephen R. Lord, Falls, Balance and Injury Research Centre, Neuroscience Research Australia, Sydney, NSW, Australia and School of Public Health and Community Medicine, UNSW Sydney, Sydney, NSW, Australia

Lulu Ma, Department of Geriatric Medicine, Prince of Wales Hospital, Sydney, NSW, Australia

Jasmine C. Menant, Falls, Balance and Injury Research Centre, Neuroscience Research Australia, Sydney, NSW, Australia and School of Public Health and Community Medicine, UNSW Sydney, Sydney, NSW, Australia

Hylton B. Menz, La Trobe Sport and Exercise Medicine Research Centre and School of Allied Health, Human Services and Sport, College of Science, Health and Engineering, La Trobe University, Melbourne, Victoria, Australia

Vasi Naganathan, Centre for Education and Research on Ageing, The University of Sydney, Sydney, NSW, Australia and Concord Repatriation General Hospital, Sydney, NSW, Australia

Naomi Noguchi, School of Public Health, Faculty of Medicine and Health, The University of Sydney, Sydney, New South Wales, Australia

Yoshiro Okubo, Falls, Balance and Injury Research Centre, Neuroscience Research Australia, Sydney, NSW, Australia and School of Public Health and Community Medicine, UNSW Sydney, Sydney, NSW, Australia

Alison Pighills, Mackay Institute of Research and Innovation, Mackay Hospital and Health Service and the College of Healthcare Sciences, James Cook University, Townsville, Qld, Australia

Kilian Rapp, Department of Clinical Gerontology, Robert-Bosch-Hospital, Auerbachstr. 110, 70376 Stuttgart, Germany

Patrick Roigk, Department of Clinical Gerontology, Robert-Bosch-Hospital, Auerbachstr. 110, 70376 Stuttgart, Germany

Daniel S. Schoene, Institute of Medical Physics, Friedrich-Alexander-Universität Erlangen-Nürnberg, Erlangen, Bayern, Germany

Catherine Sherrington, Institute for Musculoskeletal Health, School of Public Health, Sydney Medical School, The University of Sydney, Sydney, NSW, Australia

Kathryn M. Sibley, Department of Community Health Sciences, University of Manitoba, Winnipeg, Canada, and Toronto Rehabilitation Institute- University Health Network, Toronto, Canada

Daina L. Sturnieks, Falls, Balance and Injury Research Centre, Neuroscience Research Australia, Sydney, NSW, Australia and School of Public Health and Community Medicine, UNSW Sydney, Sydney NSW, Australia

Morag E. Taylor, Falls, Balance and Injury Research Centre, Neuroscience Research Australia, Sydney, NSW, Australia and Prince of Wales Clinical School, Medicine, UNSW Sydney, Sydney, NSW, Australia

Anne Tiedemann, Institute for Musculoskeletal Health, School of Public Health, Sydney Medical School, The University of Sydney, Sydney, NSW, Australia

Alexie J. Touchette, Department of Community Health Sciences Rady Faculty of Health Sciences, University of Manitoba, Winnipeg, Canada

Kimberley S. van Schooten, Falls, Balance and Injury Research Centre, Neuroscience Research Australia, Sydney, NSW, Australia and School of Public Health and Community Medicine, UNSW Sydney, Sydney, NSW, Australia

Julie Whitney, School of Population Health and Environmental Sciences, King's College London, London, UK and Department of Clinical Gerontology, King's College Hospital, London, UK

G.A. Rixt Zijlstra, Department of Health Services Research, Care and Public Health Research Institute (CAPHRI), Maastricht University, Maastricht, The Netherlands

Part I

Epidemiology and Risk Factors for Falls

Epidemiology of Falls and Fall-Related Injuries

Stephen R. Lord, Catherine Sherrington, and Cameron Hicks

In this chapter, we examine the epidemiology of falls in older people. We review the major studies that have described the incidence of falls, the locations where falls occur, and falls sequelae. We also examine the costs required to treat and manage fall-related injuries. Before addressing these issues, however, it is helpful to briefly discuss three important methodological considerations that are relevant to all research studies of falls in older people: how falls are defined, how falls are counted, and what constitutes an older person.

The Definition of a Fall

In 1987, the Kellogg International Working Group on the Prevention of Falls in the Elderly defined a fall as 'unintentionally coming to the ground or some lower level and other than as a consequence of sustaining a violent blow, loss of consciousness, sudden onset of paralysis as in stroke or an epileptic seizure' [1]. Since then, many researchers have used this or very similar definitions of a fall. The Kellogg definition is appropriate for studies aimed at identifying factors that impair sensorimotor function and balance control, whereas broader definitions that include dizziness and loss of consciousness are appropriate for studies that also address cardiovascular and neurological causes of falls such as syncope, postural hypotension, and transient ischaemic attacks.

The Prevention of Falls Network Europe (ProFaNE) collaborators, in conjunction with international experts in the field and using consensus methodology, adopted a simpler definition to include falls that occur from all causes, i.e. 'an unexpected event in which the participant comes to rest on the ground, floor or lower level' [2]. A comparable definition has also been adopted by the World Health Organization.[1] This simple definition is appropriate for multi-centre studies requiring a core data set or for situations where details of falls are

---

[1] www.who.int/news-room/fact-sheets/detail/falls

unrecorded (routine surveillance data/accident records) or where a high proportion of participants cannot provide reliable information about their falls (i.e. those with delirium and cognitive impairment).

Although falls are often referred to as accidents, it has been shown statistically that fall incidence differs significantly from a Poisson distribution [3]. This implies that causal processes are involved in falls and that they are not merely random events.

Falls Ascertainment

The earliest published studies on falls were retrospective in design, in that they asked participants whether and/or how many times they had fallen over a defined period of time – usually 12 months. This approach has limitations in that participants have only limited accuracy in remembering falls over a prolonged period [4]. Prospective designs, in which participants are followed up for a period, again usually 12 months, to more accurately determine the incidence of falling, have also been conducted. Not surprisingly, these studies have usually reported higher rates of falling. In community studies, despite new technologies designed to detect falls (see Chapter 13), ascertaining falls by self-report remains the most feasible method. Methods used to record falls in prospective follow-up periods include monthly or bi-monthly mail-out questionnaires [5, 6], weekly [7] or monthly falls calendars [8], and monthly telephone interviews [9].

The ProFaNE collaborators recommend that falls should be recorded using prospective daily recording and a notification system with a minimum of monthly reporting [2]. Telephone or face-to-face interview should be used to obtain missing data and to ascertain further details of falls and injuries. Specific information about the circumstances of any falls can also be determined with additional questions on falls diary forms. Current studies are providing the option for calendars to be completed online. Telephone interviews gain the same information as mail-out questionnaires and falls diaries but may require many calls to contact active older people. In research studies fall data should be summarized as: number of falls, number of fallers/non-fallers/frequent fallers, and fall rate per person years [2] with the rate of falls often being used as the primary outcome. In trials it is recommended that staff collecting fall data be masked to group allocation.

However, even with the most rigorous reporting methodology, it is quite likely that falls are under-reported and that data regarding circumstances surrounding falls are sometimes incomplete or inaccurate. After a fall, older people are often shocked and distressed and may not remember the predisposing factors that led to the fall. Denial is also a factor in under-reporting, as it is common for older people to lay blame on external factors for their fall, and not count it as a 'true' one. Simply forgetting falls leads to further under-reporting, especially in those with cognitive impairment. New technologies now allow for automatic detection of falls and remote monitoring of fall risk in daily life. However, despite encouraging results in controlled settings, these technologies are not yet ready for clinical use – see Chapter 13.

In residential aged care settings, the use of online incident monitoring systems maintained by nursing staff can provide an ancillary method for improving the accuracy of recording falls. In a study of intermediate care (hostel) residents in Sydney, Lord et al. [5] found that systematic recording of falls by nurses increased the number of falls reported by 32%. In hospitals, falls monitoring systems are now commonly used, but trials of fall prevention intervention often supplement these with additional methods such as medical records audits and verbal reports from staff [10].

The Definition of a Fall-Related Injury

The definitions of injurious falls have differed considerably in the literature, due primarily to whether or not minor injuries such as bruises, cuts, and abrasions have been classified as fall-related injuries. The ProFaNE collaborators recommend that due to difficulties in standardizing definitions and classifications of falls injury types, the most rigorous definition of a fall-related injury is radiologically confirmed peripheral fractures, i.e. fractures of the limbs and limb girdles [2]. More recently, it has been acknowledged that the definition of an injurious fall should be expanded to include traumatic brain injury. In recent years traumatic brain injuries due to falls have increased significantly, with associated increases in hospitalizations, disability and death [11].

The Definition of the Older Person

There is no consistency among studies as to what demographic group constitutes older people. The term is used for age groups starting from as low as 50 years. However, the most frequently used definition is people aged 65 years and over. Within this age band, commonly accepted subgroups are those aged 65–74 years, 75–84 years, and 85 years and older.

The Incidence of Falls in Older People

Community-Dwelling Older People

In 1977, Exton-Smith examined the yearly incidence of falls in 963 people over the age of 65 years living in England [12]. He found that in women, the proportion that fell increased with age from 30% in the 65 to 69 years age group to over 50% in those over the age of 85. In men, the proportion that fell increased from 13% in the 65 to 69 years age group to approximately 30% in those aged 80 years and over.

Retrospective community studies in primarily Caucasian populations undertaken since Exton-Smith's work have reported similar findings, i.e. approximately 30% of older adults experience one or more falls per year [13–15]. Campbell et al. [13] analysed a stratified population sample of 533 participants aged 65 years and over and found that 33% experienced one or more falls in the previous year. Blake et al. [15] reported a similar incidence (35%) in a study of 1042 participants aged 65 years and over. In a large study of 2793 participants aged 65 years and over, Prudham and Grimley-Evans [14] estimated an annual incidence for accidental falls of 28%, a figure identical to that found in the Australian Dubbo Osteoporosis Epidemiology Study of 1762 older people aged 60 years and over [16].

Prospective studies undertaken in community settings have found higher fall incidence rates. In the Randwick Falls and Fractures Study conducted in Australia, Lord et al. [17] found that 39% of 341 community-dwelling women aged 65 years and over reported one or more falls in a one-year follow-up period. In a large study of 761 participants aged 70 years and over undertaken in New Zealand, Campbell et al. [18] found that 40% of the 465 women and 28% of the 296 men fell at least once in the study period of one year, an overall incidence rate of 35%. In the United States, Tinetti et al. [8] found an incidence rate of one or more falls of 32% in 336 participants aged 75 years and over. Similar rates have been reported in Canada by O'Loughlin et al. [9] in a 48-week prospective study of a random sample of 409 community-dwelling people aged 65 years and over (29%), and in Finland by Luukinen et al. [19] in 833 community-dwelling people aged 70 years and over from five rural districts (30%).

Fall rates also increase beyond the age of 65 years. Figure 1.1 shows the proportion of women who took part in the Randwick Falls and Fractures Study [17] who reported falling once, twice, or three or more times in a 12 month period.

The prospective studies that have reported the incidence of multiple or recurrent falls are also in agreement. The incidence of two or more falls in a follow-up year reported in five studies ranges between 11 and 21% (average 15%). Three studies have reported data for three or more falls, and all report an incidence of 8%.

Rigorous data regarding fall incidence in older people from non-Caucasian populations are now also available. Aoyaga et al. [20] studied falls and related conditions among 1534 (624 men, 910 women) community-dwelling people aged 65 years and over in Japan. They found that only 9% of the men and 19% of the women reported one or more falls in the previous year and similarly low incidence

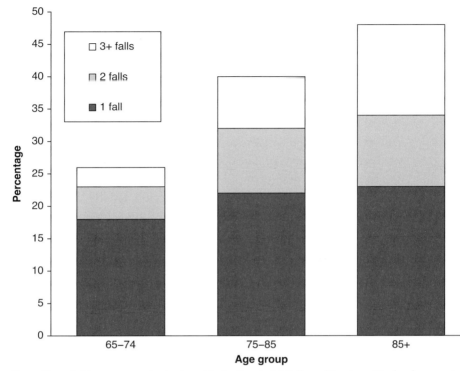

Figure 1.1   Proportion of older women who took part in the Randwick Falls and Fractures Study who reported falling, once, twice, or three or more times in a 12 month period. Diagram adapted from Lord SR, Ward JA, Williams P et al. An epidemiological study of falls in older community-dwelling women: the Randwick Falls and Fractures Study. *Aust J Public Health.* 1993;17:240–245.

rates have also been found in seven other large community studies undertaken in Japan [21]. As part of the Hawaii Osteoporosis Study, Davis et al. [22] attempted to identify neuromuscular performance measures and functional disabilities that could account for such differences in fall rates. They found that the Japanese women had faster walking speeds, chair stands, and performed better on a series of balance tests. On the other hand, the Caucasian women had greater strength, particularly at the quadriceps, and faster hand and foot reaction times. After adjusting for the neuromuscular test results and the number of functional disabilities, the odds ratio for the risk of falls remained essentially the same. It is possible that the better performances in the more functional strength and balance tests that translate more directly to activities of daily living could explain the lower risk of falls among Japanese women.

Kwan et al. [23] conducted a systematic review of fall incidence and fall risk factors in Chinese people living in China, Hong Kong, Macao, Singapore, and Taiwan. In the included 21 studies involving 25,629 people, fall rates ranged between 14.7% and 34% per annum (median 18%), i.e. a consistently lower incidence of self-reported falls than in Caucasian older people. Subsequently, Kwan et al. [24] investigated why fall rates differ between Chinese and Caucasian older people. Falls were recorded prospectively in large community-dwelling samples of Chinese older people living in Taiwan, Hong Kong, and Australia, as well as Caucasian older people living in Australia. The standardized annual fall rates for the three Chinese cohorts were 0.21 in Hong Kong, 0.26 in Taiwan, and 0.36 in Australia, which were significantly lower than that of the Caucasian cohort at 0.70. The difference in fall rates was not due to better physical ability in the Chinese cohorts. However, the Chinese cohorts expressed more concern about falling and did more planned activity. These findings suggest increased concern is protective for falls in Chinese older people and manifest as more behaviours to lessen fall risk. Interestingly, such adaptations were partially lost in the Chinese older people who migrated to a 'Westernized' country.

Ellis and Trent [25] compared risks for falls and their consequences among 104,902 people from four major race/ethnic groups who were admitted to non-federal hospitals in California from 1995 to 1997. Rates per 100,000 for same-level hospitalized fall injuries for Caucasians (161) were distinctively higher than for African-Americans (64), Hispanics (43), and Asian/Pacific Islanders (35). Caucasians were also more likely to have suffered a fracture and to be discharged to long-term care, suggesting poorer outcomes and greater injury severity.

Finally, Hanlon et al. [26] found that the hazard ratio of risk of fracture for people with more than two falls was significantly greater for African-American and American-Indian women compared to Caucasians, Hispanics and Asians, perhaps reflecting greater vitamin D deficiency. It is possible that differing levels of bone density, medical insurance, and family support may account for some of these differences observed among the groups or that despite no differences in the rate of falling between Caucasians and African-American women, ethnic differences in fracture risk may be due in part to the different ways in which they fall [27].

Seasonal Variations in Falls Frequency

It is possible that the ambient temperature may lead to a seasonal variation in the incidence of falls. People tend to hurry more in colder weather and mild hypothermia and slowed responses are more common. Equally, people tend to be less active in winter, the hours of daylight are shorter and vitamin D deficiency is more likely. There appears to be a seasonal variation in deaths from accidental falls, as illustrated in Figure 1.2 which shows annualized monthly ratios in England and Wales for 1993–1997 [27].

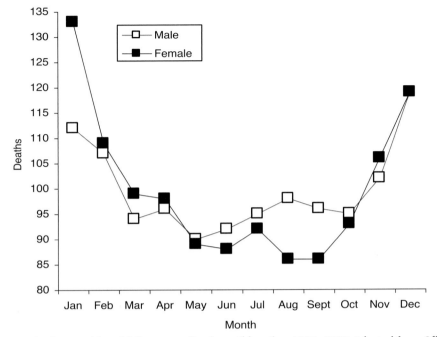

Figure 1.2   Deaths from accidental falls – annualized monthly ratios, 1993–1997. Adapted from Office for National Statistics. *1997 Mortality Statistics: Injury and Poisons.* 1999. London, The Stationery Office.

In a Finnish study, Luukinen et al. [28] found that the incidence of outdoor falls was higher in periods of extreme cold. However, there was no association between indoor falls and temperature, which they attributed to adequately heated houses. A similar study in the UK found that apart from the presence of ground frost, there was no significant association between the prevailing weather conditions and the incidence of hip fractures [29]. The precise effect of seasonal change on the epidemiology of falls is therefore somewhat unclear.

Secular Trends in Fall Injuries

Recent studies have examined routinely collected fall injury and death data as a means of assessing secular trends in fall incidence. In Australia, it has been reported that age-standardized hospitalization rates due to falls increased significantly by 3% per year for men and 2% for women over the 11 years between 2007 and 2017 [30]. Complementary studies have examined secular changes in fall injuries. These have found a decrease in the age-standardized rate of hip fractures of around 1% between 2007 and 2017 and a 7% annual increase in the age-standardized rate of traumatic brain injury over the same period [30]. US data also indicate that the age-adjusted death rate due to falls for people aged over 65 years increased by 31% between 2007 and 2016 and that age-standardized rates of traumatic brain injury are increasing [31]. Further research is required to elucidate why such secular trends in fall injury rates are occurring.

Residents of Residential Aged Care Facilities

Studies on the prevalence of falls have also been conducted in residential aged care facilities, where the reported frequency of falling is considerably higher than among those living in their own homes. For example, Luukinen et al. [32] estimate that among people aged 70 and over in Finland, the rate of falling in the residential care population is three times higher than that among those living independently in the community.

Prospective studies conducted in nursing homes have found 12-month fall incidence rates ranging from 30% to 56%. In an early study, Fernie et al. [33] studied 205 nursing home residents for 12 months and found 30% of the men and 42% of the women had one or more falls. Other studies have reported higher fall incidence rates in older people living in residential care facilities. Lipsitz et al. [34] found that 40% of 901 ambulatory nursing home residents fell two or more times in six months, and Yip et al. [35] found that 56% of 126 nursing home residents fell at least once in a year.

Two other studies have calculated fall incidence rates across a number of nursing homes. Rubenstein et al. [36] summarized the findings from five published and two unpublished studies on the incidence of falls in long-term care facilities. They calculated that the incidence rate ranged between 60% and 290% per bed, with a mean fall incidence rate of 170% or 1.7 falls per person per year. Thapa et al. [37] conducted a 12-month prospective study in 12 nursing homes involving 1228 residents. They report that during the 1003 person-years of follow-up, 548 residents suffered 1585 falls.

Fall rates are also high in residents living in intermediate-care hostels. Lord et al. [5] found a yearly fall incidence rate for one or more falls of 52%, and for two or more falls of 39% in a hostel population of older people. Tinetti et al. [38] also found a high incidence of falling in 79 persons admitted consecutively to intermediate care facilities – 32% fell two or more times in a three-month period.

In the Fracture Risk Epidemiology in the Elderly (FREE) study, 1000 residents from 26 nursing homes and 17 intermediate-care hostels were followed prospectively for a mean period of 15 months to ascertain risk factors for falls [39]. In this period, 621 residents fell at least once: 214 fell once only, 102 fell twice, 77 fell three times, 55 fell four times, and 173 fell five or more times. There were 2554 falls in all (5.45 falls/1000 resident bed days), with 786 falls (30.9%) resulting in an injury. Interestingly, there were non-linear associations between physical functioning and falls in this group, and the fall rate was significantly higher in intermediate-care residents (65%) compared with the nursing home residents (58%).

Other studies have examined fall incidence in residents of apartment-style retirement villages. Liu et al. [40] found a relatively high proportion (61%) of 96 residents fell over a 12-month period. In a randomized controlled trial examining the effects of group exercise on fall incidence, Lord et al. [41] found that 44% of 199 residents of self-care apartments in the control arm of the study fell on one or more occasions during the one-year trial – a rate that is comparable to community-dwelling people of similar age (age range: 62–92 years, mean: 77 years).

Particular Groups

Older people who have suffered a fall are at increased risk of falling again. In a prospective study of 325 community-dwelling persons who had fallen in the previous year, Nevitt et al. [7] found that 57% experienced at least one fall in a 12-month follow-up period and 31% had two or more falls. Not surprisingly, falls are also more prevalent in frail older people, in those who have difficulties undertaking activities of daily living, and in those with particular medical conditions that affect posture, balance, and gait. Northridge et al. [42] reported that when community-dwelling persons were classified as either frail or vigorous, frailer people were more than twice as likely to fall as vigorous people. Similarly, Speechley and Tinetti [43] reported 52% of a frail group fell in a one-year prospective period compared with only 17% of a vigorous group.

Falls are a common presenting condition in hospital emergency departments. Close et al. [44] found 20% of patients aged 65 years and over attending an emergency department had a primary diagnosis of a fall, and Davies et al. [45] reported an even higher percentage (44%) for this age group. Falls also occur frequently when older people are in hospital. Rates vary from approximately 2% in general hospitals where lengths of stay are relatively short [46, 47] to 27% in an acute hospital geriatrics ward [48].

With regard to medical conditions, Mahoney et al. [49] found that 14% of older patients fell in the first month after discharge from hospital following a medical illness. Fall rates are also increased in people with diseases that result in sensory and motor impairments such as stroke, Parkinson's disease, and cognitive impairment. Forster and Young [50] found that 73% of older stroke patients fell within six months of hospital discharge. Jorgensen et al. also present evidence that fall rates remain high in this group [51]. In a prospective study, they found that 23% of 111 community-dwelling people with long-standing stroke fell one or more times in a four-month period, and that this rate was double that found in 143 age- and sex-matched controls. Annual fall incidence rates above 60% in community-dwelling people with Parkinson's disease have been reported in several studies

[52–54]. It has also been noted that frequent falls are a problem in Parkinson's disease patients, with 13% reporting falling more than once a week [55]. Twelve-month fall incidence rates above 60% have also been reported for community-living people with cognitive impairment [56], and that fall rates in nursing home residents with dementia are double that of that for nursing home residents without dementia [57]. These high incidence rates appear to be accurate estimates as cognitive impairment has been found to be a strong independent risk factor for falls in many prospective studies (see Chapter 8).

Increased fall incidence is also evident in persons with arthritis. Sturnieks et al. [58] conducted a study of 684 community-dwelling men and women aged 75–98 years, of which 283 reported lower limb osteoarthritis; 137 participants with arthritis (48.4%) fell in the previous year, compared with 157 (39.2%) participants without arthritis (sex-adjusted RR: 1.22, 95% CI: 1.03,1.46).

Finally, fall incidence in older people with diabetes has been reported as part of the Study of Osteoporotic Fractures [59]. This prospective cohort study included 9249 women aged 67 years and over, of which 629 (6.8%) had diabetes, including 99 who used insulin. During an average of 7.2 years, 1640 women (18%) fell more than once a year. Fall rates were lowest in those without diabetes (17%), intermediate in those with non-insulin treated diabetes (26%) and highest in those with insulin-treated diabetes (34%). The authors found that the women with diabetes were at increased risk of falling due in part to increased rates of known fall risk factors such as poor lower limb sensation and balance.

Falls Location

In older community-dwelling people, about 50% of falls occur within their homes and immediate home surroundings (see Figure 1.3) [19, 60]. Most falls occur on level surfaces within commonly used rooms such as the bedroom, lounge-room, and kitchen. Comparatively few falls occur in the bathroom, on stairs or from ladders and stools. While a proportion of falls involve a hazard such as a loose rug or a slippery floor, many do not involve obvious environmental hazards [60]. The remaining falls occur in public places and other people's homes. Commonly reported environmental factors involved in falls in public places include pavement cracks and misalignments, gutters, steps, construction works, uneven ground, and slippery surfaces.

The location of falls is related to age, sex, and frailty. In community-dwelling older women, Lord et al. [2] found that the number of falls occurring outside the home decreased with age, with a corresponding increase in the number of falls occurring inside the home on a level surface (see Figure 1.4). Campbell et al. [60] found that fewer men than women fell inside the home (44% versus 65%) and

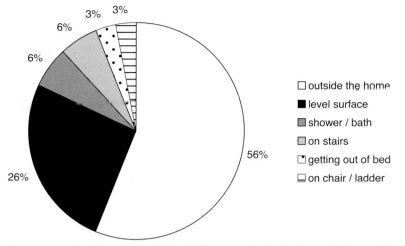

Figure 1.3   Location of falls: 56% of falls occur outside the home (in the garden, street, footpath, or shops), with the remainder (44%) occurring at various locations in the home. Adapted from Lord SR, Ward JA, Williams P, Anstey KJ. Physiological factors associated with falls in older community-dwelling women. *Australian Journal of Public Health* 1993;17:240-245.

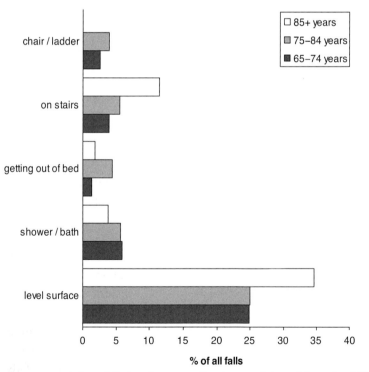

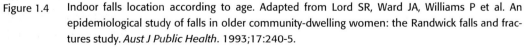

Figure 1.4   Indoor falls location according to age. Adapted from Lord SR, Ward JA, Williams P et al. An epidemiological study of falls in older community-dwelling women: the Randwick falls and fractures study. *Aust J Public Health*. 1993;17:240-5.

more men fell in the garden (25% versus 11%). Frailer groups with limited mobility suffer most falls within the home. These findings indicate that the occurrence of falls is strongly related to exposure, that is, they occur in situations where older people are undertaking their usual daily activities. Furthermore, most falls occur during periods of maximum activity in the morning or afternoon, and only about 20% occur between 9 pm and 7 am [60].

Consequences of Falls

Falls are the leading cause of injury-related hospitalization in persons aged 65 years and over, and account for 14% of emergency admissions [44] and 4% of all hospital admissions in this age group [61]. Hospital admissions resulting from falls are uncommon in young adulthood, but with advancing age, the incidence of fall-related admissions increases dramatically. Beyond 65 years, the admission rate due to falls increases exponentially for both sexes, with a ninefold increase in the rate in males and females between the ages of 65 and 85 plus years [62] (see Figure 1.5). Falls also account for 40% of injury-related deaths, and 1% of total deaths in this age group [63].

Depending on the population studied, anywhere between 22% and 60% of older people suffer injuries from falls, 10–15% suffer serious injuries, 2–6% suffer

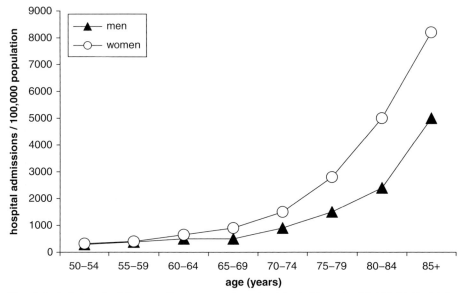

Figure 1.5   Hospital admissions for falls according to age and gender. Adapted from: Kreisfeld R, Moller J. *Injury Amongst Women in Australia*. Australian Injury Prevention Bulletin 12. Adelaide: National Injury Surveillance Unit, 1996.

fractures and 0.2–1.5% suffer hip fractures. The most commonly self-reported injuries include superficial cuts and abrasions, bruises, and sprains. The most common injuries that require hospitalization comprise traumatic brain injuries [11], hip fractures, pelvic fractures, other fractures of the leg, fractures of radius, ulna, or humerus, and fractures of the neck and trunk [1, 62, 63].

In terms of morbidity and mortality, one of the most serious fall-related injuries is fracture of the hip. Older people often recover slowly from hip fractures and are vulnerable to post-operative complications. In many cases, hip fractures result in death and of those who survive, many never regain complete mobility. Marottoli et al. [64] analysed the outcomes of 120 participants from a cohort study who suffered a hip fracture over a six-year period. They found that before their fractures, 86% could dress independently, 75% could walk independently, and 63% could climb a flight of stairs. Six months after their injuries, these percentages had fallen to 49%, 15%, and 8%, respectively.

Another consequence of falling is the 'long lie' – remaining on the ground or floor for more than an hour after a fall. The long lie is a marker of weakness, illness, and social isolation, and is associated with high mortality rates among older people. Time spent on the floor is associated with fear of falling, muscle damage, pneumonia, pressure sores, dehydration, and hypothermia [7, 65, 66]. Wild et al. [67] found that half of those who lie on the floor for an hour or longer die within six months, even if there is no direct injury from the fall. Vellas [68] found that more than 20% of patients admitted to hospital as a result of a fall had been on the ground for an hour or more. Such a figure could be expected as Tinetti et al. [69] found that up to 47% of non-injured fallers are unable to get up off the floor without assistance.

Falls can result in restriction of activity and fear of falling (see Chapter 9), reduced quality of life and loss of independence. In a study of 5093 older people, Kiel et al. [70] found that fallers, and especially recurrent fallers, were at greater risk of reporting subsequent difficulties with activities of daily living, instrumental activities of daily living, and more physically demanding activities, after controlling for age, sex, self-perceived health status, and pre-existing difficulties with activities of daily living. Tinetti et al. [71] found similar associations in a study involving 957 community-dwelling persons over the age of 71 years. They found that after adjusting for potential confounding factors, both non-injurious and injurious falls were associated with declines in basic and instrumental activities of daily living over a three-year prospective period. Furthermore, those who suffered two or more non-injurious falls reported declines in social activities and those who suffered one or more injurious falls reported reduced physical activity levels.

Falls can lead to an excessive fear of falling, sometimes referred to as the 'post-fall syndrome' which is manifest as a loss of confidence, hesitancy, tentativeness, with resultant loss of mobility and independence. It has been found that after falling, many older people report a fear of falling [71, 72] and curtailing activities due to a fear of further falls [7, 73].

Finally, falls can also lead to disability and decreased mobility which often results in dependency on others and hence an increased probability of requiring residential care [74, 75].

The Economic Cost of Falls

As indicated above, falls in older people are common and can lead to numerous disabling conditions, extensive hospital stays, and death. Indeed, as outlined in Figure 1.6, fall-related injuries incur the biggest direct cost of all injury categories. Fall-related costs can include the direct costs such as doctor visits, acute hospital and nursing home care, outpatient clinics, rehabilitation stays, diagnostic tests, medications, home care, home modifications, equipment, and residential care. Indirect costs include carer and patient morbidity and mortality costs. There are many difficulties and limitations involved in estimating the economic cost of any disease or condition. Problems exist because cost data are only estimates, and many costs are only relevant to the country in which they are incurred. Furthermore, because of inflation and other economic and health care factors, costs are outdated soon after they are published.

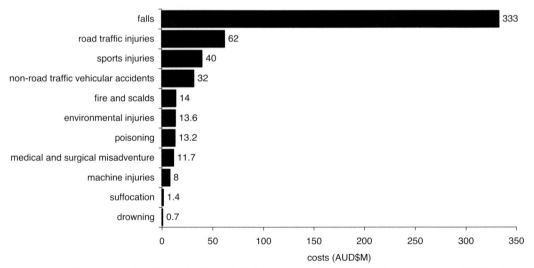

Figure 1.6   Direct costs for 11 unintentional falls injury categories. Falls injuries account for 62.8% of total direct costs. Adapted from Potter-Forbes M, Aisbett C. *Injury Costs! A Valuation of the Burden of Injury in New South Wales in 1998–1999*. NSW Injury Risk Management Research Centre, University of New South Wales, 2003.

A number of researchers have estimated the hospital costs of an injurious fall in absolute terms and as a proportion of health budgets. Englander et al. [76] projected the cost of falls to the US health care system in 1994 to total US$20.2 billion, with the cost per injured person being US$7399. The authors further extrapolated these figures to the year 2020 and estimated the cost of falls injuries at US$32.4 billion. Recent studies have shown that these costs were underestimations. Burns et al. [77] found that in 2015 the cost of a medically treated non-fatal fall was US$9780 and a fatal fall was US$26340, and the total cost of fatal and non-fatal falls for Medicare was US$32 billion. Furthermore, this figure increased to US$50.0 billion when Medicaid and out-of-pocket expenses were also included [78].

In Australia, there were 1.4 million patient days for hospital care related to injurious falls by people aged 65 years and older in 2013 [79], and it has been estimated the ageing of the Australian population will have a significant impact on the Australian health system due to the increased number of older people suffering fall-related injuries [80]. By 2051, the total health cost attributable to fall-related injury is predicted to increase almost threefold from current levels to AUD$1375 million per annum if age-specific fall rates remain unchanged; 886 000 additional hospital bed days or the equivalent of 2500 additional beds permanently allocated to falls injury treatment will be required for the increased demand and 3320 additional nursing home places will be required. These projections indicate prevention strategies will need to deliver approximately a 66% reduction in fall incidence to maintain cost parity over this period.

Conclusions

Despite the disparate methodologies of falls ascertainment used in the above studies, the incidence rates reported are quite similar. Approximately one-third of older Caucasian people living in the community fall at least once a year, with many suffering multiple falls. Fall rates are lower in Japanese, Chinese, African Americans, Hispanics, and Pacific Islanders. There appears to be a seasonal variation in the rate of falls in countries with cold climates and there is some evidence that fall incidence has been increasing over the past one or two decades. Fall rates are higher in older community-dwelling women (40%) than in older men (28%) and continue to increase with age above 65 years. The incidence of falls is increased in people living in retirement villages, hostels, and nursing homes, in those who have fallen in the past year, and in those with particular medical conditions that affect muscle strength, balance, and gait. In community-dwelling older people, about 50% of falls occur within the home and 50% in public places. Falls account for 4% of hospital admissions, 40% of injury-related deaths and 1% of total deaths in persons aged 65 years and over. The major serious injuries that result from falls include traumatic brain injuries and fractures of the wrist, neck, trunk, and hip. Falls can also result in disability, restriction of activity and fear of falling, which can reduce quality of life and independence, and contribute to an older person being admitted to a nursing home. Finally, as many fall-related injuries require medical treatment including hospitalization, falls constitute a condition requiring considerable health care expenditure.

REFERENCES

1. Gibson MJ, Andres RO, Kennedy TE et al. The prevention of falls in later life: a report of the Kellogg International Work Group on the Prevention of Falls by the Elderly. *Dan Med Bull.* 1987;34:1–24.
2. Lamb SE, Jørstad-Stein EC, Hauer K et al. Development of a common outcome data set for fall injury prevention trials: the Prevention of Falls Network Europe consensus. *J Am Geriatr Soc.* 2005;53:1618–22.
3. Evans JG. Fallers, non-fallers and Poisson. *Age Ageing.* 1990;19:268–9.
4. Cummings SR, Nevitt MC, Kidd S. Forgetting falls: the limited accuracy of recall of falls in the elderly. *J Am Geriatr Soc.* 1988;36:613–16.
5. Lord SR, Clark RD, Webster IW. Physiological factors associated with falls in an elderly population. *J Am Geriatr Soc.* 1991;39:1194–200.
6. Lord SR, Ward JA, Williams P et al. Physiological factors associated with falls in older community-dwelling women. *J Am Geriatr Soc.* 1994;42:1110–17.
7. Nevitt MC, Cummings SR, Kidd S et al. Risk factors for recurrent nonsyncopal falls: a prospective study. *J Am Med Assoc.* 1989;261:2663–8.
8. Tinetti ME, Speechley M, Ginter SF. Risk factors for falls among elderly persons living in the community. *N Engl J Med.* 1988;319:1701–7.
9. O'Loughlin JL, Robitaille Y, Boivin JF et al. Incidence of and risk factors for falls and injurious falls among the community-dwelling elderly. *Am J Epidemiol.* 1993;137:342–54.
10. Barker AL, Morello RT, Wolfe R et al. 6-PACK programme to decrease fall injuries in acute hospitals: cluster randomised controlled trial. *BMJ Clin Res.* 2016;352:h6781.
11. Harvey LA, Close JCT. Traumatic brain injury in older adults: characteristics, causes and consequences. *Injury.* 2012;43:1821–6.
12. Exton-Smith AN. Functional consequences of ageing: clinical manifestations. In: Exton-Smith AN, Grimley-Evans J, Eds. *Care of the Elderly: Meeting the Challenge of Dependency.* London: Academic Press; 1977.
13. Campbell AJ, Reinken J, Allan B et al. Falls in old age: a study of frequency and related clinical factors. *Age Ageing.* 1981;10:264–70.
14. Prudham D, Evans JG. Factors associated with falls in the elderly: a community study. *Age Ageing.* 1981;10:141–6.
15. Blake A, Morgan K, Bendall M et al. Falls by elderly people at home: prevalence and associated factors. *Age Ageing.* 1988;17:365–72.

16. Lord SR, Webster IW, Sambrook PN et al. Postural stability, falls and fractures in the elderly: results from the Dubbo Osteoporosis Epidemiology Study. *Med J Aust.* 1994;160:684–91.

17. Lord SR, Ward JA, Williams P et al. An epidemiological study of falls in older community-dwelling women: the Randwick falls and fractures study. *Aust J Public Health* 1993;17:240–5.

18. Campbell AJ, Borrie MJ, Spears GF. Risk factors for falls in a community-based prospective study of people 70 years and older. *J Gerontol.* 1989;44:M112–7.

19. Luukinen H, Koski K, Laippala P et al. Predictors for recurrent falls among the home-dwelling elderly. *Scand J Prim Health Care.* 1995;13:294–9.

20. Aoyagi K, Ross PD, Davis JW et al. Falls among community-dwelling elderly in Japan. *J Bone Miner Res.* 1998;13:1468–74.

21. Yasumura S. Frequency of falls and bone fractures in the elderly. *Japan Med Assoc J.* 2001;44:192–7.

22. Davis JW, Nevitt MC, Wasnich RD et al. A cross-cultural comparison of neuromuscular performance, functional status, and falls between Japanese and white women. *J Gerontol A Biol Sci Med Sci.* 1999;54:M288–92.

23. Kwan MMS, Close JC, Wong AKW et al. Falls incidence, risk factors, and consequences in Chinese older people: a systematic review. *J Am Geriatr Soc.* 2011;59:536–43.

24. Kwan MMS, Tsang WWN, Lin S-I et al. Increased concern is protective for falls in Chinese older people: the Chopstix Fall Risk Study. *J Gerontol A Biol Sci Med Sci.* 2013;68:946–53.

25. Ellis AA, Trent RB. Hospitalized fall injuries and race in California. *Inj Prev.* 2001;7:316–20.

26. Cauley JA, Wu L, Wampler NS et al. Clinical risk factors for fractures in multi-ethnic women: the Women's Health Initiative. *J Bone Miner Res.* 2007;22:1816–26.

27. Faulkner KA, Cauley JA, Zmuda JM et al. Ethnic differences in the frequency and circumstances of falling in older community-dwelling women. *J Am Geriatr Soc.* 2005;53:1774–9.

28. Luukinen H, Koski K, Kivelä S. The relationship between outdoor temperature and the frequency of falls among the elderly in Finland. *J Epidemiol Community Health.* 1996;50:107.

29. Parker MJ, Martin S. Falls, hip fractures and the weather. *Eur J Epidemiol.* 1994;10:441–2.

30. Pointer S. Trends in hospitalised injury due to falls in older people, 2007–08 to 2016–17. Canberra: Australia Institute of Health and Welfare; 2019.

31. Burns E, Kakara R. Deaths from falls among persons aged≥ 65 years: United States, 2007–2016. *Morb Mortal Wkly Rep.* 2018;67:509.

32. Luukinen H, Koski K, Hiltunen L et al. Incidence rate of falls in an aged population in Northern Finland. *J Clin Epidemiol.* 1994;47:843–50.

33. Fernie GR, Gryfe C, Holliday PJ et al. The relationship of postural sway in standing to the incidence of falls in geriatric subjects. *Age Ageing.* 1982;11:11–16.

34. Lipsitz LA, Jonsson PV, Kelley MM et al. Causes and correlates of recurrent falls in ambulatory frail elderly. J Gerontol. 1991;46:M114–22.

35. Yip YB, Cumming RG. The association between medications and falls in Australian nursing-home residents. *Med J Aust.* 1994;160:14–18.

36. Rubenstein LZ, Robbins AS, Schulman BL et al. Falls and instability in the elderly. *J Am Geriatr Soc.* 1988;36:266–78.

37. Thapa PB, Brockman KG, Gideon P et al. Injurious falls in nonambulatory nursing home residents: a comparative study of circumstances, incidence, and risk factors. *J Am Geriatr Soc.* 1996;44:273–8.

38. Tinetti ME, Williams TF, Mayewski R. Fall risk index for elderly patients based on number of chronic disabilities. *Am J Med.* 1986;80:429–34.

39. Lord SR, March LM, Cameron ID et al. Differing risk factors for falls in nursing home and intermediate-care residents who can and cannot stand unaided. *J Am Geriatr Soc.* 2003;51:1645–50.

40. Liu BA, Topper AK, Reeves RA et al. Falls among older people: relationship to medication use and orthostatic hypotension. *J Am Geriatr Soc.* 1995;43:1141–5.

41. Lord SR, Castell S, Corcoran J et al. The effect of group exercise on physical functioning and falls in frail older people living in retirement villages: a randomized, controlled trial. *J Am Geriatr Soc.* 2003;51:1685–92.

42. Northridge ME, Nevitt MC, Kelsey JL et al. Home hazards and falls in the elderly: the role of health and functional status. *Am J Public Health.* 1995;85:509–15.

43. Speechley M, Tinetti M. Falls and injuries in frail and vigorous community elderly persons. *J Am Geriatr Soc.* 1991;39:46–52.

44. Close J, Ellis M, Hooper R et al. Prevention of falls in the elderly trial (PROFET): a randomised controlled trial. *Lancet.* 1999;353:93–7.

45. Davies A, Kenny R. Falls presenting to the accident and emergency department: types of presentation and risk factor profile. *Age Ageing.* 1996;25:362–6.

46. Clark G. A study of falls among elderly hospitalized patients. *Aust J Adv Nurs.* 1984;2:34–44.

47. Donham J, Sadewhite C, Seltzer M et al. Identifying characteristics of the fall-prone medical-surgical patient. *Kans Nurse.* 1987;62:5–6.

48. Oliver D, Britton M, Seed P, Martin FC, Hopper AH. Development and evaluation of evidence based risk assessment tool (STRATIFY) to predict which elderly inpatients will fall: case-control and cohort studies. *Br Med J.* 1997;315:1049–53.

49. Mahoney J, Sager M, Dunham NC et al. Risk of falls after hospital discharge. *J Am Geriatr Soc.* 1994;42:269–74.

50. Forster A, Young J. Incidence and consequences of falls due to stroke: a systematic inquiry. *Br Med J.* 1995;311:83–6.

51. Jørgensen L, Engstad T, Jacobsen BK. Higher incidence of falls in long-term stroke survivors than in population controls: depressive symptoms predict falls after stroke. *Stroke.* 2002;33:542–7.

52. Schrag A, Ben-Shlomo Y, Quinn N. How common are complications of Parkinson's disease? *J Neurol.* 2002;249:419–23.

53. Wood BH, Bilclough JA, Bowron A et al. Incidence and prediction of falls in Parkinson's disease: a prospective multidisciplinary study. *J Neurol Neurosurg Psychiatry.* 2002;72:721–5.

54. Ashburn A, Stack E, Pickering RM et al. A community-dwelling sample of people with Parkinson's disease: characteristics of fallers and non-fallers. *Age Ageing.* 2001;30:47–52.

55. Koller WC, Glatt S, Vetere-Overfield B et al. Falls and Parkinson's disease. *Clin Neuropharmacol.* 1989;12:98–105.

56. Taylor ME, Delbaere K, Lord SR et al. Neuropsychological, physical, and functional mobility measures associated with falls in cognitively impaired older adults. *J Gerontol A Biol Sci Med Sci.* 2013;69:987–95.

57. Van Doorn C, Gruber-Baldini AL, Zimmerman S et al. Dementia as a risk factor for falls and fall injuries among nursing home residents. *J Am Geriatr Soc.* 2003;51:1213–18.

58. Sturnieks DL, Tiedemann A, Chapman K et al. Physiological risk factors for falls in older people with lower limb arthritis. *J Rheumatol.* 2004;31:2272–9.

59. Schwartz AV, Hillier TA, Sellmeyer DE et al. Older women with diabetes have a higher risk of falls: a prospective study. *Diabetes Care.* 2002;25:1749–54.

60. Campbell A, Borrie MJ, Spears GF et al. Circumstances and consequences of falls experienced by a community population 70 years and over during a prospective study. *Age Ageing.* 1990;19:136–41.

61. Baker SP, Harvey AH. Fall injuries in the elderly. *Clin Geriatr Med.* 1985;1:501–12.

62. Cripps R, Carman J. *Falls by the Elderly in Australia: Trends and Data for 1998.* Adelaide: Australian Institute of Health and Welfare; 2001.

63. NSW Department of Health: *The Epidemiology of Falls in Older People in NSW.* North Sydney; 1994.

64. Marottoli RA, Berkman LF, Cooney Jr LM. Decline in physical function following hip fracture. *J Am Geriatr Soc.* 1992;40:861–6.

65. Mallinson W, Green MF. Covert muscle injury in aged patients admitted to hospital following falls. *Age Ageing.* 1985;14:174–8.

66. King MB, Tineti ME. Falls in community-dwelling older persons. *J Am Geriatr Soc.* 1995;43:1146–54.

67. Wild D, Nayak U, Isaacs B. How dangerous are falls in old people at home? *Br Med J (Clin Res Ed).* 1981;282:266–8.

68. Vellas B, Cayla F, Bocquet H et al. Prospective study of restriction of activity in old people after falls. *Age Ageing.* 1987;16:189–93.

69. Tinetti ME, Liu W-L, Claus EB. Predictors and prognosis of inability to get up after falls among elderly persons. *J Am Med Assoc.* 1993;269:65–70.

70. Kiel DP, O'Sullivan P, Teno JM et al. Health care utilization and functional status in the aged following a fall. *Med Care.* 1991:221–8.

71. Tinetti ME, Williams CS. The effect of falls and fall injuries on functioning in community-dwelling older persons. *J Gerontol A Biol Sci Med Sci.* 1998;53:M112–19.

72. Tinetti ME, De Leon CFM, Doucette JT et al. Fear of falling and fall-related efficacy in relationship to functioning among community-living elders. *J Gerontol.* 1994;49:M140–7.

73. Vellas BJ, Wayne SJ, Romero LJ et al. Fear of falling and restriction of mobility in elderly fallers. *Age Ageing.* 1997;26:189–93.

74. Lord SR. Predictors of nursing home placement and mortality of residents in intermediate care. *Age Ageing.* 1994;23:499–504.

75. Tinetti ME, Williams CS. Falls, injuries due to falls, and the risk of admission to a nursing home. *New Engl J Med.* 1997;337:1279–84.

76. Englander F, Hodson TJ, Terregrossa RA. Economic dimensions of slip and fall injuries. *J Forensic Sci.* 1996;41:733–46.

77. Burns ER, Stevens JA, Lee R. The direct costs of fatal and non-fatal falls among older adults: United States. *J Safety Res.* 2016;58:99–103.

78. Florence CS, Bergen G, Atherly A et al. Medical costs of fatal and nonfatal falls in older adults. *J Am Geriatr Soc.* 2018;66:693–8.

79. Kreisfeld R, Pointer S, Bradley C. Trends in Hospitalisations due to Falls by Older People, Australia 2002–03 to 2012–13. Canberra: Australian Institute of Health and Welfare; 2017.

80. Moller J. Projected Cots of Fall Related Injury to Older Persons due to Demographic Change in Australia. Canberra: The Commonwealth Department of Health and Ageing; 2003.

2

Postural Stability and Falls

Jasmine C. Menant, Yoshiro Okubo, and Hylton B. Menz

Introduction

Postural stability can be defined as the ability of an individual to maintain the position of the body, or more specifically, its centre of mass, within specific boundaries of space, referred to as *stability limits*. Stability limits are boundaries in which the body can maintain its position without changing the base of support [1]. This definition of postural stability is useful as it highlights the need to discuss stability in the context of a particular task or activity. For example, the stability limit of normal relaxed standing is the area bounded by the two feet on the ground, whereas the stability limit of unipedal stance is reduced to the area covered by the single foot in contact with the ground. Due to this reduction in the size of the stability limit, unipedal stance is an inherently more challenging task requiring greater postural control.

Regardless of the task being performed, maintaining postural stability requires the complex integration of sensory information regarding the position of the body relative to the surroundings, and the ability to generate forces to control body movement. Thus, postural stability requires the interaction of musculoskeletal and sensory systems. The musculoskeletal component of postural stability encompasses the biomechanical properties of body segments, muscles, and joints. The sensory components include vision, vestibular function, and somatosensation which act to inform the brain of the position and movement of the body in three-dimensional space. Linking these two components together are the higher-level neurological processes enabling anticipatory mechanisms responsible for planning a movement, and adaptive mechanisms responsible for the ability to react to changing demands of the particular task [1].

Normal ageing is associated with cognitive decline and changes in function of each of the sub-components of musculoskeletal and sensory systems which contribute to postural stability [2–7]. Consequently, ageing may manifest as a measurable deficit in any task involving maintaining postural stability, such as quiet standing, performing voluntary movements, and responding to external perturbations.

Standing

Normal relaxed standing is characterized by small amounts of *postural sway*, which has been defined by Sheldon as 'the constant small deviations from the vertical and their subsequent correction to which all human beings are subject when standing upright' [8]. Control of postural sway when standing involves continual muscle activity (primarily of the calf muscles) and requires an integrated reflex response to visual, vestibular, and somatosensory inputs [9]. The relative contribution of each of these systems has been determined by experimentally blocking each of the inputs and measuring the subsequent increase in postural sway. The role of vision has been assessed by simply asking people to close their eyes, vestibular input has been minimized by tilting the head [10] or assessing the ability to balance an equivalent mechanical body [11], and somatosensory input has been blocked by ischaemia [9], standing on compliant surfaces [12, 13] and immersing the feet in cold water [14–16]. Such investigations have revealed that if any of these inputs are removed, postural sway increases. Although the extent to which one input can compensate for the loss of another is still unclear, peripheral sensation appears to be the most important sensory system in the regulation of standing balance in older adults [13].

Visual-field dependency, as assessed using the Roll Vection Test (i.e. attempt to align a rod to the vertical while exposed to a rotating visual field) has been associated with *reduced* sway. Although this appears counterintuitive, it is postulated that it might be due to a stiffening strategy to maintain stance [17]. Similar reductions in postural sway responses have also been reported in fear-inducing environmental conditions, at elevated height for example [18]. In response to a postural threat (standing on a 65-cm-high platform), non-anxious older participants showed an adaptive tightening of balance control, effectively reducing sway range in the elevated condition, whereas the anxious participants increased their sway frequency but did not reduce sway range. These findings suggest that generalized anxiety in older adults appears to differentially affect postural control strategies under threatening conditions [18].

The generalized decline in sensory functions due to normal ageing and its contribution to increased postural sway have been widely evaluated in the literature. Although interest in the measurement of sway dates back to the classic studies on tabes dorsalis by Romberg in 1853 [19], the first attempt to assess age-related changes in postural sway was conducted by Hellbrandt and Braun in 1939 [20], who measured sway in people aged from three to 86 years. The results showed that the magnitude of sway was largest in the very young and very old participants. A similar study by Boman and Javalisto [21] measured sway with an overhead camera in people aged 18–30 and 61–88 years, and reported that sway was greater in the older group, particularly in those aged over 80 years. Since these early investigations, many studies have reported age-associated increases in standing postural sway after the age of 30 years using various swaymeters, optical systems, force platforms, and accelerometers, particularly with the eyes closed [8, 22–45]. There is no clear consensus in the literature regarding sex differences in sway; although some studies report higher postural sway values in women compared to men across a range of age groups [22, 25, 28, 45], other authors have reported no significant differences [31, 33, 38, 46].

Factors found to be highly correlated with increased sway include reduced lower-extremity muscle strength [13, 47–50], reduced peripheral sensation [26, 48, 51–54], poor near visual acuity [13, 55], and slowed reaction time [13, 56]. Lord et al. [13] found that while reaction time is not associated with sway when standing on a firm surface, when participants stand on a compliant foam rubber surface a significant association between sway and reaction time is evident. This suggests that people can perceive large amounts of sway and consciously control their body movements. Smaller associations between vestibular function and sway have been reported [10, 13, 26, 57], and postural sway does not appear to be strongly associated with anthropometric measures. Danis et al. [58] reported that skeletal alignment was not associated with postural sway on a force plate, however Lichtenstein et al. [55] and Era et al. [48] reported that low body mass is associated with greater sway in both men and women. Kejonen et al. [59] measured a broad range of anthropometric parameters in 100 people aged 31–80 years, and found that few measures were strongly correlated with body displacement when standing. More recently, Reynart et al. [45] recorded postural sway during 12 quiet standing tasks with an accelerometer fixed onto the sternum on 100 men and women aged 20 to 60 years. They found no significant effect of height or weight on the average amplitude of the acceleration signal (root mean square) that they defined as an indirect measure of thorax sway.

Measurement of postural sway when standing has been reported to be a useful predictor of falls in older people. Although the evidence is not entirely consistent, a number of cross-sectional studies have reported significantly greater sway in older people with a history of falling compared to those without such a history [25, 46, 60, 61]. Similarly, numerous prospective studies have revealed that the measurement of an individual's sway is a useful predictor of falls during follow-up periods [62–67]. Despite using a range of sway measurements of varying complexity, encompassing balance boards [68], inertial sensors [69], and force platforms [70], findings from recent large studies concur. In studies by Lord et al. [62, 71–73], people with a history of falls showed greater sway in four test conditions: standing on a firm base with the eyes open; standing on a firm base with the eyes closed; standing on a 15-cm thick high-density foam rubber mat with the eyes open; and standing on the foam rubber with the eyes closed. In each of these studies, a validated, portable 'sway-meter' was used to record displacements of the body at the level of the waist (see Figure 2.1) [74].

In addition to the investigation of standing postural sway, several other standing tests have been developed which provide a greater challenge to the postural control system. One technique is to simply alter the foot position, thereby decreasing the size of the stability limit. This concept was first explored by Romberg [19], who assessed balance by observing the ability of patients to stand with their feet together. The effect of foot position on sway has more recently been evaluated in detail by numerous authors [45, 75–78], who evaluated postural stability on a force plate or with trunk inertial sensors with participants standing with their feet in varying positions (i.e. toe-in, toe-out, variations in space between the heels, and tandem stance). Increased sway was apparent with the more challenging conditions due to the reduction in the size of the stability limit. In accordance with investigations into normal bipedal standing, ageing is also associated with poorer performance in tandem standing [49, 79–83] and unipedal stance [27, 28, 45, 79–82, 84–88] with no significant effect of leg dominance [45]. Lord et al. [89] has also reported that older people with a history of falls had increased lateral sway with the eyes open and closed when undertaking a Near Tandem Stability Test. Those who had fallen were also significantly more likely to take a protective step when undertaking the test with the eyes closed. Consistent with this finding, a study of 439 older people in the Netherlands found that an inability to stand in the tandem position for at least 10 seconds was a significant independent predictor of recurrent falls in a 12-month follow-up period [67]. Similarly, three studies have reported that performance in the Unipedal Standing Test can predict falls in older people [88, 90, 91]; however, the utility of timed unipedal standing as a falls predictor is limited, as many frail older people are unable to attempt this test.

Leaning

Another approach to challenge postural control is to measure sway when the participant is placed at the perimeter of their stability limit, or to measure the

A

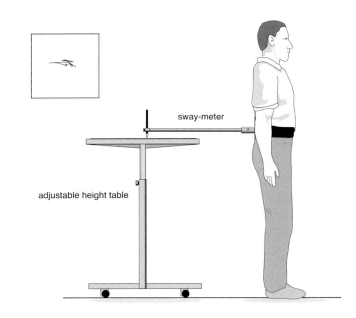

B

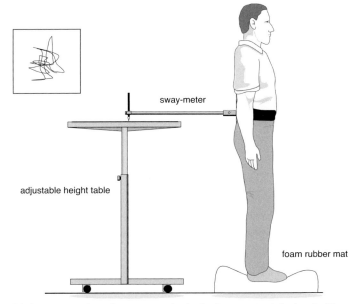

Figure 2.1   The portable 'sway meter' used to measure body displacements at the level of the waist. A: sway on the floor, B: sway on a foam rubber mat.

dimensions of the stability limit itself. Hasselkus and Shambes [24] assessed postural sway in young and older women in normal relaxed stance and when the participants leaned forward at the waist approximately 45°. The results revealed that sway was greater in the older group in both conditions, but particularly so when leaning forward, suggesting that the older women were less able to stabilize their posture when approaching the perimeter of their stability limit. King et al. [92] evaluated the ability of women aged 20 to 91 years to reach as far forward and backward as possible when standing, in order to establish age-related differences in functional base of support. Decreased functional base of support was evident after the age of 60 years and declined 16% per decade thereafter.

A similar technique is the *Functional Reach Test*, which involves the measurement of the ability to reach forward as far as possible with the arm positioned at 90° of shoulder flexion. This test was first described by Duncan et al. [93], who evaluated participants aged 21 to 87 years and reported a significant age-related decline in functional reach. Similar results were reported by Hagemon et al. [38], who reported that older people exhibited a smaller mean reach than younger people. Even though subsequent investigations of functional reach have shown the test to be correlated with performance in activities of daily living [94] and sensitive to improvements in function following rehabilitation [95], it does not appear to be a valid indicator of dynamic balance, due to the variety of strategies that can be used to extend the arm from the shoulder [96].

Furthermore, according to a recent systematic review and meta-analysis [97], performance in the Functional Reach Test is not predictive of falls: data from five prospective studies showed that older non-fallers could reach on average only 2.30 cm further (95% CI: –0.43,5.04) than older fallers, and two out of three additional studies, which were not included in the meta-analysis (n = 1373 and n = 1200, respectively), supported these findings [98, 99], suggesting that their inclusion would not have changed the findings.

Two variations on this test have also been proposed – the *Lateral Reach Test* [100] and the *Multi-Direction Reach Test* [101]. The Lateral Reach Test involves the clinical measurement of maximal excursion of the extended arm in conjunction with laboratory measures of centre of pressure displacement when participants lean as far as possible to the right and left sides [100]. The Multi-Direction Reach Test involves participants leaning forward, to the right, to the left and leaning backwards while the excursion of their arm is measured [101]. Despite their theoretical advantages over the Functional Reach Test, neither test has been found to be an accurate predictor of falls [101, 102].

Lord et al. [103] developed two additional leaning tests as measures of postural stability. The *Maximum Balance Range Test* involves the participant leaning forward and backward from the ankles as far as possible (without moving their feet or bending at the hips). Maximal antero-posterior distance moved is measured using a pen attached to a rod extending anteriorly from the participant's waist. This technique provides some benefits over the Functional Reach Test, as it avoids problems associated with variations in shoulder movement when extending the arm. The pen records the anterior and posterior movements on a sheet of graph paper which is fastened to the top of an adjustable height table. Using a similar apparatus, an additional test of *coordinated stability* can be performed in which the participant is asked to bend and rotate their hips without moving the feet so that the pen on the end of the rod follows and remains within a convoluted track which is marked on a piece of paper attached to the top of an adjustable height table. To complete the test without errors, participants have to ensure the pen remains within the track, which is 1.5 cm wide, and be capable of adjusting the position of the pen 29 cm laterally and 18 cm in the antero-posterior plane. A total error score is calculated by summing the number of occasions that the pen on the sway meter failed to stay within the path. Both the Maximal Balance Range and Coordinated Stability Tests (Figure 2.2) have been found to be reliable [103], predictive of falls [104–108], and sensitive to improvement following exercise intervention in older people [103, 109–113] from a range of settings, and physical and cognitive capacities. An example of the Coordinated Stability Test is shown in Figure 2.2.

Voluntary Stepping

Voluntary execution of fast, timely, accurate, and well-directed steps is critical to prevent falls in daily life where a balance disturbance can be anticipated [114]. Voluntary execution of protective stepping involves the following three-stage response [115, 116]: (i) perception of a postural threat, (ii) selection of an appropriate corrective response, and (iii) proper response execution. To gain a single measure of this complex, multi-system response, Lord et al. [105] devised a test of choice stepping reaction time that requires participants to perform quick, correctly targeted steps in response to visual cues. They found that among 510 retirement village residents aged 62–95 years, those with a history of falls had significantly increased choice reaction stepping times compared with those who reported no falls. Furthermore, ability to perform this test well was dependent upon adequate visual contrast sensitivity, lower limb extension strength, simple reaction time, and standing and leaning balance control. These measures, which have all been shown to be important risk factors for falls in previous studies [117], accounted for much of the variance in choice stepping reaction time (multiple r^2: 0.42). This suggests that this test may provide a composite measure of falls risk in older people. Subsequently,

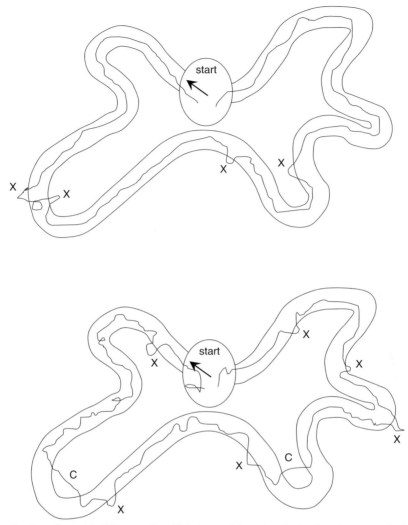

Figure 2.2   The Coordinated Stability Test, in which the participant is asked to bend or rotate the body without moving the feet so that the pen on the end of a rod follows and remains within a convoluted track which is marked on a piece of paper attached to the top of an adjustable height table. Leaving the track scores 1 error point, while failing to navigate a corner scores 5 error points. In the top diagram, the error score is 4, while in the bottom diagram the error score is 16.

a portable version of this tool has been developed (see Figure 2.3) and found to be a valid and reliable tool for assessing stepping ability in community-dwelling older people [118]. In subsequent trials, choice-stepping reaction time perform-ance has been shown to be associated with falls in prospective follow-ups [119, 120], improved following exercise interventions in older people, whether trad-itional (balance and strength) [103, 109–111] or specific (step training) [121,

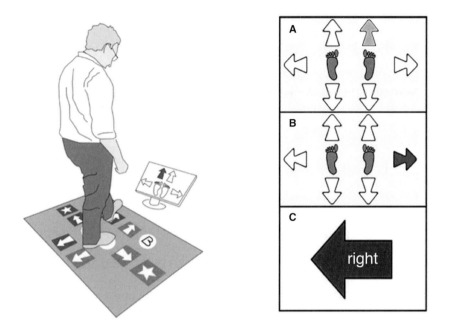

Figure 2.3   Left: The portable version of the stepping mat. Participants stood on the computerized mat (150 ×
90 cm) in front of a computer screen. The mat comprises eight panels: two central stance panels,
a left panel, a right panel, two front panels and two back panels. Right: Stepping reaction time tasks.
A: The Choice Stepping Reaction Time Test. Participants are asked to stand on the two central
panels. They are then instructed to step onto a target panel as quickly as possible when the
corresponding arrow on the screen changes colour from white to green. Participants first undertake
four practice trials followed by 24 randomly presented trials (four trials each for the six stepping
panels). An error is defined as a step to an incorrect panel. B: The Inhibitory Choice Stepping
Reaction Time Test. This is similar to the Choice Stepping Reaction Time Test (go trials indicated by
green); however, no-go trials are also presented as purple arrows. Participants are instructed to
step as quickly as possible to the indicated green arrows but not to step if a purple arrow is
presented. Participants complete six practice trials followed by 24 randomly presented trials (four
trials for each of the six panels, including green and purple arrows). C: The Stroop Stepping Test.
A large arrow is presented in the centre of the screen pointing in one of four directions (up, down,
left and right) that match the four possible step directions (forward, backward, left and right).
A word indicating a different direction is written inside the arrow. Participants are instructed to 'step
by the word' and therefore have to inhibit the response indicated by the arrow's orientation. Four
practice trials, followed by 20 randomly presented trials (five trials for each direction) are
administered.

122]. To explore further the interaction between cognitive function and balance,
stepping tests that examine the inhibitory functions of cognition have also been
devised, the Stroop Stepping Test [123] and the Inhibitory Stepping Test [121]
(see Figure 2.3), and these assessments of cognitive-motor stepping performance have been predictive of falls [123, 124]. A simple 'low-tech' version of the

system that requires only a stopwatch and a rubber mat with six rectangular standing and stepping panels has been shown to valid and reliable measure of fall risk in a prospective cohort study [125].

Other voluntary stepping tests have also been suggested. The Maximal Step Length Test assesses the ability to take the longest forward step possible and has been commonly used in community [126–131] and institutional settings [132] for its simplicity and reliability. Studies in older adults have reported that performance in the Maximal Step Length Test is associated with past [128, 129, 131–133] and future [126, 127, 130] falls, and is likely a stronger fall risk factor when normalized to the participant's body height [130, 131]. Dite and Temple [134] proposed the Four Square Step Test which evaluated time taken to step to the right, backwards, to the left and forwards over four walking canes placed on the floor in 81 older people, and found that those who had experienced multiple falls in the previous six months were significantly slower than non-fallers. The predictive value of the test was also found to be superior to the Timed Up and Go Test and the Functional Reach Test. Melzer et al. investigated the ability of the Voluntary Step Execution Test to discriminate between past fallers and non-fallers among a sample of 100 older people living in residential care. This test required participants to generate 30-cm-long steps as fast as possible on a force platform, following a tap on the heel. Longer mean step execution times ($\geq$1100 ms) across nine trials in forward, sideways, and backward directions while performing a distracting modified Stroop task were associated with an increased risk of falling [135], injurious falls [136], and recurrent falls [137]. More recently, a prospective study of 124 adults aged 60–85 years investigated gait initiation time, defined as the median time between a start stimulus (a randomly timed buzzer) and time to complete the first step across six trials [138]. Slower gait initiation times under both single- and dual-task conditions were associated with increased risk of multiple falls over a 12-month period.

The Alternate Stepping Test evaluates the ability to step alternately with each leg eight times onto a raised (19 cm high) platform and was initially found to correlate with foot problems in 135 community-dwelling older adults [106]. Subsequent researchers have also measured the time to complete five [139, 140], eight [141–143], or ten [144] alternate steps onto a platform and reported its association with past [141, 142, 144] and future falls [139, 143] in community-dwelling older adults. The Hill Step Test measures the number of steps onto 7 cm and 15 cm blocks in 15 s without alternating the feet and has been studied among geriatric and rehabilitation inpatients. Test performance was not significantly associated with prospective falls, likely due to multi-factorial nature of falls in this frail population [98, 145].

The Multi-Target Stepping Test developed by Yamada et al. [146] involves walking on a 10 m long mat with 45 coloured (red, blue, or yellow) squares arranged in three rows of 15. Failure to step on target colours, avoid distractor colours and the time to complete the MTS test have been associated with history of falls in community dwelling older adults [146, 147].

Each of these voluntary stepping tests would appear to have some value in the assessment of falls risk, as they mimic the response required to avoid a fall, and emphasize the reaction time component of balance preservation movements. They also have practical benefits over laboratory tests in that they require little or no equipment to undertake.

Internal Perturbations Generated by Functional Tasks

Leaning and stepping can be regarded as perturbations of an internal (i.e. self-generated) origin. A range of other functional tasks also represent internal perturbations which may result in loss of balance in a compromised postural control system. These include turning, bending, standing up from a chair, and walking (see Chapter 3 for a more complete discussion of gait characteristics and falls). A wide range of clinical rating scales and functional tests have now been evaluated in older people to determine their ability to predict falls. These include sit-to-stand ability [148–152], turning [151], bending down [153], tandem walking [150], and the Tinetti Balance [154] and Mobility [155, 156] Scales.

One of the most commonly used balance assessment scales, the Performance Oriented Balance and Mobility Assessment (POMA) scale is a simple clinical scale that grades performance on 14 balance items and ten gait items as normal, adaptive or abnormal [157]. The POMA has been shown to be correlated with the Berg Balance Scale [158] and laboratory measures of postural sway [159, 160], and is a moderately good predictor of falls. In a prospective study of 225 people aged over 75, Raiche et al. [161] found that a cut-off score of 36 on the POMA scale provides falls prediction with 70% sensitivity, but only moderate specificity (52%).

The Berg Balance Scale (BBS) consists of 14 items that are scored on a scale of 0 to 4. For each item a score of 0 is given if the participant is unable to do the task for that item, and a score of 4 is given if the participant is able to complete the task based on the criterion that has been assigned to it. The maximum total score on the test is 56. The items include mobility tasks such as transfers, standing unsupported, sit-to-stand, tandem standing, turning 360° and single-leg stance [162]. While some authors have found the BBS to be a useful predictor of falls [162–166], others have not [102, 167]. Overall, it would appear that the BBS has moderate-good specificity, but low sensitivity in predicting falls [168]. However, the addition of self-reported history of falling to the BBS score has been shown to enhance both the sensitivity and specificity of the instrument [169].

The Timed Up and Go Test (TUGT), derived from the original Up and Go Test [170], is an indicator of basic mobility and measures the time required for a person to rise from a chair, walk three metres, turn, walk back, and sit down. The tool was originally validated on 60 day hospital patients, where it was found that a poor performance was significantly correlated with slow gait speed, low BBS performance, and low Barthel Index scores [171]. A systematic review and meta-analysis involving 12,832 people aged 60 years and older living independently or in institutions drawn from 53 studies (25 with prospective designs) has been conducted to determine the discriminative ability and predictive validity of the Timed Up and Go Test in identifying older people who fall. The results showed that the Timed Up and Go Test discriminates better between faller and non-faller groups in lower-functioning populations from institutionalized settings (pooled mean difference: 3.59 s, 95% CI: 2.18,4.99) than in prospective studies of healthy older people, among whom it is not a useful test to predict falls (pooled mean difference: 0.63 (95% CI: 0.14,1.12). Because cut-points to discriminate between older fallers and non-fallers differed greatly between studies, it was not possible to recommend a specific threshold. As a result, the Timed-Up and Go test should not be used as a simple fall screening tool but should be supplemented with multi-factorial fall risk screening tools. The utility of this test may also be further limited in very frail older people due to floor effects – a population-based study of 2305 older people in Canada found that 30% were unable to perform the test [172]. Furthermore, it is important that clinicians follow standardized testing procedures when applying the Timed Up and Go Test as performance can be significantly influenced by chair height [173].

The benefit of clinical tests is that they require little or no equipment and are quick and easy to perform. However, the predictive validity of these tests varies between studies, possibly due to differences in the interpretation of some of the more subjective items, or, in the case of the Timed Up and Go Test, measurement errors [174, 175], variation in equipment used [173], and poor test–retest reliability [172]. The other limitation of this approach to fall risk assessment is that, if performed in isolation, they offer only limited insight into the specific physiological risk factors present in an individual, and as such, offer little guidance in relation to targeted fall prevention programmes. Therefore, such tests are useful as population-based screening tools, but need to be supplemented with more detailed assessment procedures to elucidate underlying physiological impairments that increase fall risk.

Responding to External Perturbations

Although evaluation of standing sway, reach, and functional tasks has provided useful information regarding the interaction of musculoskeletal and sensory components of postural stability, it provides only limited information regarding the ability to react to changing demands of a particular task. To more closely assess this component of postural stability, several investigations have mechanically perturbed participants by applying a direct force to their body, or by tilting or translating the surface upon which they stand. These techniques provide useful information regarding how effectively the sensory and motor systems respond to external stimuli.

Perhaps the simplest technique for assessing postural responses to perturbation is by applying a direct force to the body and measuring the ability to regain stability. This technique, sometimes referred to as the *Postural Stress Test*, was first described by Wolfson et al. [176] and involves a simple pulley-weight apparatus which displaces the centre of mass behind the stability limit. Performance on this task is rated on a nine-point ordinal scale which ranges from 'covert reactions' (score 9), in which the participant remains stable with little observable body displacement, and 'absent reactions' (score 0) in which the participant experiences a backwards fall. Wolfson et al. [176] reported that nursing-home-dwelling older people scored much lower scores on the Postural Stress Test than younger people, and that older fallers performed significantly worse on the test than non-fallers. Subsequent investigations by Chandler et al. [177] and Studenski et al. [90] achieved similar results in community-dwelling individuals with respect to fallers versus non-fallers. A clinical version of this test, in which the clinician directly exerts a force on the participant and observes their postural response, has also been found to be associated with falls in several prospective studies [151, 155, 178]; however, it is difficult to compare results across studies due to the inability to accurately standardize the force applied.

More recent investigations into responses to perturbation have used specialized platforms which translate in the antero-posterior and medio-lateral planes or rotate co-axially with the ankle joints. The use of platform rotation as a postural perturbation was first described by Nashner [179], and was subsequently developed into the *Sensory Organization Test*. This technique involves the modification of visual and support surface conditions; for the visual perturbation, the enclosure in which the participant is tested is rotated, while for the support surface perturbation, the platform upon which the participant stands is rotated according to their degree of postural sway [180]. Numerous investigations utilizing this technique have reported that older adults are less able to compensate for the altered visual and support surface conditions compared to younger adults [180–182], due to significantly slower lower-limb muscle reflex responses to rotational perturbation [180, 183, 184].

Pioneering work into translational postural perturbations was undertaken by Nashner [179, 185, 186], who established normal electromyographic responses to perturbation referred to as *muscle synergies*, in addition to describing three stereotypical *postural strategies* to compensate for different velocity perturbations. The *ankle strategy*, thought to be the most common response to standing perturbation, describes the reaction in which the participant leans forward from the ankle in response to small antero-posterior translations of the supporting surface, while the *hip strategy* involves forward trunk leaning at the level of the hip joint and occurs in response to larger perturbations. A further strategy, the *stepping strategy*, is characterized by rapid steps, hops, or stumbles which occur in order to shift the base of support under the falling centre of mass when the ankle or hip strategies have failed to compensate for very large or rapid perturbations [187].

As with rotational perturbations, older people are less able to maintain stability in response to translational perturbations compared to younger adults [30, 56, 63, 188–190]. This has been explained by the observation that older people have slower muscle reflex responses to translational perturbation [41, 191] and tend to utilize the hip strategy rather than the ankle strategy to maintain balance [189, 192]. Due to the increased challenge to the postural control system, translational perturbations reveal more pronounced age-related differences than unperturbed postural sway [30]. However, although differences in responses to translational perturbation have also been used to predict falls in older people [30, 63, 116], two investigations have revealed that measures of unperturbed sway may be better able to distinguish fallers from non-fallers than measures of response to perturbations [30, 63]. This may be because sway is a better overall indicator of physiological decline, or that platform perturbation is an unnatural movement unrelated to the context of falls in most real-life circumstances.

More recently, the *stepping strategy* has been investigated in more detail, based on the suggestion that the ability to control the centre of mass when the stability limit is moved is likely to be quite distinct from the ability to maintain balance within a stationary stability limit [193]. Luchies et al. [194] assessed the responses of young and older people when they were subjected to sudden backward waist pulls. Young participants responded to the perturbation by taking a single step, while older participants took multiple shorter steps, suggesting a decreased ability to re-establish postural stability in response to centre of mass displacement. Similarly, McIlroy and Maki [195] assessed stepping responses in young and older people when an antero-posterior perturbation was applied to the platform on which they stood. Although both performed similarly with regard to the characteristics of the first step, older people were twice as likely to take additional steps to maintain stability. Furthermore, these additional steps were laterally directed in 30% of cases, suggesting the need to control for lateral instability arising after the first compensatory stepping manoeuvre. A subsequent study utilizing medio-lateral platform perturbation revealed that older people not only took more steps, but were also more likely to contact the contralateral limb when doing so, possibly increasing the risk of a fall [196].

Rogers et al. [197] used a waist-pull apparatus to displace the centre of mass in an anterior direction at different velocities. Compared to young people and older people without a history of falling, older people with recurrent falls exhibited increased lateral motion and increased lateral foot placement when taking a first protective step. These results were consistent with a number of previous studies indicating that older people with balance problems have difficulty stabilizing the body in the medio-lateral direction when standing [63, 89, 198] and when responding to antero-posterior perturbations [195]. Another study utilizing both anterior and posterior waist pulls found that young people tended to resist the perturbation by extending or flexing their torso, whereas older people were more likely to initiate a compensatory step. Furthermore, the compensatory step initiated by balance-impaired older people failed to properly arrest their momentum due to inadequate control of torso inclination before the step, and inadequate control of linear momentum once the step was initiated, partly due to the more lateral foot placement [199]. A prospective cohort study [200] using force-controlled waist-pull perturbations also found reduced ability to withstand the perturbation with ankle and hip strategies without taking a step was associated with increased risk of future falls among 242 older people. This ability was related to better executive functioning and lower limb strength indicating that balance, strength, and agility training, in addition to cognitive exercises, may enhance the ability to withstand unexpected balance perturbations and reduce the risk of falls in older people [201].

Owings et al. [202] used a slightly different model. In this study, participants stood on a motorized treadmill and were instructed to maintain their balance in response to a posterior translation of the treadmill, then continue walking forwards. The magnitude of the backward translation was sufficient to cause some participants to fall. In this way, the responses more accurately represented those that occur when recovering from a trip when walking. Those who failed to recover from the perturbation had slower reaction times, shorter step lengths, and greater trunk flexion.

Another method for studying balance recovery in older adults involves simulating forward loss of balance by placing participants into a static forward lean position via the use of a horizontal tether, which is subsequently suddenly released after a random time delay [203]. To recover balance, participants must take one or more rapid forward steps. The stepping response characteristics such as step length, step timing, and joint kinematics and kinetics are altered in ageing and are associated with balance recovery ability [204]. Compared to older adults who can recover from the forward loss of balance in a single step, those who take multiple steps have lower limb muscle weakness [205–207] and are more likely to experience falls in the following year [208]. While this tether-release system is limited to laboratory use, a clinical tether-release assessment tool, the Spring Scale Test was developed by DePasquale et al. [209]. This test consists of a spring scale device attached to a belt around the person's waist and held by an examiner at the other end, with repeated incremental rounds of predictable loading and unpredictable unloading in anterior and posterior directions. The percentage of total body weight participants could withstand when loaded and recover when unloaded has been shown reliable and valid in distinguishing fallers from non-fallers [209].

Madigan et al. [210] recently devised a scale to assess stepping and trunk control necessary to prevent a fall following a trip-like perturbation generated by a sudden backwards acceleration of the treadmill belt. Thirty-five participants, fitted with a harness, stood on a stationary treadmill belt and were instructed to start walking and clear a foam obstacle placed in front of them on treadmill start-up. In a series of trials, the treadmill belt was suddenly accelerated to three different speeds, and a reactive balance rating scale (0 (worst) to 12 (best)) was used to rate the amount of support required by participants (from 0 (substantial harness/spotter support) to 2 (minimal support)) and the quality of participants' stepping responses (from 0 (no step) to 2 (correct clearance of the foam block)). Reactive balance rating scale scores were positively associated with kinematic measures of reactive balance (step length, step lift-off time, step touchdown time and maximum trunk angle as well as with performance in clinical tests of balance. Thus, this test may provide a valid low-tech measure of reactive balance performance and fall risk.

Conclusions

The maintenance of postural stability is a highly complex skill which is dependent on the coordination of a vast number of neurophysiological and biomechanical variables. Normal ageing is associated with decreased ability to maintain postural stability in standing (both bipedally and unipedally), when responding to unexpected perturbations and during voluntary stepping. This decrease in postural stability in older people may be explained by deficits in muscle strength, peripheral sensation, visual acuity, vestibular function, and central processing of afferent inputs. Although numerous studies have reported impaired performance on a range of balance tests in fallers compared to non-fallers, the ability of balance tests to predict falls when used in isolation is mixed. For this reason, falls assessment tools that incorporate a range of physiological tests in addition to a balance component will provide additional information.

REFERENCES

1. Shumway-Cook A, Woollacott M. *Motor Control: Theory and Practical Applications.* Baltimore: Williams and Wilkins; 1995.
2. Kaplan FS, Nixon JE, Reitz M et al. Age-related changes in proprioception and sensation of joint position. *Acta Orthop Scand.* 1985;56:72–4.
3. Kokmen E, Bossemeyer Jr RW, Barney J et al. Neurological manifestations of aging. *J Gerontol.* 1977;32:411–19.
4. Lord SR, Ward JA. Age-associated differences in sensori-motor function and balance in community dwelling women. *Age Ageing.* 1994;23:452–60.
5. Proske U, Gandevia SC. The proprioceptive senses: their roles in signaling body shape, body position and movement, and muscle force. *Physiol Rev.* 2012;92:1651–97.
6. Thornbury JM, Mistretta CM. Tactile sensitivity as a function of age. *J Gerontol.* 1981;36:34–9.
7. Li KZH, Bherer L, Mirelman A et al. Cognitive involvement in balance, gait and dual-tasking in aging: a focused review from a neuroscience of aging perspective. *Front Neurol.* 2018;9:913.
8. Sheldon JH. The effect of age on the control of sway. *Gerontology Clinics.* 1963;5:129–38.
9. Fitzpatrick R, Rogers DK, McClosky DI. Stable human standing with lower-limb muscle afferents providing the only sensory input. *J Physiol.* 1994;480:395–403.
10. Simoneau GG, Leibowitz HW, Ulbrecht JS et al. The effects of visual factors and head orientation on postural steadiness in women 55 to 70 years of age. *J Gerontol.* 1992;47:M151-8.
11. Fitzpatrick R, McCloskey D. Proprioceptive, visual and vestibular thresholds for the perception of sway during standing in humans. *J Physiol.* 1994;478:173–86.
12. Shumway-Cook A, Horak FB. Assessing the influence of sensory interaction on balance: suggestion from the field. *Phys Ther.* 1986;66:1548–50.
13. Lord SR, Clark RD, Webster IW. Postural stability and associated physiological factors in a population of aged persons. *J Gerontol.* 1991;46A:M69–76.
14. Orma EJ. The effects of cooling the feet and closing the eyes on standing equilibrium: different patterns of standing equilibrium in young men and women. *Acta Physiol Scand.* 1957;38:288–97.
15. Magnusson M, Enbom H, Johansson R et al. Significance of pressor input from the human feet in lateral postural control: the effect of hypothermia on galvanically induced body-sway. *Acta Otolaryngol.* 1990;110:321–7.

16. Magnusson M, Enbom H, Johansson R et al. Significance of pressor input from the human feet in anterior-posterior postural control: the effect of hypothermia on vibration-induced body-sway. *Acta Otolaryngol.* 1990;110:182–8.

17. Barr CJ, McLoughlin JV, van den Berg ME et al. Visual field dependence is associated with reduced postural sway, dizziness and falls in older people attending a falls clinic. *J Nutr Health Aging.* 2016;20:671–6.

18. Sturnieks DL, Delbaere K, Brodie MA et al. The influence of age, anxiety and concern about falling on postural sway when standing at an elevated level. *Hum Mov Sci.* 2016;49:206–15.

19. Romberg MH. *A Manual of the Nervous Diseases of Man.* Sydenham, England: Sydenham Society; 1853;2:396.

20. Hellbrandt FA, Braun GL. The influence of sex and age on the postural sway of man. *Am J Phys Anthropol.* 1939;XXIV:347–60.

21. Boman K, Jalavisto E. Standing steadiness in old and young persons. *Ann Med Exp Biol Fenn.* 1953;31:447–55.

22. Fregly AR, Graybiel A. An ataxia test battery not requiring rails. *Aerosp Med.* 1968;39:277–82.

23. Murray MP, Seireg AA, Sepic SB. Normal postural stability and steadiness: quantitative assessment. *J Bone Joint Surg Am.* 1975;57:510–16.

24. Hasselkus BR, Shambes GM. Aging and postural sway in women. *J Gerontol.* 1975;30:661–7.

25. Overstall PW, Exton-Smith AN, Imms FJ et al. Falls in the elderly related to postural imbalance. *Br Med J.* 1977;1:261–4.

26. Brocklehurst JC, Robertson D, James-Groom P. Clinical correlates of sway in old age: sensory modalities. *Age Ageing.* 1982;11:1–10.

27. Era P, Heikkinen E. Postural sway during standing and unexpected disturbance of balance in random samples of men of different ages. *J Gerontol.* 1985;40:287–95.

28. Ekdahl C, Jarnlo GB, Andersson SI. Standing balance in healthy subjects: evaluation of a quantitative test battery on a force platform. *Scand J Rehabil Med.* 1989;21:187–95.

29. Ring C, Nayak US, Isaacs B. The effect of visual deprivation and proprioceptive change on postural sway in healthy adults. *J Am Geriatr Soc.* 1989;37:745–9.

30. Maki BE, Holliday PJ, Fernie GR. Aging and postural control: a comparison of spontaneous- and induced-sway balance tests. *J Am Geriatr Soc.* 1990;38:1–9.

31. Pyykko I, Jantti P, Aalto H. Postural control in elderly subjects. *Age Ageing.* 1990;19:215–21.

32. Peterka RJ, Black FO. Age-related changes in human posture control: sensory organization tests. *J Vestib Res.* 1990;1:73–85.

33. Colledge NR, Cantley P, Peaston I et al. Ageing and balance: the measurement of spontaneous sway by posturography. *Gerontology.* 1994;40:273–8.

34. Baloh RW, Fife TD, Zwerling L et al. Comparison of static and dynamic posturography in young and older normal people. *J Am Geriatr Soc.* 1994;42:405–12.

35. Okuzumi H, Tanaka A, Haishi K et al. Age-related changes in postural control and locomotion. *Percept Mot Skills.* 1995;81:991–4.

36. Collins JJ, De Luca CJ, Burrows A et al. Age-related changes in open-loop and closed-loop postural control mechanisms. *Exp Brain Res*. 1995;104:480–92.

37. McClenaghan B, Williams H, Dickerson J et al. Spectral characteristics of ageing postural control. *Gait Posture*. 1995;3:123–31.

38. Hageman PA, Leibowitz JM, Blanke D. Age and gender effects on postural control measures. *Arch Phys Med Rehabil*. 1995;76:961–5.

39. Kamen G, Patten C, Du CD et al. An accelerometry-based system for the assessment of balance and postural sway. *Gerontology*. 1995;44:40–5.

40. Hay L, Bard C, Fleury M et al. Availability of visual and proprioceptive afferent messages and postural control in elderly adults. *Exp Brain Res*. 1996;108:129–39.

41. Perrin PP, Jeandel C, Perrin CA et al. Influence of visual control, conduction, and central integration on static and dynamic balance in healthy older adults. *Gerontology*. 1997;43:223–31.

42. Slobounov SM, Moss SA, Slobounova ES et al. Aging and time to instability in posture. *J Gerontol A Biol Sci Med Sci*. 1998;53A:B71-8.

43. Baloh RW, Corona S, Jacobson KM et al. A prospective study of posturography in normal older people. *J Am Geriatr Soc*. 1998;46:438–43.

44. Choy NL, Brauer S, Nitz J. Changes in postural stability in women aged 20 to 80 years. *J Gerontol*. 2003;58A:525–30.

45. Reynard F, Christe D, Terrier P. Postural control in healthy adults: determinants of trunk sway assessed with a chest-worn accelerometer in 12 quiet standing tasks. *PloS One*. 2019;14:e0211051.

46. Fernie GR, Gryfe CI, Holliday PJ et al. The relationship of postural sway in standing to the incidence of falls in geriatric subjects. *Age Ageing*. 1982;11:11–16.

47. Judge JO, King MB, Whipple R et al. Dynamic balance in older persons: effects of reduced visual and proprioceptive input. *J Gerontol A Biol Sci Med Sci*. 1995;50A:M263–70.

48. Era P, Schroll M, Ytting H et al. Postural balance and its sensory-motor correlates in 75-year-old men and women: a cross-national comparative study. *J Gerontol A Biol Sci Med Sci*. 1996;51A:M53–63.

49. Satariano WA, DeLorenze GN, Reed D et al. Imbalance in an older population: an epidemiological analysis. *J Aging Health*. 1996;8:334–58.

50. Carter ND, Khan KM, Mallinson A et al. Knee strength is a significant determinant of static and dynamic balance as well as quality of life in older community-dwelling women with osteoporosis. *Gerontology*. 2002;48:360–8.

51. MacLennan WJ, Timothy JI, Hall MRP. Vibration sense, proprioception and ankle reflexes in old age. *J Clin Exp Gerontol*. 1980;2:159–71.

52. Duncan G, Wilson JA, MacLennan WJ et al. Clinical correlates of sway in elderly people living at home. *Gerontology*. 1992;38:160–6.

53. Anacker SL, Di Fabio RP. Influence of sensory inputs on standing balance in community-dwelling elders with a recent history of falling. *Phys Ther*. 1992;72:575–81; discussion 81–4.

54. Kristinsdottir EK, Jarnlo GB, Magnusson M. Aberrations in postural control, vibration sensation and some vestibular findings in healthy 64–92-year-old subjects. *Scand J Rehabil Med.* 1997;29:257–65.

55. Lichtenstein MJ, Shields SL, Shiavi RG et al. Clinical determinants of biomechanics platform measures of balance in aged women. *J Am Geriatr Soc.* 1988;36:996–1002.

56. Stelmach GE, Phillips J, DiFabio RP et al. Age, functional postural reflexes, and voluntary sway. *J Gerontol.* 1989;44:B100–6.

57. Cohen H, Heaton LG, Congdon SL et al. Changes in sensory organization test scores with age. *Age Ageing.* 1996;25:39–44.

58. Danis CG, Krebs DE, Gill-Body KM et al. Relationship between standing posture and stability. *Phys Ther.* 1998;78:502–17.

59. Kejonen P, Kauranen K, Vanharanta H. The relationship between anthropometric factors and body-balancing movement in postural balance. *Arch Phys Med Rehabil.* 2003;84:17–22.

60. Woolley SM, Czaja SJ, Drury CG. An assessment of falls in elderly men and women. *J Gerontol A Biol Sci Med Sci.* 1997;52A:M80–7.

61. Cho CY, Kamen G. Detecting balance deficits in frequent fallers using clinical and quantitative evaluation tools. *J Am Geriatr Soc.* 1998;46:426–30.

62. Lord SR, Clark RD, Webster IW. Physiological factors associated with falls in an elderly population. *J Am Geriatr Soc.* 1991;39:1194–200.

63. Maki BE, Holliday PJ, Topper AK. A prospective study of postural balance and risk of falling in an ambulatory and independent elderly population. *J Gerontol.* 1994;49:M72–84.

64. Lord SR, Lloyd DG, Li SK. Sensori-motor function, gait patterns and falls in community-dwelling women. *Age Ageing.* 1996;25:292–9.

65. Lord SR, Clark RD. Simple physiological and clinical tests for the accurate prediction of falling in older people. *Gerontology.* 1996;42:199–203.

66. Thapa PB, Gideon P, Brockman KG et al. Clinical and biomechanical measures of balance as fall predictors in ambulatory nursing home residents. *J Gerontol A Biol Sci Med Sci.* 1996;51A:M239–46.

67. Stel VS, Smit JH, Pluijm SMF et al. Balance and mobility performance as treatable risk factors for recurrent falling in older persons. *J Clin Epidemiol.* 2003;56:659–68.

68. Johansson J, Nordstrom A, Gustafson Y et al. Increased postural sway during quiet stance as a risk factor for prospective falls in community-dwelling elderly individuals. *Age Ageing.* 2017;46:964–70.

69. Mahoney JR, Oh-Park M, Ayers E et al. Quantitative trunk sway and prediction of incident falls in older adults. *Gait Posture.* 2017;58:183–7.

70. Zhou J, Habtemariam D, Iloputaife I et al. The complexity of standing postural sway associates with future falls in community-dwelling older adults: the MOBILIZE Boston Study. *Sci Rep.* 2017;7:2924.

71. Lord SR, Sambrook PN, Gilbert C et al. Postural stability, falls and fractures in the elderly: results from the Dubbo Osteoporosis Epidemiology Study. *Med J Aust.* 1994;160:684–5, 688–91.

72. Lord SR, McLean D, Stathers G. Physiological factors associated with injurious falls in older people living in the community. *Gerontology.* 1992;38:338–46.

73. Lord SR, Ward JA, Williams P et al. Physiological factors associated with falls in older community-dwelling women. *J Am Geriatr Soc.* 1994;42:1110–17.

74. Sturnieks DL, Arnold R, Lord SR. Validity and reliability of the Swaymeter device for measuring postural sway. *BMC Geriatrics.* 2011;11:63.

75. Kirby RL, Price NA, MacLeod DA. Influence of foot position on standing balance. *J Biomech.* 1987;20:423–7.

76. Goldie PA, Bach TM, Evans OM. Force platform measures for evaluating postural control: reliability and validity. *Arch Phys Med Rehabil.* 1989;70:510–17.

77. Kollegger H, Wober C, Baumgartner C et al. Stabilizing and destabilizing effects of vision and foot position on body sway of healthy young subjects: a posturographic study. *Eur Neurol.* 1989;29:241–5.

78. Day BL, Steiger MJ, Thompson PD et al. Effect of vision and stance width on human body motion when standing: implications for afferent control of lateral sway. *J Physiol.* 1993;469:479–99.

79. Fregly AR, Smith MJ, Graybiel A. Revised normative standards of performance of men on a quantitative ataxia test battery. *Acta Otolaryngol.* 1973;75:10–16.

80. Bohannon RW, Larkin PA, Cook AC et al. Decrease in timed balance test scores with aging. *Phys Ther.* 1984;64:1067–70.

81. Heitmann DK, Gossman MR, Shaddeau SA et al. Balance performance and step width in noninstitutionalized, elderly, female fallers and nonfallers. *Phys Ther.* 1989;69:923–31.

82. Iverson BD, Gossman MR, Shaddeau SA et al. Balance performance, force production, and activity levels in noninstitutionalized men 60 to 90 years of age. *Phys Ther.* 1990;70:348–55.

83. Speers RA, Ashton-Miller JA, Schultz AB et al. Age differences in abilities to perform tandem stand and walk tasks of graded difficulty. *Gait Posture.* 1998;7:207–13.

84. Crosbie WJ, Nimmo MA, Banks MA et al. Standing balance responses in two populations of elderly women: a pilot study. *Arch Phys Med Rehabil.* 1989;70:751–4.

85. Briggs RC, Gossman MR, Birch R et al. Balance performance among noninstitutionalized elderly women. *Phys Ther.* 1989;69:748–56.

86. Maki BE, Holliday PJ, Topper AK. Fear of falling and postural performance in the elderly. *J Gerontol.* 1991;46:M123–31.

87. Balogun JA, Akindele KA, Nihinlola JO et al. Age-related changes in balance performance. *Disabil Rehabil.* 1994;16:58–62.

88. Vellas BJ, Wayne SJ, Romero L et al. One-leg balance is an important predictor of injurious falls in older persons. *J Am Geriatr Soc.* 1997;45:735–8.

89. Lord SR, Rogers MW, Howland A et al. Lateral stability, sensorimotor function and falls in older people. *J Am Geriatr Soc.* 1999;47:1077–81.

90. Studenski S, Duncan PW, Chandler J. Postural responses and effector factors in persons with unexplained falls: results and methodologic issues. *J Am Geriatr Soc.* 1991;39:229–34.

91. Hurvitz E, Richardson J, Werner R et al. Unipedal stance testing as an indicator of fall risk among older outpatients. *Arch Phys Med Rehabil.* 2000;81:587–91.

92. King MB, Judge JO, Wolfson L. Functional base of support decreases with age. *J Gerontol.* 1994;49:M258–63.

93. Duncan PW, Weiner DK, Chandler J et al. Functional reach: a new clinical measure of balance. *J Gerontol.* 1990;45:M192–7.

94. Weiner DK, Duncan PW, Chandler J et al. Functional reach: a marker of physical frailty. *J Am Geriatr Soc.* 1992;40:203–7.

95. Weiner DK, Bongiorni DR, Studenski SA et al. Does functional reach improve with rehabilitation? *Arch Phys Med Rehabil.* 1993;74:796–800.

96. Wernick-Robinson M, Krebs DE, Giorgetti MM. Functional reach: does it really measure dynamic balance? *Arch Phys Med Rehabil.* 1999;80:262–9.

97. Rosa MV, Perracini MR, Ricci NA. Usefulness, assessment and normative data of the Functional Reach Test in older adults: a systematic review and meta-analysis. *Arch Gerontol Geriatr.* 2018;81:149–70.

98. Haines T, Kuys SS, Morrison G et al. Balance impairment not predictive of falls in geriatric rehabilitation wards. *J Gerontol A Biol Sci Med Sci.* 2008;63:523–8.

99. Lin MR, Hwang HF, Hu MH et al. Psychometric comparisons of the timed up and go, one-leg stand, functional reach, and Tinetti balance measures in community-dwelling older people. *J Am Geriatr Soc.* 2004;52:1343–8.

100. Brauer S, Burns Y, Galley P. Lateral reach: a clinical measure of medio-lateral postural stability. *Physiother Res Int.* 1999;4:81–8.

101. Newton R. Validity of the multi-directional reach test: a practical measure for limits of stability in older adults. *J Gerontol A Biol Sci Med Sci.* 2001;56A:M248–52.

102. Brauer S, Burns Y, Galley P. A prospective study of laboratory and clinical measures of postural stability to predict community dwelling fallers. *J Gerontol A Biol Sci Med Sci.* 2000;55A:M469–76.

103. Lord SR, Ward JA, Williams P. Exercise effect on dynamic stability in older women: a randomized controlled trial. *Arch Phys Med Rehabil.* 1996;77:232–6.

104. Delbaere K, Close JC, Heim J et al. A multifactorial approach to understanding fall risk in older people. *J Am Geriatr Soc.* 2010;58:1679–85.

105. Lord SR, Fitzpatrick RC. Choice stepping reaction time: a composite measure of falls risk in older people. *J Gerontol.* 2001;56A:M627–32.

106. Menz HB, Lord SR. The contribution of foot problems to mobility impairment and falls in community-dwelling older people. *J Am Geriatr Soc.* 2001;49:1651–6.

107. Sturnieks DL, Tiedemann A, Chapman K et al. Physiological risk factors for falls in older people with lower limb arthritis. *J Rheumatol.* 2004;31:2272–9.

108. Taylor ME, Lord SR, Delbaere K et al. Physiological fall risk factors in cognitively impaired older people: a one-year prospective study. *Dement Geriatr Cogn Disord.* 2012;34:181–9.

109. Day L, Fildes B, Gordon I et al. A randomized factorial trial of falls prevention among older people living in their own homes. *Br Med J.* 2002;325:128–33.

110. Barnett A, Smith B, Lord SR et al. Community-based group exercise improves balance and reduces falls in at-risk older people: a randomised controlled trial. *Age Ageing*. 2003;32:407–14.

111. Lord SR, Castell S, Corcoran J et al. The effect of group exercise on physical functioning and falls in frail older people living in retirement villages: a randomised controlled trials. *J Am Geriatr Soc*. 2003;51:1685–92.

112. Vogler CM, Sherrington C, Ogle SJ et al. Reducing risk of falling in older people discharged from hospital: a randomized controlled trial comparing seated exercises, weight-bearing exercises, and social visits. *Arch Phys Med Rehabil*. 2009;90:1317–24.

113. Sherrington C, Lord SR, Vogler CM et al. A post-hospital home exercise program improved mobility but increased falls in older people: a randomised controlled trial. *PloS One*. 2014;9:e104412.

114. Patla AE. Strategies for dynamic stability during adaptive human locomotion. *IEEE Eng Med Biol Mag*. 2003;22:48–52.

115. Stelmach GE, Worringham CJ. Sensorimotor deficits related to postural stability. Implications for falling in the elderly. *Clin Geriatr Med*. 1985;1:679–94.

116. Grabiner MD, Jahnigen DW. Modeling recovery from stumbles: preliminary data on variable selection and classification efficacy. *J Am Geriatr Soc*. 1992;40:910–3.

117. Lord SR, Menz HB, Tiedemann A. A physiological profile approach to falls risk assessment and prevention. *Phys Ther*. 2003;83:237.

118. Schoene D, Lord SR, Verhoef P et al. A novel video game-based device for measuring stepping performance and fall risk in older people. *Arch Phys Med Rehabil*. 2011;92:947–53.

119. Pijnappels M, Delbaere K, Sturnieks DL et al. The association between choice stepping reaction time and falls in older adults: a path analysis model. *Age Ageing*. 2010;39:99–104.

120. Bunce D, Haynes BI, Lord SR et al. Intraindividual stepping reaction time variability predicts falls in older adults with mild cognitive impairment. *J Gerontol A Biol Sci Med Sci*. 2017;72:832–7.

121. Schoene D, Lord SR, Delbaere K et al. A randomized controlled pilot study of home-based step training in older people using videogame technology. *PloS One*. 2013;8:e57734.

122. Schoene D, Valenzuela T, Toson B et al. Interactive cognitive-motor step training improves cognitive risk factors of falling in older adults: a randomized controlled trial. *PloS One*. 2015;10:e0145161.

123. Schoene D, Smith ST, Davies TA et al. A Stroop Stepping Test (SST) using low-cost computer game technology discriminates between older fallers and non-fallers. *Age Ageing*. 2014;43:285–9.

124. Schoene D, Delbaere K, Lord SR. Impaired response selection during stepping predicts falls in older people – a cohort study. *J Am Med Dir Assoc*. 2017;18:719–25.

125. Delbaere K, Gschwind YJ, Sherrington C et al. Validity and reliability of a simple 'low-tech' test for measuring choice stepping reaction time in older people. *Clin Rehabil*. 2016;30:1128–35.

126.   Bongers KT, Schoon Y, Graauwmans, MJ et al. Safety, feasibility, and reliability of the maximal step length, gait speed, and chair test measured by seniors themselves: the Senior Step Study. *J Aging Phys Act*. 2015;23:438–43.

127.   Fujimoto A, Hori H, Tamura T et al. Relationships between estimation errors and falls in healthy aged dwellers. *Gerontology*. 2015;61:109–15.

128.   Goldberg A, Schepens S, Wallace M. Concurrent validity and reliability of the Maximum Step Length Test in older adults. *J Geriatr Phys Ther*. 2010;33:122–7.

129.   Hiura M, Nemoto H, Nishisaka K et al. The association between walking ability and falls in elderly Japanese living in the community using a path analysis. *J Community Health*. 2012;37:957–62.

130.   Lindemann U, Lundin-Olsson L, Hauer K et al. Maximum step length as a potential screening tool for falls in non-disabled older adults living in the community. *Aging Clin Exp Res*. 2008;20:394–9.

131.   Schulz BW, Jongprasithporn M, Hart-Hughes SJ, Bulat T. Effects of step length, age, and fall history on hip and knee kinetics and knee co-contraction during the maximum step length test. *Clin Biomech (Bristol, Avon)*. 2013;28:933–40.

132.   Cho B, Scarpace D, Alexander NB. Tests of stepping as indicators of mobility, balance, and fall risk in balance-impaired older adults. *J Am Geriatr Soc*. 2004;52:1168–73.

133.   Medell JL, Alexander NB. A clinical measure of maximal and rapid stepping in older women. *J Gerontol A Biol Sci Med Sci*. 2000;55A:M424–8.

134.   Dite W, Temple V. A clinical test of stepping and change of direction to identify multiple falling older adults. *Arch Phys Med Rehabil*. 2002;83:1566–71.

135.   Melzer I, Kurz I, Shahar D et al. Application of the voluntary step execution test to identify elderly fallers. *Age Ageing*. 2007;36:532–7.

136.   Melzer I, Kurz I, Shahar D et al. Predicting injury from falls in older adults: comparison of voluntary step reaction times in injured and noninjured fallers. A prospective study. *J Am Geriatr Soc*. 2009;57:743–5.

137.   Melzer I, Kurz I, Shahar D et al. Do voluntary step reactions in dual task conditions have an added value over single task for fall prediction? A prospective study. *Aging Clin Exp Res*. 2010;22:360–6.

138.   Callisaya ML, Blizzard L, Martin K et al. Gait initiation time is associated with the risk of multiple falls: a population-based study. *Gait Posture*. 2016;49:19–24.

139.   Murphy MA, Olson SL, Protas EJ et al. Screening for falls in community-dwelling elderly. *J Aging Phys Act*. 2003;11:66–80.

140.   Aslan UB, Cavlak U, Yagci N et al. Balance performance, aging and falling: a comparative study based on a Turkish sample. *Arch Gerontol Geriatr*. 2008;46:283–92.

141.   Kwan MM, Lin S-I, Chen C-H et al. Minimal chair height standing ability is independently associated with falls in Taiwanese older people. *Arch Phys Med Rehabil*. 2011;92:1080–5.

142.   Seino S, Yabushita N, Kim M-J et al. Physical performance measures as a useful indicator of multiple geriatric syndromes in women aged 75 years and older. *Geriatr Gerontol Int*. 2013;13:901–10.

143. Tiedemann A, Shimada H, Sherrington C et al. The comparative ability of eight functional mobility tests for predicting falls in community-dwelling older people. *Age Ageing.* 2008;37:430–5.

144. Miyamoto K, Takebayashi H, Takimoto K et al. A new simple performance test focused on agility in elderly people: the Ten Step Test. *Gerontology.* 2008;54:365–72.

145. Sherrington C, Lord SR, Close JCT et al. Development of a tool for prediction of falls in rehabilitation settings (Predict FIRST): a prospective cohort study. *J Rehabil Med.* 2010;42:482–8.

146. Yamada M, Higuchi T, Tanaka B et al. Measurements of stepping accuracy in a multitarget stepping task as a potential indicator of fall risk in elderly individuals. *J Gerontol A Biol Sci Med Sci.* 2011;66:994–1000.

147. Yamada M, Higuchi T, Mori S et al. Maladaptive turning and gaze behavior induces impaired stepping on multiple footfall targets during gait in older individuals who are at high risk of falling. *Arch Gerontol Geriatr.* 2012;54:e102–8.

148. Davis JW, Ross PD, Nevitt MC et al. Risk factors for falls and for serious injuries on falling among older Japanese women in Hawaii. *J Am Geriatr Soc.* 1999;47:792–8.

149. Campbell AJ, Borrie MJ, Spears GF. Risk factors for falls in a community-based prospective study of people 70 years and older. *J Gerontol.* 1989;44:M112–7.

150. Nevitt M, Cummings S, Kidd S et al. Risk factors for recurrent non-syncopal falls. *J Am Geriatr Soc.* 1989;261:2663–8.

151. Lipsitz LA, Jonsson PV, Kelley MM et al. Causes and correlates of recurrent falls in ambulatory frail elderly. *J Gerontol.* 1991;46:M114–22.

152. Schwartz AV, Villa ML, Prill M et al. Falls in older Mexican American women. *J Am Geriatr Soc.* 1999;47:1371–8.

153. O'Loughlin JL, Robitaille Y, Boivin JF et al. Incidence of and risk factors for falls and injurious falls among the community-dwelling elderly. *Am J Epidemiol.* 1993;137:342–54.

154. Thapa PB, Gideon P, Fought RL et al. Psychotropic drugs and risk of recurrent falls in ambulatory nursing home residents. *Am J Epidemiol.* 1995;142:202–11.

155. Tinetti ME, Speechley M, Ginter SF. Risk factors for falls among elderly persons living in the community. *N Engl J Med.* 1988;319:1701–7.

156. Robbins AS, Rubenstein LZ, Josephson KR et al. Predictors of falls among elderly people: results of two population-based studies. *Arch Intern Med.* 1989;149:1628–33.

157. Tinetti ME. Performance-oriented assessment of mobility problems in elderly patients. *J Am Geriatr Soc.* 1986;34:119–26.

158. Berg KO, Maki BE, Williams JI et al. Clinical and laboratory measures of postural balance in an elderly population. *Arch Phys Med Rehabil.* 1992;73:1073–80.

159. Lichtenstein MJ, Burger MC, Shields SL et al. Comparison of biomechanics platform measures of balance and videotaped measures of gait with a clinical mobility scale in elderly women. *J Gerontol.* 1990;45:M49–54.

160. Laughton CA, Slavin M, Katdare K et al. Aging, muscle activity, and balance control: physiologic changes associated with balance impairment. *Gait Posture.* 2003;18:101–8.

161.   Raiche M, Hebert R, Prince F et al. Screening older adults at risk of falling with the Tinetti balance scale. *Lancet.* 2000;356:1001.

162.   Berg KO, Wood-Dauphinee SL, Williams JI et al. Measuring balance in the elderly: validation of an instrument. *Can J Public Health.* 1992;83:S7–11.

163.   Thorbahn LD, Newton RA. Use of the Berg Balance Test to predict falls in elderly persons. *Phys Ther.* 1996;76:576–83; discussion 84–5.

164.   Shumway-Cook A, Baldwin M, Polissar NL et al. Predicting the probability for falls in community-dwelling older adults. *Phys Ther.* 1997;77:812–19.

165.   O'Brien K, Culham E, Pickles B. Balance and skeletal alignment in a group of elderly female fallers and nonfallers. *J Gerontol A Biol Sci Med Sci.* 1997;52A:B221–6.

166.   Chiu AY, Au-Yeung SS, Lo SK. A comparison of four functional tests in discriminating fallers from non-fallers in older people. *Disabil Rehabil.* 2003;25:45–50.

167.   Daubney ME, Culham EG. Lower-extremity muscle force and balance performance in adults aged 65 years and older. *Phys Ther.* 1999;79:1177–85.

168.   Riddle DL, Stratford PW. Interpreting validity indexes for diagnostic tests: an illustration using the Berg balance test. *Phys Ther.* 1999;79:939–48.

169.   Shumway-Cook A, Woollacott M, Kerns KA et al. The effects of two types of cognitive tasks on postural stability in older adults with and without a history of falls. *J Gerontol A Biol Sci Med Sci.* 1997;52A:M232–40.

170.   Mathias S, Nayak USL, Isaacs B. Balance in elderly patients: the "Get-up and Go" test. *Arch Phys Med Rehabil.* 1986;67:387–9.

171.   Podsiadlo D, Richardson S. The timed "Up & Go": a test of basic functional mobility for frail elderly persons. *J Am Geriatr Soc.* 1991;39:142–8.

172.   Rockwood K, Awalt E, Carver D et al. Feasibility and measurement properties of the Functional Reach and the Timed Up and Go tests in the Canadian Study of Health and Aging. *J Gerontol A Biol Sci Med Sci.* 2000;55A:M70–3.

173.   Siggeirsdottir K, Jonsson B, Jonsson H et al. The timed 'Up & Go' is dependent on chair type. *Clin Rehabil.* 2002;16:609–16.

174.   van Iersel MB, Munneke M, Esselink RA et al. Gait velocity and the Timed-Up-and-Go test were sensitive to changes in mobility in frail elderly patients. *J Clin Epidemiol.* 2008;61:186–91.

175.   Nordin E, Rosendahl E, Lundin-Olsson L. Timed "Up & Go" test: reliability in older people dependent in activities of daily living – focus on cognitive state. *Phys Ther.* 2006;86:646–55.

176.   Wolfson LI, Whipple R, Amerman P et al. Stressing the postural response: a quantitative method for testing balance. *J Am Geriatr Soc.* 1986;34:845–50.

177.   Chandler JM, Duncan PW, Studenski SA. Balance performance on the postural stress test: comparison of young adults, healthy elderly, and fallers. *Phys Ther.* 1990;70:410–15.

178.   Clark RD, Lord SR, Webster IW. Clinical parameters associated with falls in an elderly population. *Gerontology.* 1993;39:117–23.

179.   Nashner LM. Adaptation of movement to altered environments. *Trends Neurosci.* 1982;5:358–61.

180. Woollacott MH, Shumway-Cook A, Nashner LM. Aging and posture control: changes in sensory organization and muscular coordination. *Int J Aging Hum Dev*. 1986;23:97–114.

181. Wolfson L, Whipple R, Derby CA et al. A dynamic posturography study of balance in healthy elderly. *Neurology*. 1992;42:2069–75.

182. Whipple R, Wolfson L, Derby C et al. Altered sensory function and balance in older persons. *J Gerontol*. 1993;48:71–6.

183. Keshner EA, Allum JH, Honegger F. Predictors of less stable postural responses to support surface rotations in healthy human elderly. *J Vestib Res*. 1993;3:419–29.

184. Nardone A, Siliotto R, Grasso M et al. Influence of aging on leg muscle reflex responses to stance perturbation. *Arch Phys Med Rehabil*. 1995;76:158–65.

185. Nashner LM. Fixed patterns of rapid postural responses among leg muscles during stance. *Exp Brain Res*. 1977;30:13–24.

186. Nashner LM, Woollacott M, Tuma G. Organization of rapid responses to postural and locomotor-like perturbations of standing man. *Exp Brain Res*. 1979;36:463–76.

187. Horak FB, Shupert CL, Mirka A. Components of postural dyscontrol in the elderly: a review. *Neurobiol Aging*. 1989;10:727–38.

188. Maki BE, Holliday PJ, Fernie GR. A posture control model and balance test for the prediction of relative postural stability. *IEEE Trans Biomed Eng*. 1987;34:797–810.

189. Manchester D, Woollacott M, Zederbauer-Hylton N et al. Visual, vestibular and somatosensory contributions to balance control in the older adult. *J Gerontol*. 1989;44: M118–27.

190. Camicioli R, Panzer VP, Kaye J. Balance in the healthy elderly: posturography and clinical assessment. *Arch Neurol*. 1997;54:976–81.

191. Peterka RJ, Black FO. Age-related changes in human posture control: motor coordination tests. *J Vestib Res*. 1990;1:87–96.

192. Gu MJ, Schultz AB, Shepard NT et al. Postural control in young and elderly adults when stance is perturbed: dynamics. *J Biomech*. 1996;29:319–29.

193. Maki BE, McIlroy WE. The role of limb movements in maintaining upright stance: the "change-in-support" strategy. *Phys Ther*. 1997;77:488–507.

194. Luchies CW, Alexander NB, Schultz AB et al. Stepping responses of young and old adults to postural disturbances: kinematics. *J Am Geriatr Soc*. 1994;42:506–12.

195. McIlroy WE, Maki BE. Age-related changes in compensatory stepping in response to unpredictable perturbations. *J Gerontol A Biol Sci Med Sci*. 1996;51A:M289–96.

196. Maki BE, Edmonstone MA, McIlroy WE. Age-related differences in laterally directed compensatory stepping behavior. *J Gerontol A Biol Sci Med Sci*. 2000;55A: M270–7.

197. Rogers M, Hedman L, Johnson M et al. Lateral stability during forward-induced stepping for dynamic balance recovery in young and older adults. *J Gerontol A Biol Sci Med Sci*. 2001;56A:M589–94.

198. Williams HG, McClenaghan BA, Dickerson J. Spectral characteristics of postural control in elderly individuals. *Arch Phys Med Rehabil*. 1997;78:737–44.

199. Schulz BW, Ashton-Miller JA, Alexander NB. Compensatory stepping in response to waist pulls in balance-impaired and unimpaired women. *Gait Posture*. 2005;22:198–209.

200. Sturnieks DL, Menant J, Delbaere K et al. Force-controlled balance perturbations associated with falls in older people: a prospective cohort study. *PloS One.* 2013;8:e70981.

201. Sturnieks DL, Menant J, Vanrenterghem J et al. Sensorimotor and neuropsychological correlates of force perturbations that induce stepping in older adults. *Gait Posture.* 2012;36:356–60.

202. Owings TM, Pavol MJ, Grabiner MD. Mechanisms of failed recovery following postural perturbations on a motorised treadmill mimic those associated with an actual forward trip. *Clinical Biomech (Bristol, Avon).* 2001;16:813–19.

203. Do MC, Breniere Y, Brenguier P. A biomechanical study of balance recovery during the fall forward. *J Biomech.* 1982;15:933–9.

204. Hsiao-Wecksler ET. Biomechanical and age-related differences in balance recovery using the tether-release method. *J Electromyogr Kinesiol.* 2008;18:179–87.

205. Carty CP, Barrett RS, Cronin NJ et al. Lower limb muscle weakness predicts use of a multiple- versus single-step strategy to recover from forward loss of balance in older adults. *J Gerontol A Biol Sci Med Sci.* 2012;67:1246–52.

206. Cronin NJ, Barrett RS, Lichtwark G et al. Decreased lower limb muscle recruitment contributes to the inability of older adults to recover with a single step following a forward loss of balance. *J Electromyogr Kinesiol.* 2013;23:1139–44.

207. Graham DF, Carty CP, Lloyd DG et al. Biomechanical predictors of maximal balance recovery performance amongst community-dwelling older adults. *Exp Gerontol.* 2015;66:39–46.

208. Carty CP, Cronin NJ, Nicholson D et al. Reactive stepping behaviour in response to forward loss of balance predicts future falls in community-dwelling older adults. *Age Ageing.* 2015;44:109–15.

209. DePasquale L, Toscano L. The Spring Scale Test: a reliable and valid tool for explaining fall history. *J Geriatr Phys Ther.* 2009;32:159–67.

210. Madigan ML, Aviles J, Allin LJ et al. A reactive balance rating method that correlates with kinematics after trip-like perturbations on a treadmill and fall risk among residents of older adult congregate housing. *J Gerontol A Biol Sci Med Sci.* 2018;73:1222–8.

3

Gait Characteristics and Falls

Jasmine C. Menant, Hylton B. Menz, and Carly Chaplain

Habitual upright walking is a characteristically human trait that provides a challenging set of physiological challenges. When standing erect, two-thirds of the body's mass is located two-thirds of body height from the ground, precariously balanced on two narrow legs with the only direct contact with the ground provided by the feet [1]. Such a structure challenges the basic principles of mechanical engineering and requires a highly developed postural control system to ensure that the body remains upright. However, in order to progress forwards, it is necessary to repeatedly initiate a forward fall and then 're-capture' this momentum by the appropriate placement of the leading limb. The potential for a loss of balance when performing an apparently simple task such as walking is considerable. It is therefore not surprising that between 50 and 70% of falls in older people occur when walking [2–4]. The aim of this chapter is to provide an overview of the literature pertaining to gait patterns in older people and their relationship to falls. Specifically, this chapter will address gait characteristics during level walking, when distracted by secondary tasks, when stepping over, avoiding, and approaching obstacles, during turning, stair walking, and the ability to respond to trips and slips.

Level Walking

Many kinematic and kinetic studies have been undertaken to evaluate differences in gait patterns between young people and older people. The most consistent finding of these studies is that older people walk more slowly than young people [5–20], across a range of tasks of increasing complexity [21]. This has been found to be a function of both a shorter step length [5–7, 11, 12, 15, 16, 18, 19, 22–24], reduced cadence, and increased time spent in double limb support [6, 7, 19, 23, 24]. These spatio-temporal differences would appear to be a direct result of variation in self-selected walking speed, as when older people and younger people are instructed to walk at a specified fixed velocity, no significant differences are apparent [25]. Consensus guidelines for the assessment of gait and reference values for spatio-temporal gait parameters in older people have been proposed by a consortium of international experts in gait disorders, and recommend that gait be assessed at slow, comfortable, and fast speeds to address this [26].

Other gait alterations apparent in older people include reduced hip motion [6, 12, 22, 27], reduced angular velocity of the lower trunk [28], reduced ankle power generation [23, 27, 29] and range of motion [11], increased anterior pelvic tilt [23, 27], increased hip extension moment during swing phase [30], increased mechanical energy demands of lower limb musculature [31–33], and reduced toe pressure [34]. Studies which have assessed foot placement have also reported that older people walk with a larger degree of out-toeing [5, 6, 23].

Age-related changes in spatio-temporal gait parameters have generally been interpreted as indicating the adoption of a more conservative, or less destabilizing gait [35–39], and a number of investigations have revealed that certain changes in gait patterns may be predictive of falling in older people [40]. Gait velocity has been consistently reported to differentiate between older fallers and non-fallers [41], with single fallers [42] and multiple fallers [43] found to walk significantly more slowly. In a large prospective falls study of 597 adults aged 70 years and over [42], each 10 cm/s decrease in gait speed was associated with a 7% increased risk for falls, and those with moderately slow (between 70 and 100 cm/s) and very slow gait speeds (<70 cm/s) had 1.3 to 1.5 times the risk of falling than those with gait speeds more than 100 cm/s, even after accounting for well-documented fall risk factors (e.g. age, gender, years of education, etc). A smaller prospective falls study with a six-month follow-up based on fortnightly phone interviews, found no significant differences in any mean spatio-temporal variables at self-selected comfortable and fast speed between fallers (n = 31) and non-fallers (n = 94). A small sample size, resulting in a small number of fallers and the need to collapse single fallers with multiple fallers, might have contributed to the absence of difference in gait measures at baseline [44].

Gait Variability

Depending on the assessment conditions (e.g. hazardous forest paths versus unobstructed, flat corridors), increased variability of gait may reflect successful adaptability or be a sign of impaired balance control. A number of prospective fall studies have shown that older people who fall in the follow-up period exhibit increased variability in speed [45], cadence [19, 45–47], step length [43, 46, 48, 49], stride length [42], swing time [42], double-support time [43], and step width [50].

Gait Assessments to Predict Falls: Influence of Gait Speed

While gait is usually tested at comfortable speed, this paradigm might not be sufficiently sensitive to capture risk of falls in healthy older adults. Hence, assessments of fast gait speed have been used in some studies, with no clear conclusion about the clinical utility of such assessment. According to recent prospective falls studies, shorter step length (normalized to leg length) at fast walking speeds was associated with future falls [51], whereas gait variability assessed at three different speeds was not [44]. In a population-based study of over 150 older people aged between 60 and 86 years, Callisaya et al. [52] found that a lower walk ratio (step length divided by cadence, due here to smaller steps and increased cadence) during fast walking and a greater reduction in walk ratio from preferred to fast walking was associated with an increased risk of multiple falls. In addition, risk of multiple falls was increased in those walking at lowest walking speeds and those walking at fastest speeds, suggesting different fall mechanisms. These later findings support the postulate of a 'u-shaped' relationship between those at the slow and fast ends of the gait-speed spectrum, with frailty and age-related decline in cognitive and sensorimotor function at one extremity and, at the other, high physical and cognitive function with greater exposure to risky situations or individuals who overestimate their physical capacities and walk too quickly [53]. In a large longitudinal study of prospective falls of 763 older people aged 64–97 years (Mobilize Boston Study), Quach reported a u-shaped relationship whereby those with the slowest (<0.6 m/s) and fastest (>1.3 m/s) gait speeds had higher rates of falls and higher risk of all falls after adjusting for a range of potential confounders compared with those who walked at speeds classified as mildly abnormal (0.6 <1 m/s) and normal (1 m/s to 1.3 m/s). Interestingly, those walking the slowest had twice the risk of experiencing indoor falls and those walking the fastest had twice the risk of experiencing outdoor falls. This study also reported that a decline of more than 0.15 m/s in gait speed per year was predictive of falls [53]. Given that gait speed is an easily tested measure, tracking gait speed over time and identifying decline might be a useful marker for assessing at-risk individuals.

The functional importance and predictive value of step width (also referred to as base of support) is unclear. Some studies report that step width increases significantly with normal ageing [6], while others do not [54]. Similarly, a history of falling in older people has been associated with a narrower step width [55, 56], an increased step width [46, 57, 58], or no difference in step width [59, 60]. It is likely that different techniques have been used to measure step width that may not be directly comparable.

Kinematic Patterns

Although the evidence indicates that older people who fall walk with a characteristic 'conservative' gait pattern, only a limited number of biomechanical investigations have measured variables that more directly represent instability during gait [61–63]. After controlling for walking speed, kinematic gait patterns do not appear to differ greatly between fallers and non-fallers [64], although Kerrigan et al. [63] did find that fallers exhibited reduced peak hip extension irrespective of velocity. A kinetic study by Lee and Kerrigan [61] reported that fallers walked with decreased ankle plantar flexor torque but increased hip flexion, hip adduction, knee extension, knee varum, ankle dorsiflexion, and ankle eversion torques compared to an age-matched control group with no history of falls. However, after controlling for differences in walking speed, differences were only apparent for the sagittal plane parameters [62]. Additionally, there is some evidence indicating that restricted joint range of motion both at the knee [65] and the hip [27, 63, 65] may play a role in altering gait patterns in older fallers; however, at least for the hip joint, these contractures might be improved with a stretching programme [66].

Gait Stability Assessed with Accelerometers

Over the last two decades, the increasing use of body-worn sensors recording accelerations while individuals are ambulating has not only allowed us to measure gait stability in a more direct manner than via centre of mass models obtained from kinematics, but has also opened doors to assessing fall risk in the field. Initially, Yack and Berger [67] fixed a 3D accelerometer to individuals' torsos and found that older people who reported balance problems exhibited less smooth acceleration patterns in the upper trunk. Recording from the lower back, Moe-Nilssen and Helbostad also reported that compared with fit older people, frail ones exhibited greater anterior-posterior (AP) and vertical trunk variability but small medio-lateral (ML) trunk variability during walking [68]. Using a similar technique of assessing gait stability, but adding an accelerometer on the head, Menz et al. [69] found that older people with a low risk of falling were able to maintain equivalent stability to young people by reducing their velocity and cadence. However, older people with a high risk of falling, despite adopting a slower velocity, cadence, and step length, demonstrated less rhythmic acceleration patterns at the head and pelvis in the vertical and antero-posterior direction, particularly when walking on an irregular surface [70]. Doi et al. [71] also showed that measures of acceleration smoothness, upper trunk harmonic ratios in the vertical plane, were independently associated with the incidence of falls among 93 older people, after adjusting for confounders. The erratic acceleration patterns evident in high fall-risk older people suggest that they have difficulty controlling the momentum of their trunk. There is also the possibility that the erratic movements of the head may interfere with normal gaze stability, as it has been shown that older people exhibit larger eye movements when the head is perturbed due to suppression of the vestibulo-ocular reflex [72, 73].

Among the new parameters of gait stability that have been developed from accelerometers [74], a measure of medio-lateral dynamic stability, the short-term Lyapunov exponent (LE) computed from upper trunk acceleration has been found to show age-related changes, displaying reduced gait stability in the ML plane as early as the fourth and fifth decades [75]. Nonetheless, its clinical utility as a fall risk predictor remains to be demonstrated. Bizovska found poor predictive ability of trunk local dynamic stability for multiple falls (AUC: 0.673) recorded over a 12-month period among 131 older people [76]. A very limited sample of multiple fallers (n = 15) compared with non-fallers (n = 81) could have contributed to the null findings.

Daily Life Gait

Daily life gait recordings derived from a single accelerometer worn on the trunk have shown promising findings relative to the prediction of falls in older adults. Measures of walking speed, stride length, stride frequency, intensity, variability, smoothness, symmetry, and complexity, derived from one week of field data from waist-worn accelerometers were predictive of falls among 319 older people. In that study, gait quality in daily life, expressed by separate characteristics or a composite factor based on these highly related variables, was predictive for both time-to-first and time-to-second falls in both univariate and multi-variate models [77]. In another prospective falls study of 160 community-dwellers monitored with smartphone technology, those who fell in the one-year follow-up turned less frequently, took longer to turn, and were less consistent in turn angle than those who did not fall [78]. Importantly, daily-life walking bouts revealed significantly worse gait stability than that observed during single and dual-task walking trials performed in the laboratory [79]; as such, daily life recordings appear to have potential to predict fall risk in older people, but further validation studies are still required. For more detailed discussion on this topic, refer to Chapter 13.

Physiological and Psychological Factors Associated with Gait Changes

A summary of gait changes during level walking found to be associated with falls is shown in Figure 3.1. There are a range of possible explanations for the gait changes observed in older fallers. A number of studies have shown that reductions in the basic spatio-temporal parameters of gait (i.e. velocity and step length) are significantly associated with the same physiological factors found to be risk factors for falls, including reduced lower limb strength [19, 80–82], slow reaction time

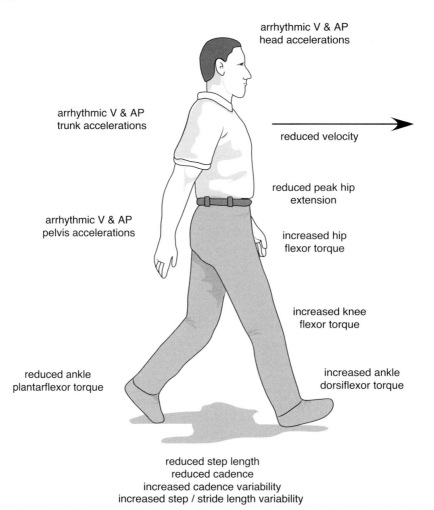

arrhythmic V & AP
head accelerations

arrhythmic V & AP
trunk accelerations

reduced velocity

reduced peak hip
extension

arrhythmic V & AP
pelvis accelerations

increased hip
flexor torque

increased knee
flexor torque

reduced ankle
plantarflexor torque

increased ankle
dorsiflexor torque

reduced step length
reduced cadence
increased cadence variability
increased step / stride length variability

Figure 3.1   Changes in gait patterns during level walking that have been found to be associated with increased risk of falling.

[19, 80], increased postural sway [8, 19], impaired peripheral sensation [19], and poor vision [83]. However, as these gait parameters can also be modified by cognitive influences, psychological factors such as anxiety and fear of falling may also alter gait patterns, i.e. these changes may reflect a *reluctance* rather than an *inability* to walk more quickly in some people [45, 84]. In a group of older people with gait disorders not attributed to specific diseases or medical conditions, Herman et al. [85] found that stride-to-stride variations in gait cycle timing were significantly associated with fear of falling, and suggested that these gait changes may be an appropriate response to unsteadiness. An alternative view is that fear of falling may lead to gait instability. Menz et al. [86] developed a structural equation

model to examine the relationships between physiological ability, fear of falling, and stability of the head and pelvis, based on gait analyses of 100 people aged 75 and over, which suggested reduced sensorimotor function and fear of falling are both correlated with shorter step length, which in turn lead to less stable pelvis accelerations and larger accelerations of the head relative to the pelvis, and these variables in turn lead to impaired head stability. This model indicates that fear of falling may make older people less stable when walking, primarily by promoting a 'guarded' stepping pattern which impairs the rhythmic movement of the upper body. An early study [87] demonstrated the detrimental impact that postural threat inducing heightened anxiety had on lower limb kinematics during virtual obstacle crossing; even though all participants adopted conservative strategies to minimize loss of balance and successfully clear the obstacle, compared with younger adults, older ones showed significantly greater reductions in lead and trail limbs crossing velocity and centre of mass velocity between the safest condition and the one inducing the greatest postural threat. Subsequently, Delbaere et al. [88] reported disproportionate gait adjustments (e.g. excessive gait slowing) displayed by fearful older adults walking on a 60 cm elevated walkway versus the floor illustrates the disabling impact that concern about falling can have on ambulation. Recent studies have employed a similar paradigm in which walkway width and height could be manipulated to induce postural threat. The first study required young adults equipped with an eye-tracker to perform a stepping precision task while walking on the floor and while walking on an elevated 1.1 m high walkway. The results revealed that when concerned about falling, the participants tended to focus gaze on immediate threats to balance followed by conscious visual monitoring of each individual step at the expense of planning ahead and transferring gaze towards the next steps [89]. Findings from the second study revealed older people allocate insufficient attention to carrying out secondary tasks (here an arithmetic task) when required to walk in a postural-threat-inducing situation or when asked to consciously attend to movement during gait [90]. Taken together, these studies suggest that anxious walkers adopt an internal focus of attention which leads to inefficient attentional processing and in consequence increased risk of falls.

Sensorimotor and psychological determinants of gait also appear to vary according to the requirements of the task [91]. Findings from a cross-sectional study of 720 older adults suggested that somatosensory function was particularly important for performing walking tasks requiring accurate foot placement, i.e. narrow beam walking and obstacle crossing, and together with lower limb strength was also associated with fast walking. In contrast, the contribution of general cognition became more apparent in a 'talking while walking' test and personal mastery was related to performance in all four adaptive walking tasks.

Physical Fatigue

A limited number of studies have investigated how muscle fatigue might affect gait patterns in older people [92–94]. Overall, it seems that lower-limb muscle fatigue from repeating sit-to-stand exercises until exhaustion [92, 93] or isokinetic contractions [94] does not affect gait speed or step/stride length [93, 94] but impairs medio-lateral stability (increased step width and medio-lateral trunk accelerations) during simple overground walking [93] and leads to slower gait and shorter strides under dual-task overground conditions [94], as well as reduced lower limb control (increased lead limb vertical loading rate) after crossing a small obstacle (height of 10% leg length) [92]. Given that most ambulation tasks in daily life involve the negotiation of secondary tasks and/or obstacles, it is likely that these small fatigue-related changes in gait patterns make older adults more susceptible to falling.

Non-Modifiable Factors Associated with Gait Speed

According to a large cohort study of 703 Mexican Americans and European Americans, Mexican Americans were approximately 2 to 2.6 times more likely than European Americans to have walking speed in the abnormal ranges (<1 m/s) [95]. In this study, contextual factors including ethnicity, education, age, sex, and socio-economic status explained approximately 20% of the variance in walking speed of the sample. Another large cross-sectional study also reported that education significantly influenced the age–walking-speed association in women younger than 55 years as well as women aged 55 years and older [96] These findings therefore indicate that some non-modifiable factors related to socio-economic status and education need to be considered by therapists and clinicians during assessments of physical function and prescription of rehabilitation/exercise plans.

Gait and Cognition

Substantial research effort in the past two decades has been focused on the cortical control of gait, demonstrating links between cognitive capacity, slow gait, and increased risk of falling (e.g. reviews [97–99]). Even though free walking implies some level of automaticity, cognitive processing from higher-order structures is required to navigate safely through the environment. This reliance on cognitive resources for safe ambulation becomes more apparent in ageing (and pathological populations) as well as in more challenging walking conditions.

Several studies have demonstrated the relationship between poor executive function and attention, and impaired gait parameters in ageing [100–102]. A seminal study of physically and cognitively healthy older adults [100] showed that slower and less stable gait (increased stride time variability) was not associated with performance in an automated, well learned finger tapping task; instead it was related to a complex motor task, ball catching. This link (or lack of) was further supported by significant associations between shorter stride time and reduced stride time variability and superior performance in the Stroop Test, a measure of processing speed, decision-making, and inhibition. No significant associations were found between gait parameters and general cognitive function or memory. Given the other well-established evidence that executive function deficits are predictive of falls [103, 104] (see Chapter 8 for more details), it has been posited that impaired cognition predicts mobility decline and falls, and mobility decline and slow gait predict cognitive deterioration and falls, with each of these phenomena occurring concurrently [105].

Dual-Tasking During Gait

Most daily life ambulatory tasks present a cognitive-motor inference resulting from having to walk while concurrently performing another task, be it motor (e.g. carrying a cup of tea) or cognitive (e.g. looking for the correct bus number). Recent findings that gait parameters recorded during long bouts of daily-living walking are more similar to laboratory-recorded gait during dual-task paradigms, support this [79]. Such cognitive-motor challenges are likely to place an older person at increased risk of falling. Slow gait speed in dual-task paradigms is predictive of falls in older people, though not to a greater extent than simple slow gait speed [41]. According to a published systematic review, other spatio-temporal gait variables (e.g. cadence, step length) might be more strongly associated with table wal falls or fall risk when assessed in dual-task walking paradigms as opposed to simple walking paradigms, though no formal meta-analysis was undertaken to support this finding [106]. There is good meta-analysis evidence that secondary tasks interfering with internal processing (e.g. mental tracking) impair gait to a greater extent than do tasks calling upon external interfering factors (e.g. reaction time) [107]. It is possible that secondary tasks that require visuo-spatial processing might interfere with balance control more so than others during walking, increasing the risk of falls. For example, Menant et al. [108] showed that older people adopt a slower, more variable, and less smooth gait pattern when required to concurrently perform a visuo-spatial processing task requiring them to imagine a star moving through labelled boxes, compared with an arithmetic task of similar difficulty. Conversely, walking while concurrently performing a secondary task is detrimental to performance in cognitive secondary tasks, confirming that gait requires attention, even in young healthy adults [109].

Mechanisms underlying age-related decrements in dual-task gait paradigms are still unclear, with a recent functional magnetic resonance study demonstrating a lack of relationship between age-related dual-task difficulties and structural interference (competition for shared brain regions) [110]. Instead, the central bottleneck theory whereby participants would have to rapidly switch between tasks, or the cross-talk model which is 'dependent on the content-based overlap between task and stimulus-response modalities' [110] might contribute to age-related differences in dual-task performances. Future studies using imaging technology might help clarify this debate.

The development of freely worn imaging technologies has allowed further examination of the cortical control of gait. Functional near-infrared spectroscopy (fNIRS), for example, is increasingly being used to investigate patterns of cortical activation during motor tasks in various populations. In gait, the prefrontal cortex has by far been the cortical region of interest most frequently investigated, due to its role in attention and executive functions [111]. Recent systematic reviews have synthesized these findings [112–115], and have shown that the majority of studies involving young people, older people, and clinical groups report increased prefrontal cortex activation associated with walking tasks of increasing complexity, either through the addition of a secondary cognitive (e.g. verbal fluency, counting backwards, dual-task paradigm) or the negotiation of an obstacle [114]. One study has also reported increased prefrontal cortex activity when performing an arithmetic task while walking predicted falls over three years in high-functioning older people (n = 166) [116]. Although promising, these findings need to be replicated in larger samples of older people and using shorter periods of falls follow-up (e.g. six months to one year).

Stepping Over and Avoiding Obstacles

During normal daily activities, it is not uncommon for us to step over obstacles as we walk. This poses a greater threat to the postural control system than level walking for two main reasons: first, the task of stepping over an obstacle requires a longer period of time spent standing on one leg, and second, there is a risk of the lead or trailing limb making contact with the obstacle and leading to a loss of balance. Indeed, a large proportion of falls in older people are attributed to tripping [117–119], and experiencing multiple stumbles has been found to be a predictor of falls over a 12-month prospective period [120]. Assessment of level walking therefore provides only limited information regarding an individual's ability to navigate the range of environments traversed in daily activities.

Biomechanics of Obstacle Crossing

Successful negotiation of an obstacle requires precise planning of the crossing step and the ability to maintain balance while allowing sufficient clearance of the leading and trailing limbs. Stepping over an obstacle involves reducing the hip flexor activity during toe-off and increasing knee flexion to enable clearance of the leading limb [121]. However, the characteristics of the crossing step are strongly influenced by the height of the obstacle. With increasing obstacle height, the speed of the crossing step decreases and the foot clearance distance increases [122]. In addition, higher obstacles require greater vertical and antero-posterior displacement of the centre of mass [123], greater muscular activity of hip abductors, external hip rotators and ankle plantar flexors of the leading limb [124, 125], and increased knee flexion of the trailing limb [126].

Systematic review evidence indicates that when crossing an obstacle, older adults show increases in hip flexion during swing and hip flexion, hip adduction, and ankle dorsiflexion during stance as well as reduced internal moments across the hip and ankle in specific phases of the obstacle crossing cycle, for both the lead and trail limb [127]. Older adults also consistently adopt more conservative lower limb kinematic strategies than young adults under time constraints, likely to promote safe clearing of the obstacle and to reduce balance loss [127]. For example, older adults tend to adopt greater mean toe clearance over obstacles compared with younger adults [128]. In addition, Chen et al. [122] assessed lower extremity kinematics when young and older participants stepped over obstacles of 0, 25, 51 and 152 mm in height, with a 4 m approach distance. Older people used a more conservative strategy when stepping over obstacles, exhibiting a slower crossing speed, shorter step length, and a smaller distance between the obstacle and the subsequent heel strike. Although none of the older participants tripped over the obstacles, 25% stepped onto the obstacle itself. A subsequent study assessed age-associated differences in the ability to step over a virtual obstacle (a band of light) which appeared in a variety of locations along an eight-metre walkway. The virtual obstacle was designed to appear at the predicted location of the next heel strike at a range of available response times (in 50 ms increments). Older participants were more likely to contact the obstacle than younger participants, particularly when the available response time was decreased [129]. Subsequently, Chen et al. [130] evaluated the effects of dividing attention on the ability to step over an obstacle in young and older people. The study utilized the same virtual obstacle and walkway as the previous study; however, in addition, participants were asked to respond verbally when they saw a red light at the end of the room. The performance of the additional task significantly increased the likelihood of stepping on the obstacle in both groups, but was particularly evident in older people, suggesting an increased risk of tripping when attention is directed elsewhere.

Obstacle Avoidance

In addition to stepping over obstacles, successful avoidance of obstacles may also play a role in preventing falls. Cao et al. [131] assessed the ability of young and older people to suddenly turn 90° when presented with a visual stimulus along a walkway, and reported that older people were less able to complete the turn when provided with smaller response times. A similar study by Gilchrist [132] assessed the ability of young and older women to side step to the left or right when walking after they were presented with a visual stimulus at the end of a walkway; 58% of the younger participants could perform the task with a single sideways step, compared to only 26% of the older participants. In addition, older participants' walking speed decreased significantly after the side-step manoeuvre, suggesting that even when avoidance of an obstacle is successful, they were less able to incorporate the manoeuvre into their normal over-ground walking pattern. Tirosh and Sparrow [133] also found that despite walking more slowly, older people take relatively longer to stop walking in response to a visual cue than younger people, and their braking response was more likely to involve more than one step. These results indicate that some older people may be at greater risk of falls as they have difficulty establishing proactive and reactive strategies to avoid obstacles altogether. There is also some preliminary evidence [134] that some older people actively modulate the width of their steps to avoid small obstacles placed along a footpath even though these hazards are unlikely to substantially affect their gait. It is unclear whether this obstacle negotiation approach is safe and appropriate or maladaptive and the reflection of an inefficient gait strategy.

Gait Adaptability

The emergence of new technologies that allow the projection of virtual obstacles on a pathway or a treadmill to provide endless combinations of obstacle negotiation paradigms have given rise to a number of investigations on gait adaptability. Older adults appear to walk significantly slower during visually guided walking conditions, whether overground or on the treadmill, which requires stepping on targets compared to unobstructed walking. This is also verified when the target location pattern matches the participants' own comfortable walking speed [135]. Deficits in executive function appear to contribute to poor gait adaptability to a path with irregular appearance of stepping targets, possibly because older adults with lower executive function are already using a significant amount of attentional resources during uncued walking on a treadmill compared with those with higher executive function [136].

Caetano et al. [137] recently devised an overground walking task to assess gait adaptation strategies in response to obstacles needed to be avoided and targets requiring precision stepping, both virtual hazards appearing on the walkway two

steps ahead of the person walking. Increased age significantly impaired performance in this test of gait adaptability, whereby older adults (n = 50) made more
mistakes and were less accurate stepping on the targets, despite walking slower,
and taking more and shorter steps than the young adults (n = 21). Deficits in
executive function, particularly inhibitory control, slow processing speed, weak
knee extensor muscles, and poor reactive balance were significant determinants of
the ability to avoid obstacles and/or step accurately on others [138]. A visually
cued stepping task on a treadmill requiring participants to make step adjustments
in response to stepping targets shifting forward, backward or sideways under time
pressure yielded similar results. Older adults undershot the targets and/or made
more errors than younger adults, especially when concurrently performing an
auditory Stroop task [139]. Of note, older adults also prioritized the secondary
task performance over the step adjustment which in a real-life situation could be
a fall catalyst. In the overground gait adaptability task, Caetano et al. [140] found
that older people who made more errors were four times more likely to be a high-
risk faller, i.e. have an increased physiological risk of falling and a history of falls.
Decline in executive function, weak lower limbs (knee extensors), and increased
concern about falling appeared to contribute to the relationship between poor gait
adaptability and an increased risk of falling.

The approach to an obstacle might also prove a sensitive paradigm to identify
older people at high risk of falling. Interestingly, a recent study showed that older
people identified as fallers (n = 27) had higher variability in step time and step
length when approaching an obstacle compared with non-fallers (n = 110),
although groups had comparable gait performance during unobstructed walking
[141]. Despite a retrospective design and limited number of trials (n = 2) and steps
(n = 7), this work suggests stepping adjustments ahead of obstacle negotiation
might be over-amplified to the point of perturbing gait stability in people at high
risk of falls.

Mechanisms for Age-Related Differences in Obstacle Negotiation

Among the underlying mechanisms responsible for these age-related differences,
visual processing is likely to play an important role in implementing avoidance
strategies and en-route planning of preparatory steps [142], while reaction time
and lower limb strength contribute to the ability to maintain balance when
stepping over the obstacle [124, 126, 143]. Thus, deficits in vision, reaction time
and lower limb strength associated with ageing or disease may be responsible for
impaired obstacle navigation or avoidance. Regarding visual contributions to
obstacle negotiation, a large body of work has reported that age-related changes
in gaze behaviour during locomotion, particularly during negotiation of stepping
targets and obstacles, stairs, and unexpected perturbations, are likely to put older

people at increased risk of falling (see Uiga et al. [144] for a review). For example, the work of Hollands et al. [145] clearly established that suboptimal visual sampling strategies in older adults and particularly those at increased risk of falls, impairs stepping precision. These researchers first showed that compared with young adults, older people prematurely transfer their gaze away from the target they are stepping on to fixate further potential hazards, and that this visual strategy resulted in less accurate and more variable subsequent steps. This hazardous gaze behaviour was particularly evident in older people at high risk of falls negotiating a path with multiple obstacles [146]. Older adults at high risk of falls also took significantly longer time than older adults at low risk of falls and younger adults to view and subsequently execute mediolateral stepping adjustments, similar to those that would be required to avoid a hazard on the walking path within short time constraints [147]. In parallel, they later demonstrated that inciting older people to keep fixating the stepping target for longer, that is, after heel contact, significantly reduced stepping errors [148]. More recent work by this research group [149] showed that when given the opportunity to preview a challenging route (comprising either one stepping target or one or two obstacles to cross) for 10 s compared to having to immediately start walking, older adults reported increased self-confidence, fixated the target for longer (a safety strategy), and improved their stepping performance, as indicated by reduced medio-lateral foot placement variability and reduced anterior-posterior foot placement error. In relation to obstacle crossing, these study findings confirm that information from the lower visual field is used from two steps ahead to adjust the leading foot position to the height of the obstacle [128, 150, 151] but not to maintain medio-lateral stability throughout the obstacle-crossing task [128]. Balance during obstacle crossing is more likely to be related to lower limb strength and position sense.

Interestingly, the use of antidepressant medication [87] may also detrimentally affect obstacle crossing in older people. In one study, 12 older people were given single doses of amitriptyline or a placebo four hours before being asked to step over an obstacle. When under the influence of the antidepressant, participants reduced their velocity, cadence, and angular velocity of knee flexion of the trailing limb, indicating that the use of these medications may increase risk of tripping [152].

Turning

Almost every activity of daily living involves some degree of steering. This complex motor task requires planning, tight balance control, and fine spatial coordination of the lower limbs, and is a well-documented trigger of freezing of gait in people with Parkinson's disease [153]. Turning during standing and walking contributed to 13% of real-life falls captured on a video system in a residential setting [154]. Nevertheless, the potential for a turning assessment to predict falls has been scarcely investigated, except in the context of the Timed Up and Go Test, which is discussed in Chapter 2. A small prospective falls study of 35 older people used accelerometers placed around the lower back and the feet to investigate which characteristics of turning quality recorded during a week-long daily-life recording and during a standard prescribed test were associated with falls [155]. Past recurrent fallers recorded the same number of turns during the week of activity monitoring, but turning duration was longer, speed slower and the turn angle was less variable compared with single- and non-fallers. In addition, variability in the number of steps per turn was larger in the fallers. In contrast, turn duration and peak velocity during the prescribed task did not differentiate between fallers and non-fallers. A larger prospective study of falls in 160 community-dwelling older adults used a tri-axial accelerometer embedded in a smartphone worn on the lower back to record turns during a week. Even though only seven older people were identified as fallers (more than one fall) during the 12-month prospective follow-up, the results confirmed that longer turning duration and more variable turning angle were associated with falls [78].

Some other work has focused on walking along curved trajectories (see [153] for a review), reporting that older adults with poor mobility and slow gait (<0.9 m/s) further reduced their walking speed by 5% [156] to 15% [157] when walking along a curved path. Among 414 older participants of the Boston RISE study [156], determinants of time to complete at usual gait speed a 4 m straight course compared with time taken to walk around a figure-of-eight pattern around two cones placed 1.5 m apart differed. While cognitive processing speed (from the Trails-Making A test), self-efficacy, finger-press reaction time, and heel-to-floor time (a seated test of rapid leg coordination) were independently associated with figure-of-eight test performance, pain severity, and peak leg press strength were determinants of performance on the straight gait test. The complementary underlying sensorimotor, psychological, and cognitive contributors addressed by these tests again emphasize the need to conduct gait assessments beyond gait speed alone when aiming to understand fall risk during ambulation.

Stair Walking

Older people frequently report difficulties in stair walking [158]. Approximately 10% of fatal falls in older people occur when walking on stairs [159] and 51% of fall-related traumatic brain injuries occur on stairs in older adults [160], indicating that age-related declines in physical ability may predispose to severe fall-related accidents when performing this common task. There are two likely mechanisms for falls on stairs: slipping (typically during stair descent), and inappropriate foot placement on the edge of the step (either during stair ascent or descent). Falls studies indicate that stair descent poses a greater risk of falling than stair ascent [161, 162], and it is clear that the movement patterns associated with these two tasks are quite different [159, 163–166]. Slipping is probably an uncommon cause of falls when descending stairs without surface contaminants, as the required coefficient of friction when walking on stairs has been found to be no different to level walking [167]. Loss of balance due to inappropriate foot place-ment appears more likely, as the margin for error is very small – the clearance between the swing foot and the step edge can be as little as 4 mm [168].

Biomechanics

A number of studies have been performed in an attempt to delineate the mechan-ical parameters that may predispose older people to falling when negotiating stairs. Williams [169, 170] found only small differences in limb movement patterns between young and older women when descending stairs, while Christina and Cavanagh [167] reported less vigorous push-off and heel strike in older people, indicating the adoption of a more cautious gait pattern. Hortobagyi and DeVita [171, 172] found that older people demonstrated greater lower limb stiffness of the landing limb when stepping down, due to a more vertical lower limb alignment at contact and greater anticipatory muscle activation. Lark et al. [173] focused on the mechanics of the single support limb prior to step descent, and reported that older people remained in a flat-foot position for a longer period of time before rising onto the ball of the foot, and exhibited less dynamic ankle stiffness than younger participants. Zietz et al. [174] also reported that during stair descent, older adults at high risk of falls based on balance performance, fear of falling, and confidence in stair walking, cleared the stair edges with less vertical distance than their older peers at low risk of falls, and with less horizontal distance than both their healthy older counterparts and young adults. This stepping pattern would increase the risk of catching the heel on the stair edge and losing balance. The older participants at risk of falls also displayed more variability in anterior-posterior and medio-lateral centre-of-mass acceleration than young adults at initial contact with the stairs, indicative of increased instability [174]. Of note, when grabbing a handrail, older adults at high risk of falls reduced variability in vertical centre-of-mass acceleration, indicative of balance improve-ment. Similar cautious strategies, i.e. reducing the centre-of-mass peak velocity and acceleration when descending steps, and increasing lead limb eccentric plantarflexion at larger riser heights to control the increased downward velocity and accelerating the COM during landing have also been reported in older adults in other studies [175]. When stepping up onto a raised surface, older people positioned both the leading and trailing feet further from the edge of the step. Due to the larger distance between the step edge and the trailing foot, the leading foot must be placed on the step at a later period of the stride. This may be a more hazardous strategy, as in the event of obstacle contact or other postural disturbance, there would be less time for a corrective response [176].

Interestingly, dimming the light had no effect on the stepping strategies of young and older adults in a stair descent experiment, however, the addition of a high-contrast step edge improved balance and posture variables (e.g. reduced variability in the vertical COM acceleration) but did not affect stepping strategies [174]. Adding a horizontal-vertical illusion (several 'T' letters in which the vertical line appears longer than the horizontal line) to the bottom and/or top step of a three-step staircase increased foot clearance over the step's edge without compromising postural stability [177]. The inclusion of such optical illusion to curbs, stairs, and other raised surfaces may be a promising way of enhancing older people's safety during raised surface/stair negotiation.

Some work has also focused on negotiation of surface height changes. Lythgo et al. [178] examined the approach and accommodation of a known surface change in 48 young and 48 older community-dwelling women. Age-related biomechanical differences were more evident during descent negotiation, as 67% of the older women used a short step strategy which is more likely to lead to a misstep because the foot is brought closer to the obstacle/step. In contrast, the majority of young women used a long or normal step strategy. The older group also took shorter steps and had smaller foot clearances, and their feet landed closer to the obstacle, preferably on the forefoot. Overall the older adults adopted earlier and larger adjustments than their younger counterparts.

Vision

Research into stair negotiation in ageing has also addressed the role of vision when negotiating stairs, as it is likely that visual impairment contributes to inappropriate selection of foot placement. Zietz and Hollands [179] described the gaze behaviour when walking up and down stairs and reported that even though both young and older adults looked approximately three steps ahead and fixated steps for shorter times when descending stairs, older adults fixated the steps for longer before stepping onto them and were less variable in the extent to which they looked ahead compared with their younger counterparts. A kinematic analysis of stair descent on older women by Simoneau et al. [168] found that impaired visual acuity was associated with increased foot clearance and a decreased distance between the descending foot and the previous step. Buckley et al. [180] evaluated the mechanics of older people stepping down from a range of step heights with and without light-scattering lenses which altered contrast sensitivity to a level similar to dense cataracts. When wearing the lenses, participants adopted a more cautious stepping down strategy, characterized by increased step execution time, increased knee flexion and ankle plantarflexion, and increased weight bearing in the contralateral limb. The authors attributed this altered strategy to the participants 'feeling' their way to the floor in an attempt to increase sensory input from the lower limb. A subsequent study [181] provided further explanation as to how this altered strategy could be detrimental to balance. Mediolateral stability (assessed by comparing the position of the centre of mass relative to the centre of pressure) was found to be impaired in both step ascent and descent when wearing the lenses, but this was particularly evident when stepping down. These results help to explain findings from a prospective study in which Lord et al. found that older subjects who wore bi- and multi-focal glasses were more likely to fall when walking on stairs than those who did not wear these glasses [182]. This is because the lower lenses of these glasses impair depth perception and edge-contrast sensitivity at critical distances for detecting obstacles in the environment, such as the edges of stairs [182].

Tripping Responses

Mechanisms Whereby Older People Trip

Epidemiological studies reveal that up to 53% of falls in older people result from tripping [118, 183–186]. Subsequently, a series of studies have been performed to elucidate the mechanisms responsible for tripping [173, 176, 180] and to determine whether ageing is associated with inadequate responses to induced trips [187–191]. Pavol et al. [187] induced trips in older people during gait using a concealed, mechanical obstacle, and found that although the majority of the perturbation trials did not cause them to fall, older women fell more than four times as frequently as older men. Somewhat surprisingly, women aged 70 years or younger were more likely to fall than women aged over 70 years, which may be explained by the older subjects adopting a more protective, less destabilizing gait pattern. However, this finding may also have been due to the small sample size (only five women were aged over 80 years).

A follow-up investigation [188] identified two different strategies to compensate for an induced trip: (i) a *lowering* strategy, in which the tripped foot is quickly lowered to the ground and the contralateral foot initiates a recovery step, and (ii) an *elevating* strategy, in which the tripped limb is elevated over the obstacle in an attempt to continue the step. Irrespective of which strategy was adopted, those who fell in response to the trip walked more quickly than those who did not fall, suggesting that walking speed may be more important than foot placement. However, a subsequent mathematical modelling paper by these authors reported that although reducing walking speed would decrease the likelihood of a fall, improving response times would be more effective [191]. Leg strength is also likely to play an important role in recovering from a trip. Smeesters et al. [190] administered trips of increasing duration until recovery was no longer possible, using a cable attached to the lower leg of healthy young participants. The threshold trip duration was significantly associated with both hip flexor strength and volitional step reaction time, indicating that trip-related falls may be due to slower reaction time and muscle weakness.

Mechanisms of Recovery from Trip Perturbations

Pijnappels et al. [192] studied push-off reactions of the support limb following an induced trip in young and older people, and found that older people who fell in response to the trip exhibited insufficient reduction in angular momentum during push-off, and reduced moment generation at the ankle, knee, and hip joints. These findings suggested that lower limb muscle weakness may be partly responsible for inadequate trip responses. A follow-up study by these authors found that the magnitude and rate of development of lower-limb muscle activity were significantly lower in older people following a trip [193], indicating that differences in motor control also play a role. More recently, Epro et al. [194] demonstrated that compared with their stronger counterparts, older women with lower triceps surae strength and reduced Achilles tendon stiffness had significantly worse ability to recover dynamic stability when walking on a treadmill following unexpected tripping perturbations from a cable attached to their right leg. However, both weak and strong older women eventually managed to adapt their reactive motor response to the perturbation. A small study involving 10 young adults, 20 older adults with (n = 10) and without (n = 10) a history of falls, and 5 stroke survivors, showed that participants who tripped several times in an obstacle paradigm had reduced knee range of motion but showed no difference in peak knee flexion during swing in a normal treadmill walking task [195].

There is substantial evidence from various tripping paradigms that adaptive strategies, both proactive and reactive, occur in response to repeated exposures to the trip perturbations [196]. Using a walkway which can deliver unexpected trips from a 14 cm high board springing up as participants walk along, Okubo et al. [197] showed that in the absence of predictive gait alterations (no slowing of gait or changes in step length/cadence), 10 young adults improved balance recovery following repeated exposure to unpredictable trips (interspersed with slips), as indicated by increases in margin of stability (anterior-posterior distance between the toe of the leading leg at touchdown and the velocity-corrected extrapolated position of the centre of mass in the anterior-posterior plane), anterior displacement of the centre of mass, and step length. Regarding balance recovery strategies, while a lowering-contact strategy was observed in 90% of participants after the first trip, it was progressively replaced by either an elevating-contact strategy or an elevating-cross strategy, respectively noted in 50% and 40% of participants by the 12th trial.

The tripping paradigms used in these studies have enabled greater insights into the mechanisms responsible for impaired responses to walking perturbations; however, more research is required to fully explain why some older people are more likely to trip. In particular, the underlying physiological contributions to maintaining stability in response to a trip (i.e. vision, sensation, strength, and reaction time) are yet to be fully explained in older people, although there is some preliminary evidence that reaction time [190, 198] and strength [190] may play a major role in young people. Furthermore, the ability of these tests to predict falls in real life is yet to be confirmed and may be limited, as the probability of tripping depends not only on the ability to respond to the perturbation, but also on the level of exposure to tripping hazards and the probability of seeing them in advance [199].

Emerging work on the benefits of training balance recovery to obstacle-induced trip perturbation through proactive and reactive adaptions among older adults is promising, although questions remain regarding the transfer of skills from treadmill-induced perturbations to over-ground real falls [200] (see Chapter 17 for more details).

Slipping Responses

Slips are the second most common gait-related mechanism of falls in older people [186, 201], and often result in injury due to the large impact forces that are generated when falling backwards or sideways [202]. Slips are most likely to occur shortly after heel strike, as during this period of the gait cycle a large proportion of bodyweight is placed on the very small heel region, and the direction of force applied to the heel promotes forward sliding unless sufficient frictional forces are generated at the foot– or shoe–ground interface [203]. Recovery from forward sliding after heel contact requires complex neural control mechanisms to detect the sliding motion, rapidly plan a response strategy, and generate a corrective step or steps [204].

During normal gait on non-slippery surfaces, the heel may slide forwards between 1 and 3 cm without being perceived and without requiring any corrective postural responses [203]. On slippery surfaces, however, forward displacements of the heel are much larger and also occur at higher velocity, thereby requiring coordinated responses to avoid falling backwards. The likelihood of falling following a slip depends on both the biomechanics of the slip event itself, and the efficacy and timing of the individual's response to the slip. Falling is more likely to occur with increased gait speed [205–207], longer steps [206], increased forward heel displacement [208–210], increased posterior displacement of the body's centre of mass relative to the base of support [211], and the larger the angle of the leg relative to the ground (representative of a longer step length prior to the slip) [210]. Other factors relating to anthropometrics and sex have also been investigated. Among a large group of older adults (n = 187), anthropometric and demographic factors including female sex, shorter stature, smaller foot size, and BMI were associated with falls from slips induced by unlocking a low-friction section of a walkway [212]. Among young and older adults walking across an oily vinyl surface, obesity was also associated with increased slip severity, specifically increased mean slip speed, as well as over eight times increased odds of falling after adjusting for age group, gender, and gait speed [207].

A number of studies have evaluated the biomechanics and physiology of slip responses. When exposed to an unexpected slip, young adults generate an extremely rapid (60–90 ms onset) postural response involving large bursts of muscle activity, typically consisting of early activation of tibialis anterior, biceps femoris, and rectus femoris on the slipping leg [213]. These muscle activation patterns are accompanied by increased flexion torque at the knee and extensor activity at the hip 190–350 ms after heel contact [214]. In older people, a similar response strategy is observed, but the response is characterized by relatively slower onset, smaller magnitude, and longer duration of muscle activity [208], all of which may contribute to an inability to reduce the forward sliding of the heel [209]. In addition, older subjects exhibit more exaggerated secondary strategies such as greater trunk hyperextension, larger arm elevation, and a shorter response step [215], all considered indicative of a less efficient response. Nonetheless, older age is not consistently associated with increased slip severity, as in Allin's study [207] where markers of slip severity (peak and mean slip speed, slip duration, and slip distance) did not differ between young and older people who experienced a single slip from walking at self-selected slightly hurried pace across a contaminated vinyl surface [207].

Yang et al. [216] investigated strategies adopted by the trailing (recovery) limb of 174 older people exposed to unexpected slip perturbations induced by a platform sliding upon foot contact. They noted that both unilateral slips resulted in 'splits' falls whereas bilateral slips were more likely to lead to 'feet forward' falls; yet both types of slips had a comparable likelihood of causing falls.

Allin et al. [206] investigated which foot kinematics discriminated between slip recoveries and three types of slips leading to a fall (feet-split falls, feet-forward falls, and lateral falls) using data from single unexpected slips over an oily surface among adults aged 18–66 years. Overall, placing the trailing foot 0–10% of body height anterior to the sacrum (too forward would induce feet-forward fall and posterior to the sacrum increased the likelihood of a feet-split or lateral fall) and rapidly arresting slipping foot motion at touch down (a more anterior position of this foot was associated with impaired recovery) were key to recovering balance successfully following a slip.

Technological developments in recent years have seen the growing use of split-belt treadmills to deliver unexpected slips and trips. Yoo et al. [217] recently showed that using this setup, slip perturbations required larger compensatory muscle moments of the hip extensors, flexors, knee flexors, and ankle plantar flexors than trip perturbations during the first stepping response. This finding appears in line with those of Patel and Bhatt [218] who reported that among young healthy people, stroke survivors, and healthy aged-matched, postural stability was significantly more affected by slips compared with trips of similar intensities, and subsequently concluded that the likelihood of backward falls might be higher than that of forward falls.

The likelihood of slipping also depends on a person's knowledge of the surface condition prior to walking over it. When study participants are told that they will be walking over a slippery surface, they adopt a more cautious gait pattern, with shorter step lengths, reduced angular velocity at heel contact and a shift in mediolateral centre of mass towards the supporting limb [219–221]. Heiden et al. [221] went one step further, differentiating biomechanical slip responses between participants with prior knowledge of the existence of a slippery surface and/or knowledge of its slipperiness. They showed that awareness in isolation only resulted in adopting a flatter foot strike but was insufficient to induce changes in ground reaction forces or lower-limb muscle activity which would hamper slip initiation. Experiencing a single slip, however, led to large adaptations in lower limb muscle activity, kinematics, and kinetics which changed foot/floor inter-actions to reduce slip severity. These beneficial biomechanical adaptations seem to occur consistently across slipping paradigms. For example, both young and older people reduce the likelihood of slipping with repeated trials of performing a sit-to-stand task on a sliding platform [213, 214]. Repeated exposures to slips appear to reduce the likelihood of balance loss through generation of adaptive strategies in adjusting centre-of-mass position and step length, as well as adopting a flatter foot strike and increasing knee flexion to improve pre-slip stability and change slip intensity to 'skate-over' or 'walk-over' strategies [222]. Using their slip and trip walkway in a protocol that precluded predictive gait alterations (metronome and stepping targets set at participants' mean step length), Okubo et al. [197] also found that repeated exposures to unexpected slips delivered by a slipping tile placed at various locations on the walkway resulted in reductions in slip speed and post-slip anterior-posterior displacement of the centre of mass, indicative of improvements in balance recovery response. However, these beneficial motor response adaptations appeared to occur at a slower rate than those noted in response to unexpected trip perturbations; backward balance loss was only reduced by 40% in the first eight slips. Taken together, these results suggest that the unexpected nature of slippery conditions contributes to the likelihood of falling in real life, but also raise the possibility that older people can be trained to develop protective slip responses [200, 223, 224] (see Chapter 17).

Despite these advances in understanding, the biomechanics and psychology of slipping, the generalizability of laboratory-based experimental findings to real-life slipping events remains unclear. During daily activities, a vast number of movements are performed on a range of surfaces when wearing a range of different shoes, and given that there are likely to be numerous subject-specific factors influencing slip responses, it is unlikely that laboratory techniques will be able to accurately predict real-life slips in older people. Indeed, Bhatt et al. [225] investigated laboratory-based falls among older adults and how they relate to clinical tests of balance and fall-risk assessment, and found that among 119 older community-dwellers, approximately half of them fell in response to a single unexpected slip delivered from slipping tiles following 9 to 12 walking trials at natural pace on a walkway. In that study, Timed Up and Go Test performance significantly discriminated between fallers and non-fallers, with those slower on the clinical test more likely to fall in response to a single slip. Interestingly, isometric knee extension and flexion strength were not associated with falls, however, the dynamic gait stability measurement, which takes into account the centre of mass position and its instantaneous velocity relative the moving base of support (feet) during unperturbed gait, was predictive of the laboratory-based slip-related falls. Further research is therefore required to elucidate the participant-specific factors that may predispose to slips and subsequent falls and injuries.

Conclusions

Human walking places considerable demands on the body's postural control system, and the complexity of the walking task makes it difficult to develop valid measures of stability for what is an inherently unstable activity. Techniques to assess walking stability on level ground have provided useful information, but each has limitations. Basic parameters of gait may be useful global measures of mobility but do not provide any information about the stability of the body. In contrast, movement patterns of the head and pelvis provide a more direct indicator of the stability of the body during gait, and suggest that older people at high risk of falls exhibit erratic, arrhythmic movement patterns which may interfere with stable vision, thereby increasing the risk of obstacle contact.

The recent development of daily-life gait assessments using body-worn sensors appears promising in the context of fall prediction in older adults.

There is now strong evidence of the cognitive control of gait and its implications for safe ambulation in an everyday environment. In addition, several studies have shown ageing is associated with compromised gait adaptability, suboptimal movement strategies when stepping over or avoiding obstacles, walking on stairs, and responding to trips and slips. Further research is now required to determine whether these movement patterns are capable of predicting who is likely to fall, which physiological, cognitive, and neural factors are responsible for these aberrant patterns, and whether targeted interventions are effective in improving responses to postural challenges and preventing falls and associated injuries.

REFERENCES

1. Winter DA, Patla AE, Frank JS. Assessment of balance control in humans. *Med Prog Technol*. 1990;16:31–51.
2. Cali CM, Kiel DP. An epidemiologic study of fall-related fractures among institutionalized older people. *J Am Geriatr Soc*. 1995;43:1336–40.
3. Berg WP, Alessio HM, Mills EM et al. Circumstances and consequences of falls in independent community-dwelling older adults. *Age Ageing*. 1997;26:261–8.
4. Norton R, Campbell AJ, Lee-Joe T et al. Circumstances of falls resulting in hip fractures among older people. *J Am Geriatr Soc*. 1997;45:1108–12.
5. Murray MP, Drought AB, Kory RC. Walking patterns of normal men. *J Bone Joint Surg Am*. 1964;46A:335–60.
6. Murray MP, Kory RC, Clarkson BH. Walking patterns in healthy old men. *J Gerontol*. 1969;24:169–78.
7. Finley FR, Cody KA, Finizie RV. Locomotion patterns in elderly women. *Arch Phys Med Rehabil*. 1969;50:140–6.
8. Imms FJ, Edholm OG. Studies of gait and mobility in the elderly. *Age Ageing*. 1981;10:147–56.
9. Cunningham DA, Rechnitzer PA, Pearce ME et al. Determinants of self-selected walking pace across ages 19 to 66. *J Gerontol*. 1982;37:560–4.
10. O'Brien M, Power K, Sanford S et al. Temporal gait patterns in healthy young and elderly females. *Physiother Can*. 1983;35:323–6.
11. Hagemon PA, Blanke DJ. Comparison of gait of young women and elderly women. *Phys Ther*. 1986;66:1382–7.
12. Elble RJ, Thomas SS, Higgins C et al. Stride-dependent changes in gait of older people. *J Neurol*. 1991;238:1–5.
13. Dobbs RJ, Lubel DD, Charlett A et al. Hypothesis: age-associated changes in gait represent, in part, a tendency towards Parkinsonism. *Age Ageing*. 1992;21:221–5.
14. Dobbs RJ, Charlett A, Bowles SG et al. Is this walk normal? *Age Ageing*. 1993;22:27–30.

15. Oberg T, Karsznia A, Oberg K. Basic gait parameters: reference data for normal subjects, 10–79 years of age. *J Rehabil Res Dev*. 1993;30:210–23.

16. Fransen M, Heussler J, Margiotta E et al. Quantitative gait analysis – comparison of rheumatoid arthritic and non-arthritic subjects. *Aust J Physiother*. 1994;40:191–9.

17. Buchner DM, Cress ME, Esselman PC et al. Factors associated with changes in gait speed in older adults. *J Gerontol A Biol Sci Med Sci*. 1996;51A:M297–302.

18. Lajoie Y, Teasdale N, Bard C et al. Upright standing and gait: are there changes in attentional requirements related to normal aging? *Exp Aging Res*. 1996;22:185–98.

19. Lord SR, Lloyd DG, Li SK. Sensori-motor function, gait patterns and falls in community-dwelling women. *Age Ageing*. 1996;25:292–9.

20. Bohannon RW. Comfortable and maximum walking speed of adults aged 20–79 years: reference values and determinants. *Age Ageing*. 1997;26:15–19.

21. Shumway-Cook A, Guralnik JM, Phillips CL et al. Age-associated declines in complex walking task performance: the Walking InCHIANTI toolkit. *J Am Geriatr Soc*. 2007;55:58–65.

22. Crowinshield RD, Brand RA, Johnston RC. The effects of walking velocity and age on hip kinematics and kinetics. *Clin Orthop Relat Res*. 1978;132:140–4.

23. Winter DA, Patla AE, Frank JS et al. Biomechanical walking pattern changes in the fit and healthy elderly. *Phys Ther*. 1990;70:340–7.

24. Ferrandez A-M, Pailhous J, Durup M. Slowness in elderly gait. *Exp Aging Res*. 1990;16:79–89.

25. Jansen EC, Vittas D, Hellberg S et al. Normal gait of young and old men and women. *Acta Orthop Scand*. 1982;53:193–6.

26. Beauchet O, Allali G, Sekhon H et al. Guidelines for Assessment of Gait and Reference Values for Spatiotemporal Gait Parameters in Older Adults: The Biomathics and Canadian Gait Consortiums Initiative. *Front Hum Neurosci*. 2017;11:353.

27. Kerrigan DC, Todd MK, Croce UD et al. Biomechanical gait alterations independent of speed in the healthy elderly: evidence for specific limiting impairments. *Arch Phys Med Rehabil*. 1998;79:317–22.

28. Gill J, Allum J, Carpenter M et al. Trunk sway measures of postural stability during clinical balance tests: effects of age. *J Gerontol A Biol Sci Med Sci*. 2001;56A:M438–47.

29. Judge JO, Davis RB, Ounpuu S. Step length reductions in advanced age: the role of ankle and hip kinetics. *J Gerontol A Biol Sci Med Sci*. 1996;51A:M303–12.

30. Mills P, Barrett R. Swing phase mechanics of healthy young and elderly men. *Hum Mov Sci*. 2001;20:427–46.

31. McGibbon C, Krebs D. Age-related changes in lower trunk coordination and energy transfer during gait. *J Neurophysiol*. 2001;85:1923–31.

32. McGibbon CA, Krebs DE, Puniello MS. Mechanical energy analysis identifies compensatory strategies in disabled elders' gait. *J Biomech*. 2001;34:481–90.

33. McGibbon C, Puniello M, Krebs D. Mechanical energy transfer during gait in relation to strength impairment and pathology in elderly women. *Clin Biomech*. 2001;16:324–33.

34. Kernozek TW, LaMott EE. Comparisons of plantar pressures between the elderly and young adults. *Gait Posture*. 1995;3:143–8.

35. Prakash C, Stern G. Neurological signs in the elderly. *Age Ageing.* 1973;2:24–7.

36. Sudarsky L. Geriatrics: gait disorders in the elderly. *N Engl J Med.* 1990;322:1441–6.

37. Sudarsky L, Ronthal M. Gait disorders in the elderly: assessing the risk for falls. In: Vellas B, Toupet M, Rubenstein L, et al., Eds. *Falls, Balance and Gait Disorders in the Elderly.* Paris: Elsevier; 1992:117–27.

38. Woollacott MH, Tang P-F. Balance control during walking in the older adult: research and its implications. *Phys Ther.* 1997;77:646–60.

39. Menz HB, Lord SR, Fitzpatrick RC. Age-related differences in walking stability. *Age Ageing.* 2003;32:137–42.

40. Hamacher D, Singh NB, Van Dieen JH et al. Kinematic measures for assessing gait stability in elderly individuals: a systematic review. *J R Soc Interface.* 2011;8:1682–98.

41. Menant JC, Schoene D, Sarofim M et al. Single and dual task tests of gait speed are equivalent in the prediction of falls in older people: a systematic review and meta-analysis. *Ageing Res Rev.* 2014;16:83–104.

42. Verghese J, Holtzer R, Lipton RB et al. Quantitative gait markers and incident fall risk in older adults. *J Gerontol A Biol Sci Med Sci.* 2009;64:896–901.

43. Callisaya ML, Blizzard L, Schmidt MD et al. Gait, gait variability and the risk of multiple incident falls in older people: a population-based study. *Age Ageing.* 2011;40:481–7.

44. Svoboda Z, Bizovska L, Janura M et al. Variability of spatial temporal gait parameters and center of pressure displacements during gait in elderly fallers and nonfallers: a 6-month prospective study. *PLoS One.* 2017;12:e0171997.

45. Maki BE. Gait changes in older adults: predictors of falls or indicators of fear? *J Am Geriatr Soc.* 1997;45:313–20.

46. Clark RD, Lord SR, Webster IW. Clinical parameters associated with falls in an elderly population. *Gerontology.* 1993;39:117–23.

47. Hausdorff JM, Rios DA, Edelberg HK. Gait variability and fall risk in community-living older adults: a 1-year prospective study. *Arch Phys Med Rehabil.* 2001;82:1050–6.

48. Hill K, Schwarz J, Flicker L et al. Falls among healthy, community-dwelling, older women: a prospective study of frequency, circumstances, consequences and prediction accuracy. *Aust NZ J Public Health.* 1999;23:41–8.

49. Lord SR, Clark RD. Simple physiological and clinical tests for the accurate prediction of falling in older people. *Gerontology.* 1996;42:199–203.

50. Johansson J, Nordström A, Nordström P. Greater fall risk in elderly women than in men is associated with increased gait variability during multitasking. *J Am Med Dir Assoc.* 2016;17:535–40.

51. Gillain S, Boutaayamou M, Schwartz C et al. Gait symmetry in the dual task condition as a predictor of future falls among independent older adults: a 2-year longitudinal study. *Aging Clin Exp Res.* 2019;31:1057–67.

52. Callisaya ML, Blizzard L, McGinley JL et al. Risk of falls in older people during fast-walking: the TASCOG study. *Gait Posture.* 2012;36:510–15.

53. Quach L, Galica AM, Jones RN et al. The nonlinear relationship between gait speed and falls: the Maintenance of Balance, Independent Living, Intellect, and Zest in the Elderly of Boston Study. *J Am Geriatr Soc.* 2011;59:1069–73.

54. Gabell A, Nayak USL. The effect of age on variability in gait. *J Gerontol.* 1984;39:662–6.

55. Guimaraes RM, Isaacs B. Characteristics of the gait in old people who fall. *Int Rehabil Med.* 1980;2:177–80.

56. Weller C, Humphrey SJE, Kirollos C et al. Gait on a shoestring: falls and foot separation in Parkinsonism. *Age Ageing.* 1992;21:242–4.

57. Gehlsen GM, Whaley MH. Falls in the elderly: Part I, Gait. *Arch Phys Med Rehabil.* 1990;71:735–8.

58. Nelson A, Certo L, Lembo L et al. The functional ambulation performance of elderly fallers and non-fallers walking at their preferred velocity. *NeuroRehabil.* 1999;13:141–6.

59. Heitmann DK, Gossman MR, Shaddeau SA et al. Balance performance and step width in noninstitutionalized, elderly, female fallers and nonfallers. *Phys Ther.* 1989;69:923–31.

60. Rodriguez-Molinero A, Herrero-Larrea A, Minarro A et al. The spatial parameters of gait and their association with falls, functional decline and death in older adults: a prospective study. *Sci Rep.* 2019;9:8813.

61. Lee LW, Kerrigan DC. Identification of kinetic differences between fallers and nonfallers in the elderly. *Am J Phys Med Rehabil.* 1999;78:242–6.

62. Kerrigan DC, Lee LW, Nieto TJ et al. Kinetic alterations independent of walking speed in elderly fallers. *Arch Phys Med Rehabil.* 2000;81:730–5.

63. Kerrigan DC, Lee LW, Collins JJ et al. Reduced hip extension during walking: healthy elderly and fallers versus young adults. *Arch Phys Med Rehabil.* 2001;82:26–30.

64. Feltner ME, MacRae PG, McNitt-Gray JL. Quantitative gait assessment as a predictor of prospective and retrospective falls in community-dwelling older women. *Arch Phys Med Rehabil.* 1994;75:447–53.

65. Escalante A, Lichtenstein MJ, Hazuda HP. Walking velocity in aged persons: its association with lower extremity joint range of motion. *Arthritis Rheum.* 2001;45:287–94.

66. Kerrigan D, Xenopoulos-Oddsson A, Sullivan M et al. Effect of a hip flexor stretching program on gait in the elderly. *Arch Phys Med Rehabil.* 2003;84:1–6.

67. Yack HJ, Berger RC. Dynamic stability in the elderly: identifying a possible measure. *J Gerontol.* 1993;48:M225–30.

68. Moe-Nilssen R, Helbostad JL. Interstride trunk acceleration variability but not step width variability can differentiate between fit and frail older adults. *Gait Posture.* 2005;21:164–70.

69. Menz HB, Lord SR, Fitzpatrick RC. Acceleration patterns of the head and pelvis when walking on level and irregular surfaces. *Gait Posture.* 2003;18:35–46.

70. Menz HB, Lord SR, Fitzpatrick RC. Acceleration patterns of the head and pelvis when walking are associated with risk of falling in community-dwelling older people. *J Gerontol A Biol Sci Med Sci.* 2003;58:M446–52.

71. Doi T, Hirata S, Ono R et al. The harmonic ratio of trunk acceleration predicts falling among older people: results of a 1-year prospective study. *J Neuroeng Rehabil.* 2013;10:7.

72. DiFabio RP, Emasithi A, Greany JF et al. Supression of the vertical vesibulo-ocular reflex in older persons at risk of falling. *Acta Otolaryngol.* 2001;121:707–14.

73. DiFabio RP, Greany JF, Emasithi A et al. Eye-head coordination during postural perturbation as a predictor of falls in community-dwelling elderly women. *Arch Phys Med Rehabil.* 2002;83:942–51.

74. Bruijn SM, Meijer OG, Beek PJ et al. Assessing the stability of human locomotion: a review of current measures. *J R Soc Interface.* 2013;10:20120999.

75. Terrier P, Reynard F. Effect of age on the variability and stability of gait: a cross-sectional treadmill study in healthy individuals between 20 and 69 years of age. *Gait Posture.* 2015;41:170–4.

76. Bizovska L, Svoboda Z, Janura M et al. Local dynamic stability during gait for predicting falls in elderly people: a one-year prospective study. *PLoS One.* 2018;13:e0197091.

77. van Schooten KS, Pijnappels M, Rispens SM et al. Daily-life gait quality as predictor of falls in older people: a 1-year prospective cohort study. *PLoS One.* 2016;11:e0158623.

78. Leach JM, Mellone S, Palumbo P et al. Natural turn measures predict recurrent falls in community-dwelling older adults: a longitudinal cohort study. *Sci Rep.* 2018;8:4316.

79. Hillel I, Gazit E, Nieuwboer A et al. Is every-day walking in older adults more analogous to dual-task walking or to usual walking? Elucidating the gaps between gait performance in the lab and during 24/7 monitoring. *Eur Rev Aging Phys Act.* 2019;16:6.

80. Duncan PW, Chandler J, Studenski S et al. How do physiological components of balance affect mobility in elderly men? *Arch Phys Med Rehabil.* 1993;74:1343–9.

81. Bassey EJ, Bendall MJ, Pearson M. Muscle strength in the triceps surae and objectively measured customary walking activity in men and women over 65 years of age. *Clin Sci.* 1988;74:85–9.

82. Buchner DM, Larson EB, Wagner EH et al. Evidence for a non-linear relationship between leg strength and gait speed. *Age Ageing.* 1996;25:386–91.

83. Saucedo F, Yang F. Effects of visual deprivation on stability among young and older adults during treadmill walking. *Gait Posture.* 2017;54:106–11.

84. Brown L, Gage W, Polych M et al. Central set influences on gait: age-dependent effects of postural threat. *Exp Aging Res.* 2002;145:286–96.

85. Herman T, Giladi N, Gurevich T et al. Gait instability and fractal dynamics of older adults with a "cautious" gait: why do certain older adults walk fearfully? *Gait Posture.* 2005;21:178–85.

86. Menz HB, Lord SR, Fitzpatrick RC. A structural equation model relating sensori-motor function, fear of falling and gait patterns in older people. *Gait Posture.* 2005;25:243–9.

87. McKenzie NC, Brown LA. Obstacle negotiation kinematics: age-dependent effects of postural threat. *Gait Posture.* 2004;19:226–34.

88. Delbaere K, Sturnieks DL, Crombez G et al. Concern about falls elicits changes in gait parameters in conditions of postural threat in older people. *J Gerontol A Biol Sci Med Sci.* 2009;64:237–42.

89. Ellmers TJ, Cocks AJ, Young WR. Exploring attentional focus of older adult fallers during heightened postural threat. *Psychol Res.* 2019;84:1877–89.

90. Ellmers TJ, Young WR. Conscious motor control impairs attentional processing efficiency during precision stepping. *Gait Posture.* 2018;63:58–62.

91. Deshpande N, Metter EJ, Ferrucci L. Sensorimotor and psychosocial correlates of adaptive locomotor performance in older adults. *Arch Phys Med Rehabil.* 2011;92:1074–9.

92. Hatton AL, Menant JC, Lord SR et al. The effect of lower limb muscle fatigue on obstacle negotiation during walking in older adults. *Gait Posture.* 2013;37:506–10.

93. Helbostad JL, Leirfall S, Moe-Nilssen R et al. Physical fatigue affects gait characteristics in older persons. *J Gerontol A Biol Sci Med Sci.* 2007;62:1010–15.

94. Morrison S, Colberg SR, Parson HK et al. Walking-induced fatigue leads to increased falls risk in older adults. *J Am Med Dir Assoc.* 2016;17:402–9.

95. Quiben MU, Hazuda HP. Factors contributing to 50-ft walking speed and observed ethnic differences in older community-dwelling Mexican Americans and European Americans. *Phys Ther.* 2015;95:871–83.

96. Tolea MI, Costa PT, Terracciano A et al. Sex-specific correlates of walking speed in a wide age-ranged population. *J Gerontol B Psychol Sci Soc Sci.* 2010;65b:174–84.

97. Amboni M, Barone P, Hausdorff JM. Cognitive contributions to gait and falls: evidence and implications. *Mov Disord.* 2013;28:1520–33.

98. Li KZH, Bherer L, Mirelman A et al. Cognitive involvement in balance, gait and dual-tasking in aging: a focused review from a neuroscience of aging perspective. *Front Neurol.* 2018;9:913.

99. Morris R, Lord S, Bunce J et al. Gait and cognition: mapping the global and discrete relationships in ageing and neurodegenerative disease. *Neurosci Biobehav Rev.* 2016;64:326–45.

100. Hausdorff JM, Yogev G, Springer S et al. Walking is more like catching than tapping: gait in the elderly as a complex cognitive task. *Exp Aging Res.* 2005;164:541–8.

101. Holtzer R, Verghese J, Xue X et al. Cognitive processes related to gait velocity: results from the Einstein Aging Study. *Neuropsychology.* 2006;20:215–23.

102. Beauchet O, Annweiler C, Montero-Odasso M et al. Gait control: a specific subdomain of executive function? *J Neuroeng Rehabil.* 2012;9:12.

103. Herman T, Mirelman A, Giladi N et al. Executive control deficits as a prodrome to falls in healthy older adults: a prospective study linking thinking, walking, and falling. *J Gerontol A Biol Sci Med Sci.* 2010;65:1086–92.

104. Muir SW, Gopaul K, Montero Odasso MM. The role of cognitive impairment in fall risk among older adults: a systematic review and meta-analysis. *Age Ageing.* 2012;41:299–308.

105. Montero-Odasso M, Verghese J, Beauchet O et al. Gait and cognition: a complementary approach to understanding brain function and the risk of falling. *J Am Geriatr Soc.* 2012;60:2127–36.

106. Muir-Hunter SW, Wittwer JE. Dual-task testing to predict falls in community-dwelling older adults: a systematic review. *Physiotherapy.* 2016;102:29–40.

107. Al-Yahya E, Dawes H, Smith L et al. Cognitive motor interference while walking: a systematic review and meta-analysis. *Neurosci Biobehav Rev.* 2011;35:715–28.

108. Menant JC, Sturnieks DL, Brodie MA et al. Visuospatial tasks affect locomotor control more than nonspatial tasks in older people. *PLoS One.* 2014;9:e109802.

109. Srygley JM, Mirelman A, Herman T et al. When does walking alter thinking? Age and task associated findings. *Brain Res.* 2009;1253:92–9.

110. Papegaaij S, Hortobagyi T, Godde B et al. Neural correlates of motor-cognitive dual-tasking in young and old adults. *PLoS One.* 2017;12:e0189025.

111. Mirelman A, Shema S, Maidan I et al. Gait. *Handb Clin Neurol.* 2018;159:119–34.

112. Gramigna V, Pellegrino G, Cerasa A et al. Near-infrared spectroscopy in gait disorders: is it time to begin? *Neurorehabil Neural Repair.* 2017;31:402–12.

113. Hamacher D, Herold F, Wiegel P et al. Brain activity during walking: a systematic review. *Neurosci Biobehav Rev.* 2015;57:310–27.

114. Pelicioni PHS, Tijsma M, Lord SR et al. Prefrontal cortical activation measured by fNIRS during walking: effects of age, disease and secondary task. *PeerJ.* 2019;7: e6833.

115. Stuart S, Vitorio R, Morris R et al. Cortical activity during walking and balance tasks in older adults and in people with Parkinson's disease: a structured review. *Maturitas.* 2018;113:53–72.

116. Verghese J, Wang C, Ayers E et al. Brain activation in high-functioning older adults and falls: prospective cohort study. *Neurology.* 2017;88:191–7.

117. Overstall PW, Exton-Smith AN, Imms FJ et al. Falls in the elderly related to postural imbalance. *Br Med J.* 1977;1:261–4.

118. Blake A, Morgan K, Bendall M et al. Falls by elderly people at home - prevalence and associated factors. *Age Ageing.* 1988;17:365–72.

119. Campbell AJ, Borrie MJ, Spears GF et al. Circumstances and consequences of falls experienced by a community population 70 years and over during a prospective study. *Age Ageing.* 1990;19:136–41.

120. Teno J, Kiel DP, Mor V. Multiple stumbles: a risk factor for falls in community-dwelling elderly. A prospective study. *J Am Geriatr Soc.* 1990;38:1321–5.

121. McFadyen BJ, Winter DA. Anticipatory locomotor adjustments during obstructed human walking. *Neurosci Res Commun.* 1991;9:37–44.

122. Chen H-C, Ashton-Miller JA, Alexander NB et al. Stepping over obstacles: gait patterns of healthy young and old adults. *J Gerontol.* 1991;46:M196–203.

123. Chou L-S, Kaufman KR, Brey RH et al. Motion of the whole body's center of mass when stepping over obstacles of different heights. *Gait Posture.* 2001;13:17–26.

124. Chou L-S, Draganich LF. Increasing obstacle height and decreasing toe-obstacle distance affect the joint moments of the stance limb differently when stepping over an obstacle. *Gait Posture.* 1998;8:186–204.

125. Begg R, Sparrow W, Lythgo N. Time-domain analysis of foot-ground reaction forces in negotiating obstacles. *Gait Posture.* 1998;7:99–109.

126. Chou L, Draganich L. Stepping over an obstacle increases the motions and moments of the joints of the trailing limb in young adults. *J Biomech.* 1997;30:331–7.

127. Galna B, Peters A, Murphy AT et al. Obstacle crossing deficits in older adults: a systematic review. *Gait Posture.* 2009;30:270–5.

128. Kunimune S, Okada S. Contribution of vision and its age-related changes to postural stability in obstacle crossing during locomotion. *Gait Posture.* 2019;70:284–8.

129. Chen H-C, Ashton-Miller JA, Alexander NB et al. Effects of age and available response time on ability to step over an obstacle. *J Gerontol*. 1994;49:M227–33.

130. Chen H-C, Schultz AB, Ashton-Miller JA et al. Stepping over obstacles: dividing attention impairs performance of old more than young adults. *J Gerontol*. 1996;51A:M116–22.

131. Cao C, Ashton-Miller JA, Schultz AB et al. Abilities to turn suddenly while walking: effects of age, gender, and available response time. *J Gerontol A Biol Sci Med Sci*. 1997;52A:M88–93.

132. Gilchrist LA. Age-related changes in the ability to side-step during gait. *Clin Biomech*. 1998;13:91–7.

133. Tirosh O, Sparrow WA. Gait termination in young and older adults: effects of stopping stimulus probability and stimulus delay. *Gait Posture*. 2004;19:243–51.

134. Schulz BW. Healthy younger and older adults control foot placement to avoid small obstacles during gait primarily by modulating step width. *J Neuroeng Rehabil*. 2012;9:69.

135. Peper CL, de Dreu MJ, Roerdink M. Attuning one's steps to visual targets reduces comfortable walking speed in both young and older adults. *Gait Posture*. 2015;41:830–4.

136. Mazaheri M, Roerdink M, Bood RJ et al. Attentional costs of visually guided walking: effects of age, executive function and stepping-task demands. *Gait Posture*. 2014;40:182–6.

137. Caetano MJ, Lord SR, Schoene D et al. Age-related changes in gait adaptability in response to unpredictable obstacles and stepping targets. *Gait Posture*. 2016;46:35–41.

138. Caetano MJD, Menant JC, Schoene D et al. Sensorimotor and cognitive predictors of impaired gait adaptability in older people. *J Gerontol A Biol Sci Med Sci*. 2017;72:1257–63.

139. Mazaheri M, Hoogkamer W, Potocanac Z et al. Effects of aging and dual tasking on step adjustments to perturbations in visually cued walking. *Exp Aging Res*. 2015;233:3467–74.

140. Caetano MJD, Lord SR, Brodie MA et al. Executive functioning, concern about falling and quadriceps strength mediate the relationship between impaired gait adaptability and fall risk in older people. *Gait Posture*. 2018;59:188–92.

141. Pieruccini-Faria F, Montero-Odasso M. Obstacle negotiation, gait variability, and risk of falling: results from the "Gait and Brain Study". *J Gerontol A Biol Sci Med Sci*. 2019;74:1422–8.

142. Patla AE. Understanding the role of vision in the control of human locomotion. *Gait Posture*. 1997;5:54–69.

143. Lamoureux EL, Sparrow WA, Murphy A et al. The relationship between lower body strength and obstructed gait in community-dwelling older adults. *J Am Geriatr Soc*. 2002;50:468–73.

144. Uiga L, Cheng KC, Wilson MR et al. Acquiring visual information for locomotion by older adults: a systematic review. *Ageing Res Rev*. 2015;20:24–34.

145. Chapman GJ, Hollands MA. Evidence for a link between changes to gaze behaviour and risk of falling in older adults during adaptive locomotion. *Gait Posture*. 2006;24:288–94.

146. Chapman GJ, Hollands MA. Evidence that older adult fallers prioritise the planning of future stepping actions over the accurate execution of ongoing steps during complex locomotor tasks. *Gait Posture*. 2007;26:59–67.

147. Chapman GJ, Hollands MA. Age-related differences in visual sampling requirements during adaptive locomotion. *Exp Aging Res.* 2010;201:467–78.

148. Young WR, Hollands MA. Can telling older adults where to look reduce falls? Evidence for a causal link between inappropriate visual sampling and suboptimal stepping performance. *Exp Aging Res.* 2010;204:103–13.

149. Curzon-Jones BT, Hollands MA. Route previewing results in altered gaze behaviour, increased self-confidence and improved stepping safety in both young and older adults during adaptive locomotion. *Exp Aging Res.* 2018;236:1077–89.

150. Kunimune S, Okada S. The effects of object height and visual information on the control of obstacle crossing during locomotion in healthy older adults. *Gait Posture.* 2017;55:126–30.

151. Timmis MA, Buckley JG. Obstacle crossing during locomotion: visual exproprioceptive information is used in an online mode to update foot placement before the obstacle but not swing trajectory over it. *Gait Posture.* 2012;36:160–2.

152. Draganich L, Zacny J, Klafta J et al. The effects of antidepressants on obstructed and unobstructed gait in healthy elderly people. *J Gerontol A Biol Sci Med Sci.* 2001;56A:M36–41.

153. Godi M, Giardini M, Schieppati M. Walking along curved trajectories: changes with age and Parkinson's disease. Hints to rehabilitation. *Front Neurol.* 2019;10:532.

154. Robinovitch SN, Feldman F, Yang Y et al. Video capture of the circumstances of falls in elderly people residing in long-term care: an observational study. *Lancet.* 2013;381:47–54.

155. Mancini M, Schlueter H, El-Gohary M et al. Continuous monitoring of turning mobility and its association to falls and cognitive function: a pilot study. *J Gerontol A Biol Sci Med Sci.* 2016;71:1102–8.

156. Odonkor CA, Thomas JC, Holt N et al. A comparison of straight- and curved-path walking tests among mobility-limited older adults. *J Gerontol A Biol Sci Med Sci.* 2013;68:1532–9.

157. Hess RJ, Brach JS, Piva SR et al. Walking skill can be assessed in older adults: validity of the Figure-of-8 Walk Test. *Phys Ther.* 2010;90:89–99.

158. Williamson J, Fried L. Characterization of older adults who attribute functional decrements to "old age". *J Am Geriatr Soc.* 1996;44:1429–34.

159. Startzell JK, Owens DA, Mulfinger LM et al. Stair negotiation in older people: a review. *J Am Geriatr Soc.* 2000;48:567–80.

160. Boye ND, Mattace-Raso FU, Van der Velde N et al. Circumstances leading to injurious falls in older men and women in the Netherlands. *Injury.* 2014;45:1224–30.

161. Cohen HH, Templer J, Archea J. An analysis of occupational stair accident patterns. *J Safety Res.* 1985;16:178–81.

162. Tinetti ME. Factors associated with serious injury during falls by ambulatory nursing home residents. *J Am Geriatr Soc.* 1987;35:644–8.

163. Andriacchi TP, Andersson GBJ, Fermier RW, Stern D, Galante JO. A study of lower-limb mechanics during stair climbing. *J Bone Joint Surg Am.* 1980;62A:749–57.

164. Lyons K, Perry J, Gronley JK et al. Timing and relative intensity of hip extensor and abductor muscle action during level and stair ambulation. *Phys Ther.* 1983;63:1597–605.

165. McFadyen BJ, Winter DA. An integrated biomechanical analysis of normal stair ascent and descent. *J Biomech.* 1988;21:733–44.

166. Zachazewski JE, Riley PO, Krebs DE. Biomechanical analysis of body mass transfer during stair ascent and descent of healthy subjects. *J Rehabil Res Dev.* 1993;30:412–22.

167. Christina K, Cavanagh P. Ground reaction forces and frictional demands during stair descent: effects of age and illumination. *Gait Posture.* 2002;15:153–8.

168. Simoneau GG, Cavanagh PR, Ulbrecht JS et al. The influence of visual factors on fall-related kinematic variables during stair descent by older women. *J Gerontol.* 1991;46:M188–95.

169. Williams K. Intralimb coordination of older adults during locomotion: stair climbing. *J Hum Mov Stud.* 1996;30:269–84.

170. Williams K. Intralimb coordination of older adults during locomotion: stair descent. *J Hum Mov Stud.* 1998;34:96–117.

171. Hortobagyi T, DeVita P. Altered movement strategy increases lower extremity stiffness during stepping down in the aged. *J Gerontol A Biol Sci Med Sci.* 1999;54A:B63–70.

172. Hortobagyi T, DeVita P. Muscle pre- and coactivity during downward stepping are associated with leg stiffness in aging. *J Electromyogr Kinesiol.* 2000;10:117–26.

173. Lark SD, Buckley JG, Bennett S et al. Joint torques and dynamic joint stiffness in elderly and young men during stepping down. *Clin Biomech.* 2003;18:848–55.

174. Zietz D, Johannsen L, Hollands M. Stepping characteristics and centre of mass control during stair descent: effects of age, fall risk and visual factors. *Gait Posture.* 2011;34:279–84.

175. Foster RJ, Maganaris CN, Reeves ND et al. Centre of mass control is reduced in older people when descending stairs at an increased riser height. *Gait Posture.* 2019;73:305–14.

176. Begg R, Sparrow W. Gait characteristics of young and older individuals negotiating a raised surface: implications for the prevention of falls. *J Gerontol A Biol Sci Med Sci.* 2000;55A:M147–54.

177. Foster RJ, Whitaker D, Scally AJ et al. What you see is what you step: the horizontal-vertical illusion increases toe clearance in older adults during stair ascent. *Invest Ophthalmol Vis Sci.* 2015;56:2950–7.

178. Lythgo N, Begg R, Best R. Stepping responses made by elderly and young female adults to approach and accommodate known surface height changes. *Gait Posture.* 2007;26:82–9.

179. Zietz D, Hollands M. Gaze behavior of young and older adults during stair walking. *J Mot Behav.* 2009;41:357–65.

180. Buckley JG, Heasley KJ, Twigg P et al. The effects of blurred vision on the mechanics of landing during stepping down by the elderly. *Gait Posture.* 2005;21:65–71.

181. Buckley JG, Heasley K, Scally A et al. The effects of blurring vision on medio-lateral balance during stepping up or down to a new level in the elderly. *Gait Posture.* 2005;22:146–53.

182. Lord SR, Dayhew J, Howland A. Multifocal glasses impair edge-contrast sensitivity and depth perception and increase the risk of falls in older people. *J Am Geriatr Soc.* 2002;50:1760–6.

183. Prudham D, Evans JG. Factors associated with falls in the elderly: a community study. *Age Ageing.* 1981;10:141–6.

184. Campbell AJ, Reinken J, Allan BC et al. Falls in old age: a study of frequency and related clinical factors. *Age Ageing.* 1981;10:264–70.

185. Tinetti ME, Speechley M, Ginter SF. Risk factors for falls among elderly persons living in the community. *N Engl J Med.* 1988;319:1701–7.

186. Lord SR, Ward JA, Williams P et al. An epidemiological study of falls in older community-dwelling women: the Randwick falls and fractures study. *Aust J Public Health.* 1993;17:240–54.

187. Pavol M, Owings T, Foley K et al. Gait characteristics as risk factors for falling from trips induced in older adults. *J Gerontol A Biol Sci Med Sci.* 1999;54A:M583–90.

188. Pavol M, Owings T, Foley K et al. Mechanisms leading to a fall from an induced trip in healthy older adults. *J Gerontol A Biol Sci Med Sci.* 2001;56:M428–37.

189. Pavol MJ, Owings TM, Foley KT et al. The sex and age of older adults influence the outcome of induced trips. *J Gerontol A Biol Sci Med Sci.* 1999;54A:M103–8.

190. Smeesters C, Hayes WC, McMahon TA. The threshold trip duration for which recovery is no longer possible is associated with strength and reaction time. *J Biomech.* 2001;34:589–95.

191. van den Bogert AJ, Pavol MJ, Grabiner MD. Response time is more important than walking speed for the ability of older adults to avoid a fall after a trip. *J Biomech.* 2002;35:199–205.

192. Pijnappels M, Bobbert MF, van Dieën JH. Push-off reactions in recovery after tripping discriminate young subjects, older non-fallers and older fallers. *Gait Posture.* 2005;21:388–94.

193. Pijnappels M, Bobbert MF, van Dieën JH. Control of support limb muscles in recovery after tripping in young and older subjects. *Exp Aging Res.* 2005;160:326–33.

194. Epro G, McCrum C, Mierau A et al. Effects of triceps surae muscle strength and tendon stiffness on the reactive dynamic stability and adaptability of older female adults during perturbed walking. *J Appl Physiol (1985).* 2018;124:1541–9.

195. Benson LC, Cobb SC, Hyngstrom AS et al. Identifying trippers and non-trippers based on knee kinematics during obstacle-free walking. *Hum Mov Sci.* 2018;62:58–66.

196. Wang Y, Wang S, Bolton R Kaur T, Bhatt T. Effects of task-specific obstacle-induced trip-perturbation training: proactive and reactive adaptation to reduce fall-risk in community-dwelling older adults. *Aging Clin Exp Res.* 2019;32:893–905.

197. Okubo Y, Brodie MA, Sturnieks DL et al. Exposure to trips and slips with increasing unpredictability while walking can improve balance recovery responses with minimum predictive gait alterations. *PLoS One.* 2018;13:e0202913.

198. Owings T, Pavol M, Grabiner M. Mechanisms of failed recovery following postural perturbations on a motorized treadmill mimic those associated with an actual forward trip. *Clin Biomech.* 2001;16:813–19.

199. Best R, Begg R. A method for calculating the probability of tripping while walking. *J Biomech*. 2008;41:1147–51.

200. Wang Y, Bhatt T, Liu X et al. Can treadmill-slip perturbation training reduce immediate risk of over-ground-slip induced fall among community-dwelling older adults? *J Biomech*. 2019;84:58–66.

201. Gabell A, Simons MA, Nayak USL. Falls in the healthy elderly: predisposing causes. *Ergonomics*. 1985;28:965–75.

202. Smeesters C, Hayes WC, McMahon TA. Disturbance type and gait speed affect fall direction and impact location. *J Biomech*. 2001;34:309–17.

203. Redfern M, Cham R, Gielo-Perczak K et al. Biomechanics of slips. *Ergonomics*. 2001;44:1138–66.

204. Pai YC, Iqbal K. Simulated movement termination for balance recovery: can movement strategies be sought to maintain stability in the presence of slipping or forced sliding? *J Biomech*. 1999;32:779–86.

205. Bhatt T, Wening JD, Pai YC. Influence of gait speed on stability: recovery from anterior slips and compensatory stepping. *Gait Posture*. 2005;21:146–56.

206. Allin LJ, Nussbaum MA, Madigan ML. Feet kinematics upon slipping discriminate between recoveries and three types of slip-induced falls. *Ergonomics*. 2018;61:866–76.

207. Allin LJ, Wu X, Nussbaum MA et al. Falls resulting from a laboratory-induced slip occur at a higher rate among individuals who are obese. *J Biomech*. 2016;49:678–83.

208. Strandberg L, Lanshammar H. The dynamics of slipping accidents. *J Occup Accid*. 1981;3:153–62.

209. Strandberg L. On accident analysis and slip resistance measurement. *Ergonomics*. 1983;26:11–32.

210. Brady R, Pavol M, Owings T et al. Foot displacement but not velocity predicts the outcome of a slip induced in young subjects while walking. *J Biomech*. 2000;33:803–8.

211. You J-Y, Chou Y-L, Lin C-J et al. Effect of slip on movement of body center of mass relative to base of support. *Clin Biomech*. 2001;16:167–73.

212. Zhang MZ, Yang F, Wang E et al. Association between anthropometric factors and falls in community-dwelling older adults during a simulated slip while walking. *J Am Geriatr Soc*. 2014;62:1808–10.

213. Tang P-F, Woollacott MH, Chong RKY. Control of reactive balance adjustments in perturbed human walking: roles of proximal and distal postural muscle activity. *Exp Aging Res*. 1998;119:141–52.

214. Cham R, Redfern M. Lower extremity corrective reactions to slip events. *J Biomech*. 2001;34:1439–45.

215. Tang P-F, Woollacott MH. Inefficient postural responses to unexpected slips during walking in older adults. *J Gerontol A Biol Sci Med Sci*. 1998;53A:M471–80.

216. Yang F, Espy D, Bhatt T et al. Two types of slip-induced falls among community dwelling older adults. *J Biomech*. 2012;45:1259–64.

217. Yoo D, Seo KH, Lee BC. The effect of the most common gait perturbations on the compensatory limb's ankle, knee, and hip moments during the first stepping response. *Gait Posture*. 2019;71:98–104.

218. Patel PJ, Bhatt T. Fall risk during opposing stance perturbations among healthy adults and chronic stroke survivors. *Exp Aging Res.* 2018;236:619–28.

219. Cham R, Redfern M. Changes in gait when anticipating slippery floors. *Gait Posture.* 2002;15:159–71.

220. Marigold D, Patla A. Strategies for dynamic stability during locomotion on a slippery surface: effects of prior experience and knowledge. *J Neurophysiol.* 2002;88:339–53.

221. Heiden TL, Sanderson DJ, Inglis JT et al. Adaptations to normal human gait on potentially slippery surfaces: the effects of awareness and prior slip experience. *Gait Posture.* 2006;24:237–46.

222. Bhatt T, Wening JD, Pai YC. Adaptive control of gait stability in reducing slip-related backward loss of balance. *Exp Aging Res.* 2006;170:61–73.

223. Gerards MHG, McCrum C, Mansfield A et al. Perturbation-based balance training for falls reduction among older adults: current evidence and implications for clinical practice. *Geriatr Gerontol Int.* 2017;17:2294–303.

224. Pai YC, Bhatt TS. Repeated-slip training: an emerging paradigm for prevention of slip-related falls among older adults. *Phys Ther.* 2007;87:1478–91.

225. Bhatt T, Espy D, Yang F et al. Dynamic gait stability, clinical correlates, and prognosis of falls among community-dwelling older adults. *Arch Phys Med Rehabil.* 2011;92:799–805.

4

Sensory and Neuromuscular Risk Factors for Falls

Stephen R. Lord

Chapter 2 outlined how human balance is dependent on the interactions of multiple sensory, motor, and integrative systems. This chapter focuses on age-related changes in key sensory and motor systems involved in balance control, and the associations between impairments in these systems and falls in older people. Specific topics of review include vision, somatosensory and vestibular acuity, and muscle strength, power, and endurance.

Age-Related Changes in Sensorimotor Function

The physiological systems that are the primary contributors to postural stability are shown in Figure 4.1. Numerous studies have found significantly reduced function of sensory, motor, and integration systems with age and that an impairment in any of these systems is associated with falls in older people. Investigators have also noted that many people experience age-related declines in sensorimotor function and increased fall risk, even in the absence of overt disease. As indicated in Figure 4.2, these people mostly cite trips, slips, loss of balance, and muscle weakness as the causes of their falls.

Figure 4.3 shows the 'normal' age-related decline in function in a sensorimotor system that contributes to stability. The figure shows that up until age 55 there is little change in function, but beyond this age there is a progressive decline. This decline occurs in all people but the variability in function becomes greater as age increases. If the criterion level for a loss of balance and subsequent fall is 50 units, it can be seen that people on the lower band reach this level by age 65, whereas those towards the upper band are still above the criterion level at 80 years of age. The figure also depicts a situation in which the onset of chronic disease such as a stroke can rapidly change functional performance and result in performance levels below the criterion level at any age. Acute illness may also result in a temporary decline in functional performance.

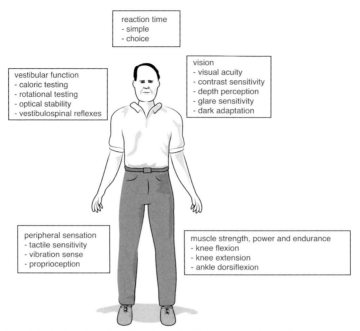

Figure 4.1   Physiological systems involved in maintaining postural stability.

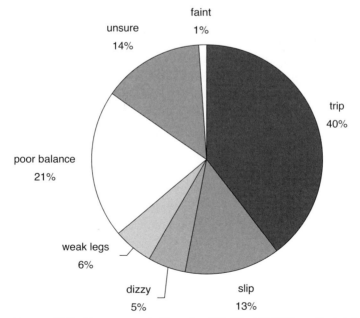

Figure 4.2   Causes of falls. Diagram adapted from Lord SR, Ward JA, Williams P, et al. An epidemiological study of falls in older community-dwelling women: the Randwick Falls and Fractures Study. *Aust J Public Health*. 1993; 17: 240–245.

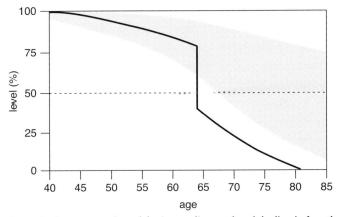

Figure 4.3   Theoretical representation of the 'normal' age-related decline in function in a sensorimotor system that contributes to stability (grey shaded area represents upper and lower boundaries). The figure shows that up until age 55 there is little change in function, but beyond this age there is a progressive decline. This decline occurs in all persons but the range in function becomes greater as age increases. The figure also depicts a situation in which the onset of disease such as a stroke (dark line) can rapidly change functional performance and result in performance levels below the criterion (dashed line) at any age.

Vision

Studies have found that distance-related visual acuity can impact fall risk for those living in aged care facilities [1] and those living at home, independently in the community [2–7]. Despite this, other studies have failed to show an association between reduced visual acuity and fall risk, particularly after adjusting for age [8–15]. Kulmala et al. [16] found impaired visual acuity increased fall risk but only in those with commitment hearing impairment. An early study by Koski et al. [17] may help to partly explain this discrepancy. They found that while visual acuity related strongly to risk of falls among those in assisted living, there was no significant relationship among those living independently in the community. Thus, visual acuity may interact with other functional domains among those already otherwise impaired. Visual acuity loss has also been shown to be an independent predictor of fall-related injuries in two of three prospective studies [18–20], as well as one large case-control study [12]. In the Blue Mountains Eye Study (which involved 3299 people aged over 49 years old), hip fractures were 8.4 times more likely among those with visual acuity worse than 6/18 [21].

Contrast sensitivity is the ability to detect subtle differences between objects in the environment. It allows for differentiation between patterns and shades, and therefore changes in terrain (steps, street kerbs, pavement cracks, and misalignments) over which people may trip. Some studies have found that reduced contrast sensitivity is not a predictor of falls after adjusting for age and confounding factors such as cognition [7, 10, 11, 22]. However, several studies have found that poor edge-contrast sensitivity significantly increases fall risk in older people [23, 24], as well as the risk of multiple falls and fractures [25]. In the Blue Mountains Eye Study, contrast sensitivity was a stronger predictor for falls than visual acuity or visual field loss [2]. In the Beaver Dam Eye Study, there was a non-significant association between retrospective falls and contrast sensitivity, as measured by the Pelli–Robson Test; however, their five-year follow-up study revealed a significant association [5]. A possible explanation for the diverse literature is the inconsistency of measures. Few of the studies examining contrast sensitivity use a range of spatial frequencies (mostly using the Melbourne Edge and Pelli–Robson Tests that examine contrast sensitivity at only a single spatial frequency) [26]. Since hazards which may lead to trips or falls in everyday life comprise a variety of spatial frequencies, it is important that future research should examine the predictive power of tests incorporating a range of spatial frequencies.

Binocular depth perception (stereopsis) is the ability to accurately judge distances and to correctly perceive spatial relationships among objects, which suggests it should be important in visually guided locomotion in the environment. Multiple studies have shown that reductions in binocular depth perception increase the risk of multiple falls [7, 23] as well as fall-related injuries [12, 20]. Those exhibiting good vision in both eyes also have a lower rate of falls, compared to those who have good vision in one eye but moderate or poor vision in the other [23]. Similarly, older people with good vision in one eye, but only moderately good vision in the other, have been shown to have an elevated hip fracture risk [20]. Only one study [11] has reported a non-significant association between binocular depth perception and falls.

Visual field loss has been less extensively examined than either visual acuity or contrast sensitivity; however, the results available indicate a strong association with falls. Although two early studies reported weak associations between visual field size and falls [7, 27], more recent studies have found visual field loss to be a significant risk factor for falls [2, 4, 28, 29], multiple falls [5, 10], and fractures [5, 24, 30]. It has also been reported that this risk remains significant when adjusting for demographic and health measures [10, 11], with one exception [31]. Notably the Beaver Dam Eye Study found that visual field loss almost doubled the risk of falls and fractures [5, 22]. While the measures of visual field loss used across the studies have not been consistent [26], the overall findings suggest that screening for visual field loss is a useful component of visual fall risk assessments in older people.

Peripheral Sensation

Interest in the topic of peripheral sensation can be dated to 1830 when Mueller referred to vibration sense in a physiology text book [32]. In the early twentieth century, several clinicians noted that vibration sense was inferior in older people compared to their younger counterparts. However, it was not until 1928 that Pearson documented that vibration sense decreases significantly with age [33]. Since then, researchers, using various vibration stimuli on different parts of the body, have consistently found age-related declines in vibration sense to frequencies above 50 Hz [34–48]. Many studies have also found vibration sense is poorer in the lower limb compared with the upper limb at all ages and shows a greater age-related decline [36–40, 45, 47].

Literature on tactile sensitivity can also be traced back to the nineteenth century, though there are comparatively fewer studies on the effect of age on this sensory modality. Similar to vibration sense, tactile sensitivity decreases with age [24, 30, 47, 49–52] and is reduced in the lower limb compared with the upper limb [47, 49, 51, 53], when measured by aesthesiometers or tests of two-point discrimination.

Even fewer studies have explored the effect of age on joint position [54]. In 1937, Laidlaw and Hamilton reported participants aged 17 to 35 years were better able to detect directions of hip, knee, and ankle movements than those aged 50 to 80 years [55]. Subsequent studies have found significant age-related declines in position sense at the knee [56–59], ankle [60–62], and metatarsophalangeal joints [63]. However, clinical studies which have investigated whether there is a decline in joint position sense beyond 65 years of age have produced inconsistent results. This may in part be due to the poor reliability of the assessments used, particularly those that rely on participant's ability to identify experimenter-induced movement of body parts [8, 64, 65].

Stelmach and Worringham have suggested caution is required in interpreting lower-limb joint position sense assessments conducted with participants in the seated position [66], because due to greater engagement of the leg muscles [67] in standing, thresholds measured at the knee and ankle are much lower [68, 69]. For example, Bullock-Saxton et al. [69] compared the effect of age on the accuracy of knee-joint repositioning during partial and full weight-bearing conditions in three groups of healthy, pain-free participants (n = 60, young: 20–35 years, middle-aged: 40–55 years and older: 60–75 years). They found that participants in all three groups performed better when full weight bearing than when partial weight bearing, and significant age-related increases were found only in the partial weight-bearing condition. However, other studies assessing position sense of the ankle joint when weight bearing, have reported increased thresholds with age. For example, Thelen et al. [70] compared the ability of young and older women to detect dorsiflexion and plantarflexion movements of the foot when weight bearing on a moveable platform, and reported that the threshold for movement detection was three to four times larger in the older group. Higher detection thresholds for ankle inversion and eversion during unipedal or bipedal stance on a rotating platform have also been found in older people [71] and those with a peripheral neuropathy [72]. Finally, Blaszczyk et al. [73] reported the older participants were significantly worse that younger participants in reproducing ankle joint positions when standing on a rotating platform.

Reduced peripheral sensation or neuropathy has also been documented as the cause of instability and falls. Hurley et al. [59] found that reduced proprioceptive acuity at the knee was significantly associated with an increased aggregate time to perform a series of functional tasks comprising a timed walk, the Get Up and Go Test, and stair ascent and descent in a combined group of young, middle-aged, and older people. Lord et al. [74] found that older people with diabetes had significantly greater postural sway when standing on firm and compliant surfaces compared with their non-diabetic counterparts. Sensory abnormalities in the lower limb and peripheral neuropathy have also been identified as fall risk factors in older people living in residential aged care [14] and older people with Alzheimer's disease [75]. In contrast, Brocklehurst et al. reported a significant association between impaired proprioception in the ankle and/or great toe, and falls in only one (75–84 years) of three age groups above 65 years of age [8], and Nevitt et al. [76], Fukagawa et al. [77], and Grisso et al. [78] found no significant associations between measures of decreased peripheral sensation and falls.

More recent studies have found stronger associations between electromyographically documented neuropathy in the lower limbs and falls [79], and have identified sensory loss to be an independent risk factor for falls in older people. Luukinen et al. [80] found that peripheral neuropathy was an independent risk factor for recurrent falling in 1016 community-dwelling persons aged 70 years or older, and Lord et al. reported vibration sense measured with a calibrated vibrator at the knee and tactile sensitivity measured with a Semmes–Weinstein aesthesiometer at the ankle were inferior in fallers compared to non-fallers in both community [81–83] and institutional settings [84, 85]. Reduced proprioception assessed with a quantitative lower-limb matching assessment has also been identified as a falls risk factor in older people living in the community [81], retirement village [86], and intermediate hostel care [84].

Thus, it seems that sensory loss is associated with falls, but that such an association only emerges when the measures of peripheral sensation are precisely and quantitatively ascertained.

Vestibular Sense

As with other sensory systems, the vestibular system shows age-related changes [87], with changes in the peripheral apparatus, brainstem, cerebellum, or cerebral cortex likely to contribute to vestibular impairment in many older people [88]. In a study of over 1000 people aged 70 years or older, more than one-third had impaired vestibular function [89]. Despite these apparent age-related changes, early reports did not draw links between reduced vestibular sense and instability or falls in older people.

The vestibular system elicits corrective movements via its vestibulo-ocular [90–92] and vestibulo-spinal [93] pathways to maintain head and neck posture during movement [66]. Ability to augment or suppress the vestibulo-ocular reflex (VOR) with horizontal rotation about the head [94], as well as reactivity to caloric and rotational stimulation [95, 96], tends to diminish with age. Vestibular sense, measured by responses to a slow head tilt, had no [8, 97] or some [98] significant association to sway or falls. And even though age-related changes in otolith function have been consistently identified [99, 100], otoliths were found to play no role in the initial detection of body sway [101].

More recent studies that have included more precise assessments of vestibular function have reported significant associations between vestibular impairment and falls and fractures. In a series of studies, Kristinsdottir et al. [102, 103] have used a head-shaking stimulus applied when participants were in a supine position to induce nystagmus – a sign indicating pathology and asymmetry of the vestibular reflexes. In two case-control studies they assessed whether vestibular asymmetry induced using this technique was associated with fall-related fractures in older people. The initial study comprised 19 participants (mean age: 72 years) with hip fracture (which occurred 12–33 months earlier) and 28 aged-matched controls [102]. They found that 13 of the hip-fracture participants (68%) demonstrated a nystagmus following the head-shake stimulus compared with 10 (36%) of the controls (OR: 3.90, 95% CI: 0.97,16.38). The second study involved 66 participants (mean age: 68 years) who had suffered a fall-related wrist fracture during a 10-month period and 49 control participants comprising healthy community-dwelling people (mean age: 75 years) [103]. They found that 50 (76%) of the wrist-fracture participants demonstrated nystagmus compared to 18 (37%) of the healthy participants (OR: 5.38, 95% CI: 2.23,13.11).

In related studies, vestibular input and its contribution to falls in older people has been examined via measures of VOR suppression [104, 105]. The control of gaze during head movement requires input from the vestibular system, known as the vestibulo-ocular reflex. However, during the performance of many well-practiced familiar tasks such as standing and walking, the VOR needs to be suppressed when both eye and head movements are used to stabilize images on the retina [106]. In a case-control study involving 36 older people categorized as being at either high or low risk of falls (18 participants per group), VOR suppression was assessed by measuring eye-movements using electro-oculography during a stand–walk task [104]. While the majority of participants showed some counter-rotation of the eyes with head pitch, a greater percentage of participants in the high-risk group did not suppress this response and consequently gaze and gaze velocity overcompensated for head pitch. In a subsequent study of 38 women (mean age: 82 years; 11 fallers), they found that participants who failed to suppress the VOR gain when subjected to a two-handed nudge to the scapulae were 18 times more likely to have fallen in the past year compared with participants who showed VOR suppression (OR:18.00, 95% CI: 1.63,198.42) [105]. Due to small sample sizes, these results need to be interpreted with caution, though they do suggest that inadequate VOR suppression following a postural perturbation or during a stand–walk task may predispose older people to falls.

Compared to peripheral sensation, assessment of vestibular sense is not as receptive to simple screening tests. However, the available data indicate that if assessed with greater precision, impaired vestibular function may be an important risk factor for falls and fall-related fractures in older people. Further research is required to elucidate the significance of vestibular input in maintaining a stable retinal image for clear vision during head movement and otolithic functioning for balance control and safe mobility.

Muscle Strength, Power, and Endurance

Loss of isometric and dynamic muscle strength with age is well documented [107–113]. Muscle strength in men decreases only slightly between 20 and 40 years, but at a more accelerated pace after the age of 40, such that hand grip strength is reduced by 5–15% [107, 108] and leg strength by 20–40% [109, 112] in men aged 60–69 compared to men aged 20–29. In women, muscle strength tends to decline from an earlier age and at a greater rate, so that over the same age range, hand grip strength declines by 10–25% [107, 108] and leg strength by 30–50% [110, 111]. It has also been shown that muscle strength continues to decline significantly beyond the sixties in both sexes [113]. Muscle strength in women is reported to be about 50–70% of that in men [107–113].

Leg extensor power (the product of force and the rate of force generation) appears to decline at an even greater rate with age than does isometric strength. In a cross-sectional study of 100 healthy people aged 65–89, Skelton et al. [114] found a 1.8% and 2% loss of isometric knee extension strength per annum compared to a 3.7% and 3.2% loss of leg extensor power per annum in men and women, respectively. A reduced capacity to rapidly generate force also limits the ability to respond quickly to a loss of balance [115], has been shown to increase laboratory-induced falls [116] and is therefore likely to increase the risk of falling in daily life.

Isometric and dynamic endurance when assessed in absolute terms also decline significantly with age. However, when endurance is measured in relation to maximal strength (i.e. 50% of maximal contraction), and therefore controlled for individual differences, no decline with age is evident [107, 117–119] – a finding that suggests that sub-maximal muscle strength is less affected by ageing than maximal muscle strength.

Lower-limb muscle weakness has significant practical implications for older people. Pearson et al. [120] found that in 14% of women aged 75 years and over living in the community, the calf muscle was not able to exert sufficient force to support the body weight. This indicates that these women would be at risk of falling in situations where they place their total body weight on one leg only, i.e. when undertaking everyday activities like stepping up a step. Similarly, Vandervoot and Hayes [121] found impaired ankle plantar flexor muscle force and power in residents of geriatric care facilities who were capable of independently performing activities of daily living. They found that the ankle plantar flexor muscles in these women exhibited considerable impairment in ability to generate stabilizing torques about the ankle joint. Inability or difficulty in rising from a chair without the use of hands is also a reflection of reduced strength and has been found to be a significant risk factor of falls in older people living in both community [76, 122] and institutional settings [123, 124].

Strength in specific lower-limb muscle groups has also been found to be inferior in fallers compared with non-fallers. Lord et al. have reported increased fall risk is associated with reduced isometric strength of the knee extensors [81, 82] and ankle dorsiflexors [81], with reduced isometric knee extension strength also increasing the risk of fractures [125]. Reduced knee extensor strength has also been identified as a risk factor for falls in other studies of older community dwellers, including participants of a large longitudinal study [126], residents of retirement villages [85], older people who require day-care [127], and those with vitamin D deficiency [128].

Lower-limb muscle weakness has been found to be associated with falls in nursing home and intermediate-care hostel residents. Whipple et al. [129] and Studenski et al. [130] compared strength measures of the knee extensors, knee flexors, ankle plantar flexors, and ankle dorsiflexors in nursing home residents with and without a history of falls. Both studies found that fallers were weaker than non-fallers in all four muscle groups, with ankle muscle weakness particularly evident in the faller groups. Their findings are consistent with other studies that have attributed an increased risk of falls to decreased ankle dorsiflexion [84], knee extension [85, 124, 131], and hip [14] strength in older people living in residential-care institutions.

Reduced muscle power and endurance are also contributors to fall risk that have been examined in two retrospective studies. A case-control study of 30 older women, half who suffered three or more falls in the past year and half who did not, found a greater asymmetry in muscle strength and power in fallers [132]. When the less powerful legs were compared, Skelton et al. also found that for fallers, it was significantly less than for non-fallers. Schwendner et al. [133] used an isokinetic dynamometer to assess endurance of the quadriceps muscle in 26 older women who reported falls within the last 18 months (mean age: 73 years), 27 older women with no history of falls (mean age: 71 years), and 29 younger women (mean age: 22 years). They found that the fallers demonstrated a much shorter time to fatigue than the non-fallers and younger women, where no difference was evident among them.

Key findings from all these studies indicate that limitations of muscle performance in the lower limb is a major risk factor for falls in older people.

Integration, Interaction, and Summation

The above studies indicate that impairment in a number of the primary physiological systems that contribute to stability is associated with falls in older people. With such an array of inputs there is also little doubt interactions occur between the various stages in the processing of a response to a fall, i.e. sensory input and feed-forward, response selection, and response execution [66, 134]. Vision for instance, has been shown to compensate for diminished peripheral input that was either experimentally induced or a result of disease and trauma [68, 135, 136].

Although marked impairment of just one of these physiological systems is sufficient to increase the risk of falls, multiple impairments of moderate severity can have the same effect. For example, in the case of a trip, reduced vision and slow reaction times may both be necessary for a fall to occur. Thus, it seems that adequate visual, somatosensory, and vestibular acuity contribute to the detection of postural disturbances and environmental hazards, while adequate strength and reaction time permit appropriate corrections to postural imbalance.

Conclusions

There is strong evidence that the sensorimotor factors that contribute to balance control show age-related declines and many studies have shown that over and above the effect of ageing, older people who fall demonstrate impaired function in these measures when compared with age- and sex-matched non-fallers. Physiological systems identified as impaired in older fallers include visual functions such as contrast sensitivity and depth perception, peripheral sensation, strength in the lower limb muscle groups, and reaction time. There is also emerging evidence that impaired vestibular functioning, and reduced muscle power and endurance are also important risk factors for falls.

REFERENCES

1. Tinetti ME, Williams TF, Mayewski R. Fall risk index for elderly patients based on number of chronic disabilities. *Am J Med.* 1986;80:429–34.
2. Ivers RQ, Cumming RG, Mitchell P et al. Visual impairment and falls in older adults: the Blue Mountains eye study. *J Am Geriatr Soc.* 1998;46:58–64.
3. Yip JLY, Khawaja AP, Broadway D et al. Visual acuity, self-reported vision and falls in the EPIC-Norfolk Eye study. *Br J Ophthalmol.* 2014;98:377–82.
4. Patino CM, McKean-Cowdin R, Azen SP et al. Central and peripheral visual impairment and the risk of falls and falls with injury. *Ophthalmology.* 2010;117:199–206.
5. Klein BEK, Moss SE, Klein R et al. Associations of visual function with physical outcomes and limitations 5 years later in an older population: the Beaver Dam Eye Study. *Ophthalmology.* 2003;110:644–50.
6. Lord SR, Menz HB. Visual contributions to postural stability in older adults. *Gerontology.* 2000;46:306–10.
7. Nevitt MC, Cummings SR, Kidd S et al. Risk factors for recurrent nonsyncopal falls: a prospective study. *J Am Med Assoc.* 1989;261:2663–8.
8. Brocklehurst JC, Robertson D, Jamesgroom P. Clinical correlates of sway in old-age – sensory modalities. *Age Ageing.* 1982;11:1–10.
9. Campbell AJ, Borrie MJ, Spears GF. Risk factors for falls in a community-based prospective study of people 70 years and older. *J Gerontol.* 1989;44:M112–17.
10. Coleman AL, Cummings SR, Yu F et al. Binocular visual-field loss increases the risk of future falls in older white women. *J Am Geriatr Soc.* 2007;55:357–64.
11. Freeman EE, Munoz B, Rubin G et al. Visual field loss increases the risk of falls in older adults: the Salisbury eye evaluation. *Invest Ophthalmol Vis Sci.* 2007;48:4445–50.
12. Ivers RQ, Norton R, Cumming RG et al. Visual impairment and risk of hip fracture. *Am J Epidemiol.* 2000;152:633–9.
13. Lord SR, Clark RD, Webster IW. Postural stability and associated physiological factors in a population of aged persons. *J Gerontol.* 1991;46:M69–76.

14. Robbins AS, Rubenstein LZ, Josephson KR et al. Predictors of falls among elderly people: results of two population-based studies. *Arch Intern Med.* 1989;149:1628–33.

15. Tinetti ME, Speechley M, Ginter SF. Risk factors for falls among elderly persons living in the community. *New Engl J Med.* 1988;319:1701–7.

16. Kulmala J, Viljanen A, Sipila S et al. Poor vision accompanied with other sensory impairments as a predictor of falls in older women. *Age Ageing.* 2009;38:162–7.

17. Koski K, Luukinen H, Laippala P et al. Risk factors for major injurious falls among the home-dwelling elderly by functional abilities. A prospective population-based study. *Gerontology.* 1998;44:232–8.

18. Cummings SR, Nevitt MC, Browner WS et al. Risk factors for hip fracture in white women. *New Engl J Med.* 1995;332:767–73.

19. Dargent-Molina P, Favier F, Grandjean H et al. Fall-related factors and risk of hip fracture: the EPIDOS prospective study. *Lancet.* 1996;348:145–9.

20. Felson DT, Anderson JJ, Hannan MT et al. Impaired vision and hip fracture: the Framingham Study. *J Am Geriatr Soc.* 1989;37:495–500.

21. Ivers RQ, Cumming RG, Mitchell P et al. Visual risk factors for hip fracture in older people. *J Am Geriatr Soc.* 2003;51:356–63.

22. Klein BEK, Klein R, Lee KE et al. Performance-based and self-assessed measures of visual function as related to history of falls, hip fractures, and measured gait time: the Beaver Dam Eye Study. *Ophthalmology.* 1998;105:160–4.

23. Lord SR, Dayhew J. Visual risk factors for falls in older people. *J Am Geriatr Soc.* 2001;49:508–15.

24. Lord SR, Ward JA. Age-associated differences in sensorimotor function and balance in community-dwelling women. *Age Ageing.* 1994;23:452–60.

25. de Boer MR, Pluijm SM, Lips P et al. Different aspects of visual impairment as risk factors for falls and fractures in older men and women. *J Bone Miner Res.* 2004;19:1539–47.

26. Black AA, Wood JM. Vision and falls. *Clin Exp Optom.* 2005;88:212–22.

27. Glynn RJ, Seddon JM, Krug JH et al. Falls in elderly patients with glaucoma. *Arch Ophthalmol.* 1991;109:205–10.

28. Ramrattan RS, Wolfs RC, Panda-Jonas S et al. Prevalence and causes of visual field loss in the elderly and associations with impairment in daily functioning: the Rotterdam Study. *Arch Ophthalmol.* 2001;119:1788–94.

29. Black AA, Wood JM, Lovie-Kitchin JE. Inferior field loss increases rate of falls in older adults with glaucoma. *Optom Vis Sci.* 2011;88:1275–82.

30. Axelrod S, Cohen LD. Senescence and embedded-figure performance in vision and touch. *Percept Mot Skills.* 1961;12:283–8.

31. Friedman SM, Munoz B, West SK et al. Falls and fear of falling: which comes first? A longitudinal prediction model suggests strategies for primary and secondary prevention. *J Am Geriatr Soc.* 2002;50:1329–35.

32. Fox JC, Klemperer WW. Vibratory sensibility: a quantitative study of its thresholds in nervous disorders. *Arch Neurol Psy.* 1942;48:622–45.

33. Pearson GHJ. Effect of age on vibratory sensibility. *Arch Neurol Psy.* 1928;20:482–96.

34. Gray RC. A quantitative study of vibration sense in normal and pernicious anaemia cases. *Minn Med*. 1932;15:674–91.

35. Newman HW, Corbin KB. Quantitative determination of vibratory sensibility. *Proc Soc Exp Biol Med*. 1936;35:273–6.

36. Laidlaw RW. Thresholds of vibratory sensibility as determined by the pallesthesiometer: a study of sixty normal subjects. *Bull Neurol Inst NY*. 1937;6:493–503.

37. Cosh JA. Studies on the nature of vibration sense. *Clin Sci*. 1953;12:131–51.

38. Mirsky IA, Futterman P, Broh-Kahn RH. The quantitative measurement of vibratory perception in subjects with and without diabetes mellitus. *J Lab Clin Med*. 1953;41:221–35.

39. Steiness IB. Vibratory perception in normal subjects: a biothesionietric study. *Acta Med Scand*. 1957;158:315–25.

40. Rosenberg G, Adams A. Effect of age on peripheral vibratory perception. *J Am Geriatr Soc*. 1958;6:471–81.

41. Steinberg FU, Graber AL. The effect of age and peripheral circulation on the perception of vibration. *Arch Phys Med Rehab*. 1963;44:645–50.

42. Whanger AD, Wang HS. Clinical correlates of the vibratory sense in elderly psychiatric patients. *J Gerontol*. 1974;29:39–45.

43. Plumb CS, Meigs JW. Human vibration perception: Part I. Vibration perception at different ages (normal ranges). *Arch Gen Psychiatry*. 1961;4:611–14.

44. Goff GD, Rosner BS, Detre T, Kennard D. Vibration perception in normal man and medical patients. *J Neurol Neurosurg Psychiatry*. 1965;28:503.

45. Perret E, Regli F. Age and the perceptual threshold for vibratory stimuli. *Eur Neurol*. 1970;4:65–76.

46. Verrillo RT. Comparison of vibrotactile threshold and suprathreshold responses in men and women. *Percept Psychophys*. 1979;26:20–4.

47. Kenshalo DR, Sr. Somesthetic sensitivity in young and elderly humans. *J Gerontol*. 1986;41:732–42.

48. Era P, Jokela J, Suominen H et al. Correlates of vibrotactile thresholds in men of different ages. *Acta Neurol Scand*. 1986;74:210–17.

49. Dyck PJ, Schultz PW, O'Brien PC. Quantitation of touch-pressure sensation. *Arch Neurol*. 1972;26:465–73.

50. Gescheider GA, Bolanowski SJ, Hall KL et al. The effects of aging on information-processing channels in the sense of touch: I. Absolute sensitivity. *Somatosens Mot Res*. 1994;11:345–57.

51. Bolton CF, Winkelmann RK, Dyck PJ. A quantitative study of Meissner's corpuscles in man. *Neurology*. 1966;16:1–9.

52. Stevens JC, Choo KK. Spatial acuity of the body surface over the life span. *Somatosens Mot Res*. 1996;13:153–66.

53. Halar EM, Hammond MC, LaCava EC et al. Sensory perception threshold measurement: an evaluation of semiobjective testing devices. *Arch Phys Med Rehab*. 1987;68:499–507.

54. Goble DJ, Coxon JP, Wenderoth N et al. Proprioceptive sensibility in the elderly: degeneration, functional consequences and plastic-adaptive processes. *Neurosci Biobehav Rev.* 2009;33:271–8.

55. Laidlaw RW, Hamilton MA. A study of thresholds in apperception of passive movement among normal control subjects. *Bull Neurol Inst NY.* 1937;6:268–340.

56. Skinner HB, Barrack RL, Cook SD. Age-related decline in proprioception. *Clin Orthop Relat Res.* 1984:208–11.

57. Kaplan FS, Nixon JE, Reitz M et al. Age-related changes in proprioception and sensation of joint position. *Acta Orthop Scand.* 1985;56:72–4.

58. Petrella RJ, Lattanzio PJ, Nelson MG. Effect of age and activity on knee joint proprioception. *Am J Phys Med Rehabil.* 1997;76:235–41.

59. Hurley MV, Rees J, Newham DJ. Quadriceps function, proprioceptive acuity and functional performance in healthy young, middle-aged and elderly subjects. *Age Ageing.* 1998;27:55–62.

60. Deshpande N, Patla AE. Visual-vestibular interaction during goal directed locomotion: effects of aging and blurring vision. *Exp Aging Res.* 2007;176:43–53.

61. You SH. Joint position sense in elderly fallers: a preliminary investigation of the validity and reliability of the SENSERite measure. *Arch Phys Med Rehabil.* 2005;86:346–52.

62. Westlake KP, Culham EG. Sensory-specific balance training in older adults: effect on proprioceptive reintegration and cognitive demands. *Phys Ther.* 2007;87:1274–83.

63. Kokmen E, Bossemeyer RW, Jr, Williams WJ. Quantitative evaluation of joint motion sensation in an aging population. *J Gerontol.* 1978;33:62–7.

64. MacLennan WJ, Timothy JI, Hall MRP. Vibration sense, proprioception and ankle reflexes in old age. *J Clin Exp Gerontol.* 1980;2:159–71.

65. Howell TH. Senile deterioration of the central nervous system. *Br Med J.* 1949;1:56–8.

66. Stelmach GE, Worringham CJ. Sensorimotor deficits related to postural stability: implications for falling in the elderly. *Clin Geriatr Med.* 1985;1:679–94.

67. Refshauge KM, Fitzpatrick RC. Perception of movement at the human ankle: effects of leg position. *J Physiol.* 1995;488:243–8.

68. Gurfinkel VS, Lipshits MI, Popov KE. Thresholds of kinesthetic sensation in the vertical posture. *Hum Physiol.* 1982;8:439–45.

69. Bullock-Saxton JE, Wong WJ, Hogan N. The influence of age on weight-bearing joint reposition sense of the knee. *Exp Brain Res.* 2001;136:400–6.

70. Thelen DG, Brockmiller C, Ashton-Miller JA et al. Thresholds for sensing foot dorsi- and plantarflexion during upright stance: effects of age and velocity. *J Gerontol A Biol Sci Med Sci.* 1998;53A:M33–8.

71. Gilsing MG, Van den Bosch CG, Lee S-G et al. Association of age with the threshold for detecting ankle inversion and eversion in upright stance. *Age Ageing.* 1995;24:58–66.

72. Van den Bosch CG, Gilsing MG, Lee S-G et al. Peripheral neuropathy effect on ankle inversion and eversion detection thresholds. *Arch Phys Med Rehab.* 1995;76:850–6.

73. Blaszczyk JW, Hansen PD, Lowe DL. Accuracy of passive ankle joint positioning during quiet stance in young and elderly subjects. *Gait Posture.* 1993;1:211–15.

74. Lord SR, Caplan GA, Colagiuri R et al. Sensori-motor function in older persons with diabetes. *Diabet Med.* 1993;10:614–18.

75. Buchner DM, Larson EB. Falls and fractures in patients with Alzheimer-type dementia. *J Am Med Assoc.* 1987;257:1492–5.

76. Nevitt MC, Cummings SR, Kidd S et al. Risk factors for recurrent nonsyncopal falls: a prospective study. *J Am Med Assoc.* 1989;261:2663–8.

77. Fukagawa NK, Wolfson L, Judge J et al. Strength is a major factor in balance, gait, and the occurrence of falls. *J Gerontol A Biol Sci Med Sci.* 1995;50A:64–7.

78. Grisso JA, Kelsey JL, Strom BL et al. Risk factors for falls as a cause of hip fracture in women. *N Eng J Med.* 1991;324:1326–31.

79. Richardson JK, Ching C, Hurvitz EA. The relationship between electromyographically documented peripheral neuropathy and falls. *J Am Geriatr Soc.* 1992;40:1008–12.

80. Luukinen H, Koski K, Laippala P et al. Predictors for recurrent falls among the home-dwelling elderly. *Scand J Prim Health Care.* 1995;13:294–9.

81. Lord SR, Sambrook PN, Gilbert C et al. Postural stability, falls and fractures in the elderly: results from the Dubbo Osteoporosis Epidemiology Study. *Med J Aust.* 1994;160:684–91.

82. Lord SR, McLean D, Stathers G. Physiological factors associated with injurious falls in older people living in the community. *Gerontology.* 1992;38:338–46.

83. Lord SR, Ward JA, Williams P et al. Physiological factors associated with falls in older community-dwelling women. *J Am Geriatr Soc.* 1994;42:1110–17.

84. Lord SR, Clark RD, Webster IW. Physiological factors associated with falls in an elderly population. *J Am Geriatr Soc.* 1991;39:1194–200.

85. Lord SR, Clark RD. Simple physiological and clinical tests for the accurate prediction of falling in older people. *Gerontology.* 1996;42:199–203.

86. Lord SR, Fitzpatrick RC. Choice stepping reaction time: a composite measure of falls risk in older people. *J Gerontol A Biol Sci Med Sci.* 2001;56:M627–32.

87. Zalewski CK. Aging of the human vestibular system. *Semin Hear.* 2015;36:175–96.

88. Arshad Q, Seemungal BM. Age-related vestibular loss: current understanding and future research directions. *Front Neurol.* 2016;7:231.

89. Katsarkas A. Dizziness in aging: a retrospective study of 1194 cases. *Otolaryngol Head Neck Surg.* 1994;110:296–301.

90. Baloh RW, Jacobson KM, Socotch TM. The effect of aging on visual-vestibuloocular responses. *Exp Aging Res.* 1993;95:509–16.

91. Baloh RW, Enrietto J, Jacobson KM et al. Age-related changes in vestibular function: a longitudinal study. *Ann NY Acad Sci.* 2001;942:210–19.

92. Kerber KA, Ishiyama GP, Baloh RW. A longitudinal study of oculomotor function in normal older people. *Neurobiol Aging.* 2006;27:1346–53.

93. Welgampola MS, Colebatch JG. Selective effects of ageing on vestibular-dependent lower limb responses following galvanic stimulation. *Clin Neurophysiol.* 2002;113:528–34.

94. Baloh RW, Jacobson KM, Socotch TM. The effect of aging on visual-vestibuloocular responses. *Exp Brain Res.* 1993;95:509–16.

95. Karlsen EA, Hassanein RM, Goetzinger CP. The effects of age, sex, hearing loss and water temperature on caloric nystagmus. *Laryngoscope.* 1981;91:620–7.

96. Ghosh P. Aging and auditory vestibular response. *Ear Nose Throat J.* 1985;64:264–6.

97. Woolley SM, Czaja SJ, Drury CG. An assessment of falls in elderly men and women. *J Gerontol A Biol Sci Med Sci.* 1997;52A:M80–7.

98. Serrador JM, Lipsitz LA, Gopalakrishnan GS et al. Loss of otolith function with age is associated with increased postural sway measures. *Neurosci Lett.* 2009;465:10–15.

99. Brantberg K, Granath K, Schart N. Age-related changes in vestibular evoked myogenic potentials. *Audiol Neurootol.* 2007;12:247–53.

100. Li C, Layman AJ, Carey JP et al. Epidemiology of vestibular evoked myogenic potentials: data from the Baltimore Longitudinal Study of Aging. *Clin Neurophysiol.* 2015;126:2207–15.

101. Nashner LM. A model describing vestibular detection of body sway motion. *Acta Otolaryngol.* 1971;72:429–36.

102. Kristinsdottir EK, Jarnlo G-B, Magnusson M. Asymmetric vestibular function in the elderly might be a significant contributor to hip fractures. *Scand J Rehabil Med.* 2000;32:56–60.

103. Kristinsdottir EK, Nordell E, Jarnlo G-B et al. Observation of vestibular asymmetry in a majority of patients over 50 years with fall-related wrist fractures. *Acta Otolaryngol.* 2001;121:481–5.

104. Di Fabio RP, Emasithi A, Greany JF et al. Suppression of the vertical vestibulo-ocular reflex in older persons at risk of falling. *Acta Otolaryngol.* 2001;121:707–14.

105. Di Fabio RP, Greany JF, Emasithi A et al. Eye-head coordination during postural perturbation as a predictor of falls in community-dwelling elderly women. *Arch Phys Med Rehab.* 2002;83:942–51.

106. Collins CJS, Barnes GR. Independent control of head and gaze movements during head-free pursuit in humans. *J Physiol.* 1999;515:299–314.

107. Petrofsky JS, Burse RL, Lind AR. Comparison of physiological responses of women and men to isometric exercise. *J Appl Physiol.* 1975;38:863–8.

108. Montoye HJ, Lamphiear DE. Grip and arm strength in males and females, age 10 to 69. *Res Q.* 1977;48:109–20.

109. Murray MP, Gardner GM, Mollinger LA et al. Strength of isometric and isokinetic contractions: knee muscles of men aged 20 to 86. *Phys Ther.* 1980;60:412–19.

110. Murray MP, Duthie EH, Gambert SR et al. Age-related differences in knee muscle strength in normal women. *J Gerontol.* 1985;40:275–80.

111. Frontera WR, Hughes VA, Lutz KJ et al. A cross-sectional study of muscle strength and mass in 45-to 78-yr-old men and women. *J Appl Physiol.* 1991;71:644–50.

112. Stålberg E, Borges O, Ericsson M et al. The quadriceps femoris muscle in 20–70-year-old subjects: relationship between knee extension torque, electrophysiological parameters, and muscle fiber characteristics. *Muscle Nerve.* 1989;12:382–9.

113. MacLennan WJ, Hall MRP, Timothy JI et al. Is weakness in old age due to muscle wasting? *Age Ageing.* 1980;9:188–92.

114. Skelton DA, Greig CA, Davies JM et al. Strength, power and related functional ability of healthy people aged 65–89 years. *Age Ageing.* 1994;23:371–7.

115. Pijnappels M, Bobbert MF, van Dieen JH. Contribution of the support limb in control of angular momentum after tripping. *J Biomech.* 2004;37:1811–18.

116. Pijnappels M, Bobbert MF, van Dieen JH. Push-off reactions in recovery after tripping discriminate young subjects, older non-fallers and older fallers. *Gait Posture.* 2005;21:388–94.

117. Larsson L, Karlsson J. Isometric and dynamic endurance as a function of age and skeletal muscle characteristics. *Acta Physiol Scand.* 1978;104:129–36.

118. Johnson T. Age-related differences in isometric and dynamic strength and endurance. *Phys Ther.* 1982;62:985–9.

119. Davies CTM, White MJ. Effects of dynamic exercise on muscle function in elderly men, aged 70 years. *Gerontology.* 1983;29:26–31.

120. Pearson MB, Bassey EJ, Bendall MJ. Muscle strength and anthropometric indices in elderly men and women. *Age Ageing.* 1985;14:49–54.

121. Vandervoort AA, Hayes KC. Plantarflexor muscle function in young and elderly women. *Eur J Appl Physiol Occup Physiol.* 1989;58:389–94.

122. Campbell AJ, Borrie MJ, Spears GF. Risk factors for falls in a community-based prospective study of people 70 years and older. *J Gerontol.* 1989;44:M112–17.

123. Lipsitz LA, Jonsson PV, Kelley MM et al. Causes and correlates of recurrent falls in ambulatory frail elderly. *J Gerontol.* 1991;46:M114–22.

124. Lord SR, March LM, Cameron ID et al. Differing risk factors for falls in nursing home and intermediate-care residents who can and cannot stand unaided. *J Am Geriatr Soc.* 2003;51:1645–50.

125. Nguyen T, Sambrook P, Kelly P et al. Prediction of osteoporotic fractures by postural instability and bone density. *Br Med J.* 1993;307:1111–15.

126. Stel VS, Smit JH, Pluijm SMF et al. Balance and mobility performance as treatable risk factors for recurrent falling in older persons. *J Clin Epidemiol.* 2003;56:659–68.

127. Takazawa K, Arisawa K, Honda S et al. Lower-extremity muscle forces measured by a hand-held dynamometer and the risk of falls among day-care users in Japan: using multinomial logistic regression analysis. *Disabil Rehabil.* 2003;25:399–404.

128. Dhesi JK, Bearne LM, Moniz C et al. Neuromuscular and psychomotor function in elderly subjects who fall and the relationship with vitamin D status. *J Bone Miner Res.* 2002;17:891–7.

129. Whipple RH, Wolfson LI, Amerman PM. The relationship of knee and ankle weakness to falls in nursing home residents: an isokinetic study. *J Am Geriatr Soc.* 1987;35:13–20.

130. Studenski S, Duncan PW, Chandler J. Postural responses and effector factors in persons with unexplained falls: results and methodologic issues. *J Am Geriatr Soc.* 1991;39:229–34.

131. Luukinen H, Koski K, Laippala P et al. Risk factors for recurrent falls in the elderly in long-term institutional care. *Public Health.* 1995;109:57–65.

132. Skelton DA, Kennedy J, Rutherford OM. Explosive power and asymmetry in leg muscle function in frequent fallers and non-fallers aged over 65. *Age Ageing.* 2002;31:119–25.

133. Schwendner KI, Mikesky AE, Holt WS, Jr et al. Differences in muscle endurance and recovery between fallers and nonfallers, and between young and older women. *J Gerontol A Biol Sci Med Sci.* 1997;52A:M155–60.

134. Grabiner MD, Jahnigen DW. Modeling recovery from stumbles: preliminary data on variable selection and classification efficacy. *J Am Geriatr Soc*. 1992;40:910–13.

135. Diener HC, Dichgans J, Guschlbauer B et al. The significance of proprioception on postural stabilization as assessed by ischemia. *Brain Res*. 1984;296:103–9.

136. Fernie GR, Holliday PJ. Postural sway in amputees and normal subjects. *J Bone Joint Surg Am*. 1978;60:895–8.

5

Biomechanics of Balance and Falling

Daina L. Sturnieks

In biomechanical terms, balance control is the maintenance of the body's centre of mass (COM: the point around which the body's mass is equally distributed) within the limits of the base of support (BOS: the area circumscribed by parts of the body that are in contact with a support surface) in the horizontal plane. Simply put, the vertical line of gravity acting through the COM (also termed the centre of gravity), must remain within the BOS for a body to remain in postural equilibrium. Falling is the loss of balance control, i.e. when the vertical projection of the COM moves beyond the BOS. Without a successful balance-correcting response or external intervention to arrest the falling state and regain postural equilibrium, a fall (to the ground or some other lower level) will result. Biomechanical investigations have sought to understand falling by characterizing balance control while standing, walking, during postural transitions, and following unexpected perturbations. These studies complement epidemiological and physiological investigations of fall risk. Findings can help to inform the development of intervention strategies and in turn, biomechanical investigations can enable the evaluation of their effects.

Control of Standing Posture

As suggested by Hellebrandt and Braun [1], standing is to oppose the ever-present collapsing stresses of gravity. Balance control in its simplest form, during 'quiet' standing, has been intensely studied to elucidate mechanisms involved, changes with age and disease, and how poor balance might contribute to the risk of falling. Often termed static balance, standing balance is in fact, not static, rather a complex task in which the central nervous system constantly monitors and executes adjustments of the COM position to stay within the BOS. In an inverted pendulum model of balance control (see Figure 5.1a), the COM oscillates at the end of a lever that rotates about the ankles [2]. Since an inverted pendulum is

(a)   (b)

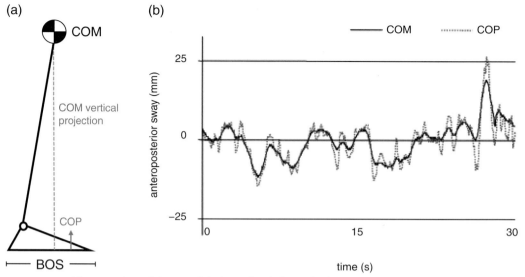

Figure 5.1   (a) Inverted pendulum model of standing balance: body centre of mass (COM) at the end of the lever that rotates about the ankle joint, upon the base of support (BOS)/foot. (b) Typical centre of pressure (COP) and centre of mass (COM) trace in the antero-posterior direction during standing balance, with the COP (controlling variable) oscillating around the COM (controlled variable).

inherently unstable, relatively minor perturbations (such as breathing) can initiate the oscillation.

The objective of the central nervous system is to maintain the vertical projection of the COM within the BOS by producing timely changes in the forces onto the support surface (underfoot). The point at which the sum of these forces acts on the support surface is the centre of pressure (COP). Shifting the COP leads to changes in the moment of force acting on the body and is achieved by changing the activity of postural muscles. For a simple example, from a state of true equilibrium where the COM is directly over the COP, activating ankle plantar flexors will shift the COP forward of the COM and accelerate the COM backward. When the backward COM motion is detected as moving towards an unsafe range (heading towards a backward fall), opposing ankle dorsiflexor activity can act to shift the COP backward to catch the COM and send it forward until the forward COM motion is detected as moving towards an unsafe range and so on. Consequently, the horizontal position of the COP oscillates around that of the COM (see Figure 5.1b). The COP, therefore, can be considered a controlling variable for balance, as it governs the horizontal acceleration of the COM [3], and this motion is known as postural sway.

Posturography, the measurement of postural sway, can be achieved in many different ways, from simple qualitative clinical tests to precise technological measurement systems often found in biomechanics laboratories today. Commonly, a force platform is used to measure the forces underfoot while the participant is standing on the platform. From these forces, the COP, or geometrical location of the centre point of the underfoot forces can be calculated for a given time period. The time series of COP values can be used to characterize postural sway. Numerous variables have been reported, although most commonly include COP magnitude measures including displacement (cm), area (cm^2), range in the antero-posterior and medio-lateral planes (cm), as well as velocity (cm/s), frequency (Hz), and variability (e.g. root mean square) measures [4]. Generally, poorer balance is indicated by a greater magnitude, faster velocity, higher frequency, and more variable postural sway [5–7]. Studies have shown force platform measures to identify differences in balance between young, middle-aged, and older people [8], in addition to age-related changes with longitudinal methods [9] and association with falls in prospective studies [6, 10].

Other systems for assessing postural sway measure motion of an estimated COM. 3D motion analysis enables the accurate measurement of coordinates of the body and an estimated body COM. Measures of the COM coordinates and its derivatives; displacement, velocity, acceleration, frequency, or other calculated indices of sway magnitude or variance have been reported. Body worn accelerometers and gyroscopes can measure changes in body segment position and angles. Combining posturography with electromyographical (EMG) studies of muscle activity provides enhanced capacity to understand balance control. In contrast to the high-tech equipment often employed, physiologists and clinicians have often characterized postural sway using simple, portable equipment, such as a pen attached to a rod extending from the waist, which traces the movements of the body onto a sheet of paper [11].

Regardless of the measurement device or technique used, the magnitude of postural sway has been repeatedly shown to increase with age in adults. Using a purposely constructed grandfather to the current day force platform, Hellebrandt and Braun [1] measured sway range and the mean position of the centre of pressure in over 100 people aged 3 to 86 years and found the line of the COM fell in front of the transverse axis of the ankle joint and slightly to the left side, regardless of age and gender. The shifts in COP averaged 3.73 cm^2, proportionately small considering the base of support area, thereby offering a liberal margin of stability. The amount of sway was found to be dependent on age, with greater sway in the young and old, compared to young and middle-aged adults, with the best postural stability seen in people aged in the third decade. From the fourth decade, a consistent loss of stability was shown and has been supported by numerous studies since [8]. In the lateral direction, this age-related change is more pronounced, suggesting the control of balance in the lateral plane is particularly problematic for older adults [6, 12].

Age-related changes in muscle function, peripheral sensation and vision lead to the reduced balance control in older age [7, 13–16], and impaired lower-limb proprioception, quadriceps strength, and reaction time have been found to be important correlates of increased sway [12]. In addition, psychological factors can influence postural sway. Maki et al. [17] found older people with a self-reported fear of falling to have increased postural sway with eyes closed compared to those without fear, despite no differences in sensorimotor performance. Conversely, experimentally induced anxiety can result in reduced amplitude of postural sway, often seen with increased postural stiffening and altered attentional focus [18], suggesting a complex interplay between physiological and psychological factors in the control of balance.

Large posturography studies show increased sway is associated with falls in older people [6, 10, 19]. Significant differences are more likely to be seen in more balance-challenging conditions, such as sensory deprivation (eyes closed or standing on a compliant surface). Multiple fallers had 33–46% greater body sway while standing on foam than those who did not experience a fall in the previous 12 months [20]. In a population of 100 older adults, Maki et al. [6] found the (root mean square) COP medio-lateral displacement, while blind-folded, to predict those people who fell over 12 months. Similarly, a prospective study of 84 aged care residents found that measures of sway in more challenging conditions (eyes closed and standing on a compliant foam mat) discriminated fallers from non-fallers, whereas sway under normal standing conditions did not [15, 21].

Perturbations to Standing Balance

In addition to sensory manipulations, mechanical disturbances have been used to better understand the loss of balance control that might contribute to falls. Mechanical perturbations displace the position of body segments and the total body COM, requiring a response to regain postural equilibrium. Such perturbations include the use of platforms that translate or rotate underfoot, with variable displacement, velocity, and acceleration profiles, from which balance control mechanisms can be investigated and an individual's balance-recovery response may be assessed. It has been shown that the postural response is scaled to the motion direction, displacement magnitude [22], and velocity of the platform [23, 24]. The platform acceleration provides the initial destabilizing input and the deceleration provides a second perturbation [25], both greatly influencing the postural response.

Following platform rotation, older adults respond with more sway compared to young [16, 26]. A prospective study monitored falls for 12 months following platform perturbation assessment and showed the amount of postural sway in response to lateral platform perturbation, while blindfolded, to predict falls with moderate accuracy [6]. Since, several studies, employing various methods of perturbing balance, including waist-pulls and release from a static body lean angle, have reported associations between measures of impaired balance recovery and falls [27–31], i.e. the use of multiple steps to recover from a forward loss of balance, poor balance-recovery behaviour in response to medio-lateral perturbations [25, 26], and lower stepping thresholds in response to lateral and posterior force-controlled waist-pulls [32–34].

Kinematic measures of the perturbation response have provided insight into the mechanisms employed to maintain stability during these postural challenges. In the antero-posterior direction (sagittal plane), small perturbations are often controlled at the ankle, i.e. ankle plantar flexion and dorsiflexion moments. Larger disturbances may involve hip and arm motion and occur with a longer delay compared to lower leg responses [35]. Reponses to lateral perturbations (frontal plane) involve the shift of loading between legs, largely due to hip and trunk muscles, to control the COM within the BOS. Maximum excursions of body segments are generally larger with age, particularly of the upper body [35].

The direction and extent of the motion of the COM are important determinants of whether balance is lost and a fall occurs. As demonstrated by Pai and Patton [36], stability of the body at any one time is dependent not only on the COM position but also its velocity, such that a COM travelling with faster velocity has a decreasing area or timeframe within which to maintain stability. Hof et al. [37] proposed that the velocity-adjusted COM be used to characterize dynamic stability. This extrapolated COM position has been used in many studies to quantify the margin of stability, defined as the distance between the closest edge of the BOS and the velocity-corrected COM position in a given plane.

As muscle activation precedes kinematic responses, electromyography (EMG), the recording of muscle activity, can provide an earlier picture of the neuromuscular response to postural perturbations. The earliest postural responses occur at latencies of 70–90 ms and are considered to be automatic, while voluntary reactions are seen at a longer latency of around 150 ms [38]. Directionally specific compensatory EMG responses are induced in synergistic leg muscles (for backward displacement, activity occurs in the gastrocnemius and biceps femoris, while for forward displacement the activity occurs in the tibialis anterior and rectus femoris) [39]. With the application of larger perturbations at the ankle, the first directionally specific, compensatory response in the prime movers is followed by an activation of the antagonist muscle and occasionally by a second burst of activity in the agonist muscle.

Perturbations of larger magnitudes that threaten to move the COM beyond the BOS limits require reconfiguring the BOS to recover balance, for example, by taking a step. Triggers of protective stepping include time and distance boundaries, i.e. the displacement of the COP relative to the BOS [40]. Successful balance recovery is dependent on timely generation of joint moments, adequate step length, and appropriate step direction. Due to slower responses and reduced force-generating capacities, older adults, particularly those with balance impairment, step more frequently in response to a given perturbation, compared to young, and often require multiple steps before balance is recovered. In taking multiple steps, older adults are more likely to contact the contralateral limb, further increasing the risk of a fall [41, 42]. The maximum lean angle from which older adults are able to recover after a sudden release is related to their ability to transfer weight and step quickly [31], highlighting the importance of the rapid development of mechanical responses in withstanding perturbations.

The ability to control balance in the lateral plane is particularly problematic for older adults [43]. Following a balance perturbation, fallers have greater COM displacement and velocity towards the stepping side at foot contact and a more laterally directed foot placement compared to younger people and older non-fallers [43]. When studying unpredictable lateral waist-pull perturbations in 50 older people, Hilliard et al. found that those who consistently responded with multiple steps were six times more likely to fall in the following year than those who did not always have a multiple step response [33]. Increased age and fall risk is associated with the use of crossover steps in responding to lateral perturbations, which is easier to initiate than sidestepping, yet requires a longer time in single stance and more complex foot trajectory, during which there is a high risk of collision with the stance limb [43].

Perturbations to Gait

While findings of studies of perturbed standing balance have advanced our understanding of unplanned postural responses, falls usually occur while moving, such as walking or during postural transitions [44]. A large proportion of falls in community-dwelling older people are attributed to tripping [45–49], and experiencing multiple 'stumbles' has been found to be a predictor of falls over a 12-month prospective period [50]. In negotiating obstacles while walking, older people have an increased risk for tripping, particularly when the available response time is decreased [51] and attention is divided [52]. Studies have shown that compared to young, older people are less adaptable to obstacles while walking, being slower to respond, with poorer stepping accuracy, and poorer clearance success rates. Poorer proactive and reactive strategies in responding to gait perturbations contribute to increased fall risk.

During a trip, obstruction of the swinging leg induces a forward rotation on the upper body over the BOS [53]. To regain balance, an effective push off of the supporting limb is required to enable a recovery step ahead of the COM to arrest the forward momentum (catch the falling upper body). Eng et al. [54] identified two main movement strategies used in response to a trip; a lowering and an elevating strategy (see Figure 5.2), which appear to be triggered depending on the timing of the trip (early or late swing phase) and the capacity of the individual to develop extensor torques. In the lowering strategy, the obstructed swing leg is lowered on the near side of the obstruction and acts as the support leg while the opposite leg clears the trip obstacle in taking the first recovery step. In the elevating strategy, the non-tripped limb remains the support leg and pushes off to elevate the body COM, giving time and space for the obstructed swing leg to overcome the trip obstacle.

Numerous studies have induced trips in the laboratory to examine successful responses and limiting factors to recovery following a trip (see van Dieën et al. [53]

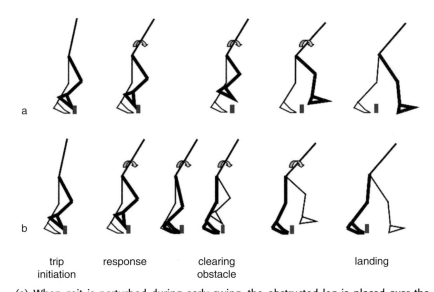

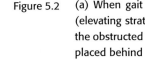

| trip initiation | response | clearing obstacle | landing |

Figure 5.2   (a) When gait is perturbed during early swing, the obstructed leg is placed over the obstacle (elevating strategy) to brake the forward rotation. (b) When gait is perturbed during late swing, the obstructed leg is placed in front of the obstacle (lowering strategy), after which the other leg is placed behind the obstacle to brake the forward rotation. Reproduced with permission from van Dieën JH, Pijnappels M, Bobbert MF. Age-related intrinsic limitations in preventing a trip and regaining balance after a trip. Saf Sci. 2005;43:437–53.

for review). A slower walking speed is associated with an improved recovery following a trip, and faster walking is associated with increased trunk flexion and greater anterior COM displacement [55]. Early work has shown that recovery requires adequate forward placement of the recovery leg, which is slower in older people and limited by lower-extremity muscular power [53, 55].

The support limb is of great importance for successful recovery of balance following a trip [56]. A strong push-off reaction, particularly at the ankle joint, enables time and clearance for correct positioning of the recovery limb and can help to arrest the forward angular momentum of the body. When properly placed, recovery-limb joint moments, together with upper body extensor moments further counteract the body's angular momentum [55]. A slower development of mechanical responses seems to be a major factor limiting an older adult's recovery from trips and other balance perturbations [53]. Older people appear to use similar strategies to young, with similar muscle activation onset times; however, their ability to produce the necessary magnitude of support limb moments in time for adequate push-off reactions appears to be reduced, due to slower rates of ankle moment generation and reduced peak joint moments in the lower limbs [57]. These limitations are particularly notable in older people with high risk of falls.

Slipping is another common cause of instability and falls. While walking, a slip occurs when the shear force at foot contact is greater than the frictional force, leading to a forward translation of the foot under the body. Due to this forward translation, the deceleration force normally occurring at foot contact is lost, and instead of the usual forward COM motion over the BOS, the COM rotates backwards. Without an appropriate response, the COM may move beyond the BOS, leading to a posterior fall. Following a slip, falling is more likely to occur with faster gait speed, increased forward foot displacement, greater posterior displacement of the body's COM relative to the BOS, and the larger the angle of the leg relative to the ground (representative of a longer step length prior to the slip) [58, 59].

To avoid a fall, the response to a slip requires a rapidly executed strategy to mitigate the slip velocity and arrest the posterior angular momentum of the upper body. A faster and/or greater generation of muscle activity may assist to control the body COM and maintain an upright posture over the BOS. Often, the slip recovery involves a backwards step to catch the destabilized body COM. Compared to young, older people slip longer and faster [60] and are more likely to fall following a slip [61], likely due to the inability to execute an effective protective backward step, which must be long enough and with sufficient extensor capacity to extend the lower limb joints and elevate the body (see Figure 5.3). Comparing older and young adult slip mechanics, Lockhart et al. found older adults' recovery process is much slower and less effective, which was associated with sensorimotor performance measures of vision, reaction time, and muscle strength [62].

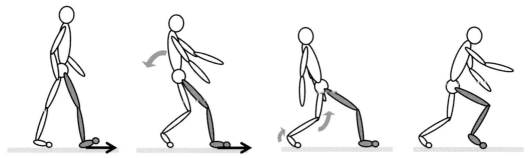

Figure 5.3   Slip event occurring at heel strike leading to backward rotation of upper body, requiring a backward step with the non-slip limb and adequate extensor moments of lower limb joints to arrest backward fall.

Movement responses following both trips and slips are rapidly altered on repeated exposure. Both young and older people are quick to adapt following repeated trials in order to improve balance recovery and avoid falling. Repeated exposure is therefore used as a training intervention for fall prevention, with promising initial findings, as outlined in Chapter 17.

Falling

The mechanisms of falling reported by older people living in the community commonly include trips, slips, and loss of balance [63–66]. For older people living in the community, falls are more likely to occur during walking [64, 65, 67] and less likely during standing and weight shifting, as is common in people living in residential care [68]. Technological advances in wearable sensors can provide detailed monitoring of daily-life activities and measure impacts associated with falls. These important factors can assist our understanding of fall events and fall risk, as described in Chapter 13.

Video recordings of 227 falls in common areas of nursing homes has provided insight into the biomechanics of falls in daily life, free from recall errors and reporting biases. Robinovitch et al. [68] reported incorrect weight shifting accounted for over 40% of falls, with half that due to a trip or stumble (21%), and half again due to COM perturbations (11%), BOS perturbations (11%), and collapses (11%), while slipping accounted for only 3% of falls. Falls occurred most commonly while walking forwards (24%), standing quietly (13%), and moving to sit down (12%).

Several studies have shown older people most commonly fall in the forward direction. A survey of older people who reported falls in the past four months revealed 60% fell in the forward direction, compared with 20% to the side and 20%

backwards. [69]. Others have reported a similarly greater proportion of forward falls, compared to other directions [67, 70]. The direction of a fall is a key predictor of injury risk. Lateral falls and slips are associated with hip injury, while forward falls and trips are associated with upper-limb injury [67, 71, 72]. For example, almost 60% of hip fractures were reportedly due to falls in the lateral direction [67]. Studies of reported falls have agreed that the hand is most commonly impacted, followed by the pelvis and head [69, 70]. Detailed video analysis of 25 falls in residential care showed all involved impact to the pelvis, 12 involved head impact, and 21 involved hand impact [73].

Avoiding harm from falls is possible with appropriate protective movements. While wrist fractures are common, it is of lesser consequence than head injuries and hip fractures, and there is some evidence that a slightly flexed elbow can reduce impact forces [74]. Trunk rotation following a lateral balance perturbation can avoid hip impact [75]. There is evidence that older people can improve their response to unexpected balance perturbations and thereby reduce injury risk, including perturbation training (repeated trip and slip simulations) [76], Tai Chi [77], and martial arts [78]. Hip protective padding might also assist in reducing impacts [79] and preventing fracture, although issues exist regarding appropriate fit and compliance with wearing them daily.

Conclusions

Biomechanics is valuable for examining both how balance is controlled and what happens when a person falls. Posturography studies have described how the brain controls balance by keeping the body COM within the BOS. Balance perturbation studies have shown reflex responses are initiated followed by direction-specific muscle activity that may enable feet-in-place responses or an appropriate step to increase the BOS and catch the body COM. Biomechanical studies have revealed tripping while walking requires a strong push-off reaction to elevate the body, with the use of different strategies that depend on the timing of the trip in the gait cycle. Adequately fast slip responses are difficult to achieve and therefore older people are more likely to fall, compared to young. Depending on the mechanism of falling, different body parts are at risk of injury, the hand being most commonly impacted as it is used to protect the head and body from impacts. The numerous and vast biomechanical analyses should inform interventions for fall prevention and fall-related injury prevention. For example, the evolution of perturbation training is improving the task specificity of fall prevention exercises and may complement traditional balance training. Biomechanical studies also suggest potential for training safer falling techniques to prevent injuries.

REFERENCES

1. Hellebrandt FA, Braun GL. The influence of sex and age on the postural sway of man. *Am J Phys Anthrolpol.* 1939;24:347–60.
2. Winter DA, Patla AE, Ishac M et al. Motor mechanisms of balance during quiet standing. *J Electromyogr Kinesiol.* 2003;13:49 56.
3. Winter DA. *The Biomechanics and Motor Control of Human Gait: Normal, Elderly and Pathological.* Waterloo, Ontario: University of Waterloo Press; 1991.
4. Piirtola M, Era P. Force platform measurements as predictors of falls among older people: a review. *Gerontology.* 2006;52:1–16.
5. Thapa PB, Gideon P, Brockman KG et al. Clinical and biomechanical measures of balance as fall predictors in ambulatory nursing home residents. *J Gerontol A Biol Sci Med Sci.* 1996;51:M239–46.
6. Maki BE, Holliday PJ, Topper AK. A prospective study of postural balance and risk of falling in an ambulatory and independent elderly population. *J Gerontol.* 1994;49:M72–84.
7. Era P, Schroll M, Ytting H et al. Postural balance and its sensory-motor correlates in 75-year-old men and women: a cross-national comparative study. *J Gerontol A Biol Sci Med Sci.* 1996;51:M53–63.
8. Era P, Heikkinen E. Postural sway during standing and unexpected disturbance of balance in random samples of men of different ages. *J Gerontol.* 1985;40:287–95.
9. Era P, Heikkinen E, Gause-Nilsson I et al. Postural balance in elderly people: changes over a five-year follow-up and its predictive value for survival. *Aging Clin Exp Res.* 2002;14:37–46.
10. Baloh RW, Corona S, Jacobson KM et al. A prospective study of posturography in normal older people. *J Am Geriatr Soc.* 1998;46:438–43.
11. Lord SR, Clark RD. Simple physiological and clinical tests for the accurate prediction of falling in older people. *Gerontology.* 1996;42:199–203.
12. Lord SR, Rogers MW, Howland A et al. Lateral stability, sensorimotor function and falls in older people. *J Am Geriatr Soc.* 1999;47:1077–81.
13. Duncan G, Wilson JA, MacLennan WJ et al. Clinical correlates of sway in elderly people living at home. *Gerontology.* 1992;38:160–6.
14. Lichtenstein MJ, Shields SL, Schiavi R et al. Clinical determinants of biomechanics platform measures of balance in aged women. *J Am Geriat Soc.* 1988;36:996–1002.
15. Lord SR, Clark RD, Webster IW. Visual acuity and contrast sensitivity in relation to falls in an elderly population. *Age Ageing.* 1991;20:175–81.
16. Stelmach GE, Phillips J, DiFabio RP et al. Age, functional postural reflexes, and voluntary sway. *J Gerontol.* 1989;44:B100–6.
17. Maki BE, Holliday PJ, Topper AK. Fear of falling and postural performance in the elderly. *J Gerontol.* 1991;46:M123–31.
18. Adkin AL, Carpenter MG. New insights on emotional contributions to human postural control. *Front Neurol.* 2018;9:789.
19. Lord SR, Sambrook PN, Gilbert C et al. Postural stability, falls and fractures in the elderly: results from the Dubbo Osteoporosis Epidemiology Study. *Med J Aust.* 1994;160:684–5, 688–91.

20. Lord SR, Castell S. Physical activity program for older persons: effect on balance, strength, neuromuscular control, and reaction time. *Arch Phys Med Rehabil.* 1994;75:648–52.

21. Lord SR, Clark RD, Webster IW. Physiological factors associated with falls in an elderly population. *J Am Geriatr Soc.* 1991;39:1194–200.

22. Horak FB, Diener HC, Nashner LM. Influence of central set on human postural responses. *J Neurophysiol.* 1989;62:841–53.

23. Bothner KE, Jensen JL. How do non-muscular torques contribute to the kinetics of postural recovery following a support surface translation? *J Biomech.* 2001;34:245–50.

24. Runge CF, Shupert CL, Horak FB et al. Ankle and hip postural strategies defined by joint torques. *Gait Posture.* 1999;10:161–70.

25. Brown LA, Jensen JL, Korff T et al. The translating platform paradigm: perturbation displacement waveform alters the postural response. *Gait Posture.* 2001;14:256–63.

26. Tokuno CD, Cresswell AG, Thorstensson A et al. Age-related changes in postural responses revealed by support-surface translations with a long acceleration-deceleration interval. *Clin Neurophysiol.* 2010;121:109–17.

27. Luchies CW, Alexander NB, Schultz AB et al. Stepping responses of young and old adults to postural disturbances: kinematics. *J Am Geriatr Soc.* 1994;42:506–12.

28. Rogers MW, Hedman LD, Johnson ME et al. Lateral stability during forward-induced stepping for dynamic balance recovery in young and older adults. *J Gerontol A Biol Sci Med Sci.* 2001;56:M589–94.

29. McIlroy WE, Maki BE. Age-related changes in compensatory stepping in response to unpredictable perturbations. *J Gerontol A Biol Sci Med Sci.* 1996;51A:M289–96.

30. Hsiao-Wecksler ET, Robinovitch SN. The effect of step length on young and elderly women's ability to recover balance. *Clin Biomech.* 2007;22:574–80.

31. Thelen DG, Wojcik LA, Schultz AB et al. Age differences in using a rapid step to regain balance during a forward fall. *J Gerontol A Biol Sci Med Sci.* 1997;52:M8–13.

32. Sturnieks DL, Menant J, Delbaere K et al. Force-controlled balance perturbations associated with falls in older people: a prospective cohort study. *PloS One.* 2013;8:e70981.

33. Hilliard MJ, Martinez KM, Janssen I et al. Lateral balance factors predict future falls in community-living older adults. *Arch Phys Med Rehabil.* 2008;89:1708–13.

34. Carty CP, Cronin NJ, Nicholson D et al. Reactive stepping behaviour in response to forward loss of balance predicts future falls in community-dwelling older adults. *Age Ageing.* 2015;44:109–15.

35. Alexander NB, Shepard N, Gu MJ et al. Postural control in young and elderly adults when stance is perturbed: kinematics. *J Gerontol.* 1992;47:M79–87.

36. Pai YC, Patton J. Center of mass velocity-position predictions for balance control. *J Biomech.* 1997;30:347–54.

37. Hof AL, Gazendam MG, Sinke WE. The condition for dynamic stability. *J Biomech.* 2005;38:1–8.

38. Rogers MW, Mille M-L. Chapter 5 – Balance perturbations. In: Day BL, Lord SR, Eds. *Handbook of Clinical Neurology.* Netherlands: Elsevier; 2018; 159:85–105.

39. Dietz V, Schubert M, Trippel M. Visually induced destabilization of human stance: neuronal control of leg muscles. *Neuroreport.* 1992;3:449–52.

40. Mille ML, Rogers MW, Martinez K et al. Thresholds for inducing protective stepping responses to external perturbations of human standing. *J Neurophysiol.* 2003;90:666–74.

41. Maki BE, Edmondstone MA, McIlroy WE. Age-related differences in laterally directed compensatory stepping behavior. *J Gerontol A Biol Sci Med Sci*. 2000;55:M270–7.

42. Mille ML, Johnson ME, Martinez KM et al. Age-dependent differences in lateral balance recovery through protective stepping. *Clin Biomech*. 2005;20:607–16.

43. Rogers MW, Mille ML. Lateral stability and falls in older people. *Exerc Sport Sci Rev*. 2003;31:182 7.

44. Talbot LA, Musiol RJ, Witham EK et al. Falls in young, middle-aged and older community dwelling adults: perceived cause, environmental factors and injury. *BMC Public Health*. 2005;5:86.

45. Prudham D, Evans JG. Factors associated with falls in the elderly: a community study. *Age Ageing*. 1981;10:141–6.

46. Campbell AJ, Reinken J, Allan BC et al. Falls in old age: a study of frequency and related clinical factors. *Age Ageing*. 1981;10:264–70.

47. Tinetti ME, Speechley M, Ginter SF. Risk factors for falls among elderly persons living in the community. *N Engl J Med*. 1988;319:1701–7.

48. Blake A, Morgan K, Bendall M et al. Falls by elderly people at home: prevalence and associated factors. *Age Ageing*. 1988;17:365–72.

49. Lord SR, Ward JA, Williams P et al. An epidemiological study of falls in older community-dwelling women: the Randwick falls and fractures study. *Aust J Public Health*. 1993;17:240–54.

50. Teno J, Kiel DP, Mor V. Multiple stumbles: a risk factor for falls in community-dwelling elderly: a prospective study. *J Am Geriatr Soc*. 1990;38:1321–5.

51. Chen HC, Ashton-Miller JA, Alexander NB et al. Effects of age and available response time on ability to step over an obstacle. *J Gerontol*. 1994;49:M227–33.

52. Chen HC, Schultz AB, Ashton-Miller JA et al. Stepping over obstacles: dividing attention impairs performance of old more than young adults. *J Gerontol A Biol Sci Med Sci*. 1996;51: M116–22.

53. van Dieën JH, Pijnappels M, Bobbert MF. Age-related intrinsic limitations in preventing a trip and regaining balance after a trip. *Safety Sci*. 2005;43:437–53.

54. Eng JJ, Winter DA, Patla AE. Strategies for recovery from a trip in early and late swing during human walking. *Exp Brain Res*. 1994;102:339–49.

55. Grabiner MD, Koh TJ, Lundin TM et al. Kinematics of recovery from a stumble. *J Gerontol*. 1993;48:M97–102.

56. Pijnappels M, Bobbert MF, van Dieen JH. Contribution of the support limb in control of angular momentum after tripping. *J Biomech*. 2004;37:1811–18.

57. Pijnappels M, Bobbert MF, van Dieen JH. Push-off reactions in recovery after tripping discriminate young subjects, older non-fallers and older fallers. *Gait Posture*. 2005;21:388–94.

58. Brady RA, Pavol MJ, Owings TM et al. Foot displacement but not velocity predicts the outcome of a slip induced in young subjects while walking. *J Biomech*. 2000;33:803–8.

59. Moyer BE, Chambers AJ, Redfern MS et al. Gait parameters as predictors of slip severity in younger and older adults. *Ergonomics*. 2006;49:329–43.

60. Lockhart TE, Woldstad JC, Smith JL. Effects of age-related gait changes on the biomechanics of slips and falls. *Ergonomics*. 2003;46:1136–60.

61. Pavol MJ, Runtz EF, Edwards BJ et al. Age influences the outcome of a slipping perturbation during initial but not repeated exposures. *J Gerontol A Biol Sci Med Sci.* 2002;57: M496–503.

62. Lockhart TE, Smith JL, Woldstad JC. Effects of aging on the biomechanics of slips and falls. *Hum Factors.* 2005;47:708–29.

63. Lord SR, Ward JA, Williams P et al. An epidemiological study of falls in older community-dwelling women: the Randwick falls and fractures study. *Aust J Public Health.* 1993;17:240–5.

64. Overstall PW, Exton-Smith AN, Imms FJ et al. Falls in the elderly related to postural imbalance. *Br Med J.* 1977;1:261–4.

65. Berg WP, Alessio HM, Mills EM et al. Circumstances and consequences of falls in independent community-dwelling older adults. *Age Ageing.* 1997;26:261–8.

66. Topper AK, Maki BE, Holliday PJ. Are activity-based assessments of balance and gait in the elderly predictive of risk of falling and/or type of fall? *J Am Geriatr Soc.* 1993;41:479–87.

67. Nevitt MC, Cummings SR. Type of fall and risk of hip and wrist fractures: the study of osteoporotic fractures. The Study of Osteoporotic Fractures Research Group. *J Am Geriatr Soc.* 1993;41:1226–34.

68. Robinovitch SN, Feldman F, Yang Y et al. Video capture of the circumstances of falls in elderly people residing in long-term care: an observational study. *Lancet.* 2013;381:47–54.

69. O'Neill TW, Varlow J, Silman AJ et al. Age and sex influences on fall characteristics. *Ann Rheum Dis.* 1994;53:773.

70. Vellas BJ, Wayne SJ, Garry PJ et al. A two-year longitudinal study of falls in 482 community-dwelling elderly adults. *J Gerontol A Biol Sci Med Sci.* 1998;53A:M264–74.

71. Palvanen M, Kannus P, Parkkari J et al. The injury mechanisms of osteoporotic upper extremity fractures among older adults: a controlled study of 287 consecutive patients and their 108 controls. *Osteoporos Int.* 2000;11:822–31.

72. Hayes WC, Myers ER, Morris JN et al. Impact near the hip dominates fracture risk in elderly nursing home residents who fall. *Calcif Tissue Int.* 1993;52:192–8.

73. Choi WJ, Wakeling JM, Robinovitch SN. Kinematic analysis of video-captured falls experienced by older adults in long-term care. *J Biomech.* 2015;48:911–20.

74. DeGoede KM, Ashton-Miller JA. Fall arrest strategy affects peak hand impact force in a forward fall. *J Biomech.* 2002;35:843–8.

75. Hsiao ET, Robinovitch SN. Common protective movements govern unexpected falls from standing height. *J Biomech.* 1998;31:1–9.

76. Pai YC, Bhatt T, Yang F et al. Perturbation training can reduce community-dwelling older adults' annual fall risk: a randomized controlled trial. *J Gerontol A Biol Sci Med Sci.* 2014;69:1586–94.

77. Gatts SK, Woollacott MH. How tai chi improves balance: biomechanics of recovery to a walking slip in impaired seniors. *Gait Posture.* 2007;25:205–14.

78. Groen BE, Smulders E, de Kam D et al. Martial arts fall training to prevent hip fractures in the elderly. *Osteoporos Int.* 2010;21:215–21.

79. Lauritzen JB, Petersen MM, Lund B. Effect of external hip protectors on hip fractures. *Lancet.* 1993;341:11–13.

6

Foot Problems, Footwear, and Falls

Hylton B. Menz

As outlined in earlier chapters, falls in older people result from the interaction between intrinsic, or physiological risk factors (such as visual impairment, muscle weakness, and slowed reaction time), and extrinsic, or environmental risk factors (such as slippery surfaces, cracked footpaths, or loose floor rugs). Because the foot is the only direct source of contact with the supporting surface when undertaking weightbearing activities, it represents an important interface between intrinsic and extrinsic falls risk factors. This interface is further modified by footwear, which can affect balance in either a beneficial or detrimental manner. As such, foot problems and footwear have a significant influence on risk of falling in older people. This chapter provides an overview of the contribution of foot problems and footwear to falls in older people, and the role of podiatry in preventing falls. The use of footwear and foot orthoses as interventions is further addressed in Chapter 22.

Foot Problems

Prevalence of Foot Problems in Older People

It has long been recognized that foot problems are common in older people [1]. A recent systematic review identified eight population-based studies of foot pain in older people with comparable case definitions, from which a pooled prevalence estimate of frequent foot pain of 24% was derived. Frequent foot pain was found to most commonly affect the forefoot and the toes, to be more prevalent in women than men, and to be at least moderately disabling in two-thirds of cases [2]. The most commonly observed and reported foot disorders resulting in foot pain in older people are keratotic lesions (corns and calluses), followed closely by nail disorders (particularly fungal nail infection), and structural deformities such as hallux valgus (bunions) and lesser toe deformities (hammertoes and clawtoes) [3–5].

Effects of Foot Problems on Balance and Gait

There is strong evidence that foot problems have a significant detrimental impact on mobility and health status in older people. Significant associations between the presence of foot problems and self-reported foot-related functional limitations [6], mobility limitations [7, 8], and inability to perform activities of daily living [4, 9, 10] (such as housework, shopping, and cooking) have been reported. Other studies have explored this relationship by conducting physical assessments in older people, and have consistently shown that foot problems are associated with reduced walking speed [4, 11–17], difficulty rising from a chair [12, 13, 15, 16], and impaired balance [13, 16].

Foot Problems and Falls

The association between foot problems and falls has been suspected for some time. In 1958, DeLargy [18] hypothesized that decreased activity associated with foot problems in older people could lead to the development of muscle weakness, thereby predisposing to falls. In 1966, Helfand [19] argued that painful lesions and structural foot deformities could *directly* lead to a fall by detrimentally altering the foot's functional base of support. Eight retrospective studies have now reported that older people who suffer from foot problems are more likely to have fallen in the previous 12 months [12, 20–26] and seven prospective studies have confirmed that foot problems are a falls risk factor [27–33]. A study of 100 older men by Gabell et al. [27] reported that undefined 'foot problems' was associated with a fourfold increased risk of falling. Tinetti et al. [28] found that the presence of a 'serious foot problem' (defined as a moderate to severe bunion, toe deformity, ulcer, or deformed nail) doubled the risk of falling in 336 people aged over 75 years, after adjusting for socio-demographic characteristics, psychological factors, and medication use. A prospective study of 979 people aged over 70 years in Finland found that older people with bunions were twice as likely to fall than those without [29]. Follow-up results from the *Women's Health and Aging Study* of 1002 older women found that foot pain was the only site of pain that was significantly associated with falls [30].

More recent prospective studies of foot problems and falls [31–33] have assessed a broader range of foot and ankle characteristics as potential risk factors. In a study of 175 retirement village residents, Menz et al. [31] found that compared to those who did not fall, fallers demonstrated decreased ankle flexibility, more severe hallux valgus deformity, decreased plantar tactile sensitivity, decreased toe plantarflexor strength, and a higher prevalence of disabling foot pain. A similar study in 312 community-dwelling older people found that fallers exhibited reduced plantar flexor strength of the hallux and higher pressures underfoot when walking, and were more likely to have foot pain, hallux valgus, and lesser toe deformity [32, 33].

Most recently, Menz et al. [34] conducted a systematic review of the 15 papers that have examined the associations between foot problems and falls. Older people who fell were more likely to have foot pain, hallux valgus, lesser toe deformity, plantar fasciitis, reduced ankle dorsiflexion range of motion, reduced toe plantar-flexion strength, impaired tactile sensitivity, and increased plantar pressures when walking. Meta-analysis indicated that fallers were more likely to have foot pain (pooled OR: 1.95, 95% CI:1.38,2.76, p: <0.001), hallux valgus (pooled OR: 1.89, 95% CI: 1.19,3.00, p: 0.007) and lesser toe deformity (pooled OR: 1.67, 95% CI: 1.07,2.59, p: 0.020). The findings of this review confirm the important role that foot problems have in predisposition to falling in older people and suggest that addressing these modifiable risk factors with targeted clinical interventions may be beneficial.

Footwear

Shoe-Wearing Habits of Older People

Footwear plays an important role in protecting the foot from extremes of temperature, moisture, and mechanical trauma. However, many older people wear suboptimal footwear [35, 36] and select their shoes based on appearance and comfort rather than safety [37]. A household survey of people aged over 80 years conducted in the United Kingdom found that most wore slippers all day, irrespective of whether they were housebound [38]. Similarly, a survey of indoor shoe-wearing habits of older people in Australia indicated that more than half spent less than $30 Australian dollars on their indoor footwear (most commonly slippers), replaced them infrequently, and often wore their indoor shoes for outdoor activities [39]. A survey of sub-acute aged care hospital patients reported that only 14% wore safe footwear, with the most commonly observed detrimental features being a lack of fastening, slippery soles, and an excessively flexible heel counter [40]. These observations were confirmed in a more recent survey of ambulant in-patients in acute and sub-acute hospital wards with a high reported rate of falls, where almost all patients wore shoes with at least one potentially hazardous feature [41].

In addition to selecting shoes with sub-optimal designs, between 26 and 50% of older people wear shoes that are too short or too narrow [42–44]. This may be due to fashion influences [45, 46], not measuring foot dimensions when purchasing shoes [39], and the limited availability of footwear that adequately caters for the altered morphology of the older foot [47, 48]. Ill-fitting footwear is strongly associated with foot pain and structural foot disorders (particularly hallux valgus and lesser toe deformity) [49], while shoes that are too tight in the forefoot or too loose in the heel may lead to reduced walking speed and gait instability [50].

Footwear Features and Their Effect on Balance

Three key footwear features have been examined for their potential detrimental effect on balance and gait: heel elevation, excessive midsole cushioning, and inadequate sole slip resistance. An overview of these findings is provided below.

Heel Elevation

Heel elevation in footwear is thought to contribute to instability by altering the body's centre of mass and the normal kinematic function of the lower limb during gait. Lord et al. [51] evaluated older women's balance (using measures of postural sway and forward leaning ability) when barefoot, wearing their own shoes, and in 6 cm high-heeled shoes, and found that the worst balance performances occurred when women wore high-heeled shoes. Similarly, Arnadottir and Mercer [52] found that performance on the Functional Reach Test, the Timed Up and Go Test and the Ten Metre Walk Test was impaired in older women when shoes with a mean heel height 5 cm compared to shoes with a mean heel height of 1 cm. In contrast to these findings, Lindemann et al. [53] found no differences in balance when older women wore shoes with a range of heel heights. The highest heel used in this study was 4 cm, suggesting that there may be a critical height at which heel elevation becomes problematic for balance. More recently, Menant et al. conducted several studies in which the elevated-heel shoes only differed to the standard control footwear with regard to heel height (4.5 cm versus 2.7 cm). These studies found that heel elevation resulted in increased postural sway when standing [54] and increased double-support time, foot clearance, and horizontal heel velocity when walking on a range of surfaces [55]. Taken together, these findings suggest that heel elevation greater than 4 cm is detrimental to balance in older people. Fortunately, however, there is some evidence that the use of high heels diminishes with age. A survey of past shoe-wearing habits in women aged 50 years and over found that the use of high heels was common between the ages of 20 to 29, but declined to less than 10% by the age of 40 years [56]. This may be indicative of a life-course trajectory in which the influence and perceived importance of fashion diminishes over time and is replaced with a greater emphasis on comfort and practicality.

Excessive Midsole Cushioning

The use of thick, soft materials in footwear midsoles may be detrimental to balance by reducing sensory input to the central nervous system regarding foot position and limiting the normal postural corrections that occur in response to this afferent feedback. Studies which have assessed standing balance in shoes with varying midsole hardness have produced inconsistent findings depending on the level of hardness tested, with only extremely soft soles (Shore A15 durometer hardness) being detrimental [54, 57–60]. However, Menant et al. [61] assessed gait stability on even and uneven surfaces when walking in shoes with standard (Shore A-40) and soft (Shore A-25) midsoles, and found that the softer sole shoes led to a greater lateral centre-of-mass–base-of-support margin than the standard shoes, with no concurrent increase in step width. This finding suggests that participants restricted the medio-lateral excursion of their centre of mass rather than pro-actively adjusting their foot placement to maintain frontal plane stability in the presence of the soft midsole. A subsequent study evaluated gait patterns on a range of different surfaces (standard, irregular, and wet), and found that wearing the soft midsole shoe on a wet surface resulted in shorter step length and a flatter foot landing compared to the standard midsole, indicative of the adoption of anticipatory gait changes to reduce the risk of slipping [55]. In summary, the available evidence suggests that although midsole hardness does not appear to influence standing balance in older people (unless it is extremely soft), softer midsoles have a detrimental effect on more challenging walking tasks, possibly by reducing foot position awareness and mechanical stability.

Inadequate Slip Resistance

Gait analysis studies have revealed that slipping is most likely to occur shortly after heel strike [62]. Therefore, the geometry and texture of the heel section of a shoe may play an important role in preventing slipping accidents. To investigate this possibility, Menz et al. [63] used a specially designed force plate apparatus and tested the slip resistance of lace-up Oxford-style shoes and women's fashion shoes with a range of heel configurations on a range of walking surfaces. Results indicated that most slip-resistant shoe was the Oxford shoe with the 10° heel bevel, which was consistent with previous reports in the occupational safety literature [64]. Bevelling the heel is thought to improve slip resistance by increasing the surface area of the plantar aspect of the sole shortly after initial heel contact. However, whether the findings of 'bench-test' studies such as these are transferrable to gait studies in older people is unclear. Two experiments by Menant et al. failed to demonstrate any benefit of shoes with a textured sole compared to a smooth sole when older people were observed walking [55] or rapidly terminating gait [65] on a wet surface. The available evidence therefore suggests that although slip-related falls are common in older people, determining the ideal slip resistance of a shoe is a somewhat difficult task. The general recommendation that slippery or worn soles should be avoided by older people at risk of falling is reasonable, given that the number of falls caused by inadequate slip resistance is likely to be far more common than those caused by excessive slip resistance. However, further research needs to be undertaken to determine whether sole designs that appear to be beneficial under mechanical testing conditions translate to the prevention of falls in real-life situations.

Footwear and Falls

The previous section has highlighted that footwear may influence balance in a beneficial or detrimental manner. However, establishing a link between footwear and falls is inherently difficult. Although several studies have implicated a wide range of shoe features which may have been responsible for an older person's fall (such as narrow heels, slippery soles, inadequate fixation, poorly fitting shoes, and soft heel counters) [35, 66–70], the wearing of a particular shoe at the time of a fall does not necessarily confirm causation. Furthermore, studies relying on older people to report the shoes they were wearing at the time of the fall are problematic, due to the limited accuracy of falls recall, particularly in the presence of cognitive impairment [71].

Stronger evidence comes from cohort studies, in which footwear characteristics are documented at baseline and incident falls are prospectively documented. Five such studies of footwear and falls have been undertaken. In a residential aged care population of 606 older people, wearing slippers rather than enclosed shoes increased the risk of *fractures* during the 12-month follow-up period. However, there was no association between footwear and *falls* once potential confounders were accounted for [72]. The remaining four studies were all conducted in community-dwelling older people. A study of 4281 people aged over 66 years by Larsen et al. [73] found that those who had fallen in the last 24 hours were four times more likely to have been wearing socks or slippers. Koepsell et al. [74] found that going barefoot or wearing stockings was associated with a tenfold increased risk of falling over a two-year period, with athletic shoes being associated with the lowest risk. Further evaluation of footwear characteristics from this study found that increased heel height was associated with an increased risk of falling, whereas greater sole contact area was associated with a decreased risk [75]. More recently, Menz et al. [76] found that being barefoot or wearing socks increased the risk of indoor falls in 176 retirement villages residents over a 12-month period. Similar results were reported by Kelsey et al. [77] who found that older people who sustained a serious fall-related injury were twice as likely to be shoeless or wearing slippers compared to those who were wearing other shoes at the time of the fall. Although each of these studies suggests that there may be a relationship between footwear, falls, and fractures, variations in falls documentation techniques, statistical adjustment for confounders, and the lack of a standard protocol when assessing footwear makes it difficult to reach firm conclusions.

Podiatry and Fall Prevention

Given that foot problems and inappropriate footwear increase the risk of falling in older people, there is increasing recognition of the role of podiatry in the prevention of falls. Three randomized trials – two undertaken in community-dwelling older people [78, 79] and one in residential aged care [80] – have demonstrated that a multi-faceted intervention consisting of routine podiatry care, a foot and ankle exercise program, foot orthoses, and footwear advice is effective in preventing falls, with a pooled risk reduction of 23% [81]. These interventions are well accepted by older people [82] and relatively inexpensive to implement, so may be cost effective when administered in primary care settings [83].

Conclusions

Foot problems are common in older people, and there is now good evidence that foot problems impair balance and gait, and increase the risk of falling in older people. In contrast, the link between footwear and falls is less clear. Although footwear may influence balance in either a beneficial or a detrimental manner, many questions remain unanswered regarding the influence of specific design features on balance and falls. Nevertheless, it would seem reasonable to suggest that older people should be advised against the wearing of high- or narrow-heeled shoes, shoes with very soft soles, and shoes with slippery soles. The potential role of specially designed footwear as an intervention to improve balance and prevent falls is discussed further in Chapter 22.

REFERENCES

1. Riccitelli ML. Foot problems of the aged and infirm. *J Am Geriatr Soc*. 1966;14:1058–61.
2. Thomas M, Roddy E, Zhang W et al. The population prevalence of foot and ankle pain in middle and old age: a systematic review. *Pain*. 2011;152:2870–80.
3. Dunn JE, Link CL, Felson DT et al. Prevalence of foot and ankle conditions in a multiethnic community sample of older adults. *Am J Epidemiol*. 2004;159:491–8.
4. Benvenuti F, Ferrucci L, Guralnik JM et al. Foot pain and disability in older persons: an epidemiologic survey. *J Am Geriatr Soc*. 1995;43:479–84.
5. Black JR, Hale WE. Prevalence of foot complaints in the elderly. *J Am Podiatr Med Assoc*. 1987;77:308–11.
6. Badlissi F, Dunn JE, Link CL et al. Foot musculoskeletal disorders, pain, and foot-related functional limitation in older persons. *J Am Geriatr Soc*. 2005;53:1029–33.
7. Keysor JJ, Dunn JE, Link CL et al. Are foot disorders associated with functional limitation and disability among community-dwelling older adults? *J Aging Health*. 2005;17:734–52.

8. Menz HB, Dufour AB, Katz P et al. Foot pain and pronated foot type are associated with self-reported mobility limitations in older adults: the Framingham Foot Study. *Gerontology.* 2016;62:289–95.

9. Gorter KJ, Kuyvenhoven MM, deMelker RA. Nontraumatic foot complaints in older people. A population-based survey of risk factors, mobility, and well-being. *J Am Podiatr Med Assoc.* 2000;90:397–402.

10. Bowling A, Grundy E. Activities of daily living: changes in functional ability in three samples of elderly and very elderly people. *Age Ageing.* 1997;26:107–14.

11. Leveille SG, Guralnik JM, Ferrucci L et al. Foot pain and disability in older women. *Am J Epidemiol.* 1998;148:657–65.

12. Barr ELM, Browning C, Lord SR et al. Foot and leg problems are important determinants of functional status in community dwelling older people. *Disabil Rehabil.* 2005;27:917–23.

13. Menz HB, Lord SR. Foot pain impairs balance and functional ability in community-dwelling older people. *J Am Podiatr Med Assoc.* 2001;91:222–9.

14. Mickle KJ, Munro BJ, Lord SR et al. Cross-sectional analysis of foot function, functional ability, and health-related quality of life in older people with disabling foot pain. *Arthritis Care Res.* 2011;63:1592–8.

15. Golightly YM, Hannan MT, Shi XA et al. Association of foot symptoms with self-reported and performance-based measures of physical function: the Johnston County Osteoarthritis Project. *Arthritis Care Res.* 2011;63:654–9.

16. Menz HB, Dufour AB, Casey VA et al. Foot pain and mobility limitations in older adults: the Framingham Foot Study. *J Gerontol A Biol Sci Med Sci.* 2013;68:1281–5.

17. Muchna A, Najafi B, Wendel CS et al. Foot problems in older adults: associations with incident falls, frailty syndrome and sensor-derived gait, balance, and physical activity measures. *J Am Podiatr Med Assoc.* 2018;108:126–39.

18. DeLargy D. Accidents in old people. *Med Press.* 1958;239:117–20.

19. Helfand AE. Foot impairment: an etiologic factor in falls in the aged. *J Am Podiatr Med Assoc.* 1966;56:326–30.

20. Wild D, Nayak U, Isaacs B. Characteristics of old people who fell at home. *J Clin Exp Gerontol.* 1980;2:271–87.

21. Blake A, Morgan K, Bendall M et al. Falls by elderly people at home: prevalence and associated factors. *Age Ageing.* 1988;17:365–72.

22. Bumin G, Uyanik M, Aki E et al. An investigation of risk factors for falls in elderly people in a Turkish rest home: a pilot study. *Aging Clin Exp Res.* 2002;14:192–6.

23. Dolinis J, Harrison JE. Factors associated with falling in older Adelaide residents. *Aust NZ J Public Health.* 1997;21:462–8.

24. Menz HB, Lord SR. The contribution of foot problems to mobility impairment and falls in older people. *J Am Geriatr Soc.* 2001;49:1651–6.

25. Chaiwanichsiri D, Janchai S, Tantisiriwat N. Foot disorders and falls in older persons. *Gerontology.* 2009;55:296–302.

26. Awale A, Hagedorn TJ, Dufour AB et al. Foot function, foot pain, and falls in older adults: The Framingham Foot Study. *Gerontology.* 2017;63:318–24.

27. Gabell A, Simons MA, Nayak USL. Falls in the healthy elderly: predisposing causes. *Ergonomics.* 1985;28:965–75.

28. Tinetti ME, Speechley M, Ginter SF. Risk factors for falls among elderly persons living in the community. *New Eng J Med.* 1988;319:1701–7.

29. Koski K, Luukinen H, Laippala P et al. Physiological factors and medications as predictors of injurious falls by elderly people: a prospective population-based study. *Age Ageing.* 1996;25:29–38.

30. Leveille SG, Bean J, Bandeen-Roche K et al. Musculoskeletal pain and risk of falls in older disabled women living in the community. *J Am Geriatr Soc.* 2002;50:671–8.

31. Menz HB, Morris ME, Lord SR. Foot and ankle risk factors for falls in older people: a prospective study. *J Gerontol A Biol Sci Med Sci.* 2006;61A:M866–70.

32. Mickle KJ, Munro BJ, Lord SR et al. ISB Clinical Biomechanics Award 2009: toe weakness and deformity increase the risk of falls in older people. *Clin Biomech.* 2009;24:787–91.

33. Mickle KJ, Munro BJ, Lord SR et al. Foot pain, plantar pressures, and falls in older people: a prospective study. *J Am Geriatr Soc.* 2010;58:1936–40.

34. Menz HB, Auhl M, Spink MJ. Foot problems as a risk factor for falls in community-dwelling older people: a systematic review and meta-analysis. *Maturitas.* 2018;118:7–14.

35. Finlay OE. Footwear management in the elderly care program. *Physiotherapy.* 1986;72:172–8.

36. Ikpeze TC, Omar A, Elfar JH. Evaluating problems with footwear in the geriatric population. *Geriatr Orthop Surg Rehabil.* 2015;6:338–40.

37. Davis A, Murphy A, Haines TP. "Good for older ladies, not me": how elderly women choose their shoes. *J Am Podiatr Med Assoc.* 2013;103:465–70.

38. White E, Mulley G. Footwear worn by the over 80s: a community survey. *Clin Rehabil.* 1989;3:23–5.

39. Munro BJ, Steele JR. Household-shoe wearing and purchasing habits: a survey of people aged 65 years and older. *J Am Podiatr Med Assoc.* 1999;89:506–14.

40. Jessup RL. Foot pathology and inappropriate footwear as risk factors for falls in a subacute aged-care hospital. *J Am Podiatr Med Assoc.* 2007;97:213–7.

41. Chari SR, McRae P, Stewart MJ et al. Point prevalence of suboptimal footwear features among ambulant older hospital patients: implications for fall prevention. *Aust Health Rev.* 2016;40:399–404.

42. Nixon BP, Armstrong DG, Wendell C et al. Do US veterans wear appropriately sized shoes? The Veteran Affairs shoe size selection study. *J Am Podiatr Med Assoc.* 2006;96:290–2.

43. Chaiwanichsiri D, Tantisiriwat N, Janchai S. Proper shoe sizes for Thai elderly. *Foot.* 2008;18:186–91.

44. McInnes AD, Hashmi F, Farndon LJ et al. Comparison of shoe-length fit between people with and without diabetic peripheral neuropathy: a case-control study. *J Foot Ankle Res.* 2012;5:9.

45. Joyce P. Women and their shoes: attitudes, influences and behaviour. *Br J Podiat.* 2000;3:111–15.

46. Seferin M, Van der Linden J. Protection or pleasure: female footwear. *Work.* 2012;41:290–4.

47. Chantelau E, Gede A. Foot dimensions of elderly people with and without diabetes mellitus: a data basis for shoe design. *Gerontology.* 2002;48:241–4.

48. Mickle KJ, Munro BJ, Lord SR et al. Foot shape of older people: implications for shoe design. *Footwear Sci.* 2010;2:131–9.

49. Buldt AK, Menz HB. Incorrectly fitted footwear, foot pain and foot disorders: a systematic search and narrative review of the literature. *J Foot Ankle Res.* 2018;11:43.

50. Doi T, Yamaguchi R, Asai T et al. The effects of shoe fit on gait in community-dwelling older adults. *Gait Posture.* 2010;32:274–8.

51. Lord SR, Bashford GM. Shoe characteristics and balance in older women. *J Am Geriatr Soc.* 1996;44:429–33.

52. Arnadottir SA, Mercer VS. Effects of footwear on measurements of balance and gait in women between the ages of 65 and 93 years. *Phys Ther.* 2000;80:17–27.

53. Lindemann U, Scheibe S, Sturm E et al. Elevated heels and adaptation to new shoes in frail elderly women. *Z Gerontol Geriatr.* 2003;36:29–34.

54. Menant JC, Steele JR, Menz HB et al. Effects of footwear features on balance and stepping in older people. *Gerontology.* 2008;54:18–23.

55. Menant JC, Steele JR, Menz HB et al. Effects of walking surfaces and footwear on temporo-spatial gait parameters in young and older people. *Gait Posture.* 2009;29:392–7.

56. Menz HB, Roddy E, Marshall M et al. Epidemiology of shoe wearing patterns over time in older women: associations with foot pain and hallux valgus. *J Gerontol A Biol Sci Med Sci.* 2016;71:1682–7.

57. Robbins SE, Gouw GJ, McClaran J. Shoe sole thickness and hardness influence balance in older men. *J Am Geriatr Soc.* 1992;40:1089–94.

58. Robbins SE, Waked E, McClaran J. Proprioception and stability: foot position awareness as a function of age and footwear. *Age Ageing.* 1995;24:67–72.

59. Robbins SE, Waked E, Allard P et al. Foot position awareness in younger and older men: the influence of footwear sole properties. *J Am Geriatr Soc.* 1997;45:61–6.

60. Lord SR, Bashford GM, Howland A et al. Effects of shoe collar height and sole hardness on balance in older women. *J Am Geriatr Soc.* 1999;47:681–4.

61. Menant JC, Perry SD, Steele JR et al. Effects of shoe characteristics on dynamic stability when walking on even and uneven surfaces in young and older people. *Arch Phys Med Rehabil.* 2008;89:1970–6.

62. Redfern M, Cham R, Gielo-Perczak K et al. Biomechanics of slips. *Ergonomics.* 2001;44:1138–66.

63. Menz HB, Lord SR. Slip resistance of casual footwear: implications for falls in older adults. *Gerontology.* 2001;47:145–9.

64. Lloyd D, Stevenson MG. Measurement of slip resistance of shoes on floor surfaces. Part 2: effect of a bevelled heel. *J Occup Health Saf.* 1989;5:229–35.

65. Menant JC, Steele JR, Menz HB et al. Rapid gait termination: effects of age, walking surfaces and footwear characteristics. *Gait Posture.* 2009;30:65–70.

66. Barbieri E. Patient falls are not patient accidents. *J Gerontol Nurs.* 1983;9:165–73.

67. Connell BR, Wolf SL. Environmental and behavioural circumstances associated with falls at home among healthy individuals. *Arch Phys Med Rehab.* 1997;78:179–86.

68. Frey CC, Kubasak M. Faulty footwear contributes to why seniors fall. *Biomechanics.* 1998;5:45–7.

69. Hourihan F, Cumming RG, Tavener-Smith KM et al. Footwear and hip fracture-related falls in the elderly. *Australas J Ageing.* 2000;19:91–3.

70. Sherrington C, Menz HB. An evaluation of footwear worn at the time of fall related hip fracture. *Age Ageing.* 2003;32:310–14.

71. Cummings SR, Nevitt MC, Kidd S. Forgetting falls: the limited accuracy of recall of falls in the elderly. *J Am Geriatr Soc.* 1988;36:613–16.

72. Kerse N, Butler M, Robinson E et al. Wearing slippers, falls and injury in residential care. *Aust NZ J Public Health.* 2004;28:180–7.

73. Larsen ER, Mosekilde L, Foldspang A. Correlates of falling during 24 h among elderly Danish community residents. *Prev Med.* 2004;39:389–98.

74. Koepsell TD, Wolf ME, Buchner DM et al. Footwear style and risk of falls in older adults. *J Am Geriatr Soc.* 2004;52:1495–501.

75. Tencer AF, Koepsell TD, Wolf ME et al. Biomechanical properties of shoes and risk of falls in older adults. *J Am Geriatr Soc.* 2004;52:1840–6.

76. Menz HB, Morris ME, Lord SR. Footwear characteristics and risk of indoor and outdoor falls in older people. *Gerontology.* 2006;52:174–80.

77. Kelsey JL, Procter-Gray E, Nguyen U-SDT et al. Footwear and falls in the home among older individuals in the MOBILIZE Boston Study. *Footwear Sci.* 2010;2:123–9.

78. Spink MJ, Menz HB, Fotoohabadi MR et al. Effectiveness of a multifaceted podiatry intervention to prevent falls in community dwelling older people with disabling foot pain: randomised controlled trial. *Br Med J.* 2011;342:d3411.

79. Cockayne S, Adamson J, Clarke A et al. Cohort randomised controlled trial of a multifaceted podiatry intervention for the prevention of falls in older people (The REFORM Trial). *PloS One.* 2017;12:e0168712.

80. Wylie G, Menz HB, McFarlane S et al. Podiatry intervention versus usual care to prevent falls in care homes: pilot randomised controlled trial (the PIRFECT study). *BMC Geriatr.* 2017;17:143.

81. Wylie G, Torrens C, Campbell P et al. Podiatry interventions to prevent falls in older people: a systematic review and meta-analysis. *Age Ageing.* 2019;48:327–36.

82. Menz HB, Spink MJ, Landorf KB et al. Older people's perceptions of a multifaceted podiatric medical intervention to prevent falls. *J Am Podiatr Med Assoc.* 2013;103:457–64.

83. Corbacho B, Cockayne S, Fairhurst C et al. Cost-effectiveness of a multifaceted podiatry intervention for the prevention of falls in older people: the Reducing Falls with Orthoses and a Multifaceted Podiatry Intervention Trial findings. *Gerontology.* 2018;64:503–12.

7

Brain Function and Falls

Michele Callisaya, Oshadi Jayakody, and Kim Delbaere

Ageing is associated with a wide range of changes in the brain, including grey and white matter atrophy, as well as markers of small vessel disease such as white matter hyperintensities, microbleeds, and infarcts. Furthermore, beta-amyloid plaques and tau (the hallmarks of Alzheimer's disease) are evident in the brain years before symptoms of dementia appear. A brain free of disease, with intact grey and white matter, is essential for the fast and efficient operation of the neural networks during daily life activities, and therefore also in reducing the risk of falling.

It is well known that brain ageing and disease can result in slowed processing speed and poorer executive function that increase a person's risk of falls. However, emerging evidence has suggested that disruption to the brain structure and function also plays an important role for motor control, even in cognitively intact older people. These recent studies build on the seminal work of Norman Geschwind who introduced the idea of the 'disconnection syndrome' in 1965, which proposed that functional deficits result not only from cortical lesions but also from ablation of white matter tracts (i.e. damaged myelin or axonal loss) between sensory and association cortices [1, 2]. This chapter will outline the evidence from neuroimaging studies showing that falls and sensorimotor risk factors of falls (such as balance and gait performance) are reliant on the structural and functional integrity of the brain.

Brain Atrophy

Brain volume declines with advancing age [3]. Loss in volume appears to occur at a greater rate in the frontal lobe, but also in the basal ganglia, temporal, and cerebellar regions [4]. This links to the commonly stated 'last in, first out' hypothesis, which suggests that structures that mature later in development are more vulnerable to the effects of ageing when compared to early maturing structures [5]. Lower volumes of total grey and white matter are associated with major risk factors for falls such as slow gait [6–9], concern about falling [10, 11], subclinical depression [12], and poorer cognitive function [13]. The cognitive domains of executive function and processing speed [14, 15] are commonly associated with increased risk of falls. Interestingly, lower frontal lobe volumes are associated with dysfunction in executive function as well as slow gait speed [6, 16], potentially suggesting shared underlying neural pathways. There is now increasing evidence that differential age effects in the prefrontal cortex may contribute to age-related declines in physical performance [16, 17], particularly when older people perform motor tasks requiring more attention (i.e. when dual tasking)[18]. Some elegant studies now show that processing speed partially mediates the association between the prefrontal cortex and slow gait [16], and that grey matter co-variance patterns in areas including the brain stem, precuneus, fusiform, motor, supplementary motor, and prefrontal regions are associated with both gait, processing speed, and executive function [19]. The control of balance and gait is likely to be more complex than just a few brain areas, and this is reflected by studies reporting associations between widespread cortical (pre-frontal, frontal, cingulate, insula, temporal, parahippocampal, parietal, occipital, and cerebellum) and subcortical (thalamus, caudate, putamen, and claustrum) areas of lower grey matter volume with slower gait speed [6, 7] and areas including the right putamen, right posterior superior parietal cortex, and bilateral cerebellum with poorer balance [7].

Few studies have examined whether there is an association between brain atrophy and actual falls. Interestingly in one study that compared those that reported having fallen over 12 months (n = 23) with those reporting no falls (n = 54), *higher* volumes in the hippocampus and somatosensory cortex were found in fallers [20]. The authors hypothesized that these higher brain volumes may be due to compensatory mechanisms when trying to integrate multiple sensory information [20]. In contrast, in a small (n = 42) prospective study of people with mild cognitive impairment, smaller volumes in the middle frontal and superior frontal gyrus were associated with increased risk of falls over 12 months [21]. These areas are important for planning, spatially orientated processing, and motor control, potentially explaining their link to falls [21]. One study in 281 older people aged 70–90 years looked at concern about falling and found that higher levels of concern were associated with reduced volumes in areas important for emotional control and for motor control, executive functions, and visual processing [11]. The authors suggested that neurodegeneration in these areas could be the results of lifelong stress and worry, and lead to subtle balance impairments in old age (independent of other sensorimotor fall risk factors).

Taken together, age- or disease-related changes in both grey and white matter contribute to impairments in risk factors for falls. There is preliminary evidence that areas of lower, but also potentially increased, brain volume are related to falls. Larger prospective studies are required to fully understand the underlying mechanisms.

White Matter Hyperintensities

White matter hyperintensities of presumed vascular origin (WMHs) are observed as hyperintense signals on T2-weighted MRI brain scans, often around the lateral ventricles but also in other areas of white matter (see Figure 7.1a) [22]. They occur to varying degrees in most older people [23]. The pathophysiology of WMHs is not well understood, but thought to be due to ischaemic damage, hypoperfusion, inflammation, gliosis, demyelination, and axonal loss [24]. WMHs are considered a form of incomplete infarction where there may be selective damage to some cellular components, in contrast to lacunar infarcts which result from more severe ischemic damage and present as small areas of necrosis. Until recently, WMHs were considered clinically irrelevant due to their high prevalence and lack of specificity with respect to the aetiology of underlying tissue changes. However, the accumulation of research findings has revealed their clinical significance in relation to a range of common geriatric syndromes. Higher levels of WMHs are associated with risk factors for falls such as slow gait [17, 25–27], gait variability [25], poor balance [28–30], depression [31], and poorer cognitive function [32–34]. In terms of cognition they are most commonly associated with poorer executive function and slower processing speed [35]. In line with these findings, both a higher burden (see Figure 7.2) and progression of WMHs are associated prospectively with increased risk of falls in both cognitively healthy people [25, 34, 36] and those with dementia [37]. Diffuse WMHs are also associated with increased risk of hip fractures over nine years in people aged 65–80 years [38] and injurious falls over one year in a cohort of 70–90-year-olds [34].

It is unclear whether the location of WMHs is important in relation to gait and falls. WMHs in frontal, corpus callosal, and periventricular regions are all associated with slow gait [39–41], and the overall burden, periventricular, and frontal deep lesions are all associated with prior falls [25, 42]. The mechanisms underlying WMHs and falls is likely due to disruption of white matter tracts that connect cortical and sub-cortical areas that are important for balance, gait, mood, and cognitive control (particularly executive function) [43].

Epidemiological studies have elucidated potential risk factors for extensive WMHs. Apart from older age, WMHs are associated with vascular risk factors and disease [24]. Hypertension is the most important modifiable WMH risk factor and has been consistently shown to be associated with WMHs. This association was first reported in the Framingham Study, where a greater burden of WMHs

(a)

(b)

(c)

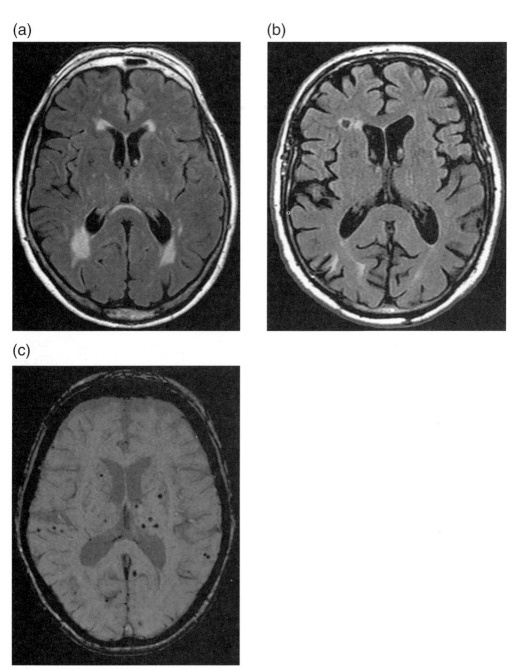

Figure 7.1   (a) White matter hyperintensities, (b) subcortical brain infarcts, and (c) cerebral microbleeds.

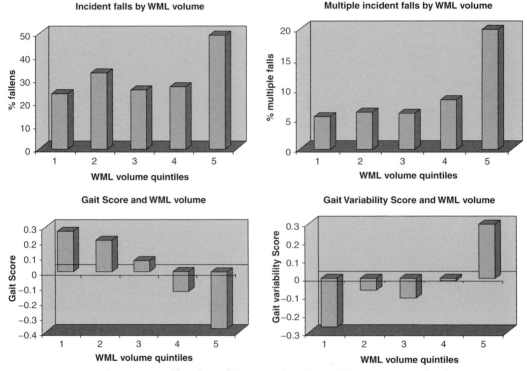

Figure 7.2   Increasing category of baseline white matter hyperintensities are associated with poorer gait, any falls, and multiple incident falls (with permission from Srikanth V, Beare R, Blizzard L et al. Cerebral white matter lesions, gait, and the risk of incident falls: a prospective population-based study. *Stroke*. 2009;40:175–80).

was associated with higher systolic blood pressure and a diagnosis of hypertension [44]. Strategies aimed at lowering blood pressure are likely to be important in slowing down WMHs, opening a vascular pathway and new targets for fall prevention in older people.

White Matter Integrity

Advanced age is associated with changes in all white matter components; however, degenerative changes are seen mostly at the microscopic level due to largely preserved white matter volumes [45]. Age-associated white matter integrity changes may therefore be best appreciated with imaging tools that can detect microstructural abnormalities. Diffuse tensor imaging (DTI) has emerged as a useful method for detecting the deterioration of white matter (axonal and myelin) integrity and is able to detect changes in the white matter earlier than occurs with white matter volume loss or WMHs [46]. Several studies have investigated age-related decreases in white matter integrity throughout the brain. Similar to the pattern for grey matter atrophy, most studies report an anterior–posterior gradient of decline in the structural integrity of white matter. Age-related differences have been shown to be greater in the genu compared to the splenium of the corpus callosum, as well as in frontal compared to temporal and occipital white matter [47].

Poorer white matter integrity, in both areas of normal-appearing white matter and WMHs, is associated with risk factors for falls such as slower gait [40, 48, 49], balance [50], and poorer cognitive functions [51]. Interestingly the strongest and most consistent association with gait appears to be in the internal capsule and corpus callosum (particularly the genu) [40, 51]. The corpus callosum is composed of the largest number of fibres in the brain, connecting each hemisphere and traversing the subcortical white matter. It is essential for motor, sensory, and cognitive processes [40]. The genu connects the prefrontal cortex, an area important for executive functions. Several studies have found a positive relationship between gait performances and white matter integrity in the genu of the corpus callosum, which supports the importance of integrated frontal executive function in the maintenance of gait and balance [48, 52]. However, in two studies that compared those that reported a fall to those that reported no falls in the past 12 months, there were no associations with white matter integrity [51, 53]. Future studies need to explore the relationship between specific white matter tracts and their integrity with prospective risk of falling.

Subcortical Infarcts and Microbleeds

Subcortical or lacunar infarcts (see Figure 7.1b) are another common sign of small vessel disease, with a prevalence of up to 20% in older people [23]. They are small areas of necrosis that result from more severe ischemic damage and can be observed as 3–10 mm and hypointense on T1-weighted and fluid attenuated inversion recovery (FLAIR) MRI sequences. Cerebral microbleeds (see Figure 7.1c) are hypointense homogenous lesions on T2-weighted gradient enhanced echo sequences that are 2–10 mm and round or oval in shape. They are evident in around 5% of healthy older people [22, 23]. Subcortical infarcts or microbleeds in combination with WMHs [54] are associated with poorer balance and gait [54], and subcortical infarcts alone are associated with poorer balance [17], gait [17], executive function, and attention [55].

One prospective study of two population-based cohorts found three or more subcortical infarcts were associated with falls, independent of WMHs suggesting independent pathways [55]. Autopsy studies have also examined associations with falls before death. In one study, which reported a 36% prevalence of microinfarcts (<1 mm on autopsy), both cortical and subcortical microinfarcts were associated with prior poor mobility and falls [56]. In a further autopsy study of people >75 years, only white matter pallor and microscopic atherosclerosis were independently associated with falls in those without dementia. In those with dementia only microinfarcts overall were associated with falls [57]. Taken together, makers of small vessel disease such as infarcts, WHMs, and microbleeds appear to disrupt both cognition and mobility, placing individuals at increased risk of falls.

Cerebral Amyloid and Tau

Amyloid-beta (Aβ) deposition and tau are the hallmarks of Alzheimer's disease [58]. Positron emission tomography (PET) imaging using the C-Pittsburgh Compound-B (PiB) is able to identify levels of Aβ. Although tau imaging is emerging [59], the most common way to measure levels of total and phosphorylated tau are in the cerebral spinal fluid via lumbar puncture. Higher burden of Aβ has been found to be associated with poorer cognitive function [60–62], slow gait speed [63, 64], and physiological falls risk as measured by the physiological profile assessment [60]. Furthermore, on autopsy (n = 86), substantia nigra neurofibrillary tangles (aggregates of hyperphosphorylated tau) were related to gait impairments [65]. In terms of falling, in cognitively normal older people (n = 125), higher PiB retention as well as cerebral spinal fluid biomarker ratios (tau/Aβ42) were associated with a shorter time to a first fall over a 12-month period [66]. These findings suggest that Alzheimer's pathology may cause more subtle changes to cognition and gait prior to dementia that result in falls.

Position Emission Tomography

Position Emission Tomography (PET) using dopamine transporter radioligands (e.g. [^{11}C] β-CFT: 2-beta-carbomethoxy-3-beta-(4-fluorophenyl) tropane), can be used to examine striatal dopaminergic transporter activity which has been found to decrease in older age [67]. Even in people free of neurological disease, striatal dopamine loss is associated with slow gait [68] and poorer postural control, particularly when visual information is perturbed [67]. It is therefore plausible that loss of dopamine in the striatum of the basal ganglia is a potential candidate in the aetiology of falls. In a study of community-dwelling people, a sub-analysis suggested lower striatal dopamine transporter activity in those who had multiple falls over six months compared to those who had zero or one falls [69]. In contrast, PET imaging of acetylcholinesterase activity suggests a link between cholinergic denervation (thalamic or cortical) and falls in people with Parkinson's disease [70].

Fludeoxyglucose (FDG) PET uses the radioactive probe ^{18}F-fludeoxyglucose to study regional cerebral glucose metabolism, a proxy for neural activity. In high-functioning older women, lower normalized cerebral metabolic values at rest (decreased neural activity) in the prefrontal, posterior cingulate, and parietal cortices was associated with slow gait speed and lower cadence when measured under maximal, but not normal-pace walking [71]. These findings are consistent with knowledge that these areas are important for cognitive functions (especially attention, executive, and visuospatial function) that are associated with poorer gait [72] and falls in older people [73].

Functional Magnetic Resonance Imaging

Brain areas do not act in isolation, but in co-ordinated networks that can be examined using functional MRI. Regions with positive correlation in blood oxygen-level dependence (BOLD) signal are likely to be functionally connected, where the BOLD signal indicates neuronal metabolism or activity [74]. Connectivity can be examined within and between networks, and functional MRI studies have found substantially different brain activation patterns when comparing older and younger adults when they perform motor tasks. Cabeza proposed a compensatory mechanism, namely the Hemispheric Asymmetry Reduction in Older Adults (HAROLD) model [75]. This model suggests increased brain activity levels are required for successful motor output in older adults to compensate for age-related peripheral sensory deficits and brain structural decline. One study found between, but not within, network differences in those who did and did not report past falls [76]. They examined four different networks (the default mode network, fronto-executive, frontoparietal, and primarysensorimotor network). Those that had fallen had greater connectivity between the default mode and frontoparietal networks during right-hand finger tapping. However, those reporting falls had less connectivity between left sensorimotor and frontoparietal networks (during rest) and between right hemisphere sensorimotor and frontoparietal networks (during rest and a left finger-tapping task) which was also associated with decline in mobility and cognition over 12 months (rest only) [76]. The authors hypothesized that disconnections between networks may increase fall risk via reduced ability to attend to external stimuli or may result in mind wandering (default mode and frontoparietal network connections) or less motor preparatory inputs before a motor performance (sensorimotor and frontoparietal network connections). This suggests that it is possible to compensate for age-related changes in brain structure by recruiting bilaterally or from additional cortical regions. However, with advancing age, severe damage of cerebral structures may influence these compensatory processes, increasing one's risk of falling.

Functional Near Infrared Spectroscopy

Functional near-infrared spectroscopy (fNIRS) is a relatively new non-invasive optical neuroimaging technique used to quantify (indirect) neural activation by measuring changes in blood flow (i.e. haemodynamic responses). fNIRS uses light with different wavelengths in the near-infrared spectrum which is transmitted through the skull. Oxy- and deoxyhaemoglobin absorb light at different wavelengths, and an increase in oxyHb and a decrease of deoxyHb is interpreted as an intensified blood flow in the active brain regions [77]. While there are still many challenges related to standardizing assessment procedures, fNIRS has one key advantage of being able to record neural activation while performing activities such as walking. The prefrontal cortex has been most commonly examined in studies of gait to examine the hypothesis that gait requires attention and executive function [78]. Generally greater activation has been found in the prefrontal cortex while walking and talking when compared to single-task walking, suggesting that it is a more attention-demanding task [79]. Only one study has examined fNIRS in relation to falls. In people with no gait abnormalities or dementia, higher prefrontal activation while walking and talking predicted an increased risk of falling [18], whereas, in the same study there was no association with mobility or the cognitive task, suggesting that increased prefrontal activation during walking while talking may occur earlier than clinical changes in gait or cognition and hence be an early early marker of fall risk.

Conclusions

Motor control and integration of sensorimotor information are achieved through the involvement of many brain structures. Neurodegenerative changes in grey and white matter, vascular lesions, altered brain connectivity, loss of neurotransmitters, and altered metabolism in the brain all appear to contribute to risk of falls. This is likely due to their effect on balance, gait, mood, and cognitive functions. Areas such as the prefrontal and motor cortex, basal ganglia, cerebellum, and parietal cortices may be particularly important due to their relationship with executive function, processing speed, and impairment in mobility. For neurodegenerative changes that are ischaemic in origin, it is possible that vascular risk modification has the potential to reduce fall risk. Reducing cardiovascular risk factors and increasing physical activity can affect the efficiency of brain metabolism in areas involved in executive function and attentional control. Furthermore, vascular treatments that have the potential to slow down the rate of development of WMHs might also have the potential to reduce the risk of falls and functional decline.

REFERENCES

1. Geschwind N. Disconnexion syndromes in animals and man. I. *Brain*. 1965;88:237–94.
2. Geschwind N. Disconnexion syndromes in animals and man. II. *Brain*. 1965;88:585–644.
3. Raz N, Rodrigue KM, Haacke EM. Brain aging and its modifiers: insights from in vivo neuromorphometry and susceptibility weighted imaging. *Ann NY Acad Sci*. 2007;1097:84–93.
4. Galluzzi S, Beltramello A, Filippi M et al. Aging. *Neurol Sci*. 2008;29:296–300.
5. Webb SJ, Monk CS, Nelson CA. Mechanisms of postnatal neurobiological development: implications for human development. *Dev Neurospcyhol*. 2001;19:147–71.
6. Callisaya ML, Beare R, Phan TG et al. Global and regional associations of smaller cerebral gray and white matter volumes with gait in older people. *PloS One*. 2014;9:e84909.
7. Rosano C, Aizenstein HJ, Studenski S et al. A regions-of-interest volumetric analysis of mobility limitations in community-dwelling older adults. *J Gerontol A Biol Sci Med Sci*. 2007;62:1048–55.
8. Callisaya ML, Beare R, Phan TG et al. Brain structural change and gait decline: a longitudinal population-based study. *J Am Geriatr Soc*. 2013;61:1074–9.
9. Rosano C, Sigurdsson S, Siggeirsdottir K et al. Magnetization transfer imaging, white matter hyperintensities, brain atrophy and slower gait in older men and women. *Neurobiol Aging*. 2010;31:1197–204.
10. Davis JC, Nagamatsu LS, Hsu CL et al. Self-efficacy is independently associated with brain volume in older women. *Age Ageing*. 2012;41:495–501.
11. Tuerk C, Zhang H, Sachdev P et al. Regional gray matter volumes are related to concern about falling in older people: a voxel-based morphometric study. *J Gerontol A Biol Sci Med Sci*. 2016;71:138–44.
12. Hayakawa YK, Sasaki H, Takao H et al. Structural brain abnormalities in women with subclinical depression, as revealed by voxel-based morphometry and diffusion tensor imaging. *J Affect Disord*. 2013;144:263–8.
13. Tabatabaei-Jafari H, Shaw ME, Cherbuin N. Cerebral atrophy in mild cognitive impairment: a systematic review with meta-analysis. *Alzheimers Dement*. 2015;1:487–504.
14. Muir SW, Gopaul K, Montero Odasso MM. The role of cognitive impairment in fall risk among older adults: a systematic review and meta-analysis. *Age Ageing*. 2012;41:299–308.
15. Davis JC, Best JR, Khan KM et al. Slow processing speed predicts falls in older adults with a falls history: 1-Year prospective cohort study. *J Am Geriatr Soc*. 2017;65:916–23.
16. Rosano C, Studenski SA, Aizenstein HJ et al. Slower gait, slower information processing and smaller prefrontal area in older adults. *Age Ageing*. 2012;41:58–64.
17. Rosano C, Brach J, Longstreth WT, Jr et al. Quantitative measures of gait characteristics indicate prevalence of underlying subclinical structural brain abnormalities in high-functioning older adults. *Neuroepidemiology*. 2006;26:52–60.

18. Verghese J, Wang C, Ayers E et al. Brain activation in high-functioning older adults and falls: prospective cohort study. *Neurology*. 2017;88:191–7.

19. Blumen HM, Brown LL, Habeck C et al. Gray matter volume covariance patterns associated with gait speed in older adults: a multi-cohort MRI study. *Brain Imaging Behav*. 2018;13:446–60.

20. Beauchet O, Launay CP, Barden J et al. Association between falls and brain subvolumes: results from a cross-sectional analysis in healthy older adults. *Brain Topogr*. 2017;30:272–80.

21. Makizako H, Shimada H, Doi T et al. Poor balance and lower gray matter volume predict falls in older adults with mild cognitive impairment. *BMC Neurol*. 2013;13:102.

22. Wardlaw JM, Smith EE, Biessels GJ et al. Neuroimaging standards for research into small vessel disease and its contribution to ageing and neurodegeneration. *Lancet Neurol*. 2013;12:822–38.

23. Moran C, Phan TG, Srikanth VK. Cerebral small vessel disease: a review of clinical, radiological, and histopathological phenotypes. *Int J Stroke*. 2012;7:36–46.

24. Wardlaw JM, Valdes Hernandez MC, Munoz-Maniega S. What are white matter hyperintensities made of? Relevance to vascular cognitive impairment. *J Am Heart Assoc*. 2015;4:001140.

25. Srikanth V, Beare R, Blizzard L et al. Cerebral white matter lesions, gait, and the risk of incident falls: a prospective population-based study. *Stroke*. 2009;40:175–80.

26. Whitman GT, Tang Y, Lin A et al. A prospective study of cerebral white matter abnormalities in older people with gait dysfunction. *Neurology*. 2001;57:990–4.

27. Baloh RW, Ying SH, Jacobson KM. A longitudinal study of gait and balance dysfunction in normal older people. *Arch Neurol*. 2003;60:835–9.

28. Zheng JJ, Delbaere K, Close JC et al. White matter hyperintensities are an independent predictor of physical decline in community-dwelling older people. *Gerontology*. 2012;58:398–406.

29. Zheng JJ, Delbaere K, Close JC et al. Impact of white matter lesions on physical functioning and fall risk in older people: a systematic review. *Stroke*. 2011;42:2086–90.

30. Baezner H, Blahak C, Poggesi A et al. Association of gait and balance disorders with age-related white matter changes: the LADIS study. *Neurology*. 2008;70:935–42.

31. de Groot JC, de Leeuw FE, Oudkerk M et al. Cerebral white matter lesions and depressive symptoms in elderly adults. *Arch Gen Psychiatry*. 2000;57:1071–6.

32. van der Flier WM, van Straaten EC, Barkhof F et al. Small vessel disease and general cognitive function in nondisabled elderly: the LADIS study. *Stroke*. 2005;36:2116–20.

33. de Groot JC, de Leeuw FE, Oudkerk M et al. Cerebral white matter lesions and cognitive function: the Rotterdam Scan Study. *Ann Neurol*. 2000;47:145–51.

34. Zheng JJ, Lord SR, Close JC et al. Brain white matter hyperintensities, executive dysfunction, instability, and falls in older people: a prospective cohort study. *J Gerontol A Biol Sci Med Sci*. 2012;67:1085–91.

35. Bolandzadeh N, Davis JC, Tam R et al. The association between cognitive function and white matter lesion location in older adults: a systematic review. *BMC Neurol*. 2012;12:126.

36. Callisaya ML, Beare R, Phan T et al. Progression of white matter hyperintensities of presumed vascular origin increases the risk of falls in older people. *J Gerontol A Biol Sci Med Sci.* 2014;70:360–6.

37. Taylor ME, Lord SR, Delbaere K et al. White matter hyperintensities are associated with falls in older people with dementia. *Brain Imaging Behav.* 2018;13:1265–72.

38. Corti MC, Baggio G, Sartori L et al. White matter lesions and the risk of incident hip fracture in older persons: results from the progetto veneto anziani study. *Arch Intern Med.* 2007;167:1745–51.

39. Srikanth V, Phan TG, Chen J et al. The location of white matter lesions and gait: a voxel-based study. *Ann Neurol.* 2010;67:265–9.

40. de Laat KF, Tuladhar AM, van Norden AG et al. Loss of white matter integrity is associated with gait disorders in cerebral small vessel disease. *Brain.* 2011;134:73–83.

41. Moscufo N, Guttmann CR, Meier D et al. Brain regional lesion burden and impaired mobility in the elderly. *Neurobiol Aging.* 2011;32:646–54.

42. Blahak C, Baezner H, Pantoni L et al. Deep frontal and periventricular age related white matter changes but not basal ganglia and infratentorial hyperintensities are associated with falls: cross sectional results from the LADIS study. *J Neurol Neurosurg Psychiatry.* 2009;80:608–13.

43. Srikanth VK, Sanders LM, Callisaya ML et al. Brain ageing and gait. *Aging Health.* 2010;6:123–31.

44. Jeerakathil T, Wolf PA, Beiser A et al. Stroke risk profile predicts white matter hyperintensity volume: the Framingham Study. *Stroke.* 2004;35:1857–61.

45. Davis SW, Dennis NA, Buchler NG et al. Assessing the effects of age on long white matter tracts using diffusion tensor tractography. *Neuroimage.* 2009;46:530–41.

46. Werring DJ, Clark CA, Barker GJ et al. Diffusion tensor imaging of lesions and normal-appearing white matter in multiple sclerosis. *Neurology.* 1999;52:1626–32.

47. Salat D, Tuch D, Greve D et al. Age-related alterations in white matter microstructure measured by diffusion tensor imaging. *Neurobiol Aging.* 2005;26:1215–27.

48. de Laat KF, van Norden AG, Gons RA et al. Diffusion tensor imaging and gait in elderly persons with cerebral small vessel disease. *Stroke.* 2011;42:373–9.

49. Ghanavati T, Smitt MS, Lord SR et al. Deep white matter hyperintensities, microstructural integrity and dual task walking in older people. *Brain Imaging Behav.* 2018;12:1488–96.

50. Van Impe A, Coxon JP, Goble DJ et al. White matter fractional anisotropy predicts balance performance in older adults. *Neurobiol Aging.* 2012;33:1900–12.

51. Ryberg C, Rostrup E, Stegmann MB et al. Clinical significance of corpus callosum atrophy in a mixed elderly population. *Neurobiol Aging.* 2007;28:955–63.

52. Bhadelia RA, Price LL, Tedesco KL et al. Diffusion tensor imaging, white matter lesions, the corpus callosum, and gait in the elderly. *Stroke.* 2009;40:3816–20.

53. Wong YQ, Tan LK, Seow P et al. Microstructural integrity of white matter tracts amongst older fallers: a DTI study. *PloS One.* 2017;12:e0179895.

54. Choi P, Ren M, Phan TG et al. Silent infarcts and cerebral microbleeds modify the associations of white matter lesions with gait and postural stability: population-based study. *Stroke.* 2012;43:1505–10.

55. Callisaya ML, Srikanth VK, Lord SR et al. Sub-cortical infarcts and the risk of falls in older people: combined results of TASCOG and Sydney MAS studies. *Int J Stroke*. 2014;9:55–60.

56. Ince PG, Minett T, Forster G et al. Microinfarcts in an older population-representative brain donor cohort (MRC CFAS): prevalence, relation to dementia and mobility, and implications for the evaluation of cerebral Small Vessel Disease. *Neuropathol Appl Neurobiol*. 2017;43:409–18.

57. Richardson K, Hunter S, Dening T et al. Neuropathological correlates of falling in the CC75C population-based sample of the older old. *Curr Alzheimer Res*. 2012;9:697–708.

58. Jack CR, Jr, Bennett DA, Blennow K et al. NIA-AA Research Framework: toward a biological definition of Alzheimer's disease. *Alzheimers Dement*. 2018;14:535–62.

59. Villemagne VL, Dore V, Bourgeat P et al. Aβ-amyloid and Tau imaging in dementia. *Semin Nucl Med*. 2017;47:75–88.

60. Dao E, Best JR, Hsiung GR et al. Associations between cerebral amyloid and changes in cognitive function and falls risk in subcortical ischemic vascular cognitive impairment. *BMC Geriatr*. 2017;17:133.

61. Pike KE, Savage G, Villemagne VL et al. Beta-amyloid imaging and memory in non-demented individuals: evidence for preclinical Alzheimer's disease. *Brain*. 2007;130:2837–44.

62. Rowe CC, Bourgeat P, Ellis KA et al. Predicting Alzheimer disease with beta-amyloid imaging: results from the Australian imaging, biomarkers, and lifestyle study of ageing. *Ann Neurol*. 2013;74:905–13.

63. Del Campo N, Payoux P, Djilali A et al. Relationship of regional brain beta-amyloid to gait speed. *Neurology*. 2016;86:36–43.

64. Nadkarni NK, Perera S, Snitz BE et al. Association of brain amyloid-beta with slow gait in elderly individuals without dementia: influence of cognition and apolipoprotein E epsilon4 genotype. *JAMA Neurol*. 2017;74:82–90.

65. Schneider JA, Li JL, Li Y et al. Substantia nigra tangles are related to gait impairment in older persons. *Ann Neurol*. 2006;59:166–73.

66. Stark SL, Roe CM, Grant EA et al. Preclinical Alzheimer disease and risk of falls. *Neurology*. 2013;81:437–43.

67. Cham R, Perera S, Studenski SA et al. Striatal dopamine denervation and sensory integration for balance in middle-aged and older adults. *Gait Posture*. 2007;26:516–25.

68. Cham R, Studenski S, Perera S et al. Striatal dopaminergic denervation and gait in healthy adults. *Exp Brain Res*. 2008;185:391–8.

69. Bohnen NI, Muller ML, Kuwabara H et al. Age-associated striatal dopaminergic denervation and falls in community-dwelling subjects. *J Rehabil Res Dev*. 2009;46:1045–52.

70. Bohnen N, Müller M, Koeppe R et al. History of falls in Parkinson disease is associated with reduced cholinergic activity. *Neurology*. 2009;73:1670–6.

71. Sakurai R, Fujiwara Y, Yasunaga M et al. Regional cerebral glucose metabolism and gait speed in healthy community-dwelling older women. *J Gerontol A Biol Sci Med Sci*. 2014;69:1519–27.

72. Martin KL, Blizzard L, Wood AG et al. Cognitive function, gait, and gait variability in older people: a population-based study. *J Gerontol A Biol Sci Med Sci*. 2013;68:726–32.

73. Martin KL, Blizzard L, Srikanth VK et al. Cognitive function modifies the effect of physiological function on the risk of multiple falls: a population-based study. *J Gerontol A Biol Sci Med Sci.* 2013;68:1091–7.

74. Glover GH. Overview of functional magnetic resonance imaging. *Neurosurg Clin N Am.* 2011;22:133–9, vii.

75. Cabeza R. Cognitive neuroscience of aging: contributions of functional neuroimaging. *Scand J Psychol.* 2001;42:277–86.

76. Hsu CL, Voss MW, Handy TC et al. Disruptions in brain networks of older fallers are associated with subsequent cognitive decline: a 12-month prospective exploratory study. *PloS One.* 2014;9:e93673.

77. Scholkmann F, Kleiser S, Metz AJ et al. A review on continuous wave functional near-infrared spectroscopy and imaging instrumentation and methodology. *NeuroImage.* 2014;85:6–27.

78. Holtzer R, Epstein N, Mahoney JR et al. Neuroimaging of mobility in aging: a targeted review. *J Gerontol A Biol Sci Med Sci.* 2014;69:1375–88.

79. Holtzer R, Mahoney JR, Izzetoglu M et al. fNIRS study of walking and walking while talking in young and old individuals. *J Gerontol A Biol Sci Med Sci.* 2011;66:879–87.

8

Impaired Cognition and Falls

Morag E. Taylor and Julie Whitney

Dementia is a progressive clinical syndrome characterized by neurocognitive domain impairment(s) (i.e. complex attention, executive function, learning and memory, language, perceptual-motor, and social cognition), with or without significant behavioural disturbances, resulting in impairments in activities of daily living [1]. Further, these signs and symptoms cannot be better explained by another medical condition and should not be solely present during delirium [1].

Currently, it is estimated 50 million people are living with dementia, which represents around 5–8% of the global population aged over 60 [2]. The incidence of dementia increases with age, with every 6.3 years amounting to a doubling of the incidence. Incidence increases from 3.9/1000-person years between the ages of 60 and 64 to 104.8/1000-person years in those aged over 90 [3]. Due to increased life expectancy, the global population is rapidly ageing and the number of people living with dementia is expected to reach 152 million by 2050 [2]. The total global cost of dementia in 2015 was $818 billion and this is expected to rise to $2 trillion by 2030.

Dementia is an umbrella term that is used to describe a range of disorders of progressive deterioration in cognition with different underlying pathophysiological mechanisms. The most common of these disorders are Alzheimer's disease (AD), vascular dementia, dementia with Lewy bodies, frontotemporal dementia, and mixed pathology. In 2013, the Diagnostic and Statistical Manual of Mental Disorders (DSM-5) renamed dementia as major neurocognitive disorder (NCD) [1]. To add complexity, the terms cognitive impairment and dementia overlap and are often used interchangeably. For simplicity, and to reflect the terminology used in the current literature, we have used the term cognitive impairment throughout this chapter.

Risk Factors for Falls

Cognitive impairment is consistently found to predict falls, with both the risk and rate of falls being at least twice as high when compared to those without cognitive impairment (see Figure 8.1) [4–9]. The presence of cognitive impairment increases

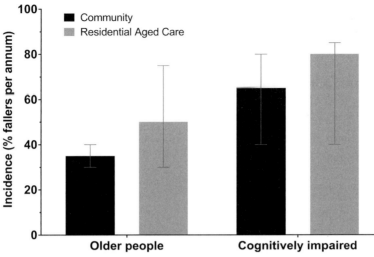

Figure 8.1   Diagrammatic representation of annual fall incidence in older people and cognitively impaired older people in the community and residential aged care settings.
Note. The error bars depict approximate ranges reported in the literature; some of the residential care 'older people' populations included people with dementia.

the risk of multiple falls [8] and injurious falls including a three- to fourfold increase in the risk of hip fractures [10–13]. The risk of poor outcomes following a fall is higher in people with cognitive impairment, with a greater likelihood of functional impairment, institutionalization, and death [10, 11, 14–18].

Research into risk factors and interventions in cognitively impaired people has been undertaken in the community, in hospitals, and in residential care settings, with the latter group exhibiting a greater degree of cognitive impairment and physical frailty, as well as increased risk and rate of falls (see Figure 8.1).

Risk factors for falls in older adults with cognitive impairment can be considered in two classes:

➢ Risk factors known to increase falls in the general population which are more pronounced and/or more prevalent in cognitive impairment
➢ Risk factors specific to cognitive impairment.

Risk Factors Known to Increase Falls that Are More Pronounced and/or More Prevalent in Cognitive Impairment
Balance

Remaining upright involves a complex process in which various sensory inputs are processed and integrated by the central nervous system (CNS) resulting in motor outputs that produce the correct amplitude, co-ordination, and timing of muscle contractions. In consequence, conditions that affect the CNS such as cognitive impairment have an impact on postural stability. Older people with cognitive impairment have poorer static and dynamic balance, and smaller limits of stability than cognitively healthy older people [8, 19–22]. Executive dysfunction has also been associated with reduced postural control and the relationship between executive function and falls is mediated in part by physical performance, including balance, in older people with cognitive impairment [23]. For these reasons, poor balance is predictive of falls in this group [24–27].

Gait (Including Dual Tasking)

As with balance control, gait requires complex integration of visual, sensory, and vestibular inputs to negotiate through the environment and complete additional tasks as required. Changes in gait occur early in the development of cognitive impairment and may even precede a clinical diagnosis [28, 29]. When compared to healthy controls, individuals with cognitive impairment demonstrate reduced gait speed, shorter step/stride length, greater gait variability, worse co-ordination and poorer obstacle clearance [19, 29, 30]. These gait variables, including reduced (estimated) lateral gait stability, also discriminate between fallers and non-fallers or are associated with a higher rate of falls in people with cognitive impairment [25, 26, 31–36].

Dual-task gait paradigms involve measuring the change in gait speed when a second, often cognitive, task is attempted, with the dual-task cost calculated as the difference between gait speed in the dual and single tasks. However, it is also important to consider the cost to the secondary task (e.g. cognitive task), which can be determined by measuring secondary task performance with and without walking. It is then possible to produce a mean dual-task cost for both gait and the secondary task [37]. People with cognitive impairment perform dual tasks more slowly, with greater gait variability, or make more errors [38–40]. It is less clear whether dual task paradigms discriminate between fallers and non-fallers in older people with cognitive impairment [31, 34, 41]. The reason for differences in findings may relate to variation in the difficulty of the additional task. It also appears likely that dual-task paradigms are more effective at highlighting fall risk in robust older adults without gait impairments [42].

Medication Use

As with cognitively intact older people, the use of multiple medications increases fall risk in people with cognitive impairment [25, 26, 35, 43]. Centrally acting medications are frequently prescribed to people with cognitive impairment [44–47], and these medications, specifically antipsychotics, anxiolytics, hypnotics, sedatives, antidepressants, and opioids, increase falls and fall-related injuries in this group [24–26, 47–52].

Other Risk Factors

Inactivity and functional impairment have been identified as risk factors for falls in people with cognitive impairment [4, 25, 53]. A sedentary lifestyle is associated with executive dysfunction, physical decline, and an increased risk of developing dementia [54–56]. Furthermore, moving into residential care, which is a common consequence of cognitive impairment and falls, is associated with a significant reduction in physical activity [57]. Fear of falling, an established fall risk factor in cognitively healthy people, is also associated with falls in people with cognitive impairment [25].

There is some evidence to suggest autonomic dysfunction, including orthostatic hypotension, is more common in older people with cognitive impairment [58] but whether these symptoms are predictive of falls in this group is less clear. One study, which used beat-to-beat blood pressure measurement was able to identify differences between fallers and non-fallers in people with cognitive impairment [4], and may relate to a common association between white matter lesions, autonomic dysfunction, and falls [24, 59, 60].

Risk Factors Specific to Cognitive Impairment
Cognition

Impaired general cognition is associated with an increased risk of falls [7, 26, 43, 56]. More specifically, impairment in executive function, processing speed, and visuospatial function are associated with falling [23, 25–27, 35, 48, 61].

Behavioural and Psychological Symptoms

The non-cognitive manifestations of dementia are sometimes referred to as behavioural and psychological symptoms (BPS) and include apathy, depression, sleep disturbance, agitation, psychosis, hallucinations, and wandering (defined as 'seemingly aimless ambulation, often with observable patterns such as lapping, pacing, or random ambulation' [62]). BPS symptoms are common with multiple contributing factors, but recently they have been considered, at least in part, to be an indicator of unmet needs (e.g. pain, thirst, and hunger).

In residential care populations with cognitive impairment, BPS such as increased Neuropsychiatric Inventory (NPI) scores, hyperactivity, restlessness, paranoia, hallucinations, and impulsivity have been associated with increased fall risk [26, 50, 63–67]. NPI scores have also been related to falls in community-dwelling people with cognitive impairment [53, 68], and 'wandering' behaviour has been connected with an increased risk of hip fracture [69].

Depression and anxiety also increase the risk of falls in people with cognitive impairment [25, 70]. The prevalence of depression in people with cognitive impairment is double that of cognitively intact older people, with more than 20–30% of people with cognitive impairment experiencing depression [71]. There is also evidence that depression is both a risk factor and a prodrome to dementia [71, 72]. Anxiety symptoms are also common with prevalence estimates up to 70% in older people with cognitive impairment [73]. Despite the limited exploration of anxiety as a risk factor for falls, evidence so far indicates it is associated with increased risk [25, 26].

Perceived versus Observed Physical Ability (Judgement Error)

Recent literature has also examined judgement error of perceived and observed physical ability as a fall risk factor, and demonstrated an independent association with falls [74], a relationship that was not demonstrated in cognitively healthy older people [75].

Fall Prevention

Fall Prevention Interventions by Settings

Community

The recently published Cochrane review on exercise and falls, which provided strong evidence that exercise is an effective intervention to prevent falls, noted that 67% of the studies excluded people with cognitive impairment [76]. Similar exclusions were noted in the recent Cochrane review of multiple and multi-factorial fall prevention interventions [77]. However, a complementary systematic review of three randomized controlled trials (RCTs) found exercise reduced fall rates by 45% in people with cognitive impairment [78], and a comparable review reached similar conclusions, i.e. a 32% reduction in falls in participants allocated to the exercise arms [79]. However, these findings should be interpreted with caution due to the small number of studies and participants. Further high-quality research is warranted.

One Finnish RCT (FINALEX trial), included in the above reviews, demon-strated that both home and group exercise effectively reduced falls in people with AD [80]. This intervention involved exercising with supervision from a qualified physiotherapist for one hour twice a week for 12 months. Exercises for endurance, muscle strength, balance, and executive function were per-formed. Functional ability deteriorated in all the groups over the follow-up period, but this deterioration was significantly slower in the home-exercise group compared to controls. The participants in this study had a mean Mini Mental State Examination (MMSE) of 18, suggesting this intervention was effective for individuals with mild to moderate AD, which is further supported by the Clinical Dementia Rating scores (82% scored 0.5–2). In a further sub-group analysis on the FINALEX trial, Öhman et al. [81] found that in individuals with mild AD, the intervention significantly slowed functional deterioration but did not reduce falls. On the other hand, in individuals with more advanced AD, the programme did not prevent functional decline, but significantly reduced falls. These findings highlight the complexity of the relationship between physical performance, cognitive function, and fall risk.

Since the Cochrane reviews and systematic review and meta-analysis by Sherrington et al. [76–78], one large high-quality RCT (i-FOCIS trial) has been conducted evaluating the fall prevention effectiveness of a tailored home-based exercise programme and occupational-therapy-led home-hazard reduction programme in community-dwelling older people with cognitive impairment [82]. This study involved 11 home visits, which were a combination of occupational therapy and physiotherapy during the 12-month study period [82]. Functional cognition was assessed using the Large Allen's Cognitive Level Scale and the findings of this assessment were used to tailor the intervention, e.g. whether supervision was required for the prescribed exercise programme, how the exercise sessions were delivered, caregiver education, and how the home safety and exercise booklet were presented. The intervention did not reduce the rate of falls (primary outcome), but did reduce the risk of multiple falls (while controlling for follow-up and baseline differences) and the rate of falls in participants with better physical function at baseline (pre-specified sub-group analysis).

Contrasting the samples from the FINALEX trial and the i-FOCIS trial identifies several differences. For example, the i-FOCIS participants were older and had poorer cognitive and physical function. Since the i-FOCIS trial prevented falls in people with better physical function, the findings from this trial taken together with the FINALEX trial suggest that exercise with or without a home-hazard reduction programme may prevent falls in people with cognitive impairment and better physical function.

An RCT analysing the effects of donepezil (anti-dementia drug) use in people with mild cognitive impairment (MCI) found a non-significant reduction in the number and rate of falls in the Donepezil arm [83]. However, due to the small sample size, this trial was underpowered for fall analyses.

Residential Aged Care Facilities

The prevalence of cognitive impairment in residential aged care facilities (RACFs) is high, with up to 70% of this population demonstrating some degree of cognitive impairment [84]. Several RCTs have effectively reduced falls either as multi-factorial or single interventions, including supervised exercise, medication review, vitamin D supplementation, continence management, and staff education [85–91]. As these studies did not exclude on the basis of cognitive impairment, it is likely these interventions are effective in people with cognitive impairment, as several trials adjusted their outcomes for cognition, which did not alter their findings [92–94]. Where trials performed a-priori sub-group analysis based on level of cognition, results are conflicting. Jensen et al. [85] found their multi-factorial intervention reduced falls in people with a higher MMSE ($\geq$19) but not in those with MMSE<19. On the other hand, Rapp et al. [87] found that their multi-factorial intervention was more effective in individuals with cognitive impairment. In the recent Cochrane review for RACFs, the effect on falls was equivocal for medication review, exercise, environmental adaptations, and multi-factorial interventions [90]. Vitamin D (in those deficient) may reduce the rate of falls [90]. Sub-group analysis of multi-factorial interventions, based on whether participants had confirmed cognitive impairment or not, did not identify efficacy differences. Since the recent Cochrane review, there has been one successful, and cost effective, cluster RCT that compared a 12-month exercise programme (two days per week) to usual care; the rate of falls and injurious falls were reduced by 55% and 54% respectively in the exercise arm [91, 95]. Fifty-five percent of the exercise arm in this trial had cognitive impairment, but a sub-group analysis was not performed. In contrast, a recent RCT in residential care in Sweden, specifically targeting older people with dementia, compared a four-month high-intensity functional exercise programme to a seated attention control activity two to three times per week for four months [96]. The high-intensity functional exercise programme did not prevent falls over six or 12 months but did prevent moderate to severe fall-related injuries over 12 months [96]. These two studies potentially indicate that the programme dose, in particular length, needs to be greater to demonstrate effect.

It is possible factors other than cognitive impairment contribute to these ambiguous findings in RACFs. It may be that the increased physical frailty, severity of cognitive impairment and/or complexity of the care setting explains the differences. Studies that have addressed risk factors identified in RACFs such as BPS using dementia care mapping have also been inconsistent [90]. More research is required to better understand the most effective interventions for people with cognitive impairment living in RACFs.

Hospitals

It is estimated that 25% of all inpatients aged over 65 have some degree of cognitive impairment [97]. During a period of acute illness and hospitalization, individuals with cognitive impairment have a higher risk of developing delirium

[98, 99]. Delirium, defined as 'recent onset of fluctuating inattention and confusion, linked to one or more triggering factors', can present as hyperactive, which manifests as agitation and restlessness, hypoactive, which presents as apathy with reduced activity levels, or a mixed type [98]. Delirium affects attention, an element of cognition known to be associated with increased likelihood of falling [26]. Delirium, and associated clinical manifestations, in conjunction with other known risk factors in the hospital setting (see Chapter 26) leads to an increased risk of falls in people with cognitive impairment [99]. Therefore, interventions to prevent falls in hospital inpatients should address risk factors relating to cognition and delirium, as well as measures to reduce the risk associated with physical, medical, medication, and environmental risk factors.

Many of the interventions that have been implemented in hospital inpatient settings have included people with cognitive impairment, but few have performed sub-group analysis between patients with and without cognitive impairment [100–102]. The most recent Cochrane review found multi-factorial interventions were effective for sub-acute settings but not acute or mixed settings (not cognitive impairment specific) [90]. The prevalence of delirium is higher in acute settings and although limited (study and participant numbers and study quality), there is evidence that multi-component interventions aimed at preventing delirium in (predominantly medical) patients considered 'at risk' also prevent falls [103]. In the acute and sub-acute (mixed) setting, Haines et al. [104] analysed the effect of an individualized multi-media education intervention with health professional follow-up; overall this programme did not reduce the rate of falls. However, in the cognitively healthy patients (Short Portable Mental Status Questionnaire; SPMSQ >7) the rate of falls was significantly lower and in the patients with cognitive impairment the rate of falls was higher, though not significantly [104]. Indirect evidence for the prevention of falls in hospital comes from an education programme and staff training programme designed for cognitively healthy patients (MMSE >23) in the sub-acute setting [105]. The intervention significantly reduced falls in the intended group of cognitively intact inpatients, and interestingly there was also a trend for fewer falls in patients with cognitive impairment. This suggests these patients may have received a small benefit from the staff education process, despite not receiving the intervention [90]. In another study that evaluated the effect of comprehensive geriatric assessment post hip fracture, sub-group analysis suggested that people with dementia experienced fewer falls as a result of the intervention. However, the numbers in the analysis were small and this evidence was regarded as low quality [90, 106]. More research is needed in determining effective fall prevention strategies in hospitalized patients with cognitive impairment. See Table 8.1 for a brief summary of the fall prevention evidence.

Table 8.1 Current recommendations for fall prevention in older people in general compared to people with cognitive impairment[a]

Setting	Community	Residential Aged Care	Hospital
Older people	(a) Exercise (b) Multi-component interventions (but these are not better than exercise alone)	Vitamin D for deficient individuals	(a) Multi-factorial in sub-acute (b) Preliminary: additional physio-therapy in sub-acute
Cognitively impaired	Preliminary: exercise with or without a home safety programme in people with better physical function	Vitamin D for deficient individuals (populations included cognitively impaired individuals)	(a) Preliminary: multi-component delirium prevention (b) Preliminary: multi-factorial in sub-acute (small effect)

Note. Preliminary indicates low-quality evidence and/or few studies/participants, therefore findings are not conclusive

[a] Based on evidence from recent Cochrane reviews, or, in their absence, systematic reviews with meta-analysis and recent randomized controlled trials [76–78, 82, 90, 103]

Conclusions

Falls are common in older people with cognitive impairment and are associated with poorer outcomes when compared to their cognitively healthy peers. Physical and cognitive impairments, and psychological and behavioural symptoms contribute to this increased risk of falls. There remains a relative paucity of evidence for fall prevention in older people with cognitive impairment. The studies available are limited in number and size and have often produced conflicting findings. With these constraints in mind: (a) exercise, with or without a home safety programme, shows promise as a fall prevention strategy in people in the community setting, particularly in individuals with better physical function, (b) in the residential care setting, vitamin D supplementation may lower the rate of falls in individuals who are vitamin D deficient (this evidence is from studies that included people with cognitive impairment), and (c) in the hospital setting, multi-component interventions aimed at preventing delirium may also prevent falls, and staff training as part of a multi-factorial intervention that involves patient education for cognitively intact patients may have a small effect on reducing fall rate in people with cognitive impairment. Overall, the fall prevention evidence is inconclusive and more high-quality research is needed.

REFERENCES

1. American Psychiatric Association. *Diagnostic and Statistical Manual of Mental Disorders. 5th Edn.* Arlington, VA: American Psychiatric Association; 2013.

2. World Health Organization. *Dementia.* 2019 www.who.int/en/news-room/fact-sheets /detail/dementia (accessed April 2021).

3. Alzheimer's Disease International, Prince M, Wimo A, Guerchet M et al. *World Alzheimer Report 2015.* www.alzint.org/resource/world-alzheimer-report-2015/ (accessed April 2021).

4. Allan LM, Ballard CG, Rowan EN et al. Incidence and prediction of falls in dementia: a prospective study in older people. *PLoS ONE.* 2009;4:e5521.

5. Tinetti ME, Speechley M, Ginter SF. Risk factors for falls among elderly persons living in the community. *N Engl J Med.* 1988;319:1701–7.

6. Anstey KJ, von Sanden C, Luszcz MA. An 8-year prospective study of the relationship between cognitive performance and falling in very old adults. *J Am Geriatr Soc.* 2006;54:1169–76.

7. Asada T, Kariya T, Kinoshita T et al. Predictors of fall-related injuries among community-dwelling elderly people with dementia. *Age Ageing.* 1996;25:22–8.

8. Taylor ME, Delbaere K, Lord SR et al. Physical impairments in cognitively impaired older people: implications for risk of falls. *Int Psychogeriatr.* 2013;25:148–56.

9. Petersen JD, Siersma VD, Christensen RD et al. The risk of fall accidents for home dwellers with dementia: a register- and population-based case-control study. *Alzheimers Dement.* 2018;10:421–8.

10. Baker NL, Cook MN, Arrighi HM et al. Hip fracture risk and subsequent mortality among Alzheimer's disease patients in the United Kingdom, 1988–2007. *Age Ageing.* 2011;40:49–54.

11. Harvey L, Mitchell R, Brodaty H et al. The influence of dementia on injury-related hospitalisations and outcomes in older adults. *Injury.* 2016;47:226–34.

12. Harvey L, Mitchell R, Brodaty H et al. Differing trends in fall-related fracture and non-fracture injuries in older people with and without dementia. *Arch Gerontol Geriatr.* 2016;67:61–7.

13. Weller I, Schatzker J. Hip fractures and Alzheimer's disease in elderly institutionalized Canadians. *Ann Epidemiol.* 2004;14:319–24.

14. Cree M, Soskolne CL, Belseck E et al. Mortality and institutionalization following hip fracture. *J Am Geriatr Soc.* 2000;48:283–8.

15. Marottoli RA, Berkman LF, Leo-Summers L et al. Predictors of mortality and institutionalization after hip fracture: the New Haven EPESE cohort. Established Populations for Epidemiologic Studies of the Elderly. *Am J Public Health.* 1994;84:1807–12.

16. Poynter L, Kwan J, Sayer AA et al. Does cognitive impairment affect rehabilitation outcome? *J Am Geriatr Soc.* 2011;59:2108–11.

17. Scandol JP, Toson B, Close JC. Fall-related hip fracture hospitalisations and the prevalence of dementia within older people in New South Wales, Australia: an analysis of linked data. *Injury.* 2012;44:776–83.

18. Gruber-Baldini AL, Zimmerman S, Morrison RS et al. Cognitive impairment in hip fracture patients: timing of detection and longitudinal follow-up. *J Am Geriatr Soc.* 2003;51:1227–36.

19. Franssen EH, Souren LE, Torossian CL et al. Equilibrium and limb coordination in mild cognitive impairment and mild Alzheimer's disease. *J Am Geriatr Soc.* 1999;47:463–9.

20. Leandri M, Cammisuli S, Cammarata S et al. Balance features in Alzheimer's disease and amnestic mild cognitive impairment. *J Alzheimers Dis.* 2009;16:113–20.

21. Suttanon P, Hill KD, Said CM et al. Balance and mobility dysfunction and falls risk in older people with mild to moderate Alzheimer disease. *Am J Phys Med Rehabil.* 2012;91:12–23.

22. Szczepańska-Gieracha J, Cieślik B, Chamela-Bilińska D et al. Postural stability of elderly people with cognitive impairments. *Am J Alzheimers Dis Other Demen.* 2016;31:241–6.

23. Taylor ME, Lord SR, Delbaere K et al. Reaction time and postural sway modify the effect of executive function on risk of falls in older people with mild to moderate cognitive impairment. *Am J Geriatr Psychiatry.* 2017;25:397–406.

24. Horikawa E, Matsui T, Arai H et al. Risk of falls in Alzheimer's disease: a prospective study. *Intern Med J.* 2005;44:717–21.

25. Taylor ME, Delbaere K, Lord SR et al. Neuropsychological, physical, and functional mobility measures associated with falls in cognitively impaired older adults. *J Gerontol A Biol Sci Med Sci.* 2014;69:987–95.

26. Whitney J, Close JC, Jackson SH et al. Understanding risk of falls in people with cognitive impairment living in residential care. *J Am Med Dir Assoc.* 2012;13:535–40.

27. Hauer K, Dutzi I, Gordt K et al. Specific motor and cognitive performances predict falls during ward-based geriatric rehabilitation in patients with dementia. *Sensors.* 2020;20:5385.

28. Beauchet O, Annweiler C, Callisaya ML et al. Poor gait performance and prediction of dementia: results from a meta-analysis. *J Am Med Dir Assoc.* 2016;17:482–90.

29. Valkanova V, Ebmeier KP. What can gait tell us about dementia? Review of epidemiological and neuropsychological evidence. *Gait Posture.* 2017;53:215–23.

30. Mc Ardle R, Morris R, Wilson J et al. What can quantitative gait analysis tell us about dementia and its subtypes? A structured review. *J Alzheimers Dis.* 2017;60:1295–312.

31. Camicioli R, Licis L. Motor impairment predicts falls in specialized Alzheimer care units. *Alzheimer Dis Assoc Disord.* 2004;18:214–18.

32. Nakamura T, Meguro K, Sasaki H. Relationship between falls and stride length variability in senile dementia of the Alzheimer type. *Gerontology.* 1996;42:108–13.

33. Sterke CS, van Beeck EF, Looman CW et al. An electronic walkway can predict short-term fall risk in nursing home residents with dementia. *Gait Posture.* 2012;36:95–101.

34. Taylor ME, Delbaere K, Mikolaizak AS et al. Gait parameter risk factors for falls under simple and dual task conditions in cognitively impaired older people. *Gait Posture.* 2013;37:126–30.

35. Taylor ME, Ketels MM, Delbaere K et al. Gait impairment and falls in cognitively impaired older adults: an explanatory model of sensorimotor and neuropsychological mediators. *Age Ageing*. 2012;41:665–9.

36. Mehdizadeh S, Dolatabadi E, Ng K-D et al. Vision-based assessment of gait features associated with falls in people with dementia. *J Gerontol A Biol Sci Med Sci* 2019;75:1148–53.

37. Beurskens R, Bock O. Age-related deficits of dual-task walking: a review. *Neural Plast.* 2012;2012:1–9.

38. Allali G, Kressig RW, Assal F et al. Changes in gait while backward counting in demented older adults with frontal lobe dysfunction. *Gait Posture*. 2007;26:572–6.

39. Lamoth CJ, van Deudekom FJ, van Campen JP et al. Gait stability and variability measures show effects of impaired cognition and dual tasking in frail people. *J Neuroeng Rehabil.* 2011;8:2.

40. Amboni M, Barone P, Hausdorff JM. Cognitive contributions to gait and falls: evidence and implications. *Mov Disord.* 2013;28:1520–33.

41. Gonçalves J, Ansai JH, Masse FAA et al. Dual-task as a predictor of falls in older people with mild cognitive impairment and mild Alzheimer's disease: a prospective cohort study. *Braz J Phys Ther.* 2018;22:417–23.

42. Booth V, Logan P, Masud T et al. Falls, gait, and dual-tasking in older adults with mild cognitive impairment: a cross-sectional study. *Eur Geriatr Med.* 2015:S32–156.

43. Eriksson S, Gustafson Y, Lundin-Olsson L. Risk factors for falls in people with and without a diagnose of dementia living in residential care facilities: a prospective study. *Arch Gerontol Geriatr.* 2008;46:293–306.

44. Forsell Y, Winblad B. Psychiatric disturbances and the use of psychotropic drugs in a population of nonagenarians. *Int J Geriatr Psychiatry.* 1997;12:533–6.

45. Giron MST, Forsell Y, Bernsten C et al. Psychotropic drug use in elderly people with and without dementia. *Int J Geriatr Psychiatry.* 2001;16:900–6.

46. Lesén E, Carlsten A, Skoog I et al. Psychotropic drug use in relation to mental disorders and institutionalization among 95-year-olds: a population-based study. *Int Psychogeriatr.* 2011;23:1270–7.

47. Torvinen-Kiiskinen S, Tolppanen AM, Koponen M et al. Antidepressant use and risk of hip fractures among community-dwelling persons with and without Alzheimer's disease. *Int J Geriatr Psychiatry.* 2017;32:e107–15.

48. Eriksson S, Lundquist A, Gustafson Y et al. Comparison of three statistical methods for analysis of fall predictors in people with dementia: negative binomial regression (NBR), regression tree (RT), and partial least squares regression (PLSR). *Arch Gerontol Geriatr.* 2009;49:383–9.

49. Kröpelin TF, Neyens JCL, Halfens RJG et al. Fall determinants in older long-term care residents with dementia: a systematic review. *Int Psychogeriatr.* 2013;25:549–63.

50. Pellfolk T, Gustafsson T, Gustafson Y et al. Risk factors for falls among residents with dementia living in group dwellings. *Int Psychogeriatr.* 2009;21:187–94.

51. Hart LA, Marcum ZA, Gray SL et al. The association between central nervous system-active medication use and fall-related injury in community-dwelling older adults with dementia. *Pharmacotherapy.* 2019;39:530–43.

52. Taipale H, Hamina A, Karttunen N et al. Incident opioid use and risk of hip fracture among persons with Alzheimer disease: a nationwide matched cohort study. *Pain.* 2019;160:417–23.

53. Salva A, Roque M, Rojano X et al. Falls and risk factors for falls in community-dwelling adults with dementia (NutriAlz Trial). *Alzheimer Dis Assoc Disord.* 2012;26:74–80.

54. Sofi F, Valecchi D, Bacci D et al. Physical activity and risk of cognitive decline: a meta-analysis of prospective studies. *J Intern Med.* 2011;269:107–17.

55. Stephen R, Hongisto K, Solomon A et al. Physical activity and Alzheimer's disease: a systematic review. *J Gerontol A Biol Sci Med Sci.* 2017;72:733–9.

56. Taylor ME, Boripuntakul S, Toson B et al. The role of cognitive function and physical activity in physical decline in older adults across the cognitive spectrum. *Aging Ment Health.* 2019;23:863–71.

57. Sackley C, Levin S, Cardoso K et al. Observations of activity levels and social interaction in a residential care setting. *Int J Ther Rehabil.* 2006;13:370–3.

58. Passant U, Warkentin S, Gustafson L. Orthostatic hypotension and low blood pressure in organic dementia: a study of prevalence and related clinical characteristics. *Int J Geriatr Psychiatry.* 1997;12:395–403.

59. Kenny RA, Shaw FE, O'Brien JT et al. Carotid sinus syndrome is common in dementia with Lewy bodies and correlates with deep white matter lesions. *J Neurol Neurosurg Psychiatry.* 2004;75:966–71.

60. Taylor ME, Lord SR, Delbaere K et al. White matter hyperintensities are associated with falls in older people with dementia. *Brain Imaging Behav.* 2019;13:1265–72.

61. Olsson RH, Jr., Wambold S, Brock B et al. Visual spatial abilities and fall risk: an assessment tool for individuals with dementia. *J Gerontol Nurs.* 2005;31:45–51;quiz 2–3.

62. Cipriani G, Lucetti C, Nuti A et al. Wandering and dementia. *Psychogeriatrics.* 2014;14:135–42.

63. Hasegawa J, Kuzuya M, Iguchi A. Urinary incontinence and behavioral symptoms are independent risk factors for recurrent and injurious falls, respectively, among residents in long-term care facilities. *Arch Gerontol Geriatr.* 2010;50:77–81.

64. Kallin K, Gustafson Y, Sandman PO et al. Factors associated with falls among older, cognitively impaired people in geriatric care settings: a population-based study. *Am J Geriatr Psychiatry.* 2005;13:501–9.

65. Stapleton C, Hough P, Oldmeadow L et al. Four-item fall risk screening tool for subacute and residential aged care: the first step in fall prevention. *Australas J Ageing.* 2009;28:139–43.

66. Thapa PB, Gideon P, Fought RL et al. Psychotropic drugs and risk of recurrent falls in ambulatory nursing home residents. *Am J Epidemiol.* 1995;142:202–11.

67. Roitto H-M, Öhman H, Salminen K et al. Neuropsychiatric symptoms as predictors of falls in long-term care residents with cognitive impairment. *J Am Med Dir Assoc.* 2020;21:1243–8.

68. Roitto HM, Kautiainen H, Ohman H et al. Relationship of neuropsychiatric symptoms with falls in Alzheimer's disease: does exercise modify the risk? *J Am Geriatr Soc.* 2018;66:2377–81.

69. Buchner DM, Larson EB. Falls and fractures in patients with Alzheimer-type dementia. *J Am Med Assoc.* 1987;257:1492–5.

70. Fernando E, Fraser M, Hendriksen J et al. Risk factors associated with falls in older adults with dementia: a systematic review. *Physiother Can.* 2017;69:161–70.

71. Enache D, Winblad B, Aarsland D. Depression in dementia: epidemiology, mechanisms, and treatment. *Curr Opin Psychiatry.* 2011;24:461–72.

72. Cherbuin N, Kim S, Anstey KJ. Dementia risk estimates associated with measures of depression: a systematic review and meta-analysis. *BMJ Open.* 2015;5:e008853.

73. Seignourel PJ, Kunik ME, Snow L et al. Anxiety in dementia: a critical review. *Clin Psychol Rev.* 2008;28:1071–82.

74. Taylor ME, Butler AA, Lord SR et al. Inaccurate judgement of reach is associated with slow reaction time, poor balance, impaired executive function and predicts prospective falls in older people with cognitive impairment. *Exp Gerontol.* 2018;114:50–6.

75. Butler AA, Lord SR, Fitzpatrick RC. Reach distance but not judgment error is associated with falls in older people. *J Gerontol A Biol Sci Med Sci.* 2011;66:896–903.

76. Sherrington C, Fairhall NJ, Wallbank GK et al. Exercise for preventing falls in older people living in the community. *Cochrane Database Syst Rev.* 2019;1:CD012424.

77. Hopewell S, Adedire O, Copsey BJ et al. Multifactorial and multiple component interventions for preventing falls in older people living in the community. *Cochrane Database Syst Rev.* 2018;7:CD012221.

78. Sherrington C, Michaleff ZA, Fairhall N et al. Exercise to prevent falls in older adults: an updated systematic review and meta-analysis. *Br J Sports Med.* 2016;51:1750–8.

79. Burton E, Cavalheri V, Adam R et al. Effectiveness of exercise programs to reduce falls in older people with dementia living in the community: a systematic review and meta-analysis. *Clin Interv Aging.* 2015;10:421–34.

80. Pitkälä KH, Pöysti MM, Laakkonen ML et al. Effects of the Finnish Alzheimer Disease Exercise Trial (FINALEX): a randomized controlled trial. *JAMA Intern Med.* 2013;173:894–901.

81. Öhman H, Savikko N, Strandberg T et al. Effects of exercise on functional performance and fall rate in subjects with mild or advanced Alzheimer's disease: secondary analyses of a randomized controlled study. *Dem Geriatr Cogn Disord.* 2016;41:233–41.

82. Taylor ME, Wesson J, Sherrington C et al. Tailored exercise and home hazard reduction for fall prevention in older people with cognitive impairment: the i-FOCIS randomized controlled trial. *J Gerontol A Biol Sci Med Sci.* 2021;76:655–65.

83. Montero-Odasso M, Speechley M, Chertkow H et al. Donepezil for gait and falls in mild cognitive impairment: a randomized controlled trial. *Eur J Neurol.* 2019;26:651–9.

84. Prince M, Knapp M, Guerchet M et al. *Dementia UK: 2nd Edn – Overview.* London: Alzheimer's Society; 2014.

85. Jensen J, Nyberg L, Gustafson Y et al. Fall and injury prevention in residential care-effects in residents with higher and lower levels of cognition. *J Am Geriatr Soc.* 2003;51:627–35.

86. Neyens JC, Dijcks BP, Twisk J et al. A multifactorial intervention for the prevention of falls in psychogeriatric nursing home patients, a randomised controlled trial (RCT). *Age Ageing.* 2009;38:194–9.

87. Rapp K, Sarah EL, Gisela B et al. Prevention of falls in nursing homes: subgroup analyses of a randomized fall prevention trial. *J Am Geriatr Soc.* 2008;56:1092–7.

88. Rosendahl E, Gustafson Y, Nordin E et al. A randomized controlled trial of fall prevention by a high-intensity functional exercise program for older people living in residential care facilities. *Aging Clin Exp Res.* 2008;20:67–75.

89. Vlaeyen E, Coussement J, Leysens G et al. Characteristics and effectiveness of fall prevention programs in nursing homes: a systematic review and meta-analysis of randomized controlled trials. *J Am Geriatr Soc.* 2015;63:211–21.

90. Cameron ID, Dyer SM, Panagoda CE et al. Interventions for preventing falls in older people in care facilities and hospitals. *Cochrane Database Syst Rev.* 2018;2018: CD005465.

91. Hewitt J, Goodall S, Clemson L et al. Progressive resistance and balance training for falls prevention in long-term residential aged care: a cluster randomized trial of the Sunbeam Program. *J Am Med Dir Assoc.* 2018;19:361–9.

92. Bouwen A, De Lepeleire J, Buntinx F. Rate of accidental falls in institutionalised older people with and without cognitive impairment halved as a result of a staff-oriented intervention. *Age Ageing.* 2008;37:306–10.

93. Flicker L, MacInnis RJ, Stein MS et al. Should older people in residential care receive vitamin D to prevent falls? Results of a randomized trial. *J Am Geriatr Soc.* 2005;53:1881–8.

94. Sakamoto Y, Ebihara S, Ebihara T et al. Fall prevention using olfactory stimulation with lavender odor in elderly nursing home residents: a randomized controlled trial. *J Am Geriatr Soc.* 2012;60:1005–11.

95. Hewitt J, Saing S, Goodall S et al. An economic evaluation of the SUNBEAM programme: a falls-prevention randomized controlled trial in residential aged care. *Clin Rehabil.* 2019;33:524–34.

96. Toots A, Wiklund R, Littbrand H et al. The effects of exercise on falls in older people with dementia living in nursing homes: a randomized controlled trial. *J Am Med Dir Assoc.* 2019;20:835–42.

97. Alzheimer's Society. *Counting the Cost: Caring for People with Dementia on Hospital Wards.* London: Alzheimer's Society; 2009.

98. Young J, Inouye SK. Delirium in older people. *Br Med J.* 2007;334:842–6.

99. Fogg C, Griffiths P, Meredith P et al. Hospital outcomes of older people with cognitive impairment: an integrative review. *Int J Geriatr Psychiatry.* 2018;33:1177–97.

100. Dykes PC, Carroll DL, Hurley A et al. Fall prevention in acute care hospitals: a randomized trial. *J Am Med Assoc.* 2010;304:1912–18.

101. Haines TP, Bennell KL, Osborne RH et al. Effectiveness of targeted falls prevention programme in subacute hospital setting: randomised controlled trial. *Br Med J.* 2004;328:676.

102. Healey F, Monro A, Cockram A et al. Using targeted risk factor reduction to prevent falls in older in-patients: a randomised controlled trial. *Age Ageing.* 2004;33:390–5.

103. Hshieh TT, Yue J, Oh E et al. Effectiveness of multicomponent nonpharmacological delirium interventions: a meta-analysis. *JAMA Intern Med.* 2015;175:512–20.

104. Haines TP, Hill AM, Hill KD et al. Patient education to prevent falls among older hospital inpatients: a randomized controlled trial. *Arch Intern Med.* 2011;171:516–24.

105. Hill AM, McPhail SM, Waldron N et al. Fall rates in hospital rehabilitation units after individualised patient and staff education programmes: a pragmatic, stepped-wedge, cluster-randomised controlled trial. *Lancet.* 2015;385:2592–9.

106. Stenvall M, Olofsson B, Lundstrom M et al. A multidisciplinary, multifactorial intervention program reduces postoperative falls and injuries after femoral neck fracture. *Osteoporos Int.* 2007;18:167–75.

9

The Psychology of Fall Risk: Fear, Anxiety, Depression, and Balance Confidence

Thomas Hadjistavropoulos and Kim Delbaere

Originally discussed in early clinical reports (e.g. [1]), the relationship between psychological factors and falls is now well supported in the literature. Specifically, fear of falling, balance confidence or fall efficacy (i.e. belief in ability to maintain one's balance),[1] and depression are well-established predictors of falls and determinants of fall risk (e.g. [4,5]). Anxiety also appears to play a role in the determination of balance performance and gait parameters [6]. These psychological variables, which can also be the consequence of or be changed by a fall, can lead to activity avoidance in an effort to prevent future injuries [7]. In this chapter, psychological risk and consequences of falls and interventions designed to address them are discussed.

Fear of Falling, Fall Efficacy, and Balance Confidence

Fear of falling refers to an ongoing and persistent state of worry about falling, while fall efficacy or balance confidence refers to a belief in one's ability to avoid a fall. The estimated prevalence of fear of falling and low fall efficacy among older persons varies widely as a function of study and methodology used, but has been estimated to be as high as 85% [5]. According to Legters [8], about one in three older people without a fall history and two in three with a fall history report a fear of falling.

There is limited empirical information on how fear of falling and fall efficacy develop, partly because this is highly dependent on the individual. Injurious falls can increase fear of falling and reduce confidence in ability to maintain one's balance [9], and it is also probable that these psychological variables are affected by self-appraisals of physical abilities so that those who know that they have physical limitations (e.g. reduced muscle strength, poor postural control, general frailty) may be less confident in their ability to maintain their balance compared to

---

[1] Given a very high correlation between measures of falls efficacy and balance confidence and the similarity of the items comprising these measures [2,3], we treat the terms 'fall efficacy' and 'balance confidence' as being interchangeable.

those who are physically strong. To the extent that physical limitations increase with age, it is not surprising that older adults in general have lower balance confidence and higher fear of falling than younger persons [10]. At the same time, in a study of persons who were being treated for musculoskeletal injuries, age differences in balance confidence were not found [11]. The presence of age differences in balance confidence in the general population and the possible absence of age differences among those with musculoskeletal injuries support the idea that balance confidence is likely influenced by self-appraisals of one's physical status and capabilities. Additionally, depression and generalized anxiety have been linked to low self-efficacy and increased levels of fear of falling [12]. Depression is also known to affect cognitive domains such as attention, executive function, and processing speed, domains which are central to gait performance and falls [13]. Specifically, psychomotor slowing is a common feature among depressive patients, and has been shown to increase fall risk. Individuals with depression were more likely to walk with a cautious gait, similar to people with fear of falling [14].

The role of fear of falling and balance confidence in fall risk has been given extensive consideration since the pioneering work of Tinetti et al. [15] who recognized the importance of measuring fear of falling and fall efficacy, not only as risk factors for falls among older persons, but also as a common outcome following a fall. These investigators conceptualized a fall efficacy questionnaire as a measure of fear of falling based on Bandura's [16] social cognitive theory of self-efficacy. Although the idea of fall efficacy as a measure of fear of falling led to numerous investigations that supported the contribution of psychological factors to fall risk, conceptualizing fall efficacy as an index of fear of falling is conceptually incorrect [2]. While fall efficacy, measured by tools such as the Falls Efficacy Scale (FES) [15] and the Activity and Balance Confidence (ABC) Scale [17] and fear of falling measured by tools such as the Survey of Activities and Fear of Falling in the Elderly (SAFFE) [18] tend to be correlated, they are distinct and possibly overlapping dimensions [19]. Self-efficacy beliefs are about one's own ability and are different from fear, which is an emotion. While low self-efficacy beliefs about balance are likely to contribute to fear of falling, fear also has physiological (e.g. increased skin conductance and heart rate) and behavioural (e.g. avoidance) components. Focusing on self-efficacy and confidence alone does not adequately capture the construct of fear. While measures of balance confidence and self-efficacy are highly correlated with one another, they are less correlated with measures of fear of falling [3]. Moreover, fall efficacy appears to make distinct contributions to the prediction of functional ability after fear of falling has been controlled for supporting the distinctiveness of the two constructs [20]. Finally, fall efficacy and fear of falling appear to have different correlates [21]. Nonetheless, both fear of falling and balance confidence have been associated with an increased risk of future falls and with reductions in quality of life [22–24] perhaps because fear of falling often leads to a reduction in activity levels and community participation [25]. Some research has suggested that balance confidence may be a mediator in the relationship between fear of falling and subsequent falls [26]. Denison et al. [20] supported this idea and demonstrated that self-efficacy was observed to be a key mediator between pain-related fear and falls. Li et al. [24] also demonstrated that self-efficacy was the mediating factor between fear of falling and functional ability. More research is needed to clarify this relationship; it is likely that low falls efficacy may precede fear of falling in at least some cases.

It is sometimes assumed that fear of falling leads to fall risk because it increases activity avoidance which in turn leads to stiffness and deconditioning (e.g. [27]). Activity avoidance and reduced engagement in physical activities are commonly observed in people with fear of falling [24]. Behavioural conceptualizations suggest that fear of falling may be maintained through reinforcement associated with short-term anxiety reduction. Moreover, by constantly avoiding fear-evoking activities, an individual is unable to learn that those activities may be performed safely, without falling [28]. As such, it has been argued that this cyclical pattern of activity avoidance, fear of falling, and physical deconditioning can result in further physical decline and falls [27]. However, the idea of avoidance as a mediator between fear of falling and falls is not well supported. Specifically, longitudinal research has established that fear of falling leads to increased activity avoidance, but increased activity avoidance has not been associated with increased probability of a fall over a six-month period [21]. It is possible that avoidance plays a role in fall prediction over a longer time period, but this possibility remains to be investigated.

An alternative explanation of the relationship between fear and falls is that fear of falling and anxiety have a direct negative effect on balance performance [2]. Fear of falling can change how people walk and cause a so-called cautious gait of shorter stride length and longer double limb support [14]. Experimental research has demonstrated that increased anxiety and fear are associated with a less stable posture and a cautious gait that, paradoxically, increases fall risk [6, 29–31]. While changes in spatial and temporal gait parameters are primarily caused by physical factors, greater levels of fear of falling can lead to additional adaptations in more challenging situations [32]. Therefore, it has been suggested that this protective strategy may reduce walking stability and directly increase fall risk as a result [33]. That said, there is also some evidence that, at least in non-fearful people, challenging walking tasks (which are accompanied by elevations in physiological indicators of anxiety) can also result in helpful gait adaptations that may help prevent falls [34].

A third possible explanation of the relationship between fear of falling and falls relates to the aforementioned possibility that both fear of falling and balance confidence are associated with awareness of one's physical limitations and that those who are fearful of falling may be more likely to have independent risk factors for falling that are difficult to measure in research studies. Nevertheless, several studies have demonstrated that fear of falling can be excessive [9], possibly due to previous negative experiences with traumatic falls [35].

Depression and Anxiety

Although a variety of biopsychosocial factors contribute to the causation of depressive and anxiety-related disorders (e.g. loneliness and social isolation, genetic factors, financial strain, chronic illness), depression and anxiety can also be the result of frailty and musculoskeletal injury resulting from falls or other accidents [36]. Specifically, depression has been identified as a consequence of falling with more depressed mood shown in people with a prolonged recovery, possibly related to reduced functional ability [37,38]. In one study, people recovering from a fall-related fracture showed a higher prevalence of depression at a four-month follow-up compared to the control group [39]. Severe depressive symptoms have been associated with an increased risk of onset of disability in activities of daily living (ADLs) as well as an increased risk of mortality and impaired psychosocial functioning [40,41].

Large studies have reported the prevalence of depressive symptoms to be about 15% in the general population and up to 35% in community-dwelling older adults [42]. Depression shows a curvilinear relationship with age, decreasing in middle age and increasing again in the 'older-old' group (85 years and over) [43]. Moreover, depressive symptoms are highly co-morbid with anxiety disorders in older adults [4]. The prevalence of anxiety-related clinical problems in older adults has been estimated as being approximately 15–17% [44,45].

Although often occurring as a consequence of falling, depression and anxiety may also be predictive of falls in community-dwelling older adults [46–51]. One contributing factor is the use of medications which are often used to treat these conditions [52–54]. More specifically, selective serotonin reuptake inhibitors (SSRIs) and tricyclic antidepressants (TCAs) have been associated with increased risk of prospective falls and fractures [55–59]. Anxiolytic medications have also been linked to an increased risk of falls [60]. There is evidence that antidepressants are a risk factor for falls independently of depressive symptoms and that antidepressants are a stronger risk factor for falls than depression [5,6,38,57]. That said, Kvelde et al. [4] showed that depression also increases fall risk, independent of antidepressant use and of the reduced executive and physical functioning that may accompany depression. Several mechanisms besides antidepressant use have been suggested as mediating the relationship between falls and depression [61]. For example, depression increases the probability of sleep difficulties and may have a negative impact on appetite. In turn, insomnia increases the risk of falls, independent of sedative use [62], and poor appetite has also be associated with weight loss and nutrient deficiencies (e.g. vitamin D) that may increase fall risk [63]. Moreover, psychomotor and gait disturbances, and slower reaction times have been observed in people with depression and may also increase fall risk [61]. In addition, depression and falls share common risk factors (e.g. chronic medical illnesses, functional disability, history of falls) that can help explain the role of depression in the prediction of falls [42,61,64–66]. Finally, people with depression tend to present with elevated fear of falling, which is not surprising given the frequent association of anxiety and depression [54,61].

Although depression has been associated with fall risk in older adults, evidence establishing anxiety-related disorders (e.g. anxiety disorders, trauma-related disorders, obsessive compulsive disorder) as a risk factor for falls (over and above anxiolytic medications) has not been found consistently [10]. However, there are possible mechanisms that anxiety-related disorders could theoretically increase fall risk. For example, people who present with agoraphobia and are afraid to leave their home may have more limited opportunity to be physically active, which could impair their balance performance. In addition, insomnia, which frequently accompanies anxiety, could lead to insufficient sleep and resultant fatigue, which could also increase fall risk [62]. Finally, anxiety may compete with attentional resources that are needed to optimize balance while walking [67]. More specifically, based on Eysenck's processing-efficiency theory, the continuous worry resulting from such disorders competes for resources in working memory and can therefore interfere with tasks requiring complex attention and co-ordination [67]. More research on the possible association between anxiety-related disorders and falls is needed. It is not clear whether certain disorders (e.g. generalized anxiety disorder) are more or less likely to predispose to falls compared to other anxiety-related conditions, such as panic disorder.

Psychological Interventions in Fall Prevention

Psychological interventions designed to overcome fear of falling have been developed. Such interventions tend to be cognitive behavioural in nature and involve challenging unrealistic beliefs about falling, promotion of physical activity, exposure therapy (i.e. exposing participants, in a graduated way, to avoided activities so that they can get accustomed to them) and goal setting [68,69]. Frequently, these interventions are combined with exercise programs. In a meta-analytic investigation, Liu et al. [68] demonstrated that cognitive behavioural therapy is effective in reducing fear of falling and improving balance. The impact of these interventions on falls, however, is not clear.

Although more research is needed, several studies have shown that appropriate exercise interventions also tend to reduce fear of falling, at least in the short-term [70]. Moreover, given overwhelming evidence that exercise has a potent positive effect on anxiety and depression in general (e.g. [71,72]), more research is needed to determine the extent to which the effect of exercise on fear of falling is mediated by increases in balance and strength versus other psychological mechanisms that may affect wellbeing and social engagement (e.g. increases in self-esteem). It is probable that the effect of exercise in improving psychological risk factors for falling is multi-factorial.

Psychological interventions such as cognitive behaviour therapy have been shown to be effective in reducing depression and anxiety among older adults [73,74]. Such interventions should be considered, not only because they can help manage a risk factor for falling, but also because they are alternatives to anxiolytic and antidepressant medications that may increase fall risk. Although psychological interventions have been shown to reduce fear of falling, anxiety, and depression, it remains to be seen whether they are also effective in preventing falls.

Conclusions

Psychological variables such as depression, anxiety, and fear of falling are common in older adults and have been identified both as a risk factor for falls and as a potential consequence of falling. Physical factors, including poor balance and slowed gait speed, are associated with depressive symptoms and fear of falling, and have also been shown to predict falls. In addition, a number of psychological outcomes of falling have been reported as consequences of falling, including depression, fear of falling, reduced self-efficacy, and activity avoidance. Although targeted psychological interventions have been shown to reduce these psychological outcomes, it remains to be seen whether they are also effective in preventing falls.

REFERENCES

1. American Psychiatric Association. *Diagnostic and Statistical Manual of Mental Disorders. 5th Edn.* Arlington, VA: American Psychiatric Association; 2013.
2. World Health Organization. *Dementia.* 2019 www.who.int/en/news-room/fact-sheets/detail/dementia (accessed April 2021).

3. Alzheimer's Disease International, Prince M, Wimo A, Guerchet M et al. *World Alzheimer Report 2015.* www.alzint.org/resource/world-alzheimer-report-2015/ (accessed April 2021).

4. Allan LM, Ballard CG, Rowan EN et al. Incidence and prediction of falls in dementia: a prospective study in older people. *PLoS ONE.* 2009;4:e5521.

5. Tinetti ME, Speechley M, Ginter SF. Risk factors for falls among elderly persons living in the community. *N Engl J Med.* 1988;319:1701–7.

6. Anstey KJ, von Sanden C, Luszcz MA. An 8-year prospective study of the relationship between cognitive performance and falling in very old adults. *J Am Geriatr Soc.* 2006;54:1169–76.

7. Asada T, Kariya T, Kinoshita T et al. Predictors of fall-related injuries among community-dwelling elderly people with dementia. *Age Ageing.* 1996;25:22–8.

8. Taylor ME, Delbaere K, Lord SR et al. Physical impairments in cognitively impaired older people: implications for risk of falls. *Int Psychogeriatr.* 2013;25:148–56.

9. Petersen JD, Siersma VD, Christensen RD et al. The risk of fall accidents for home dwellers with dementia: a register- and population-based case-control study. *Alzheimers Dement.* 2018;10:421–8.

10. Baker NL, Cook MN, Arrighi HM et al. Hip fracture risk and subsequent mortality among Alzheimer's disease patients in the United Kingdom, 1988–2007. *Age Ageing.* 2011;40:49–54.

11. Harvey L, Mitchell R, Brodaty H et al. The influence of dementia on injury-related hospitalisations and outcomes in older adults. *Injury.* 2016;47:226–34.

12. Harvey L, Mitchell R, Brodaty H et al. Differing trends in fall-related fracture and non-fracture injuries in older people with and without dementia. *Arch Gerontol Geriatr.* 2016;67:61–7.

13. Weller I, Schatzker J. Hip fractures and Alzheimer's disease in elderly institutionalized Canadians. *Ann Epidemiol.* 2004;14:319–24.

14. Cree M, Soskolne CL, Belseck E et al. Mortality and institutionalization following hip fracture. *J Am Geriatr Soc.* 2000;48:283–8.

15. Marottoli RA, Berkman LF, Leo-Summers L et al. Predictors of mortality and institutionalization after hip fracture: the New Haven EPESE cohort. Established Populations for Epidemiologic Studies of the Elderly. *Am J Public Health.* 1994;84:1807–12.

16. Poynter L, Kwan J, Sayer AA et al. Does cognitive impairment affect rehabilitation outcome? *J Am Geriatr Soc.* 2011;59:2108–11.

17. Scandol JP, Toson B, Close JC. Fall-related hip fracture hospitalisations and the prevalence of dementia within older people in New South Wales, Australia: an analysis of linked data. *Injury.* 2012;44:776–83.

18. Gruber-Baldini AL, Zimmerman S, Morrison RS et al. Cognitive impairment in hip fracture patients: timing of detection and longitudinal follow-up. *J Am Geriatr Soc.* 2003;51:1227–36.

19. Franssen EH, Souren LE, Torossian CL et al. Equilibrium and limb coordination in mild cognitive impairment and mild Alzheimer's disease. *J Am Geriatr Soc.* 1999;47:463–9.

20. Leandri M, Cammisuli S, Cammarata S et al. Balance features in Alzheimer's disease and amnestic mild cognitive impairment. *J Alzheimers Dis.* 2009;16:113–20.

21. Suttanon P, Hill KD, Said CM et al. Balance and mobility dysfunction and falls risk in older people with mild to moderate Alzheimer disease. *Am J Phys Med Rehabil.* 2012;91:12–23.

22. Szczepańska-Gieracha J, Cieślik B, Chamela-Bilińska D et al. Postural stability of elderly people with cognitive impairments. *Am J Alzheimers Dis Other Demen.* 2016;31:241–6.

23. Taylor ME, Lord SR, Delbaere K et al. Reaction time and postural sway modify the effect of executive function on risk of falls in older people with mild to moderate cognitive impairment. *Am J Geriatr Psychiatry.* 2017;25:397–406.

24. Horikawa E, Matsui T, Arai H et al. Risk of falls in Alzheimer's disease: a prospective study. *Intern Med J.* 2005;44:717–21.

25. Taylor ME, Delbaere K, Lord SR et al. Neuropsychological, physical, and functional mobility measures associated with falls in cognitively impaired older adults. *J Gerontol A Biol Sci Med Sci.* 2014;69:987–95.

26. Whitney J, Close JC, Jackson SH et al. Understanding risk of falls in people with cognitive impairment living in residential care. *J Am Med Dir Assoc.* 2012;13:535–40.

27. Hauer K, Dutzi I, Gordt K et al. Specific motor and cognitive performances predict falls during ward-based geriatric rehabilitation in patients with dementia. *Sensors.* 2020;20:5385.

28. Beauchet O, Annweiler C, Callisaya ML et al. Poor gait performance and prediction of dementia: results from a meta-analysis. *J Am Med Dir Assoc.* 2016;17:482–90.

29. Valkanova V, Ebmeier KP. What can gait tell us about dementia? Review of epidemiological and neuropsychological evidence. *Gait Posture.* 2017;53:215–23.

30. Mc Ardle R, Morris R, Wilson J et al. What can quantitative gait analysis tell us about dementia and its subtypes? A structured review. *J Alzheimers Dis.* 2017;60:1295–312.

31. Camicioli R, Licis L. Motor impairment predicts falls in specialized Alzheimer care units. *Alzheimer Dis Assoc Disord.* 2004;18:214–18.

32. Nakamura T, Meguro K, Sasaki H. Relationship between falls and stride length variability in senile dementia of the Alzheimer type. *Gerontology.* 1996;42:108–13.

33. Sterke CS, van Beeck EF, Looman CW et al. An electronic walkway can predict short-term fall risk in nursing home residents with dementia. *Gait Posture.* 2012;36:95–101.

34. Taylor ME, Delbaere K, Mikolaizak AS et al. Gait parameter risk factors for falls under simple and dual task conditions in cognitively impaired older people. *Gait Posture.* 2013;37:126–30.

35. Taylor ME, Ketels MM, Delbaere K et al. Gait impairment and falls in cognitively impaired older adults: an explanatory model of sensorimotor and neuropsychological mediators. *Age Ageing.* 2012;41:665–9.

36. Mehdizadeh S, Dolatabadi E, Ng K-D et al. Vision-based assessment of gait features associated with falls in people with dementia. *J Gerontol A Biol Sci Med Sci.* 2019;75:1148–53.

37. Beurskens R, Bock O. Age-related deficits of dual-task walking: a review. *Neural Plast.* 2012;2012:1–9.

38. Allali G, Kressig RW, Assal F et al. Changes in gait while backward counting in demented older adults with frontal lobe dysfunction. *Gait Posture.* 2007;26:572–6.

39. Lamoth CJ, van Deudekom FJ, van Campen JP et al. Gait stability and variability measures show effects of impaired cognition and dual tasking in frail people. *J Neuroeng Rehabil*. 2011;8:2.

40. Amboni M, Barone P, Hausdorff JM. Cognitive contributions to gait and falls: evidence and implications. *Mov Disord*. 2013;28:1520–33.

41. Gonçalves J, Ansai JH, Masse FAA et al. Dual-task as a predictor of falls in older people with mild cognitive impairment and mild Alzheimer's disease: a prospective cohort study. *Braz J Phys Ther*. 2018;22:417–23.

42. Booth V, Logan P, Masud T et al. Falls, gait, and dual-tasking in older adults with mild cognitive impairment: a cross-sectional study. *Eur Geriatr Med*. 2015:S32–156.

43. Eriksson S, Gustafson Y, Lundin-Olsson L. Risk factors for falls in people with and without a diagnose of dementia living in residential care facilities: a prospective study. *Arch Gerontol Geriatr*. 2008;46:293–306.

44. Forsell Y, Winblad B. Psychiatric disturbances and the use of psychotropic drugs in a population of nonagenarians. *Int J Geriatr Psychiatry*. 1997;12:533–6.

45. Giron MST, Forsell Y, Bernsten C et al. Psychotropic drug use in elderly people with and without dementia. *Int J Geriatr Psychiatry*. 2001;16:900–6.

46. Lesén E, Carlsten A, Skoog I et al. Psychotropic drug use in relation to mental disorders and institutionalization among 95-year-olds: a population-based study. *Int Psychogeriatr*. 2011;23:1270–7.

47. Torvinen-Kiiskinen S, Tolppanen AM, Koponen M et al. Antidepressant use and risk of hip fractures among community-dwelling persons with and without Alzheimer's disease. *Int J Geriatr Psychiatry*. 2017;32:e107–15.

48. Eriksson S, Lundquist A, Gustafson Y et al. Comparison of three statistical methods for analysis of fall predictors in people with dementia: negative binomial regression (NBR), regression tree (RT), and partial least squares regression (PLSR). *Arch Gerontol Geriatr*. 2009;49:383–9.

49. Kröpelin TF, Neyens JCL, Halfens RJG et al. Fall determinants in older long-term care residents with dementia: a systematic review. *Int Psychogeriatr*. 2013;25:549–63.

50. Pellfolk T, Gustafsson T, Gustafson Y et al. Risk factors for falls among residents with dementia living in group dwellings. *Int Psychogeriatr*. 2009;21:187–94.

51. Hart LA, Marcum ZA, Gray SL et al. The association between central nervous system-active medication use and fall-related injury in community-dwelling older adults with dementia. *Pharmacotherapy*. 2019;39:530–43.

52. Taipale H, Hamina A, Karttunen N et al. Incident opioid use and risk of hip fracture among persons with Alzheimer disease: a nationwide matched cohort study. *Pain*. 2019;160:417–23.

53. Salva A, Roque M, Rojano X et al. Falls and risk factors for falls in community-dwelling adults with dementia (NutriAlz Trial). *Alzheimer Dis Assoc Disord*. 2012;26:74–80.

54. Sofi F, Valecchi D, Bacci D et al. Physical activity and risk of cognitive decline: a meta-analysis of prospective studies. *J Intern Med*. 2011;269:107–17.

55. Stephen R, Hongisto K, Solomon A et al. Physical activity and Alzheimer's disease: a systematic review. *J Gerontol A Biol Sci Med Sci*. 2017;72:733–9.

56. Taylor ME, Boripuntakul S, Toson B et al. The role of cognitive function and physical activity in physical decline in older adults across the cognitive spectrum. *Aging Ment Health.* 2019;23:863–71.

57. Sackley C, Levin S, Cardoso K et al. Observations of activity levels and social interaction in a residential care setting. *Int J Ther Rehabil.* 2006;13:370–3.

58. Passant U, Warkentin S, Gustafson L. Orthostatic hypotension and low blood pressure in organic dementia: a study of prevalence and related clinical characteristics. *Int J Geriatr Psychiatry.* 1997;12:395–403.

59. Kenny RA, Shaw FE, O'Brien JT et al. Carotid sinus syndrome is common in dementia with Lewy bodies and correlates with deep white matter lesions. *J Neurol Neurosurg Psychiatry.* 2004;75:966–71.

60. Taylor ME, Lord SR, Delbaere K et al. White matter hyperintensities are associated with falls in older people with dementia. *Brain Imaging Behav.* 2019;13:1265–72.

61. Olsson RH, Jr., Wambold S, Brock B et al. Visual spatial abilities and fall risk: an assessment tool for individuals with dementia. *J Gerontol Nurs.* 2005;31:45–51;quiz 2–3.

62. Cipriani G, Lucetti C, Nuti A et al. Wandering and dementia. *Psychogeriatrics.* 2014;14:135–42.

63. Hasegawa J, Kuzuya M, Iguchi A. Urinary incontinence and behavioral symptoms are independent risk factors for recurrent and injurious falls, respectively, among residents in long-term care facilities. *Arch Gerontol Geriatr.* 2010;50:77–81.

64. Kallin K, Gustafson Y, Sandman PO et al. Factors associated with falls among older, cognitively impaired people in geriatric care settings: a population-based study. *Am J Geriatr Psychiatry.* 2005;13:501–9.

65. Stapleton C, Hough P, Oldmeadow L et al. Four-item fall risk screening tool for subacute and residential aged care: the first step in fall prevention. *Australas J Ageing.* 2009;28:139–43.

66. Thapa PB, Gideon P, Fought RL et al. Psychotropic drugs and risk of recurrent falls in ambulatory nursing home residents. *Am J Epidemiol.* 1995;142:202–11.

67. Roitto H-M, Öhman H, Salminen K et al. Neuropsychiatric symptoms as predictors of falls in long-term care residents with cognitive impairment. *J Am Med Dir Assoc.* 2020;21:1243–8.

68. Roitto HM, Kautiainen H, Ohman H et al. Relationship of neuropsychiatric symptoms with falls in Alzheimer's disease: does exercise modify the risk? *J Am Geriatr Soc.* 2018;66:2377–81.

69. Buchner DM, Larson EB. Falls and fractures in patients with Alzheimer-type dementia. *J Am Med Assoc.* 1987;257:1492–5.

70. Fernando E, Fraser M, Hendriksen J et al. Risk factors associated with falls in older adults with dementia: a systematic review. *Physiother Can.* 2017;69:161–70.

71. Enache D, Winblad B, Aarsland D. Depression in dementia: epidemiology, mechanisms, and treatment. *Curr Opin Psychiatry.* 2011;24:461–72.

72. Cherbuin N, Kim S, Anstey KJ. Dementia risk estimates associated with measures of depression: a systematic review and meta-analysis. *BMJ Open.* 2015;5:e008853.

73. Seignourel PJ, Kunik ME, Snow L et al. Anxiety in dementia: a critical review. *Clin Psychol Rev.* 2008;28:1071–82.

74. Taylor ME, Butler AA, Lord SR et al. Inaccurate judgement of reach is associated with slow reaction time, poor balance, impaired executive function and predicts prospective falls in older people with cognitive impairment. *Exp Gerontol.* 2018;114:50–6.

75. Butler AA, Lord SR, Fitzpatrick RC. Reach distance but not judgment error is associated with falls in older people. *J Gerontol A Biol Sci Med Sci.* 2011;66:896–903.

76. Sherrington C, Fairhall NJ, Wallbank GK et al. Exercise for preventing falls in older people living in the community. *Cochrane Database Syst Rev.* 2019;1:CD012424.

77. Hopewell S, Adedire O, Copsey BJ et al. Multifactorial and multiple component interventions for preventing falls in older people living in the community. *Cochrane Database Syst Rev.* 2018;7:CD012221.

78. Sherrington C, Michaleff ZA, Fairhall N et al. Exercise to prevent falls in older adults: an updated systematic review and meta-analysis. *Br J Sports Med.* 2016;51:1750–8.

79. Burton E, Cavalheri V, Adam R et al. Effectiveness of exercise programs to reduce falls in older people with dementia living in the community: a systematic review and meta-analysis. *Clin Interv Aging.* 2015;10:421–34.

80. Pitkälä KH, Pöysti MM, Laakkonen ML et al. Effects of the Finnish Alzheimer Disease Exercise Trial (FINALEX): a randomized controlled trial. *JAMA Intern Med.* 2013;173:894–901.

81. Öhman H, Savikko N, Strandberg T et al. Effects of exercise on functional performance and fall rate in subjects with mild or advanced Alzheimer's disease: secondary analyses of a randomized controlled study. *Dem Geriatr Cogn Disord.* 2016;41:233–41.

82. Taylor ME, Wesson J, Sherrington C et al. Tailored exercise and home hazard reduction for fall prevention in older people with cognitive impairment: the i-FOCIS randomized controlled trial. *J Gerontol A Biol Sci Med Sci.* 2021;76:655–65.

83. Montero-Odasso M, Speechley M, Chertkow H et al. Donepezil for gait and falls in mild cognitive impairment: a randomized controlled trial. *Eur J Neurol.* 2019;26:651–9.

84. Prince M, Knapp M, Guerchet M et al. *Dementia UK: 2nd Edn – Overview.* London: Alzheimer's Society; 2014.

85. Jensen J, Nyberg L, Gustafson Y et al. Fall and injury prevention in residential care-effects in residents with higher and lower levels of cognition. *J Am Geriatr Soc.* 2003;51:627–35.

86. Neyens JC, Dijcks BP, Twisk J et al. A multifactorial intervention for the prevention of falls in psychogeriatric nursing home patients, a randomised controlled trial (RCT). *Age Ageing.* 2009;38:194–9.

87. Rapp K, Sarah EL, Gisela B et al. Prevention of falls in nursing homes: subgroup analyses of a randomized fall prevention trial. *J Am Geriatr Soc.* 2008;56:1092–7.

88. Rosendahl E, Gustafson Y, Nordin E et al. A randomized controlled trial of fall prevention by a high-intensity functional exercise program for older people living in residential care facilities. *Aging Clin Exp Res.* 2008;20:67–75.

89. Vlaeyen E, Coussement J, Leysens G et al. Characteristics and effectiveness of fall prevention programs in nursing homes: a systematic review and meta-analysis of randomized controlled trials. *J Am Geriatr Soc.* 2015;63:211–21.

90. Cameron ID, Dyer SM, Panagoda CE et al. Interventions for preventing falls in older people in care facilities and hospitals. *Cochrane Database Syst Rev.* 2018;2018: CD005465.

91. Hewitt J, Goodall S, Clemson L et al. Progressive resistance and balance training for falls prevention in long-term residential aged care: a cluster randomized trial of the Sunbeam Program. *J Am Med Dir Assoc.* 2018;19:361–9.

92. Bouwen A, De Lepeleire J, Buntinx F. Rate of accidental falls in institutionalised older people with and without cognitive impairment halved as a result of a staff-oriented intervention. *Age Ageing.* 2008;37:306–10.

93. Flicker L, MacInnis RJ, Stein MS et al. Should older people in residential care receive vitamin D to prevent falls? Results of a randomized trial. *J Am Geriatr Soc.* 2005;53:1881–8.

94. Sakamoto Y, Ebihara S, Ebihara T et al. Fall prevention using olfactory stimulation with lavender odor in elderly nursing home residents: a randomized controlled trial. *J Am Geriatr Soc.* 2012;60:1005–11.

95. Hewitt J, Saing S, Goodall S et al. An economic evaluation of the SUNBEAM programme: a falls-prevention randomized controlled trial in residential aged care. *Clin Rehabil.* 2019;33:524–34.

96. Toots A, Wiklund R, Littbrand H et al. The effects of exercise on falls in older people with dementia living in nursing homes: a randomized controlled trial. *J Am Med Dir Assoc.* 2019;20:835–42.

97. Alzheimer's Society. *Counting the Cost: Caring for People with Dementia on Hospital Wards.* London: Alzheimer's Society; 2009.

98. Young J, Inouye SK. Delirium in older people. *Br Med J.* 2007;334:842–6.

99. Fogg C, Griffiths P, Meredith P et al. Hospital outcomes of older people with cognitive impairment: an integrative review. *Int J Geriatr Psychiatry.* 2018;33:1177–97.

100. Dykes PC, Carroll DL, Hurley A et al. Fall prevention in acute care hospitals: a randomized trial. *J Am Med Assoc.* 2010;304:1912–18.

101. Haines TP, Bennell KL, Osborne RH et al. Effectiveness of targeted falls prevention programme in subacute hospital setting: randomised controlled trial. *Br Med J.* 2004;328:676.

102. Healey F, Monro A, Cockram A et al. Using targeted risk factor reduction to prevent falls in older in-patients: a randomised controlled trial. *Age Ageing.* 2004;33:390–5.

103. Hshieh TT, Yue J, Oh E et al. Effectiveness of multicomponent nonpharmacological delirium interventions: a meta-analysis. *JAMA Intern Med.* 2015;175:512–20.

104. Haines TP, Hill AM, Hill KD et al. Patient education to prevent falls among older hospital inpatients: a randomized controlled trial. *Arch Intern Med.* 2011;171:516–24.

105. Hill AM, McPhail SM, Waldron N et al. Fall rates in hospital rehabilitation units after individualised patient and staff education programmes: a pragmatic, stepped-wedge, cluster-randomised controlled trial. *Lancet.* 2015;385:2592–9.

106. Stenvall M, Olofsson B, Lundstrom M et al. A multidisciplinary, multifactorial intervention program reduces postoperative falls and injuries after femoral neck fracture. *Osteoporos Int.* 2007;18:167–75.

10

Medical Risk Factors for Falls

Naomi Noguchi and Vasi Naganathan

The early landmark trials which showed that multi-factorial interventions were effective in preventing falls included assessments of medical risk factors for falls which were then used to guide interventions. As discussed in Chapter 20, the identification of medical risk factors can inform which of a suite of possible multi-factorial interventions a patient should receive. The maintenance of the postural stability is a complex task involving many physiological systems (Chapters 2–5). Sensory input from visual and vestibular pathways, muscle spindles, and joint proprioceptors is channelled centrally to the brain where it is rapidly processed to produce appropriate and co-ordinated motor responses [1]. The key components of this process are represented in Figure 10.1, while Table 10.1 lists some of the diseases which can impact on these systems to increase an individual's risk of falling.

Many diseases can increase the risk of falling by a direct impact on physiological systems. For an example, cataract formation leads to impaired visual acuity and contrast sensitivity. However, some intermittent pathologies are never likely to be studied in such a way as to provide evidence of being an independent predictor of falls. For example, it is difficult to show a direct cause and effect relationship between intermittent cardiac arrythmia and falls, in the absence of constant cardiac monitoring.

One of the challenges in determining causes of falls is differentiating falls from syncope, and the inherent problem of limited recall or even amnesia for a fall event. In addition, individual disease processes can lead to an increased risk of falling via more than one physiological mechanism. For example, Parkinson's disease causes problems with balance and gait but can also have a direct impact on blood pressure, potentially leading to a fall via decreased cerebral perfusion.

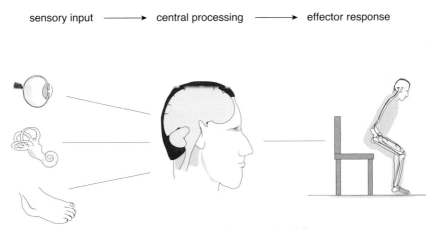

sensory input ⟶ central processing ⟶ effector response

Figure 10.1   Key components involved in maintenance of the postural stability.

Diseases Affecting Sensory Input

Vision

With ageing, the eye undergoes physiological changes which are associated with a decline in visual acuity, contrast sensitivity, depth perception, and visual field [2]. As outlined in Chapter 4, many authors have reported visual impairment, including poor visual acuity, poor contrast sensitivity, and reduced depth perception to be a strong risk factor for falls in older people [3]. Deficits in acuity and contrast sensitivity, restriction of the visual field, increased susceptibility to glare, and poor depth perception may result in misjudgement of distances and misinterpretation of spatial information such as the nature of ground surfaces. In addition to normal age-related refractive changes, older people are particularly susceptible to developing visual deficits from common eye pathologies including cataracts, macular degeneration, and glaucoma. Older people with diabetes and hypertension can also have the additional burden of associated retinopathies.

Cataracts

Cataracts affect approximately 30% of people over the age of 50 [4] and are a common cause of impaired vision in older people. The term *cataract* refers to an increase in the opacity of the lens, leading to smoky, cloudy, or hazy vision. Although cataract formation is predominantly a disease of old age, the changes in molecular structure of the lens due to the ageing process itself do not fully explain the production of cataracts. Cataracts form as a result of complex biochemical reactions which eventually lead to oxidation of the lens, membrane breakdown,

Table 10.1 Diseases having a direct impact on the maintenance of postural stability

Diseases affecting sensory input	**Vision**	Condition causing refractive error
		Age-related macular degeneration
		Glaucoma
		Cataracts
		Stroke causing visual field defect
	Proprioception	Diabetes
		Vitamin B12 deficiency
		Syphilis (rare)
		Degenerative joint disease, especially of neck and knees
	Vestibular	Age-related middle and inner ear changes
		Chronic ear infections
		Perforated ear drum
		Labyrinthitis
		Meniere's disease
Diseases affecting central processing	*Cerebrum*	Cerebrovascular disease (stroke)
		Dementia
		Brain tumour (benign and malignant)
	Cerebellum	Cerebrovascular disease (stroke)
		Long-term alcohol misuse
		Idiopathic cerebellar degeneration
	Basal ganglia	Cerebrovascular disease (stroke)
		Parkinson's disease
	Brain stem	Cerebrovascular disease (stroke)
		Postural hypotension
		Carotid sinus hypersensitivity
Diseases affecting effector response	*Spinal cord and nerves*	Any condition causing narrowing of spinal cord
		Motor neuron disease
		Multiple sclerosis
		Foot drop (common peroneal nerve)
	Muscles	Cerebrovascular disease (stroke)
		Motor neuron disease
		Muscular dystrophy
		Multiple sclerosis
		Polymyalgia rheumatica
		Polymyositis
		Hypothyroidism
		Vitamin D deficiency
		Diabetes
		Muscle disuse following fracture, injury, or prolonged immobility
	Joints	Osteoarthritis
		Rheumatoid arthritis
	Other	Foot problems
		Peripheral vascular disease
		Urinary incontinence

and eventual opacity, while ageing increases the susceptibility of the lens to the detrimental effects of these oxidative agents [5].

A number of studies have reported an association between the presence of cataracts and falls, but the majority have methodological limitations such as lack of adjustment for confounders or reliance on self-reported diagnosis of cataract [6]. The Blue Mountains Eye Study, however, had a large sample size (3654 people over the age of 49), conducted eye examinations in all participants, and took confounders into account [3]. This study found an association only between posterior subcapsular cataract and falls. This relatively uncommon cataract type is associated with systemic inflammation such as diabetes, smoking, drinking, and steroid use. Major types of cataract, such as nuclear cataract and cortical cataract, were not associated with falls.

Glaucoma

Glaucoma refers to the group of eye diseases characterized by raised intraocular pressure leading to pathological changes in the optic disc and resultant visual field defects that are irreversible. Glaucoma is a common cause of blindness in older people and affects approximately 5% of people in their seventies. Although the presence of glaucoma has not been associated with an increased risk of falls, the use of topical eye medications was associated with falling in one study [3]. The mechanism for this is unclear and may relate to glare caused by the eye drops or from orthostatic hypotension caused by systemic absorption of topical drugs that contain beta blockers.

Macular Degeneration

Several disorders can lead to degenerative lesions in the macular region of the retina. Age-related macular degeneration is the most common and serious form, affecting approximately nine percent of older people aged over 45 years with the prevalence increasing rapidly with age [7]. Age-related macular degeneration is irreversible and is recognized as the leading cause of blindness among older people in industrialized countries [8]. Despite the recognition of macular degeneration as a common and serious eye disease, few studies have assessed the role of macular degeneration as a risk factor for falls. Although one would imagine that vision problems due to macular degeneration would increase the risk of falls, the aforementioned Blue Mountains Eye Study in Australia found no such significant relationship [3].

Peripheral Sensation

The proprioceptive system contributes to stability, particularly during changes of position while walking and especially on uneven surfaces. It is of particular importance when other senses are impaired. Ageing is associated with reduced peripheral sensation, and several prospective studies have found that older people who experience falls perform worse in tests of lower limb proprioception [9], vibration sense [10], and tactile sensitivity [11, 12] (see Chapter 4). Loss of peripheral sensation can also result from a wide range of diseases, including diabetes mellitus, alcohol misuse, Vitamin B12 deficiency and chemotherapy [13]. The most common disease responsible for loss of peripheral sensation is diabetes [14]. In a landmark study of diabetic patients' prognosis, peripheral nerve damage occurred in up to 25% of people with diabetes mellitus after 10 years of being diagnosed with the disease, and up to 50% of people after 20 years disease duration [15]. People with diabetic neuropathy have impaired standing stability compared to age-matched controls [16] and perform worse in tests of foot position sense [17]. A systematic review found that older people with diabetes, especially those who are treated with insulin, are at increased risk of falls [18]. It is unclear whether this is because people on insulin are more likely to have peripheral neuropathy or because they are more likely to have other diabetic complications such as retinopathy.

Mechanoreceptors in the apophyseal joints of the cervical spine also play an important role in maintaining postural stability and damage to the cervical spine mechanoreceptors, such as degenerative joint disease, trauma, and cervical spondylosis, may also increase fall risk [19].

Vestibular Pathology

The function of the vestibular system is to generate information about head position and movement and to distribute this information to sites in the nervous system involved in the maintenance of postural stability. The vestibular system contributes to spatial orientation at rest as well as during acceleration and controls visual fixation during movement.

The three main components of vestibular function are: (i) the vestibulo-ocular reflex (VOR), which is responsible for generating eye rotations to compensate for movements of the head, (ii) the vestibulocollic (VCR) and cervicocollic (CCR) reflexes, which are responsible for stabilizing the head by initiating neck movements, and the (iii) vestibulospinal reflex (VSR), responsible for stabilizing the head and maintaining upright stance by triggering muscle activity in the neck, trunk, and extremities [20].

A wide range of conditions can impair the function of the vestibular system, including direct trauma, infection (labyrinthitis and vestibular neuritis), calcium carbonate deposition in the semi-circular canals leading to benign paroxysmal positional vertigo (BPPV), drug toxicity (aspirin, loop diuretics, aminoglycoside antibiotics, antineoplastic drugs such as cisplatin and carboplatin), vestibular migraine, cerebellar ataxia (gluten ataxia, CNS vasculitis, multiple sclerosis, infection, stroke, etc.) and auto-immune disease (ankylosing spondylitis, Behcet's disease, systemic lupus erythematosus, Sjoegren's syndrome, etc.) [21]. Depending on the site and severity of the impairment, vestibular disease may manifest as hearing loss, vertigo (an illusion of rotatory motion), and dizziness, thereby predisposing to instability and falls. The symptoms associated with vestibular pathology are discussed further in Chapter 20.

People with severe vestibular hypofunction demonstrate obvious impairments in posture and gait, characterized by postural instability and a broad-based, staggering gait pattern with unsteady turns [22] that place them at an increased risk of recurrent falls [23]. However, in cases of long-term total vestibular loss, gait may appear normal and deficits will only become apparent when the person stands in the tandem position with their eyes closed (the 'sharpened Romberg' position). This suggests that visual and somatosensory inputs are able to compensate for absence of vestibular input, and that vestibular loss may only produce overt postural instability if visual and peripheral sensation cues are altered or unavailable or if vision and peripheral sensation are also impaired.

The findings from observational studies have been inconsistent with regard to the association between impaired vestibular function and fall risk [23–25]. It appears that people with vestibular disorders are aware of their poor balance and adopt appropriate corrective strategies or reduce risk-taking behaviour. Another reason why epidemiological studies may not find the association is that for many people vestibular problems are intermittent in nature, akin to postural hypotension. No studies have examined the association between specific vestibular diseases and falls.

Diseases Affecting Central Processing

On reaching the brain, sensory information is channelled to the cerebrum, cerebellum, basal ganglia, and brain stem. Problems with balance can be experienced due to impaired central processing, despite normal sensory input and normal effector organ function. This section focuses on the common conditions that can impair central processing.

Stroke

Stroke is common in older people and represents a spectrum of symptomatology depending on the brain region affected. The severity of the symptoms also ranges from barely detectable changes in physical or cognitive functioning through to overt cognitive problems from vascular dementia or severe physical disability. Strokes are classified into two major types: brain ischemia and brain haemorrhage.

There are three main types of brain ischaemia: thrombosis (in situ obstruction of cerebral artery), emboli (debris originates elsewhere that blocks cerebral artery), and systemic hypoperfusion (due to a more general circulatory problem). Thrombotic strokes can be due to both large or small vessel disease. Brain haemorrhages account for approximately 15% of strokes and are more commonly seen in people with uncontrolled or poorly controlled hypertension. Brainstem and cerebellar strokes may cause damage to areas of the brain closely associated with balance, while sensory and visual inattention when recovering from a stroke may predispose a person to collide with objects. Parietal lobe damage may impair the planning and execution of locomotor activities, and in cases where the frontal lobes are damaged, there is the possibility that judgement may be affected, causing the older person to take risks when navigating obstacles in the environment [26].

Falls remain common for years following a stroke. In a large multi-centre study that determined the frequency of complications after strokes, 25% fell during the initial hospital admission and 45% fell between six and 18 months after discharge [27]. People who suffer falls following a stroke commonly attribute their falls to loss of balance, misjudgement/lack of concentration, or their foot dragging on the ground causing them to trip [28]. A number of studies have been performed to elucidate the potential mechanisms responsible for balance impairment in stroke patients, when standing, performing the sit-to-stand task and during walking. When lateral perturbations are applied to people with stroke when standing, they respond with a markedly abnormal postural response characterized by delayed-onset latencies and amplitudes of gluteus medius and hip adductor muscles, and increased muscle activity of the contralateral, non-paretic side [29]. During sit-to-stand, people with stroke who suffer from falls generate less force and exhibit greater medio-lateral sway than stroke patients who do not fall [30]. In addition, Brown et al. [31] assessed verbal reaction time when people with stroke and controls performed three postural tasks (sitting, standing, and standing with feet together). While the reaction times of the control participants did not differ across the three tasks, the stroke participants demonstrated a slowing of reaction time as the postural challenge increased, indicating that more attention was required for postural tasks following stroke.

A number of gait analysis studies have been performed in people who have suffered a stroke. The changes observed depend largely on the brain region affected [32]. However, in general, people with stroke exhibit an inability to generate sufficient forces in lower-limb muscles, and have difficulty co-ordinating the actions of agonist–antagonist muscle groups when walking [33]. This may result in a decreased ability to maintain the extended leg during the stance phase of walking and decreased foot clearance during the swing phase – factors that can predispose to tripping [26]. People with stroke also adopt different strategies when crossing over obstacles which may be protective of tripping, such as increasing toe clearance and step time [34].

These findings indicate that stroke is a strong predictor of falls and that the balance and gait impairments resultant from the disease are manifold and largely determined by the site and severity of the ischaemia or haemorrhage.

Parkinson's Disease

Extrapyramidal disorders lead to significant alterations in the sequencing of movement and may impair speed of a postural correction following a displacement. Parkinson's disease is characterized by the classic triad, first described by Sir James Parkinson, of bradykinesia, tremor, and muscular rigidity, and is known to affect approximately 1% of people in their seventies [35]. The disease is due to a deficiency of the neurotransmitter dopamine in the substantia nigra and associated nigra striatal pathway. It should not be confused with the syndrome of 'parkinsonism' which could be due to a number of causes, including small vessel ischaemia and adverse effects of medications.

Older people with Parkinson's disease commonly exhibit a flexed or stooped posture of both the trunk and limbs, and impaired postural equilibrium. The characteristic 'festinant' gait of the parkinsonian patient involves short, shuffling steps, lack of arm swing, loss of trunk movements, and decreased foot clearance [36]. These changes, while not associated with increased sway when standing [37], are associated with impaired responses to external perturbations [38], decreased functional reach [39], and increased variability in stride length when walking [40].

A systematic review has found that 60% of people with Parkinson's disease fall at least once per year, with 39% falling recurrently in this period, and that Parkinson's disease is a strong risk factor for falls in both community-dwelling and institutionalized older adults [41]. People with Parkinson's disease have a rigid posture, abnormal gait, and impaired ability to respond to external perturbations, factors that all predispose to falling. Finally, it has been suggested that recurrent falls may result from a loss of balance while turning or episodes of 'freezing' in which an individual attempts to overcome an inability to initiate movement and loses balance.

Cerebellar Disorders

The vestibulocerebellum and spinocerebellum regions of the brain are of particular importance to the maintenance of postural stability. Cerebellar disorders create grossly abnormal stepping patterns and impair corrective mechanisms. In addition to ischemia and haemorrhage that have been discussed in the previous section, other types of lesions in these regions as a result of drug toxicity, alcoholism, or degeneration, have also been shown to increase sway when standing [42–44]. Older people with cerebellar disorders tend to have truncal ataxia, a wide-based gait, and variable step length [45]. Although few authors have reported cerebellar dysfunction to be a risk factor for falls per se [46], two of the characteristic gait variables associated with these syndromes – wide-based gait [47] and irregular step length [48] – have been found to increase fall risk.

Dementia

Dementia affects approximately 5% of the population over the age of 60 years world-wide [49] and has been reported as a strong and consistent risk factor for falls in both community-dwelling and institutionalized adults [50]. Cognitive impairment associated with dementia may increase risk of falling by directly influencing the older person's ability to appropriately deal with environmental hazards, increasing the tendency of an older person to wander [51], and altering gait patterns [52]. In a community sample of 174 people with cognitive impairment, higher fall rates were associated with slower reaction time, impaired standing and controlled leaning balance, slower gait speed, impaired sit-to-stand ability, poorer visuospatial ability and executive functioning, and presence of depressive symptoms [53]. This pattern of findings is generally similar to that found in 109 nursing-home residents where fallers took more medications, including antidepressants, had more functional impairment, poorer balance and gait, were more impulsive and anxious, exhibited more dementia-related behaviours, and performed worse on cognitive tests involving attention and orientation, memory, and fluency [54]. Taken together, these findings indicate people with cognitive impairment who fall have significant physical risk factors in addition to disease-specific fall risk factors that impair cognition.

Falls in people with dementia are of particular concern in long-term care facilities, as cognitive impairment is one of the most common reasons for nursing home admission [55]. In institution-dwelling older adults, dementia has been shown to be associated with having at least one fall but not with serious fall-related injuries [55].

As outlined in Chapter 8, there is now some evidence of effective strategies to prevent falls in cognitively impaired people. However, few interventions have been widely implemented into clinical care and bone health in this population is often not considered because of concerns with compliance. Thus, individuals with cognitive impairment are at high-risk in terms of both falls and hip fractures [56, 57]. More trials of interventions to prevent falls in people with dementia are needed to provide greater certainty for evidenced-based approaches to prevention.

Depression

Fifteen percent of community-dwelling older people show significant depressive symptoms, with 1–2% exhibiting major depressive disorders [58]. Systematic review evidence from 25 prospective studies involving 21,455 participants has shown that for both studies reporting odds ratios and those stating relative risks, patients with baseline depressive symptoms had a greater likelihood of falling during follow-up (pooled OR: 1.46, 95% CI: 1.27,1.67 and pooled RR: 1.52, 95% CI: 1.19,1.84). In addition, depressive symptoms were equally likely to predispose to falls in community samples and those with identified healthcare needs [58].

The mechanisms underlying depressive symptoms and fall risk have not been fully evaluated; however, it has been suggested that older people who suffer from depression are less likely to be involved in physical activity, and are therefore at greater risk of falls due to reduced muscle strength, co-ordination, and balance [59]. A causal-path analytic model has also revealed the association between self-reported depression and choice stepping reaction time (a composite measure of fall risk) in older people was mediated by two paths: one through lower-imb weakness and the other through reduced executive functioning, with both mediating variables then influencing choice stepping reaction time via slow simple reaction time and impaired balance. The use of antidepressant medications has also been reported to be a risk factor for falls in community-dwelling and institutionalized older people, and while not well understood may relate to increased sedation and adverse effects on balance and gait (see Chapter 11).

Cardiovascular Problems Resulting in Neural Failure of Postural Control

The hindbrain is particularly prone to alteration in perfusion and a momentary disturbance may be sufficient to impair muscle tone long enough for a fall to occur. In addition, impaired baroreceptor function may dampen the physiological response to postural change and precipitate a fall secondary to a perfusion deficit. Any condition which has the ability to temporarily impair perfusion of the hindbrain has the potential to precipitate a fall which may or may not be associated with dizziness and/or syncope. The symptoms associated with brain hypoperfusion are further discussed in Chapter 20. The common causes of transient cerebral hypoperfusion relate to a drop in blood pressure or any tachy-/bradyarrhythmia.

Orthostatic Hypotension

Orthostatic hypotension, also known as *postural hypotension*, refers to a drop in blood pressure which occurs when transferring from a supine to an erect position. It is commonly defined as either a drop in systolic pressure of 20 mmHg or a drop in diastolic pressure of 10 mmHg on standing. *Symptomatic* orthostatic hypotension results when people report dizziness, light-headedness, or faintness at the time of the documented drop in blood pressure.

The prevalence of orthostatic hypotension in people over age 65 is about 20% [60–63]. Some of the variation that is observed between studies can be attributed to variations in the population assessed, the technique of blood pressure measurement performed, and the definitions used. In the Cardiovascular Health Study, 18% of people over the age of 65 had orthostatic hypotension, but only 2% were symptomatic [60]. Orthostatic hypotension is often due to medications that reduce blood pressure, such as antihypertensive agents, antianginals, antidepressants, antiparkinsonian medications, antipsychotics, and volume-depleting drugs such as diuretics [64]. Orthostatic hypotension is associated with heart failure, diabetes mellitus, Parkinson's disease, stroke, dementia, and depression [65]. In some diseases, such as diabetes or the Parkinson plus syndromes, orthostatic hypotension is due to autonomic nervous system failure [65].

A strong link between falls and orthostatic hypotension has not been found in longitudinal studies [66]. This relates partly to the intermittent nature of the condition, the frequent absence of symptoms and the need for long-term continuous monitoring to document blood pressure changes, including normal circadian changes [67], and post-prandial variations [68]. In clinical practice, the challenge is to determine if the finding of postural hypotension is of clinical significance in terms of fall risk. Further research may be required to determine the timing and frequency of orthostatic blood pressure measurement that is most predictive of falls [69].

Diseases Affecting Effector Response

Following central processing, efferent signals are transmitted via the spinal cord and peripheral nerves to limb and trunk muscles whereby continuous muscular correction maintains postural stability. Any disease or disability that affects the bones, muscles, and joints – the effector components of stability – may contribute to the risk of falling.

Osteoarthritis

Osteoarthritis is a common degenerative disease of articular cartilage which primarily affects the major weight-bearing joints of the body, leading to structural deformity, decreased range of motion, and pain. Older people with knee and hip osteoarthritis often suffer wasting of associated muscle groups, have difficulty rising from a chair and performing daily tasks, and tend to walk more slowly than older people without the condition [70]. There is also evidence to suggest that the presence of osteoarthritis impairs standing balance and joint position sense [71].

It has previously been shown that adequate joint range of movement in the lower limbs is essential to respond adequately to unexpected postural perturbations [72], while the presence of pain in lower limb joints may be a source of postural disturbance during voluntary movements. Thus, by reducing joint range of motion, reducing muscle strength, and causing pain in lower limb joints, osteo-arthritis can have a detrimental effect on postural stability in older people.

For these reasons, osteoarthritis has been widely assumed to be a risk factor for falls. However, a systematic review in 2013 has found that self-reported joint pain is associated with falls in older women but not in older men and that the presence of osteoarthritis was protective against fall-related fractures [73]. However, the Rotterdam Study, a large prospective cohort study involving 2773 people, showed that radiographic knee osteoarthritis was associated with both incident vertebral and non-vertebral fractures after adjusting for BMD and postural stability [74]. A number of intervention studies in patients with osteoarthritis reported improvements in strength and balance, but very few have resulted in reduced fall rates [75]. Future intervention studies need to evaluate the effect of such interventions on outcomes such as falls and fall-related injuries.

Myelopathy

Degenerative changes in the cervical spine (often referred to as cervical spondyl-osis) are common in older people. With advancing age, the spinal canal in the cervical region of the spine becomes increasingly narrow due to ligamentous hypertrophy, intervertebral disc herniation and formation of osteophytes on cervical vertebral processes. The narrowing of the spinal canal may lead to mechanical spinal cord impingement and associated postural dysfunction referred to as myelopathy [76]. Myelopathy is commonly associated with subject-ive reports of clumsiness, difficulty climbing stairs and experiences of the legs 'giving way', while objective findings include unsteadiness in standing and ataxic gait. No studies have reported myelopathy to be a prospective risk factor for falls in a large sample of older people. Nevertheless, it has been suggested that myelopathy may be under-diagnosed, and as such, may be a more common cause of falls than is widely recognized [77].

Other Diseases and Conditions

Peripheral Vascular Disease

Approximately 15% of people aged over 70 years have peripheral arterial disease (PAD) defined as ankle-brachial index (ABI) <0.90 in either leg [78]. PAD is a leading cause of mobility impairment due to its association with intermittent claudication – an intense, cramping pain in the calf muscles during exertion. People with PAD subsequently have lower levels of physical activity and may be at increased risk of falls. Gardner and Montgomery conducted the first investigation into balance and falls in older people with intermittent claudication [79]. Compared to 458 control subjects, the 367 participants with intermittent claudication exhibited 28% shorter unipedal stance time, were 86% more likely to report gait unsteadiness, and were more likely to have fallen in the last 12 months (26% versus 15% of controls) [79]. In participants with intermittent claudication, those with a history of falls exhibited 19% shorter unipedal stance time and took 14% longer to perform a sit-to-stand task [79]. Although these findings suggest an association between impaired circulation, instability, and falls, no adjustment for potential confounders was undertaken, so the relative importance of intermittent claudication compared to other fall risk factors remains unclear. Nor is it clear whether the mechanism for increased risk is solely through the effector response or whether impaired circulation can manifest itself through altered peripheral sensation.

Foot Problems

Foot problems are common in older people. The Framingham Study found in a cohort of older adults (mean age 71) that about 20% reported foot pain that limits their mobility on most days of the week [80]. Foot problems may result from osteoarthritic decreases in joint range of motion [81], dermatological conditions [82], detrimental effects of footwear such as high heels and narrow toe box [83], and systemic diseases such as peripheral vascular disease [84], diabetes mellitus [85], and osteoarthritis [86]. The most common foot problems in older people are painful corns and calluses, hallux valgus ('bunions'), and hammertoes. Women report a higher prevalence of foot problems such as bunions, corns, and calluses than men [87].

Foot problems constitute a major contributing factor to mobility impairment in older people. Older people with foot pain walk more slowly than those without and have more difficulty performing daily household tasks [88]. Twenty percent of older people who are housebound attribute their impaired mobility to foot problems [89], and there is some evidence that assessment of impaired foot and leg function can provide an accurate indicator of overall functional capability, and predict risk of nursing-home admission [90].

As the foot provides the structural foundation for both static support and progression of the body during locomotion, it is plausible that foot problems could increase the risk of falling [91]. A systematic review on the association between foot problems found that foot pain, hallux valgus, and lesser toe deformity are associated with falls [91]. However, many of the included studies defined foot problems poorly, clustering them together as 'foot problems' or 'foot disorders' or combining foot problems with leg problems [91].

A few studies that have directly investigated the role of foot problems in postural stability and falls. A study in which a detailed foot assessments of 135 older people was conducted found that a continuous score of overall foot impairment (including presence of lesions, hallux valgus, and lesser toe deformities) was a significant independent predictor of performance in a range of balance and functional tests, and discriminated between older people with and without a history of falls [92]. Of the foot problems documented in this study, the presence of foot pain and lesser toe deformity had the greatest impact on impaired balance and functional ability [92]. It has also been shown that hallux valgus, reduced ankle flexibility, reduced plantar tactile sensitivity, and toe muscle weakness are associated with impaired balance [93].

In community-dwelling older people with disabling foot pain, a multi-factorial podiatry intervention reduced the incidence of falls [94], and subsequent implementation trials lend support for this intervention as an effective fall prevention strategy (see Chapter 6).

Urinary Incontinence

Incontinence is a common and often under-diagnosed problem in older people, particularly older women. In industrialized societies, up to 34% of older men and 55% of older women suffer from an inability to control urinary functions but only a small proportion of both sexes seek medical care for their urinary incontinence [95, 96]. Both retrospective and prospective studies have consistently reported urinary incontinence to be a risk factor for falls in community-dwelling [97] older people but the excess risk was small when other fall risk factors were taken into account.

Although it has been hypothesized that incontinence leads to falls from loss of balance when rushing to the toilet, especially at night, or an increased likelihood of slipping on urine, there is some question as to whether incontinence is a primary cause of falls, or whether it is simply a marker of generalized physical frailty. While numerous falls in long-term care facilities occur when going to, or returning from the toilet [98], few falls in community-dwelling older people involve toileting. The close associations reported between incontinence, dementia, depression, falls, and level of mobility suggests that these 'geriatric syndromes' may have shared risk factors rather than causal connections [99].

Acute Illness

Acute illness may be precipitant for falls in older people and in particular those who are frail. Accordingly, fall rates in older people in acute hospitals are elevated, with national study data from England and Wales showing 83% of the falls occurred in patients aged over 65 years [100]. Acute illness can impair strength and balance, precipitate delirium and reduce blood pressure. In addition, routinely prescribed medications may have adverse effects in acute illness and newly prescribed medications may increase this risk.

Conclusions

Manifold medical conditions have been identified as risk factors for falls. These span conditions affecting sensory input, central processing, the effectors, and the cardiovascular system. Many of the diseases associated with falls manifest as physiological deficits which have been discussed in previous chapters. This diagnostic information informs medical management, as outlined in Chapter 20. However, the attribution of a degree of fall risk to a specific medical diagnosis has limitations, because the relative severity of the condition may vary considerably between individuals, and individuals may have multiple conditions. Furthermore, deficits in sensory and motor function may be evident in many older people with no recorded medical illnesses. As such, a holistic rather than a purely disease-oriented approach to fall risk assessment, which involves direct measurement of physical and mental capabilities, would appear to be a comprehensive approach to assessing risk of falling.

REFERENCES

1. Wolfson LI, Whipple R, Amerman P et al. Gait and balance in the elderly: two functional capacities that link sensory and motor ability to falls. *Clin Geriatr Med.* 1985;1:649–59.
2. Salvi SM, Akhtar S, Currie Z. Ageing changes in the eye. *Postgrad Med J.* 2006;82:581.
3. Boptom RQI, Cumming RG, Mitchell P et al. Visual impairment and falls in older adults: the Blue Mountains Eye Study. *J Am Geriatr Soc.* 1998;46:58–64.
4. Bailey RN, Zhang RW, Geiss LS et al. Visual impairment and eye care among older adults - five states, 2005. *Morb Mortal Wkly Rep.* 2006;55:1321–5.
5. Sekuler R, Kline D, Dismukes K. Aging and human visual function. *Optom Vis Sci.* 1983;60:547.
6. Herndon JG, Helmick CG, Sattin RW et al. Chronic medical conditions and risk of fall injury events at home in older adults. *J Am Geriatr Soc.* 1997;45:739–43.
7. Wong WL, Su X, Li X et al. Global prevalence of age-related macular degeneration and disease burden projection for 2020 and 2040: a systematic review and meta-analysis. *Lancet Glob Health.* 2014;2:e106–16.
8. Vingerling JR, Klaver CC, Hofman A et al. Epidemiology of age-related maculopathy. *Epidemiol Rev.* 1995;17:347.
9. Lord SR, Ward JA, Williams P et al. Physiological factors associated with falls in older community-dwelling women. *J Am Geriatr Soc.* 1994;42:1110–17.

10. Koski K, Luukinen H, Laippala P et al. Risk factors for major injurious falls among the home-dwelling elderly by functional abilities: a prospective population-based study. *Gerontology*. 1998;44:232.

11. Sorock GS, Labiner DM. Peripheral neuromuscular dysfunction and falls in an elderly cohort. *Am J Epidemiol*. 1992;136:584–91.

12. Lord S, Lloyd D, Li S. Sensori-motor function, gait patterns and falls in community-dwelling women. *Age Ageing*. 1996;25:292.

13. Sabin T. Peripheral neuropathy: disorders of proprioception. In: Masdeu J, Sudarsky L, Wolfson L, (Eds.) *Gait Disorders of Aging: Falls and Therapeutic Strategies*. Philadelphia: Lippincott-Raven; 1997.

14. Barrell K, Smith AG. Peripheral neuropathy. *Med Clin North Am*. 2019;103:383–97.

15. Pirart J. Diabetes mellitus and its degenerative complications: a prospective study of 4,400 patients observed between 1947 and 1973. *Diabetes Care*. 1978;1:168–88.

16. Simoneau GG, Ulbrecht JS, Derr JA et al. Postural instability in patients with diabetic sensory neuropathy. *Diabetes Care*. 1994;17:1411–21.

17. Simoneau GG, Derr JA, Ulbrecht JS et al. Diabetic sensory neuropathy effect on ankle joint movement perception. *Arch Phys Med Rehab*. 1996;77:453–60.

18. Yang Y, Hu X, Zhang Q et al. Diabetes mellitus and risk of falls in older adults: a systematic review and meta-analysis. *Age Ageing*. 2016;45:761–7.

19. Wyke B. Conference on the ageing brain: cervical articular contributions to posture and gait: their relation to senile disequilibrium. *Age Ageing*. 1979;8:251–8.

20. Highstein S. How does the vestibular part of the inner ear work? In: Baloh R, Halmagyi G, (Eds.) *Disorders of the Vestibular System*. New York: Oxford University Press; 1996.

21. *Disorders of the vestibular system*. Baloh RW, Halmagyi GM, (Eds.) New York: Oxford University Press; 1996.

22. Fife TD, Baloh RW. Disequilibrium of unknown cause in older people. *Ann Neurol*. 1993;34:694–702.

23. Herdman SJ, Blatt P, Schubert MC et al. Falls in patients with vestibular deficits. *Am J Otol*. 2000;21:847–51.

24. Di Fabio RP, Greany JF, Emasithi A et al. Eye-head coordination during postural perturbation as a predictor of falls in community-dwelling elderly women. *Arch Phys Med Rehab*. 2002;83:942–51.

25. Whitney SL, Hudak MT, Marchetti GF. The dynamic gait index relates to self-reported fall history in individuals with vestibular dysfunction. *J Vestib Res*. 2000;10:99–105.

26. Tideiksaar R. *Falling in Old Age: Its Prevention and Treatment*. New York: Springer Publishing Company; 1989. 196.

27. Kumar S, Selim MH, Caplan LR. Medical complications after stroke. *Lancet Neurol*. 2010;9:105–18.

28. Hyndman D, Ashburn A, Stack E. Fall events among people with stroke living in the community: circumstances of falls and characteristics of fallers. *Arch Phys Med Rehab*. 2002;83:165–70.

29. Kirker SGB, Simpson DS, Jenner JR et al. Stepping before standing: hip muscle function in stepping and standing balance after stroke. *J Neurol Neurosurg Psychiatry.* 2000;68:458–64.

30. Cheng P-T, Liaw M-Y, Wong M-K et al. The sit-to-stand movement in stroke patients and its correlation with falling. *Arch Phys Med Rehab.* 1998;79:1043–6.

31. Brown L, Gage W, Polych M et al. Central set influences on gait. *Exp Brain Res.* 2002;145:286–96.

32. Mitoma H, Hayashi R, Yanagisawa N et al. Gait disturbances in patients with pontine medial tegmental lesions: clinical characteristics and gait analysis. *Arch Neurol.* 2000;57:1048–57.

33. Lamontagne A, Richards CL, Malouin F. Coactivation during gait as an adaptive behavior after stroke. *J Electromyogr Kinesiol.* 2000;10:407–15.

34. Said CM, Goldie PA, Patla AE et al. Effect of stroke on step characteristics of obstacle crossing. *Arch Phys Med Rehab.* 2001;82:1712–19.

35. Pringsheim T, Jette N, Frolkis A et al. The prevalence of Parkinson's disease: a systematic review and meta-analysis. *Mov Disord.* 2014;29:1583–90.

36. Martin JP. *The Basal Ganglia and Posture.* Philadelphia: Lippincott; 1967. 152.

37. Schieppati M, Nardone A. Free and supported stance in Parkinson's disease: the effect of posture and 'postural set' on leg muscle responses to perturbation, and its relation to the severity of disease. *Brain.* 1991;114:1227.

38. Rogers MW. Disorders of posture, balance, and gait in Parkinson's disease. *Clin Geriatr Med.* 1996;12:825–45.

39. Schenkman M, Morey M, Kuchibhatla M. Spinal flexibility and balance control among community-dwelling adults with and without Parkinson's disease. *J Gerontol.* 2000;55: M441–5.

40. Morris ME, Iansek R, Matyas TA et al. The pathogenesis of gait hypokinesia in Parkinson's disease. *Brain.* 1994;117(5):1169.

41. Allen NE, Schwarzel AK, Canning CG. Recurrent Falls in Parkinson's disease: a systematic review. *Parkinsons Dis.* 2013;2013:906274.

42. Mauritz KH, Dichgans J, Hufschmidt A. Quantitative analysis of stance in late cortical cerebellar atrophy of the anterior lobe and other forms of cerebellar ataxia. *Brain.* 1979;102:461–82.

43. Bronstein AM, Hood JD, Gresty MA et al. Visual control of balance in cerebellar and parkinsonian syndromes. *Brain.* 1990;113(3):767.

44. Horak FB, Diener HC. Cerebellar control of postural scaling and central set in stance. *J Neurophysiol.* 1994;72:479–93.

45. Diener HC, Nutt JG. Vestibular and cerebellar disorders of equilibrium and gait. In: Masdeu JC, Sudarsky L, Wolfson L, (Eds.) *Gait Disorders of Aging: Falls and Therapeutic Strategies.* Philadelphia: Lippincott-Raven; 1997.

46. Robbins AS, Rubenstein LZ, Josephson KR et al. Predictors of falls among elderly people: results of two population-based studies. *Arch Intern Med.* 1989;149:1628–33.

47. Woolley SM, Czaja SJ, Drury CG. An assessment of falls in elderly men and women. *J Gerontol A Biol Sci Med Sci.* 1997;52:M80–7.

48. Hausdorff JM, Edelberg HK, Mitchell SL et al. Increased gait unsteadiness in community-dwelling elderly fallers. *Arch Phys Med Rehab.* 1997;78:278–83.

49. Sosa-Ortiz AL, Acosta-Castillo I, Prince MJ. Epidemiology of dementias and Alzheimer's disease. *Arch Med Res.* 2012;43:600–0.

50. Muir SW, Gopaul K, Montero Odasso MM. The role of cognitive impairment in fall risk among older adults: a systematic review and meta-analysis. *Age Ageing.* 2012;41:299–308.

51. Mossey JM. Social and psychologic factors related to falls among the elderly. *Clin Geriatr Med.* 1985;1:541–53.

52. Nakamura T, Meguro K, Sasaki H. Relationship between falls and stride length variability in senile dementia of the Alzheimer type. *Gerontology.* 1996;42:108–13.

53. Taylor ME, Delbaere K, Lord SR et al. Neuropsychological, physical, and functional mobility measures associated with falls in cognitively impaired older adults. *J Gerontol A Biol Sci Med Sci.* 2014;69:987–95.

54. Whitney J, Close JC, Jackson SH et al. Understanding risk of falls in people with cognitive impairment living in residential care. *J Am Med Dir Assoc.* 2012;13:535–40.

55. Nawrot T, Van Rensbergen G. Medical conditions of nursing home admissions. *BMC Geriatr.* 2010;10:46.

56. Hsu B, Bleicher K, Waite L et al. Community-dwelling men with dementia are at high risk of hip but not any other fracture: the Concord Health and Ageing in Men Project. *Geriatr Gerontol Int.* 2018;18:1479–84.

57. Wang H-K, Hung C-M, Lin S-H et al. Increased risk of hip fractures in patients with dementia: a nationwide population-based study. *BMC Neurol.* 2014;14:175.

58. Beekman AT, Copeland JR, Prince MJ. Review of community prevalence of depression in later life. *Br J Psychiatry.* 1999;174:307–11.

59. Kvelde T, Pijnappels M, Delbaere K et al. Physiological and cognitive mediators for the association between self-reported depressed mood and impaired choice stepping reaction time in older people. *J Gerontol A Biol Sci Med Sci.* 2010 65;(5):538–44.

60. Rutan HG, Hermanson EB, Bild JD et al. Orthostatic hypotension in older adults: the Cardiovascular Health study. *Hypertension.* 1992;19:508–19.

61. de La Iglesia B, Ong ACL, Potter JF et al. Predictors of orthostatic hypotension in patients attending a transient ischaemic attack clinic: database study. *Blood Press.* 2013;22:120–7.

62. van Hateren KJJ, Kleefstra N, Blanker MH et al. Orthostatic hypotension, diabetes, and falling in older patients: a cross-sectional study. *Br J Gen Pract.* 2012;62:e696.

63. Valbusa EF, Labat EC, Salvi EP et al. Orthostatic hypotension in very old individuals living in nursing homes: the PARTAGE study. *J Hypertens.* 2012;30:53–60.

64. Mets TF. Drug-induced orthostatic hypotension in older patients. *Drugs Aging.* 1995;6:219–28.

65. Mathias CJ. Orthostatic hypotension: causes, mechanisms, and influencing factors. *Neurology.* 1995;45:S6–11.

66. Jansen S, Bhangu J, de Rooij S et al. The association of cardiovascular disorders and falls: a systematic review. *J Am Med Dir Assoc.* 2016;17:193–9.

67. Lipsitz LA. Abnormalities in blood pressure homeostasis that contribute to falls in the elderly. *Clin Geriatr Med.* 1985;1:637–48.

68. Puisieux F, Bulckaen H, Fauchais AL et al. Ambulatory blood pressure monitoring and postprandial hypotension in elderly persons with falls or syncopes. *J Gerontol A Biol Sci Med Sci.* 2000;55:M535–40.

69. McDonald C, Pearce M, Kerr SR et al. A prospective study of the association between orthostatic hypotension and falls: definition matters. *Age Ageing.* 2017;46:439–45.

70. Hurley MV, Scott DL, Rees J et al. Sensorimotor changes and functional performance in patients with knee osteoarthritis. *Ann Rheum Dis.* 1997;56:641–8.

71. Hassan BS, Mockett S, Doherty M. Static postural sway, proprioception, and maximal voluntary quadriceps contraction in patients with knee osteoarthritis and normal control subjects. *Ann Rheum Dis.* 2001;60:612–18.

72. Whipple R, Wolfson L, Derby C et al. Altered sensory function and balance in older persons. *J Gerontol.* 1993;48:71.

73. Ng CT, Tan MP. Osteoarthritis and falls in the older person. *Age Ageing.* 2013;42:561–6.

74. Bergink AP, Van Der Klift M, Hofman A et al. Osteoarthritis of the knee is associated with vertebral and nonvertebral fractures in the elderly: the Rotterdam Study. *Arthritis Care Res.* 2003;49:648–57.

75. Gillespie LD, Robertson MC, Gillespie WJ et al. Interventions for preventing falls in older people living in the community. *Cochrane Database Syst Rev.* 2012;CD007146.

76. Brain WR, Northfield D, Wilkinson M. The neurological manifestations of cervical spondylosis. *Brain.* 1952;75:187–225.

77. Sudarsky L, Ronthal M. Gait disorders among elderly patients: a survey study of 50 patients. *Arch Neurol.* 1983;40:740–3.

78. Selvin PE, Erlinger PT. Prevalence of and risk factors for peripheral arterial disease in the United States: results from the national health and nutrition examination survey, 1999–2000. *Circulation.* 2004;110:738–43.

79. Gardner AW, Montgomery PS. Impaired balance and higher prevalence of falls in subjects with intermittent claudication. *J Gerontol A Biol Sci Med Sci.* 2001;56:M454.

80. Menz HB, Dufour AB, Casey VA et al. Foot pain and mobility limitations in older adults: the Framingham Foot study. *J Gerontol A Biol Sci Med Sci.* 2013;68:1281–5.

81. Vandervoort AA, Chesworth BM, Cunningham DA et al. Age and sex effects on mobility of the human ankle. *J Gerontol.* 1992;47:M17.

82. Schiraldi FG. Common dermatologic manifestations in the older patient. *Clin Podiatr Med Surg.* 1993;10:79–95.

83. Menz HB, Morris ME. Footwear characteristics and foot problems in older people. *Gerontology.* 2005;51:346–51.

84. Robbins JM, Austin CL. Common peripheral vascular diseases. *Clin Podiatr Med Surg.* 1993;10:205–19.

85. Hingorani A, Lamuraglia GM, Henke P et al. The management of diabetic foot: a clinical practice guideline by the Society for Vascular Surgery in collaboration with the American Podiatric Medical Association and the Society for Vascular Medicine. *J Vasc Surg.* 2016;63:3S–21.

86. Black JR. Pedal morbidity in rheumatic disease. *J Am Podiatr Med Assoc.* 1982;72:360–4.

87. Dunn JE, Link CL, Felson DT et al. Prevalence of foot and ankle conditions in a multiethnic community sample of older adults. *Am J Epidemiol.* 2004;159:491–8.

88. Benvenuti F, Ferrucci L, Guralnik JM et al. Foot pain and disability in older persons: an epidemiologic survey. *J Am Geriatr Soc.* 1995;43:479–84.

89. Gorter KJ, Kuyvenhoven MM, de Melker RA. Nontraumatic foot complaints in older people: a population-based survey of risk factors, mobility, and well-being. *J Am Podiatr Med Assoc.* 2000;90:397–402.

90. Guralnik JM, Simonsick EM, Ferrucci L et al. A short physical performance battery assessing lower extremity function: association with self-reported disability and prediction of mortality and nursing home admission. *J Gerontol.* 1994;49:M85.

91. Menz HB, Auhl M, Spink MJ. Foot problems as a risk factor for falls in community-dwelling older people: a systematic review and meta-analysis. *Maturitas.* 2018;118:7–14.

92. Menz HB, Lord SR. The contribution of foot problems to mobility impairment and falls in community-dwelling older people. *J Am Geriatr Soc.* 2001;49:1651–6.

93. Menz HB, Morris ME, Lord SR. Foot and ankle characteristics associated with impaired balance and functional ability in older people. *J Gerontol A Biol Sci Med Sci.* 2005;60:1546–52.

94. Spink MJ, Menz HB, Fotoohabadi MR et al. Effectiveness of a multifaceted podiatry intervention to prevent falls in community dwelling older people with disabling foot pain: randomised controlled trial. *Br Med J.* 2011;342:31.

95. Shamliyan TA, Wyman JF, Ping R et al. Male urinary incontinence: prevalence, risk factors, and preventive interventions. *Rev Urol.* 2009;11:145–65.

96. Minassian V, Yan X, Lichtenfeld M et al. The iceberg of health care utilization in women with urinary incontinence. *Int Urogynecol J.* 2012;23:1087–93.

97. Chiarelli PE, Mackenzie LA, Osmotherly PG. Urinary incontinence is associated with an increase in falls: a systematic review. *Aust J Physiother.* 2009;55:89–95.

98. Ashley MJ, Gryfe CI, Amies A. A longitudinal study of falls in an elderly population II: some circumstances of falling. *Age Ageing.* 1977;6:211–20.

99. Tinetti ME, Doucette J, Claus E et al. Risk factors for serious injury during falls by older persons in the community. *J Am Geriatr Soc.* 1995;43:1214–21.

100. Healey F, Scobie S, Oliver D et al. Falls in English and Welsh hospitals: a national observational study based on retrospective analysis of 12 months of patient safety incident reports. *Qual Saf Health Care.* 2008;17:424–30.

11

Medications as Risk Factors for Falls

Lulu Ma and Vasi Naganathan

Medications have long been implicated as an iatrogenic cause of falls and fractures, with several prospective cohort studies providing support for a link between medications and falls. This chapter discusses the pharmacology of ageing and the potential physiological mechanisms by which medications may impair postural stability. Specific drug classes strongly associated with falls are highlighted and the role of optimization prescribing in relation to polypharmacy is explored.

Medications, Ageing, and Falls

The ageing process is associated with an alteration of the body's ability to absorb, metabolize, distribute, and excrete drugs (pharmacokinetics) as well as an alteration of drug effects at the intended target sites (pharmacodynamics). Changes occur in body composition with age, with a reduction in total body water and lean body mass and a relative increase in body fat which impact on the pharmacokinetics of drugs. Advancing age can also be associated with an increase in the number of disease processes that can impact on the body's ability to deal with and respond to drugs.

In addition to the effects of ageing, pharmacological properties and side effect profiles help explain why certain drugs impair postural stability and predispose to falls. For example, anticholinergic burden has been shown to impair balance and mobility, slow gait speed, and impair attention and concentration [1, 2]. This is exemplified in a study of residents in aged care facilities where both dose and number of anticholinergic and sedative drugs increased falls [3]. Orthostatic hypotension [4] is also a side effect of many medications (including antihypertensives, diuretics, antidepressants, and antipsychotics). However, the association between blood pressure lowering medications and falls is less clear, where recent meta-analyses suggest antihypertensives increase fall risk on initiation [5], but not in the longer term [5–8].

The majority of evidence linking medications to falls comes from observational studies. These studies have varied in quality and methods used, with many having

Table 11.1 Pooled odds ratios for falling associated with psychoactive medication classes[a]

Drug class	Number of studies	Pooled odds ratio
Antipsychotics	33	1.48 (1.23–1.79)
Antidepressants	48	1.69 (1.52–1.88)
Tricyclic antidepressants	5	1.95 (1.79–2.13)
Selective serotonin reuptake inhibitors	5	1.98 (1.87–2.10)
Benzodiazepines	26	1.73 (1.49–2.01)
Benzodiazepines (short acting)	4	1.42 (1.22–1.65)
Benzodiazepines (long acting)	4	1.54 (1.28–1.85)

[a] Compiled from Seppala L, Wermelink A, De Vries M et al. Falls-risk-increasing drugs: A systematic review and meta-analysis: II. Psychotrophics. *J Am Med Dir Assoc* 2018;19:371. e11–.e17)

Table 11.2 Pooled odds ratios for falling associated with analgesic medications[a]

Drug class	Number of studies	Pooled odds ratio
Antiepileptics	16	1.95 (1.65–2.31)
Analgesics	13	1.16 (0.85–1.60)
Opiates	14	1.51 (1.15–1.99)
NSAIDs	17	1.31 (1.11–1.55)

[a] Compiled from Seppala L, van der Glind E, Daams J et al. Fall-risk increasing drugs: a systematic review and meta-analysis: III. Others. *J Am Med Dir Assoc* 2018;19: 372.e1–.e8.

limitations relating to confounding by indication and single time-point assessments of medication use. However, several high-quality prospective cohort studies have been undertaken and consistent patterns of evidence have emerged from comprehensive systematic reviews and meta-analyses. Tables 11.1 to 11.3 provide summaries of the findings from the most recent systematic reviews.

Psychotropic Medications

Psychotropic medications, also known as central nervous system active medications and psychoactive medications, is a collective term for centrally acting drug classes including sedatives/hypnotics, antipsychotics, and antidepressants. These medications have been implicated as a group and individually in increasing fall risk. Two large cohort studies of community dwellers [9,10] demonstrated a dose-dependent association between psychotropic drug use and impaired sensorimotor function (with measures including tactile sensitivity, lower-limb muscle strength, reaction time, and postural sway).

Table 11.3 Pooled odds ratios for falling associated with cardiac medications[a]

Drug class	Number of studies	Pooled odds ratio
Antiarrhythmics	10	1.27 (0.79–2.06)
Digoxin	4	2.06 (1.56–2.74)
ACE inhibitors	12	1.03 (0.90–1.19)
Antihypertensives	28	1.38 (1.19–1.56)
Nitrates	5	1.24 (0.79–1.95)
Thiazide diuretics	5	1.16 (0.87–1.55)
Diuretics	35	1.02 (0.90–1.15)
Loop diuretics	3	1.58 (1.52–1.65)
Calcium channel blockers	15	0.98 (0.85–1.14)
Beta blockers	16	0.96 (0.87–1.06)
Alpha adrenoceptor antagonist	7	1.20 (0.89–1.61)

[a] Compiled from De Vries M, Seppala L, Daams J et al. Falls-risk-increasing drugs: a systematic review and meta-analysis: I. Cardiovascular drugs. J Am Med Dir Assoc 2018;9:371.e1-.e9.

In meta-analyses of both unadjusted and adjusted data in a systematic review of randomized controlled trials, cohort, cross-sectional, case-control, and case-crossover studies; Seppala et al. [11] found seven classes of psychotropic medications (antipsychotics, antidepressants, tricyclics, selective serotonin re-uptake inhibitors (SSRIs), benzodiazepines, short-acting benzodiazepines, and long-acting benzodiazepines) were associated with an increased risk of falls in older adults (see Table 11.1). Furthermore, many observational studies have found dose-dependent associations between higher doses or number of psychotropic medications on the one hand and a greater risk of falls on the other. This has been shown in community, inpatient, and residential aged care settings [10–13].

Benzodiazepines and Other Sedatives

Consecutive systematic reviews have found clear associations between benzodiazepines and falls [7,11,14], that is, people taking benzodiazepines are at 1.5–2 times the risk of falls compared to non-users. This association is present in both new and chronic users [15], with the risk greatest in the first few days after people commence taking these medications [16,17]. The risk of falls in benzodiazepine users has been also shown to be dose dependent [11,17]. For example, a large cohort study in residential aged care found the risk of falling was twice as high for people taking a diazepam equivalent dose >8 mg compared to an equivalent dose of <2 mg [17]. In addition to falls, benzodiazepine initiation has been associated with increased risk of fall-related injury and hip fracture [16,18].

Benzodiazepines are classified by half-life; short, intermediate, and long acting. There is a perception that benzodiazepines with a shorter half-life may be better tolerated and thus have a reduced risk of falls, but the evidence for this is mixed. While earlier meta-analyses demonstrated no difference in fall risk between short- and long-acting preparations [14,15], the most recent review by Seppala et al. [11] suggest shorter-acting medications may convey a lower risk. Although this should not be taken to mean that short-acting benzodiazepines carry no falls risk.

Non-benzodiazepine hypnotics are also used to treat insomnia. These medications include zolpidem, zopiclone, eszopiclone, and zaleplon and are known collectively as 'Z-drugs', and thought to be safer and better tolerated. However, a recent meta-analysis found increased risk of fractures and injuries with Z-drugs, and a trend towards increased falls [16,19].

Benzodiazepines and Z-drugs may predispose older people to falls by causing sedation and impaired balance. An epidemiological study demonstrated increased falls at night in those taking benzodiazepines with a half-life of <12 hours [17]. Laboratory studies involving healthy volunteers have shown that benzodiazepines and Z-drugs increase postural sway in a dose-dependent fashion [20], although Z-drugs to a lesser extent. In an early study, Swift et al. [21] found that postural sway was greater in older compared with younger participants for the same dose of benzodiazepine, and a more recent pharmacodynamic study found that the dose needed to reach the sedative point (EC50) in older healthy participants was half that required for younger participants [22].

Antidepressants

Antidepressant medication classes include selective serotonin re-uptake inhibitors (SSRIs), serotonin and noradrenaline re-uptake inhibitors (SNRIs), tricyclic antidepressants (TCAs), and monoamine oxidase inhibitors (MOAIs). Most studies exploring the relationship between antidepressants and falls have concentrated on SSRI and TCA classes, reflecting prevalent prescribing patterns. Systematic reviews have shown consistent associations between antidepressant use and falls in older people [11,23]. This increased risk is present for both SSRI and TCA classes; however, the risk may be higher in the SSRI group [11,24]. Fall risk appears to be highest on initiation of medications [11,23], with one study demonstrating an odds ratio (OR) of 6.3 (95% CI: 2.65,14.97) for hip fracture within the first two weeks after prescription of the SSRIs (fluoxetine or paroxetine) and 4.76 (95% CI: 3.06,7.41) after prescription of TCAs [25]. However, fall risk remains elevated with chronic use in a dose-dependent manner [11,15].

The underlying mechanisms by which antidepressants lead to increased fall risk remain largely unanswered and is an area requiring further evaluation. TCAs are associated with sedative effects to a much greater degree than SSRIs, yet the epidemiological data suggest they increase the risk of falls to at least the same extent. A study of prescription event monitoring of 13,554 patients taking an atypical antidepressant (mirtazapine) found that drowsiness and lassitude were the most frequent adverse drug reactions, which were highest in the first month of treatment [26]. Studies examining the effects of TCAs and SSRIs on balance and gait have produced generally consistent findings. Draganich et al. [27] found that a single dose of the TCA amitriptyline impaired gait when stepping over obstacles in healthy older volunteers but that this was not the case with single doses of the SSRIs desipramine or paroxetine. Similarly, in a study of depressed patients on long-term antidepressant treatment, patients taking TCAs had significantly impaired balance, whereas patients taking SSRIs did not [28]. Two studies have contrasted the effect of SSRIs on postural sway in depressed older patients. The first found sertraline increased postural sway [29], and the second found paroxetine did not [30].

Major depression is a serious condition, which, as discussed in Chapter 9, is associated with an increased risk of falls [31]. The adverse effects of medications and their interactions with patient co-morbidities and medications should be considered when prescribing antidepressants. In those taking antidepressants, the long term risk of falls and other adverse effects needs weighed up against the potential benefits of continued use.

Antipsychotics

Systematic review evidence indicates antipsychotic medications increase fall risk by approximately 1.5-fold [7,11,14] in older people living in both the community and residential care settings [11,14], and that higher doses increase the fall risk more than lower doses [11].

In terms of mechanisms regarding increased fall risk, Beuzen et al. [32] demonstrated that olanzapine and haloperidol significantly increased postural sway and impaired attention and memory in healthy older volunteers. The effect on postural sway was most marked on the initial dose, and was reduced by day 4 of administration, suggesting greater fall risk on medication initiation. In contrast, a more recent study demonstrated only minor motor activity, postural stability, and information processing impairments with doses of 0.25 and 0.5 mg of risperidone [33].

Despite fewer extrapyramidal side effects, it appears fall risk is not lower with the atypical antipsychotic agents, risperidone and olanzapine [11]. For example, in a study of 2005 aged care residents, Hien et al. [34] found the hazard ratios for falls were 1.32 (95% CI: 0.57,3.06) for risperidone, and 1.74 (95% CI: 1.04,2.90) for olanzapine after adjusting for a comprehensive range of fall risk factors, which indicated these medications were not associated with fewer falls than the older, more-established antipsychotics. In contrast, one randomized controlled trial indicated quetiapine did not increase fall risk, although observational studies have found higher doses of quetiapine increase fall risk [11].

Analgesics

Analgesics are a heterogenous group of medications with narcotic analgesics and non-steroidal anti-inflammatory drugs (NSAIDs) the most studied categories in relation to falls.

Opiates

Recent meta-analyses have demonstrated opiates to be associated with an increased risk of falls with pooled ORs of 1.6 (95% CI: 1.35,1.91) [35] and 1.51 (95% CI: 1.15,1.99) [36]. Another systematic review demonstrated that opioid use was associated with falls, fall-related injuries, and fractures [36]. The mechanisms by which opiate analgesics increase the risk of falling remains unclear.

NSAIDs

The evidence for increased risk of falls in NSAID users is inconsistent and studies remain limited. However, the most recent and comprehensive systematic review found NSAID use did not increase fall risk in an adjusted analysis (OR: 1.09, 95% CI: 0.96,1.23) [36].

Cardiovascular Drugs

Antihypertensives

Antihypertensives represent a broad group of medications that are used to lower blood pressure. Some common side effects of antihypertensive agents that may increase fall risk include balance and gait impairments, dizziness, and postural hypotension. The association between antihypertensives and falls is inconsistent. However, the risk of falling with antihypertensive use appears to be highest on initiation or within the first 24 hours of a dosage adjustment, then decreases to non-significant levels afterward [5]. Overall, there is no clear evidence that chronic antihypertensive use increases the risk of falls [5–8]. It is also possible that the lack of a consistent association could be due to some observational studies excluding syncope and fainting in their definitions of a fall.

Several meta-analyses have identified a protective effect of chronic beta-blocker use on falls [5,8]. It was postulated by these study authors that this may be due to the cardioprotective effect of beta-blockers or due to selective non-prescribing of beta blockers in more frail adults [5,8]. A large cohort study of beta blockers found there was an increased risk of falling associated with non-selective beta blockers, which was not present for selective beta blockers [38].

Diuretics

Diuretics may predispose to falls by extracellular fluid shifts. Loop diuretics have been shown to be associated with risk of falling in two meta-analyses [5,8]. This risk appears to be highest on initiation and remains elevated within the first three weeks of use [5].

Antiarrhythmic Medications

Type 1A antiarrhythmic medications and digoxin have been identified among the antiarrhythmic class to increase fall risk [6,8]. Although, the associations remain inconsistent and the effect size for falls is likely to be only modest [6,8].

Anticoagulants

The use of anticoagulant agents for stroke prevention in older patients at risk of falls remains controversial. Physician attitudes towards use of warfarin in older patients remains cautious, particularly so in those with co-morbidities or at higher risk of bleeding, falling, and medication non-compliance [39].

Some studies on warfarin and bleeding risk have argued strongly that the benefit of anticoagulation outweighs the risk of intracranial bleeding following a fall [40,41], and there is evidence that prescribing of warfarin does not significantly increase baseline bleeding risk in those at high risk of recurrent falls [41]. A more recent prospective cohort study demonstrated that patients on anticoagulation had far worse bleeding injury outcomes on repeat admissions for falls, including threefold mortality rate compared with those not on anticoagulation [42]. There is an ongoing need for individualized, shared decision-making when prescribing anticoagulants, especially in patients at high risk of adverse outcomes.

Polypharmacy and Evidence-Based Prescribing

The concurrent use of multiple medications is defined as polypharmacy. This is a phenomenon that becomes more common in older people with two or more chronic conditions [43]. The increased number of medications increase the potential number of adverse reactions and drug–drug interactions. Although the number of medications used by an individual could be considered a marker of their underlying co-morbidity, the evidence suggests that poorer outcomes are independent of their co-morbidities [44,45].

It has been consistently found that polypharmacy increases the risk of falls [24,43]. In a residential aged care setting, the use of four or more drugs was associated with a fourfold increase in falls [46]. In addition, it has been found that older people taking combinations of fall-risk increasing drugs, such as psychotropics or cardiac medications have a higher risk of falling than those taking combinations of lower-risk medications [6]. The association between polypharmacy and falls highlights the need for ongoing medication review in older people, and consideration to the possible harm of prescribing fall-risk increasing drugs in at-risk older people.

Conclusions

Both the ageing process and disease affect an older person's ability to deal with and respond to drugs. A failure of clinicians to appreciate the pharmacology of ageing can lead to untoward and potentially avoidable events, including falls and fractures in older people. Certain classes of medication have been found to predispose older people to falls, with the most convincing evidence for the centrally acting medications. Even after considering underlying disease, benzodiazepines, anticonvulsants, and antidepressants remain independent predictors of falling. Methodological limitations and the multi-factorial nature of falls aetiology have made it difficult to identify causal connections between medications and falls. Nevertheless, there is now evidence that changes in the central nervous system, postural hypotension, neuromuscular incoordination, and impaired balance are physiological mechanisms that mediate the association between medication use and falls. The prescription of multiple medications to older people will become increasingly more frequent in the context of evidence-based medicine and the development of new medications for the prevention and treatment of age-related diseases. Clinicians need to 'optimize' prescribing, such that older people have access to, and can make informed choices about, the combination of medications from which they potentially stand to benefit. Further research is required to ascertain the mechanisms by which some drugs increase an individual's risk of falling, and there is a need to further investigate the risks and benefits of withdrawing medications known to increase an older person's propensity to fall.

REFERENCES

1. Hilmer S, Mager D, Simonsick E et al. A drug burden index to define the functional burden of medications in older people. *Arch Intern Med.* 2007;167:781–7.
2. Cao Y, Mager D, Simonsick E et al. Physical and cognitive performance and burden of anticholinergics, sedatives and ACE inhibitors in older women. *Clin Pharmacol Ther.* 2008;83:422–9.
3. Wilson N, Hilmer S, March L et al. Associations between drug burden index and falls in older people in residential aged care. *J Am Geriatr Soc.* 2011;59:875–80.
4. Arjen M, Hoang P, Sharmin S et al. Orthostatic hypotension and falls in older adults: a systematic review and meta-analysis. *J Am Med Dir Assoc.* 2019;20:589–97.
5. Kahlaee H, Latt M, Schneider C. Association between chronic or acute use of antihypertensive class of medications and falls in older adults. A systematic review and meta-analysis. *Am J Hypertens.* 2018;31:467–79.

6. Leipzig R, Cumming R, Tinetti M. Drugs and falls in older people: a systematic review and meta-analysis. II. Cardiac and analgesic drugs. *J Am Geriatr Soc*. 1999;47:40–50.

7. Woolcott J, Richardson K, Wiens M et al. Meta-analysis of the impact of 9 medication classes on falls in elderly persons. *Arch Intern Med*. 2009;169:1952–60.

8. De Vries M, Seppala L, Daams J et al. Falls-risk-increasing drugs: a systematic review and meta-analysis. I. Cardiovascular drugs. *J Am Med Dir Assoc*. 2018;9:371.e1–9.

9. Lord S, Webster I, Sambrook P et al. Postural stability, falls and fractures in the elderly: results from the Dubbo Osteoporosis Epidemiology Study. *Med J Aust*. 1994;160:684–91.

10. Lord S, Anstey K, Williams P et al. Psychoactive medication use, sensori-motor function and falls in older women. *Br J Clin Pharmacol*. 1995;39:227–34.

11. Seppala L, Wermelink A, De Vries M et al. Falls-risk-increasing drugs: a systematic review and meta-analysis. II. Psychotrophics. *J Am Med Dir Assoc*. 2018;19:371.e11–17.

12. Thapa P, Gideon P, Fought R et al. Psychotropic drugs and risk of recurrent falls in ambulatory nursing home residents. *Am J Epidemiol*. 1995;142:202–11.

13. Salgado R, Lord S, Packer J et al. Factors associated with falling in elderly hospital patients. *Gerontology*. 1994;40:325–31.

14. Leipzig R, Cumming R, Tinetti M. Drugs and falls in older people: a systematic review and meta-analysis. I. Psychotropic drugs. *J Am Geriatr Soc*. 1999;47:30–9.

15. Hartikainen S, Lonnroos E, Louhivuori K. Medication as a risk factor for falls: critical systematic review. *J Gerontol A Biol Sci Med Sci*. 2007;62:1172–81.

16. Donnelly K, Bracchi R, Hewitt J et al. Benzodiazepines, Z-drugs and the risk of hip fracture: a systematic review and meta-analysis. *PLoS One*. 2017;12:e0174730.

17. Ray W, Thapa P, Gideon P. Benzodiazepines and the risk of falls in nursing home residents. *J Am Geriatr Soc*. 2000;48;6:682–5.

18. Cumming R, Le Couteur D. Benzodiazepines and risk of hip fractures in older people: a review of the evidence. *CNS Drugs*. 2003;17:825–37.

19. Treves N, Perlman A, Geron L et al. Z-drugs and risk for falls and fractures in older adults: a systematic review and meta-analysis. *Age Ageing*. 2018;47:201–8.

20. Allain H, Bentue-Ferrer D, Polard E et al. Postural instability and consequent falls and hip fractures associated with use of hypnotics in the elderly. *Drugs Aging*. 2005;22:749–65.

21. Swift C, Ewen J, Clarke P et al. Responsiveness to oral diazepam in the elderly: relationship to total and free plasma concentrations. *Br J Clin Pharmacol*. 1985;20:111–18.

22. Albrecht S, Ihmsen H, Hering W et al. The effect of age on the pharmacokinetics and pharmacodynamics of midazolam. *Clin Pharmacol Ther*. 1999;65:630–9.

23. Darowski A, Chambers S-ACF, Chambers DJ. Antidepressants and falls in the elderly. *Drugs Aging*. 2009;26:381–94.

24. Park H, Satoh H, Miki A et al. Medications associated with falls in older people: systematic review of publications from a recent 5-year period. *Eur J Clin Pharmacol*. 2015;71:1429–40.

25. Ensrud KE, Blackwell T, Mangione C et al. Central nervous system active medications and risk for fractures in older women. *Arch Intern Med*. 2003;163:949–57.

26. Biswas P, Wilton L, Shakir S. The pharmacovigilance of mirtazapine: results of a prescription event monitoring study on 13,554 patients in England. *J Psychopharmacol*. 2003;17:121–26.

27. Draganich L, Zacny J, Klafta J et al. The effects of antidepressants on obstructed and unobstructed gait in healthy elderly people. *J Gerontol A Biol Sci Med Sci*. 2001;56:M36–41.

28. Li X, Hamdy R, Sandborn W et al. Long-term effects of antidepressants on balance, equilibrium, and postural reflexes. *Psychiatry Res*. 1996;63:191–6.

29. Laghrissi-Thode F, Pollock B, Miller M et al. Comparative effects of sertraline and nortriptyline on body sway in older depressed patients. *Am J Geriatr Psychiatry*. 1995;3:217–28.

30. Laghrissi-Thode F, Pollock B, Miller M et al. Double-blind comparison of paroxetine and nortriptyline on the postural stability of late-life depressed patients. *Psychopharmacol Bull*. 1995;31:659–63.

31. Laboni A, Flint A. The complex interplay of depression and falls in older adults: a clinical review. *Am J Geriatr Psychiatry*. 2013;21:484–92.

32. Beuzen J, Taylor N, Wesnes K et al. A comparison of the effects of olanzapine, haloperidol and placebo on cognitive and psychomotor functions in healthy elderly. *J Psychopharmacol*. 1999;13:152–8.

33. Allain H, Tessler C, Bentue-Ferrer D, et al. Effects of risperidone on psychometric and cognitive functions in healthy elderly volunteers. *Psychopharmacology (Berl)*. 2003;165:419–29.

34. Hien LTT, Cumming RG, Cameron ID et al. Atypical antipsychotic medications and risk of falls in residents of aged care facilities. *J Am Geriatr Soc*. 2005;53:1290–5.

35. Bloch F, Thibaud M, Dugue B et al. Psychotrophic drugs and falls in the elderly people: updated literature review and meta-analysis. *J Aging Health* 2010;23:329–46.

36. Seppala L, van der Glind E, Daams J et al. Fall-risk increasing drugs: a systematic review and meta-analysis. III. Others. *J Am Med Dir Assoc*. 2018;19: 372.e1–8.

37. Yoshikawa A, Ramirez G, Smith ML et al. Opioid use and the risk of falls, fall injuries and fractures among older adults: a systematic review and meta-analysis. *J Gerontol A Biol Sci Med Sci*. 2020;75:1989–95.

38. Ham A, van Dijk S, Swart K et al. Beta-blocker use and fall risk in older individuals: original results from two studies with meta-analysis. *Br J Clin Pharmacol*. 2017;83:2292–302.

39. Pugh D, Pugh J, Mead G. Attitudes of physicians regarding anticoagulation for atrial fibrillation: a systematic review. *Age Ageing*. 2011;40:675–83.

40. Man-Son-Hing M, Nichol G, Lau A et al. Choosing antithrombotic therapy for elderly patients with atrial fibrillation who are at risk for falls. *Arch Intern Med*. 1999;159:677–85.

41. Donzé J, Clair C, Hug B, et al. Risk of falls and major bleeds in patients on oral anticoagulation therapy. *Am J Med*. 2012;125:773–8.

42. Chiu A, Jean R, Fleming M et al. Recurrent falls among elderly patients and the impact of anticoagulation therapy. *World J Surg*. 2018;42:3932–8.

43. Fried T, O'Leary J, Towle V et al. Health outcomes associated with polypharmacy in community-dwelling older adults: a systematic review. *J Am Geriatr Soc*. 2014;62:2261–72.

44. Frazier S. Health outcomes and polypharmacy in elderly individuals: an integrated literature review. *J Geront Nurs*. 2005;31:4–11.

45. Hajjar E, Cafiero A, Hanlon J. Polypharmacy in elderly patients. *Am J Geriatr Pharmacother*. 2007;5:345–51.

46. Neutel C, Perry S, Maxwell C. Medication use and risk of falls. *Pharmacoepidemiol Drug Saf*. 2002;11:97–104.

12

Environmental Risk Factors for Falls

Alison Pighills and Lindy Clemson

In relation to falls in older people, the focus on the environment is often restricted to the individual's immediate home surroundings [1]. However, the environment can be conceptualized on three levels: the individual's immediate home surroundings, which is the home and adjoining grounds, the wider community or local neighbourhood, and the country, including the social, cultural, and political context of the society in which the person lives, including accessibility, potential hazards relating to public facilities, government policy on environmental design, housing standards, public transport, neighbourhood conditions, and social networks [2]. Within each of these levels, the environment comprises social and physical elements [3]. In this chapter, the environment in relation to falls is defined as 'the context within which the occupational performance of the person takes place. It influences behaviour and in turn is influenced by the behaviour of the person' [4, p17]. This inclusive definition is used because there have been promising study findings suggesting that fall prevention interventions are effective in the wider community [5–8]. Further, there is debate about whether research should separately address falls in the home environment and those in the wider community, because hazards and risk factor profiles of people who fall in these environments differ [9–11].

Private Residences

Between 46% and 77% of all falls occur within the home or surrounding grounds [12–15]. The most frequently cited environmental risk factors in private residences by older people are slippery surfaces, obstacles in pathways, and poor illumination [16]. The most commonly identified hazards in formal assessments are mats, floor surfaces, steps/stairs, obstacles, and the absence of grab rails in bathrooms [15, 17, 18]. These design features contribute to injurious falls and are often the focus of recommended modifications [19]. Carter et al. [20] found that 80% of older people's homes had at least one hazard and 39% had more than five.

Bathrooms were the most hazardous room, with 66% having at least one potential hazard. Of interest, among those rating their homes as very safe, 30% had more than five hazards.

Indoor falls predominantly occur in frequently used rooms, such as the lounge/dining area, bedroom, kitchen, and bathroom [21–24]. The majority of falls occur during periods of greatest activity, with over 60% occurring in the afternoon [13, 23]. Night-time falls are less prevalent, but more serious, and predominantly occur in the bathroom or on poorly lit stairs, where harder surfaces and longer falls increase the risk of injury [14, 25, 26]. In the UK, it has been reported that approximately 57,000 older people experience falls on steps and stairs each year, of whom 1000 die and 22,000 are seriously injured [27–29].

Good evidence regarding the role of the environment is provided by prospective cohort studies, in which household hazards are assessed at baseline and falls are monitored subsequently over a defined period. Of the four studies that examined a broad range of hazards, none found household hazards to be associated with falls in primary analyses (Table 12.1). One study reported tripping hazards in hallways were associated with an increased risk of falls [30]. Secondary analyses from two others highlighted interesting findings in relation to hazards and falls when participants were classified as either vigorous or frail [31, 32] – see Table 12.1.

The study by Leclerc [33], is perhaps the best to date that has examined the association between home hazards and falls as it conducted home hazard assessments at baseline and every six months over 18 months in a frail older population (community-dwelling older people requiring home-care services). In addition, the statistical analysis adjusted for time-varying exposures, multiple events, and confounding factors. They found the presence of hazards was significantly associated with falls, with the risk of falling increasing by 19% with each additional hazard [33]. This innovative approach addresses, at least in part, the transient nature and risk of home hazards, and is consistent with randomized control trial evidence that indicates removing hazards as part of comprehensive occupational therapy interventions reduces the risk of falls in at-risk older people (see Chapter 23).

Residential Aged Care Facilities

Residents in aged care facilities are generally frailer than their community-dwelling counterparts, with more physical and cognitive impairments [34]. Indeed, residents in aged care facilities experience approximately five times more falls than older people living in private residences [35]. To prevent falls and maximize mobility, aged care facilities usually have fewer environmental hazards. Generally, corridors

Table 12.1 Summary of prospective cohort studies investigating the association between environmental variables and falls

Study	Participants	Risk factor assessment	Outcome	Comments
Tinetti et al. [12], USA, 12 m follow-up	n = 336 Age ≥ 75	Checklist administered by trained assessors	No association between the number of hazards identified and falls	Secondary analysis found vigorous people more likely to have a fall associated with an environmental hazard, many of which were outside the home [32]
Nevitt et al. [52], USA, 12 m follow-up	n = 325 Age ≥ 60	Self-administered questionnaire	No association between specific hazards and falls	People reporting environmental factors interfering with ADLs had a higher rate of multiple falls in the home with OR: 3.1, 95% CI: 1.4,6.2 Secondary analysis found that hallway rugs and a composite home hazard score were significantly associated with falls in vigorous people [31]
Campbell et al. [23], New Zealand, 12 m follow-up	n = 761 Age ≥ 70	Checklist administered by OTs	Hazards identified in assessment not associated with falls. Only 4% of falls involved identified hazards	Most falls occurred usual household items not identified as potential hazards
Gill et al. [30], USA, 36 m follow-up	n = 1088 Age ≥ 72	Checklist administered by trained assessors – research nurses	No relationship between environmental hazards and falls	1 of 13 hazards (tripping hazards in hallways) associated with falls (HR: 2.3, 95% CI: 1.2,4.6)
Leclerc et al. [33], Canada, 18 m follow-up	n = 959 Age ≥ 65	Checklist administered by a trained physical rehabilitation therapist	Presence of hazards significantly associated with falls and fall related injury in older people receiving home care	Environmental hazards in 91% of homes, most commonly in the bathroom. Mean 3.3 hazards per individual

are wider and fitted with handrails, showers and toilets are equipped with grab-rails, shower chairs and toilet frames are provided, and bathrooms are lined with slip-resistant flooring. However, such equipment can also be hazardous if incorrectly fitted, in poor working order or constituting trip hazards.

In a retrospective review of residential care facility fall incident reports, environmental factors, most commonly furniture, were involved in more than 50% of falls, with the majority of falls occurring in residents' rooms (57%) [36]. However, the environmental factors identified were commonly used household items and the precipitant may well relate more to the individual's ability to function effectively in his/her environment. Another retrospective study found that bed and toilet heights were inappropriate for the majority of residents [37]. While it is difficult to distil the contribution of environmental factors to falls in residential aged care, it is clearly good practice to provide safe environments for all older people regardless of their level of frailty [38].

Public Places

Older community-dwelling people spend only 78–90 minutes per day outside on average [39, 40], yet outdoor falls account for over 50% of all falls experienced by this group. Outdoor falls are associated with more serious injuries, [9, 11, 24, 39, 41] and most commonly occur while walking, resulting in forward falls onto hard surfaces [39]. Environmental factors involved in outdoor falls include uneven and wet surfaces and trip and slip hazards [39]. Outdoor falls commonly occur in yards or gardens, footpaths, streets or curbs, on outside stairs, and in car parks [11, 39].

It has been reported that in addition to vision impairment, factors generally considered to be protective for falls (younger age, being male, being physically healthy and active, having a faster comfortable walking speed, being able to negotiate high steps) are risk factors for outdoor falls [11, 24, 39]. This indicates that active older people are more likely to fall outdoors undertaking higher-risk activities [41]. There are few validated, reliable, assessments of identify outdoor fall risk. Of these, the Outdoor Falls Questionnaire (OFQ) [42] may have potential to determine both individual and population-level needs for outdoor fall prevention.

Behavioural Factors

Brace et al. [43] conducted semi-structured interviews to elucidate how people behaved in their home environment. Of their sample, 66% reported rushing, 80% reported hoarding clutter, 54% reported changing their own light bulbs, and 43%

undertook do-it-yourself activities. Participants also commonly reported not putting lights on at night when moving between rooms, and reasons for not doing so included being able to manage without lights, not wanting to disturb others, already having adapted to the dark conditions, not having considered using the light, saving money, and completing familiar tasks for which vision was not necessary.

In another study, a survey was conducted to investigate how older people negotiated their stairs [29]. Failure to switch on stair lights when using the stairs at night was reported by 18% of people. Reasons cited included to avoid being seen naked, because glass doors at the bottom of the stairs let in sufficient light, and the fact that too much light woke them up and prevented them getting back to sleep. Objects were found on the stairs in 29% of the households and 71% of participants reported placing objects on stairs. If participants had to carry an object downstairs that would cause them difficulty, 29% reported that they would not ask for help, and descend the stairs regardless. It was concluded that reducing falls on the stairs requires a holistic approach, addressing both the environment and behaviour.

Clemson et al. [44] undertook a qualitative study in which fall events were reconstructed to place them in the context of environmental hazards and contributing behaviours. Patterns of environmental/behavioural factors that led to falls included not paying attention to the route ahead, lack of familiarity with surroundings, inappropriate walking speed, altered behaviours due to reduced mobility and impaired vision, impaired physical functioning, lack of confidence, overexertion, and unnoticed environmental factors. In a study by Connell and Wolf, participant-cited behavioural factors contributing to falls included hurrying, carelessness, and inattention [45]. These authors evaluated the environmental and behavioural circumstances associated with falls and near-falls experienced by older people with re-enactments. Seven behavioural patterns were identified: collisions in the dark, failing to avoid temporary hazards, preoccupation with temporary conditions, frictional variations between shoes and floor coverings, and excessive environmental demands. Behaviours were then categorized as habitual (did not require planning) and intentional (required intention, planning, and reflection) and attention to the environmental–behavioural interaction was suggested as an essential component of the environmental assessment in relation to fall risk.

Assessment for fall risk should take account of the relationships between intrinsic, behavioural, and environmental fall risk factors. Pure hazard reduction fails to recognize the nature of environmental hazards, which may change frequently. It is not surprising that most falls are ascribed to environmental factors because environmental hazards are too ubiquitous to be eliminated, and the environment is too fluid to make 'fall proof'. For example, a visitor may leave

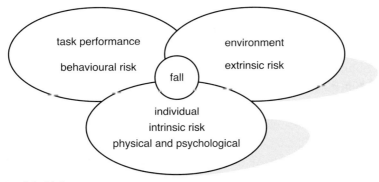

Figure 12.1   Model of falls.

a handbag strap in a walkway, posing an environmental hazard, which is removed on their departure. Figure 12.1 presents a model of falls, which depicts the nature of the relationship between the three risk categories. For example, an older person with lower-limb muscle weakness (intrinsic risk) ascending stairs lacking a handrail (environmental risk) in haste (behavioural risk) may fall. It would be inappropriate to consider any one category as the sole determining factor, without considering the impact of all three as observed during task performance.

Interaction Between the Individual, Behaviour, and the Environment

In line with the concept of environmental press [46], the relationships between physical competence, risk-taking behaviour, and environmental risk appear to play an important role in falls. Vigorous older people can withstand more demanding environmental challenges, which are more often encountered outdoors, but may fall in the presence of extreme challenges, such as slippery surfaces. Less physically able older people may limit themselves to less challenging and hazardous environments, and very frail older people may fall regardless of their environment [47]. Most robustly designed observational studies have shown that the mere presence of hazards is not associated with falling [48]. This supports the relevance of context, environment, use of environment, and a person's capacity as key features of environmental assessment for fall risk.

Conclusions

Falls within the home and surroundings are widespread, accounting for between 46% and 77% of falls experienced by community-dwelling older people. Outdoor falls are also common and are associated with more serious injuries. Despite only limited evidence for an association between environmental hazards and falls, identifying and remediating environmental hazards has good face validity [2, 49]. As fall risk involves the interplay between intrinsic, behavioural, and environmental risk factors, environmental assessment in the home should take intrinsic and behavioural risk factors into consideration in addition to the remediation of environmental hazards. Enhancing safety in public places should be conducted at the population level and focus on hazards that could be addressed through policy change (such as stair geometry and universal placement of grab bars in toilets and showers) and reducing environmental hazards through building code regulations and standardized universal design [26, 39, 50, 51].

REFERENCES

1. Lyons RA, John A, Brophy S et al. Modification of the home environment for the reduction of injuries. *Cochrane Database Syst Rev.* 2006;(4):CD003600.
2. Todd C, Ballinger C, Whitehead S. *A Global Report on Falls Prevention: Reviews of Socio-Demographic Factors Related to Falls and Environmental Interventions to Prevent Falls Amongst Older People Living in the Community.* Geneva: World Health Organisation; 2007.
3. Christiansen CH, Baum CM, (Eds.) *Occupational Therapy: Performance, Participation and Wellbeing.* Thorofare, NJ: SLACK Incorporated; 2005.
4. Law M, Cooper B, Strong S et al. The person-environment-occupation model: a transactive approach to occupational performance. *Can J Occup Ther.* 1996;63:9–22.
5. Cumming RG, Thomas M, Szonyi G et al. Home visits by an occupational therapist for assessment and modification of environmental hazards: a randomised trial of falls prevention. *J Am Geriatr Soc.* 1999;47:1397–402.
6. Nikolaus T, Bach M. Preventing falls in community dwelling frail older people using a home intervention team: results from the randomised falls-HIT trial. *J Am Geriatr Soc.* 2003;51:300–5.
7. Clemson L, Cumming RG, Kendig H et al. The effectiveness of a community-based program for reducing the incidence of falls in the elderly: a randomized trial. *J Am Geriatr Soc.* 2004;52:1487–94.
8. Campbell AJ, Robertson MC, La Grow SJ et al. Randomised controlled trial of prevention of falls in people aged 75 with severe visual impairment: the VIP trial. *Br Med J.* 2005;331:1136–43.
9. Bath PA, Morgan K. Differential risk factor profiles for indoor and outdoor falls in older people living at home in Nottingham, UK. *Eur J Epidemiol.* 1999;15:65–73.
10. Stel VS, Pluijm SMF, Deeg DJH et al. A classification tree for predicting recurrent falling in community-dwelling older persons. *J Am Geriatr Soc.* 2003;51:1356–64.
11. Kelsey JL, Berry SD, Procter-Gray E et al. Indoor and outdoor falls in older adults are different: the maintenance of balance, independent living, intellect, and zest in the elderly of Boston Study. *J Am Geriatr Soc.* 2010;58:2135–41.
12. Tinetti ME, Speechley M, Ginter SF. Risk factors for falls among elderly persons living in the community. *N Engl J Med.* 1988;319:1701–7.

13. Walker JE, Howland J. Falls and fear of falling among elderly persons living in the community: occupational therapy interventions. *Am J Occup Ther*. 1990;45:119–22.

14. Nyberg L, Gustafson Y, Breggren D et al. Falls leading to femoral neck fractures in lucid older people. *J Am Geriatr Soc*. 1996;44:156–60.

15. Peel N, Steinberg M, Williams G. Home safety assessment in the prevention of falls among older people. *Aust NZ J Public Health*. 2000;24:536–9.

16. Walker-Peterson E, Clemson L. Understanding the role of occupational therapy in fall prevention for community-dwelling older adults. *OT Pract*. 2008;13:1–8.

17. Clemson L, Roland M, Cumming RG. Types of hazards in the homes of elderly people. *OTJR*. 1997;17:200–13.

18. McNulty MC, Johnson J, Poole JL et al. Using the transtheoretical model of change to implement home safety modifications with community dwelling older adults. *Phys Occup Ther Geriatr*. 2003;21:53–66.

19. Shroyer JL. Recommendations for environmental design research correlating falls and the physical environment. *Exp Aging Res*. 1994;20:303–9.

20. Carter SE, Campbell EM, Sanson-Fisher RW et al. Environmental hazards in the homes of older people. *Age Ageing*. 1997;26:195–202.

21. Tideiksaar R. Home safe home: practical tips for fall proofing. *Geriatr Nurs*. 1989;10:280–4.

22. Sattin RW, Rodriguez JG, DeVito CA et al. Home environmental hazards and the risk of fall injury events among community dwelling older people: Study to Assess Falls Among the Elderly (SAFE) Group. *J Am Geriatr Soc*. 1998;46:669–76.

23. Campbell AJ, Borrie MJ, Spears GF et al. Circumstances and consequences of falls experienced by a community population 70 years and over during a prospective study. *Age Ageing*. 1990;19:136–41.

24. Bergland A, Jarnlo GB, Laake K. Predictors of falls in the elderly by location. *Aging Clin Exp Res*. 2003;15:43–50.

25. Nevitt M, Cummings S. Type of fall and risk of hip and wrist fractures: the study of osteoporotic fractures. *J Am Geriatr Soc*. 1993;41:1226–34.

26. Edwards N, Dulai J, Rahamn A. A scoping review of epidemiological, ergonomic and longitudinal cohort studies examining the links between stair and bathroom falls and the built environment. *Int J Environ Res Public Health*. 2019;16:1598.

27. Department of Trade and Industry. *Home Accident Surveillance System including Leisure Activities: 21st Annual Report 1997 Data*. London: Department of Trade and Industry; 1999.

28. Hill LD, Haslam RA, Brooke-Wavell K et al. *Avoiding Slips, Trips and Broken Hips: How Do Older People Use Their Stairs?* London: Department of Trade and Industry; 2000.

29. Hill LD, Haslam RA, Howarth PA et al. *Safety of Older People on Stairs: Behavioural Factors*. London: Department of Trade and Industry; 2000.

30. Gill TM, Williams CS, Tinetti ME. Environmental hazards and the risk of non syncopal falls in the homes of community-living older persons. *Med Care*. 2000;30:1174–83.

31. Northridge ME, Nevitt MC, Kelsey JL et al. Home hazards and falls in the elderly: the role of health and functional status. *Am J Public Health*. 1995;85:509–15.

32. Speechley M, Tinetti ME. Falls and injuries in frail and vigorous community elderly persons. *J Am Geriatr Soc.* 1991;39:46–52.

33. Leclerc BS, Bégin C, Cadieux E et al. Relationship between home hazards and falling among community-dwelling seniors using home-care services. *Rev Epidemiol Sante Publique.* 2010;58:3–11.

34. Andersson Å, Frank C, Willman AML et al. Factors contributing to serious adverse events in nursing homes. *J Clin Nurs.* 2018;27:e354–62.

35. Queensland Health. Stay on your feet: for hospitals and residential aged care facilities 2012. www.health.qld.gov.au/stayonyourfeet/for-hosp-facility (accessed April 2021).

36. Fleming BE, Pendergast DR. Physical condition, activity pattern, and environment as factors in falls by adult care facility residents. *Arch Phys Med Rehab.* 1993;74:627–30.

37. Capezuti E, Wagner L, Brush BL et al. Bed and toilet height as potential environmental risk factors. *Clin Nurs Res.* 2008;17:50–66.

38. Northridge M, Nevitt M, Kelsey J. Non-syncopal falls in the elderly in relation to home environments. *Osteoporos Int.* 1996;6:249–55.

39. Li W, Keegan THM, Sternfeld B et al. Outdoor falls among middle-aged and older adults: a neglected public health problem. *Am J Public Health.* 2006;96:1192–200.

40. Robinson JP, Silvers A. Measuring potential exposure to environmental pollutants: time spent with soil and time spent outdoors. *J Expo Sci Environ Epidemiol.* 2000;10:341–54.

41. O'Loughlin JL, Boivin JF, Robitaille Y et al. Falls among the elderly: distinguishing indoor and outdoor risk factors in Canada. *J Epidemiol Community Health.* 1994;48:488–9.

42. Chippendale T, Knight R-A, An MSM et al. Development and validity of the Outdoor Falls Questionnaire (OFQ). *Am J Occup Ther.* 2016;70:1–7.

43. Brace CL, Haslam RA, Brooke-Wavell K et al. *The Contribution of Behaviour to Falls Among Older People in and Around the Home.* Loughborough: Loughborough University; 2003.

44. Clemson L, Manor D, Fitzgerald MH. Behavioural factors contributing to older adults falling in public places. *OTJR.* 2003;23:107–17.

45. Connell B, Wolf S. Environmental and behavioral circumstances associated with falls at home among healthy elderly individuals. *Arch Phys Med Rehab.* 1997;78:179–86.

46. Lawton MP, Windley PG, Byers TD. *Ageing and the Environment: Theoretical Approach.* New York: Springer; 1982.

47. Lord SR, Shrerrington C, Menz HB. *Falls in Older People; Risk Factors and Strategies for Prevention.* Cambridge: Cambridge University Press; 2000.

48. Lord SR, Menz HB, Sherrington C. Home environment risk factors for falls in older people and the efficacy of home modifications. *Age Ageing.* 2006;35:55–9.

49. Lach HW, Reed AT, Arfken CL et al. Falls in the elderly: reliability of a classification system. *J Am Geriatr Soc.* 1991;39:197–202.

50. Blanchet R, Edwards N. A need to improve the assessment of environmental hazards for falls on stairs and in bathrooms: results of a scoping review. *BMC Geriatr.* 2018;18:272.

51. Edwards NC. Preventing falls among seniors: the way forward. *J Safety Res.* 2011;42:537–41.

52. Nevitt M, Cummings S, Kidd S et al. Risk factors for recurrent non-syncopal falls. *J Am Med Assoc.* 1989;261:2663–8.

13

Fall Detection and Risk Assessment with New Technologies

Kimberley S. van Schooten and Matthew A. Brodie

Recent advances in technology allow for remote fall detection and risk assessment in the home environment. Technology has the potential to contribute to the prevention of falls, and associated physical and psychological trauma, and thereby improve the lives of older people. The aim of this chapter is to provide a comprehensive overview of the fields of remote fall detection and risk assessment with a focus on wearable technology and its clinical utility.

Fall Detection

Although falls are a major health issue, most falls do not result in serious injury and when they do, medical assistance is generally prompt. Some falls, however, go unnoticed and consequences can be dire if the person is not able to get up or call for help. Previous studies report that between 50% and 80% of older people are unable to get up independently after a fall [1–3]. Common factors that increase the risk of falling, such as low muscle strength and cognitive impairment, also lead to difficulty getting up after a fall. Tinetti et al. [2] found that people who were unable to get up may spend up to two hours on the floor after a non-injurious fall, and two and a half hours in case of a injurious fall. Longer lies are associated with pressure sores, dehydration, hypothermia, and even death [2]. Even without physical consequences, long lies can lead to psychological distress, activity restriction, and subsequent functional decline. Personal response alarms can prevent some long lies, but 80% of fallers cannot or do not activate these alarms after a fall [1, 4]. Automatic fall detection could reduce long lies and their consequences by notifying a carer or call centre.

Stages of a Fall

Automatic fall detection works by detecting stages of the fall. A fall can be considered to be a cascade of five stages: (i) normal activities of daily living, (ii) critical or descent stage with a sudden free-fall motion, (iii) impact phase comprising the impact with the ground, (iv) resting stage with the person lying on the ground, and (v) recovery stage if the person is able to get up and move after the fall [5, 6]. Detection of any of these stages can be challenging because of their rarity and the diversity of daily-life behaviour, making accurate automatic fall detection a technical challenge. The following sections provide an overview of different technologies to detect falls.

Technology for Automatic Fall Detection

Automatic fall detection has been performed with environmental sensors and wearable sensors. Both approaches have their advantages and disadvantages. Environmental sensors, which can be optical, pressure, or acoustic based, generally provide rich information about not only the fall itself but also the circumstances of the fall. These technologies are unobtrusive as they do not require the user to wear a device; they are embedded in the environment.

Wu [7] describes one of the early attempts to detect falls based on video cameras. Three young participants were asked to perform daily activities (i.e. walking, transferring, stair walking, bending over) and trips, forward and backwards falls from standing. This study revealed that both vertical and horizontal velocity of the trunk increased at around 300–400 ms before the impact phase. More recent work has used advanced depth cameras and decision algorithms to automatically identify falls from camera surveillance systems. An example is the study by O'Connor et al. [8], who installed depth cameras in independent and assisted-living residences of 105 older people. The system estimated the speed of the body and acceleration prior to the person falling to the ground. Using this system, they automatically detected 64 real-world falls in 19 individuals.

Other techniques used to detect falls include instrumented floors and acoustics. Litvak et al. [9] have provided a proof-of-concept system that incorporates an accelerometer and microphone on the floor to differentiate between falls of a human-like dummy, daily activities, and dropping objects on the floor. They used a quadratic discriminant function to differentiate falls from other activities and reported a sensitivity and specificity of 95%. More recently, Minvielle et al. [10] developed pressure-sensitive flooring to detect falls. They asked 28 young volunteers to perform diverse falls and daily activities (e.g. walking, jumping, running, dropping objects on the floor) and tested various machine-learning classifiers to identify falls. They achieved an accuracy of 98.4% for falls using a random forest classifier. Environmental sensing methods are, however, limited in their range of operation and require considerable infrastructure.

Wearables for Automatic Fall Detection

Personal response alarms allow people to contact a carer or call centre for assistance in case of an emergency. These wearable devices date back to the

1970s when Wilhelm Hormann introduced the German 'Hausnotruf'-system and the American International Telephone Company introduced the 'Emergency Dialer[1]'. Automatic fall detectors were developed later, in the 1990s, after technological advances led to smaller electronic sensors. The first to report on these techniques were Lord and Colvin [11], who suggested using accelerometry to detect the impact of a fall, and Williams et al. [12], who used a piezoelectric shock sensor and a mercury tilt switch to detect the impact from a fall followed by a lying position. The field has grown considerably since then, but the concept has remained remarkably similar.

A fall is characterized by an initial rapid acceleration, followed by an almost instant deceleration when the body impacts the ground or lower level (see Figure 13.1). Early fall-detection algorithms focused on detecting this impact with the ground using a threshold on the magnitude of the acceleration signal. Once the magnitude of the acceleration signal exceeds this threshold an impact is detected and an alarm is raised. Others have combined this impact detection with detection of a change in orientation and a barometer to detect height change [13] to increase accuracy. The advantage of these methods is that they are relatively simple and have low processing requirements.

Threshold-Based Fall Detection

Bagalà et al. [14] performed a comprehensive evaluation of the accuracy of threshold-based fall detection methods on 29 real-world falls in 15 people. They captured real-world falls by monitoring a group of high-risk individuals (people with progressive supra-nuclear palsy and geriatric rehabilitation patients) during daily life using a single accelerometer worn on the lower back. While the accuracy of most fall detection algorithms was very high, exceeding 92% in 10 out of 13 algorithms [14], the sensitivity was considerably lower (median 48% of falls detected by the algorithms tested). The authors concluded that fall detection methods developed in laboratory settings did not perform well when attempting to detect real-world falls [14]. These findings highlight the need for independent validation and replication of results in real-life settings.

A major concern with detection algorithms is the number of false positives. Similar to the story of the boy who cried wolf in Aesop's fables, a high number of false positives could lead to saturation of the response to detected falls. Several common activities during daily life can lead to false positive fall alarms. Studies have reported false positives during elevator use, transport use, replacing the sensor, and putting it down [15, 16]. Bagalà et al. [14] also evaluated the rate of

---

[1] Advertised as 'Emergency Dialer' in Popular Science, October 1975, p104. https://books.google.com.au/books?id=LQEAAAAAMBAJ&lpg=PA104&dq=popular%20science%201930&pg=PA104#v=onepage&q&f=true

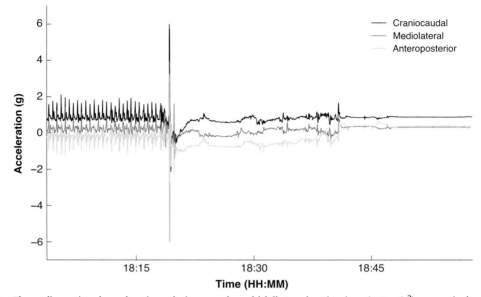

Figure 13.1   Three-dimensional accelerations during a real-world fall. Acceleration in g (9.8 m/s²) on vertical axis, time of the day on horizontal axis. The fall occurred at around 18:20 during walking, was followed by a short period of lying, transitioning to sitting, with standing up at around 18:40. Adapted from van Schooten KS, Pijnappels M, Rispens SM et al. Ambulatory fall-risk assessment: amount and quality of daily-life gait predict falls in older adults. J Gerontol A Biol Sci Med Sci. 2015;70:608-15 [40].

false positives of the investigated fall-detection algorithms during daily life in three fallers for whom they obtained 24-hour recordings. They observed false positive rates ranging between two and 84 falls per 24 hours (Figure 4 in Bagala et al. [14]), suggesting that these threshold-based algorithms are not yet suitable for daily-life use.

Pattern Recognition and Machine-Learning-Based Fall Detection

More recent fall detection development has moved from impact detection towards pattern recognition methods. The potential advantage of these methods is that they are able to detect a larger variety of falls and are less sensitive to signal noise. Zhang et al. [17] combined a support vector machine, kernel discriminant analysis, and a k-nearest neighbour classifier to identify falls. They collected data using mobile phones in 12 older adults, 20 young adults, and a dummy, who performed daily activities (e.g. walking, sitting down) and phone movement. Young adults also performed high-intensity daily activities (e.g. running, jumping), near falls and falling down on a soft surface, while the dummy was used to collect data during falling down on a hard surface. They trained the classifier on 67% of their data, and subsequently tested its accuracy on the remaining 33%.

They report sensitivity of 98% for low-impact falls and 97% for high-impact falls, with some false alarms during phone movement and the high-intensity daily activities. Kerdegari et al. [18] trained a neural network to recognise characteristics of falls. They asked 50 young adults to perform nine different activities of daily life (ADLs) and 11 types of falls inside the laboratory. They trained the neural network on 75% of their data, and subsequently tested its accuracy on the remaining 25%. They reported a sensitivity of 92%, specificity of 91% and accuracy of 92%. While high reported accuracies can be compelling, the data sets used are unlikely to be rich enough to train classifiers to detect real-world falls in clinical cohorts. In our view, orders of magnitude more data will be required to resolve this issue.

Real-World Utility of Fall Detection

Few of these more advanced techniques have been tested on real-world falls. Palmerini et al. [19] used wavelet analysis on the data reported in Bagalà et al. [14]. They created a typical fall trace by averaging the 29 real-world falls and determined the degree of similarity between real-world data and this typical fall trace. This technique achieved a sensitivity and specificity of 90%, with 0.72 false alarms per hour. The authors concluded that the wavelet analysis outperformed impact-based algorithms but cannot be used alone as a fall detector because of the high number of false alarms.

Most of these algorithms have been developed and trained on the same data set, which tends to inflate accuracy; there are, however, exceptions. Aziz et al. [20] trained a support vector machine on eight different ADLs, five near-fall activities, and seven types of falls performed by 10 young adults inside the laboratory. They then tested its accuracy on real-world data, including 10 falls, collected in 19 older people. They achieved a sensitivity of 80% and a specificity of 100%, with 0.05 to 0.15 false arms per hour.

Lipsitz et al. [21] were among the first to evaluate the accuracy of an established fall-detection algorithm in real life. They asked 62 older people living in a residential care facility to wear a commercial fall detector (Philips, the Netherlands) and compared the device to nursing staff fall-incidence reports. Concordance between these methods was low. The device detected 17 out of 89 falls within eight hours of the nursing staff report and had 111 false alarms during the monitoring period (on average 150 days per resident). Possible explanations for these findings are that the algorithm did not work well, the falls were low-impact, which the device could not detect, or that nursing staff fall incidence reports were inaccurate. Nevertheless, this clearly demonstrates that fall-detection techniques require improvement prior to real-world implementation.

Future of Automatic Fall Detection

Development of automatic fall detection algorithms is often hampered by a lack of representative and accurate data. With the increase of big data, data sharing, and initiatives such as the PROFANE fall repository [22] and the UKBiobank, this concern might be soon be one of the past. It is also anticipated that the use of biological signals and advanced processing may advance the field. To date, most wearables used for fall detection have used accelerometers, tilt sensors, gyroscopes, and barometers. Advances in technology will allow for inclusion physiological signals, such as heart rate, breathing rates, and perspiration, which may improve accuracy and reduce false alarms. Moreover, embedding these body-worn systems into a smart environment may enhance their accuracy even further.

Fall Risk Assessment

Identifying individuals at high risk for falls helps direct finite public health resources towards prevention of falls. Many low-tech fall risk assessment tools have been developed [23–25] but these tools are not always routinely integrated into clinical practice. Common explanations for their under-utilization are uncertainty about accuracy and lack of time, resources, and training. Technology has the potential to provide an accurate, relatively inexpensive and easy-to-administer assessment that could be used to track changing fall risk over years, months, hours, and minutes.

Technology for Fall Risk Assessment

A wide range of technologies have been used to estimate fall risk. Similar to techniques used for fall detection, these can be differentiated into environmental and wearable sensors. Environmental sensors for fall risk assessment usually comprise video cameras, ambient motion sensors, and/or pressure sensors. The sensors are relatively unobtrusive and can require minimal user input but are restricted in their capture volume.

Ejupi et al. [26] utilized the Xbox 360 Kinect system (Microsoft, USA) to assess five-times sit-to-stand performance as an indicator of fall risk in 94 community-living older adults. In this study, people who reported one or more falls in the past 12 months, took significantly longer to complete the five-times sit-to-stand test and moved significantly slower during the test compared to people who did not report falls over this period. Furthermore, in a sub-group of 20 people, the correlations between in-laboratory and at-home assessments were high (r ≥ 0.77), suggesting that at-home assessments are feasible. Mehdizadeh et al. [27] recently used a similar system to extract gait characteristics during everyday gait. They captured data of 52 older people with dementia, and showed that the estimated lateral margin of stability, step width, and step time variability were significantly associated with the number of falls during admission.

Other techniques to estimate fall risk include pressure sensors and sensor networks. Kwok et al. [28] used the Wii Balance Board (Nintendo, Japan) to assess postural sway as an indicator of fall risk in 73 community-living older people. They found that people with a higher anteroposterior sway velocity were more likely to experience falls in the coming year. Nait Aicha et al. [29] installed ambient sensor systems comprising motion, contact, pressure, and toilet flush sensors to create three smart homes. Movements of residents of these homes were tracked for 27 months, and their gait velocity (a measure previously related to falls, e.g. [30]) was estimated based on sequences and timing of sensor events. Using this approach, they were able to longitudinally track walking speed, which could have clinical utility, since a decline of walking speed has been associated with greater risk of falls [31].

Wearables for Fall Risk Assessment

Advances in miniature sensing and computing modules allow for registration of movement during everyday activities. Moe-Nilssen [32] was one of the first to propose the use wearable sensors for natural gait analysis. Using a series of experiments and case studies, he showed that lumbar spine inclination and acceleration root mean square (a measure of intensity) are modulated by walking speed, and illustrated that these measures are sensitive to balance impairment and walking conditions [33].

More recently, inertial sensors have been deployed for extended periods of time during daily life to gain insight into fall risk. Weiss et al. [34] were the first to show a link between daily-life gait and fall history. They asked 72 community-living older people to wear a device containing a triaxial accelerometer and gyroscope on their lower back for three days. They showed differences between people with and without a history of recurrent falls in the amount, intensity, and variability of walking bouts. Rispens et al. [35] independently confirmed that daily-life gait characteristics assessed using an accelerometer that was worn for one week, were associated with the number of falls in the past year in 114 community-dwelling older people. They further showed that measures of gait smoothness, regularity, and stability had high test–retest reliability. Similarly, Brodie et al. [36] showed that extended (eight-week) monitoring periods using a pendent accelerometer were acceptable to older people. They showed that the distribution of daily-life walking was associated with falls history [36], different from laboratory-assessed gait [37] and potentially provided a better assessment of fall risk [38]. Together these studies suggest that remote fall risk assessments based on daily-life gait could hold clinical utility.

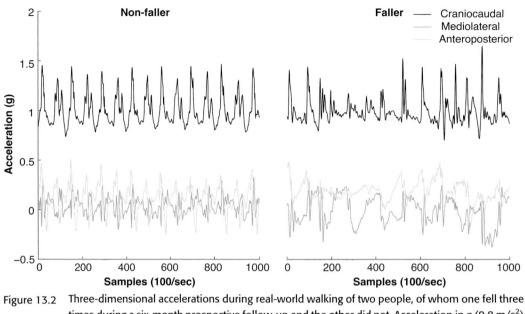

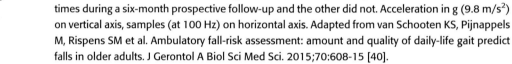

Figure 13.2   Three-dimensional accelerations during real-world walking of two people, of whom one fell three times during a six-month prospective follow-up and the other did not. Acceleration in g (9.8 m/s²) on vertical axis, samples (at 100 Hz) on horizontal axis. Adapted from van Schooten KS, Pijnappels M, Rispens SM et al. Ambulatory fall-risk assessment: amount and quality of daily-life gait predict falls in older adults. J Gerontol A Biol Sci Med Sci. 2015;70:608-15 [40].

The idea is again relatively simple; quality of gait is characterized by the smoothness, regularity, and stability of trunk movements during walking. An example of trunk movements, here linear accelerations in three directions, are provided in Figure 13.2. Both signals were captured during a single 10-second gait episode in daily life. The panel on the left depicts a person with low fall risk (no falls during the subsequent six months) and the panel on the right depicts a person with high fall risk (three falls during subsequent 6 months). The non-faller takes 15 steps and the faller takes 14 steps in 10 seconds, suggesting a small difference in step length or walking speed. The acceleration signals, especially in the transverse plane, appear smoother and more regular in the non-faller. Such characteristics of daily-life gait can differentiate between fallers and non-fallers (for review see [39]), and hence hold promise for fall risk assessment.

Quality of Daily-Life Gait as a Measure of Fall Risk

Van Schooten et al. [40] found daily-life gait characteristics obtained via accelerometry were predictive of falls and provided complementary information to commonly used clinical risk factors for falls. They asked 169 older people to wear a triaxial accelerometer on their lower back for one week and obtained clinical tests of fall risk. They developed three multi-variate models, reporting an area under the curve of 0.68 for clinical assessments, 0.71 for daily-life assessments, and a significant improvement to 0.81 when both daily-life and clinical assessments were combined. The final prediction model included history of falls, depressive symptoms, amount of walking, stability, intensity, smoothness, and complexity of gait as interactions between intensity and smoothness of gait with amount of walking. The latter interaction suggests that the amount of walking was a risk factor for falls for people with poorer gait quality. In a complementary study, Brodie et al. [41] used a multi-dimensional clustering analysis in 96 older people to identify four main risk groups according to their walking patterns: Impaired (93% fallers), Restrained (8% fallers), Active (50% fallers), and Athletic (4% fallers). Interestingly, while the amount of walking was associated with many health benefits in this study, it was also a risk factor for falls in some groups with poorer gait quality. In a follow-up study in 319 older people, Van Schooten et al. [42] confirmed that daily-life gait characteristics were predictive of falls. They further developed cross-validated prediction models for time-to-first-fall and second-fall (area under the curves of 0.66–0.72 and 0.69–0.76, respectively) comprising a composite measure of gait quality together with history of falls, alcohol consumption, and muscle strength.

Fall Risk in Clinical Groups

Several studies have explored the utility of gait monitoring for fall risk assessment in clinical groups. For example, Kikkert et al. [43] obtained clinical risk factors for falls and analysed gait in 61 older patients who were referred to a geriatric day clinic for memory complaints, mobility problems, or polypharmacy. They showed that gait characteristics related to speed, variability, and smoothness/regularity of gait provided additional predictive value over clinical risk factors such as cognitive status, use of medication, co-morbidities, muscle strength, and posture. Del Din et al. [44] monitored daily-life gait in 115 older people with and 122 without Parkinson's disease. They analysed the amount of gait (coined macro level) and quality of gait (micro level) to identify generic and disease-specific gait characteristics associated with past falls. The authors report that fallers walked in shorter bouts of less variable length with slower, shorter, and less variable steps than non-fallers. They further observed greater step length variability in fallers with Parkinson's disease, and lower step velocity variability in fallers without Parkinson's disease, compared to non-fallers. In a similar study in stroke survivors, Punt et al. [45] identified reduced gait symmetry and increased medio-lateral sway as generic fall risk factors. They further observed that gait variability and smoothness in the medio-lateral direction had a weaker association, and gait stability had a stronger association, with fall history in stroke survivors compared to older people who had not had a stroke. Such analyses eliciting generic and disease-specific gait risk factors are essential for future clinical implementation of these wearable fall risk assessments.

Quality of Daily-Life Movements, Not Only Gait, as a Predictor of Fall Risk

Despite this chapter's focus on gait, other or more-specific movements in daily life may also hold promise for fall risk assessment. For example, Mancini et al. [46] investigated turning during everyday gait in 35 older people. They showed a higher average turn duration and more steps per turn (thus slower turns) in people with a history of recurrent falls compared to people without a history of falls. The authors further observed a more variable number of steps per turn in individuals who fell during the six months after assessment. Pozaic et al. [47] utilized wrist-worn inertial sensors to analyse daily-life sit-to-stand movements. They collected data in 136 older people and investigated the predictive value of sit-to-stand characteristics for falls in the subsequent month. The authors showed that characteristics related to hand movement intensity, jerk, medio-lateral sway, smoothness, and estimated applied support were associated with fall risk. Advances in activity recognition and sensor fusion techniques will allow for more accurate extraction of specific activities and may further improve fall risk assessment.

Clinical Implementation

With wearable sensors becoming ubiquitous in our daily life, clinical use is the next frontier. Despite the potential, there are several barriers to translation related to standardization, sensitivity to change, and data security, which need to be overcome prior to clinical implementation. Although wearable sensors in research studies are commonly worn on the trunk or lower back because of their proximity to the body's centre of mass, other locations might be more clinically feasible [48], which will require new algorithms. Moreover, standardization of extracted characteristics through external validation, publicly available data repositories and algorithm transparency is essential to establish common sets of validated outcomes for clinical use, while also providing a platform for future researchers to improve on the status quo. Complicating matters is the current trend towards requiring algorithms to be registered as medical devices. Medical-device registration and distribution requires resources from companies that are unlikely to openly share developments.

In addition to standardization, sensitivity to change due to clinical interventions or age- or disease-related decline over time needs to be established. Several studies have suggested sensitivity of gait characteristics to experimental manipulations of the sensory system, medication use, fatigue, and training [49–53].

However, conclusive clinical evidence is required before implementing longitudinal use. Finally, with the current focus on protection of personal data in many Western countries, we anticipate that intensified regulation of wearable information, in particular geo-location information, will lead to ethical debate.

Future of Wearable Fall Risk Assessment

As with the development in fall detection, the addition of sensing modules (e.g. physiological signals, geo-positioning, gyroscopes, magnetometers) are likely to lead to advances in the field. Experimental studies have revealed rapid changes in brain activity following balance perturbations [54] and sudden increases in arousal, as is likely during a stumble, can elicit sympathetic nervous system activity [55]. The addition of brain activity, heart rate, and perspiration sensors might therefore lead to increased accuracy of fall risk assessments. In addition, cleaning of data based on geolocation to identify frequently travelled paths may help reduce environmental noise [56] and integration of multiple sensors may improve orientation estimation [57] and lead to more accurate fall risk assessments.

Development of novel characteristics that best differentiate fallers from nonfallers is ongoing. For example, Ihlen et al. [58] reanalysed the data by Van Schooten et al. [42], extracting a new characteristic describing gait phase-dependent regularity. They showed that this phase-dependent regularity improved the predictive ability for single and multiple falls over six months when compared to previously used gait characteristics. The authors further found that gait regularity was markedly reduced in fallers compared to nonfallers at 60% of the step cycle, which corresponds with the push-off phase during gait – a potential target of intervention [59].

Current approaches tend to focus on falls in the next months. Fall risk, however, is a dynamic process that may change over minutes or even seconds. In a recent paper, Klenk et al. [60] propose a conceptual model for dynamic fall risk that includes intrinsic risk factors that change over time and includes exposure through high-risk activities, such as walking and transferring, and environmental risk factors, such as poor lighting and tripping hazards. Recently the use of wearable devices to identify near falls has received increasing attention [61]. Weiss et al. [62] induced near falls in 15 participants by placing obstacles on a treadmill during walking. They showed that characteristics related to movement intensity and jerk obtained via trunk accelerometry were able to differentiate between near falls and normal gait. While still in its infancy, the frequency of stumbles, slips, and trips may prove a useful real-time fall risk assessment tool in the future. Further on this theme, using wearable devices to detect unstable gait patterns (such as freezing of gait in people with Parkinson's, which often precede falls) to enable real-time intervention through auditory cues has been proposed by several groups [63, 64]

Limitations of Fall Risk Assessments

While the combined results of the studies cited provide a compelling case for the benefit of fall risk assessments, it is worth considering some important limitations. While many of the univariate associations between daily-life gait characteristics and falls have been replicated, it is not known if the multi-variate models developed in specific cohorts will transfer to new cohorts. In a probabilistic model, Palumbo et al. [65] estimate the best prognostic ability of fall prediction models for any fall within the next year. Through a series of assumptions and models, they show that, because of the presence of noise and chance, the highest achievable area under the curve would be 0.80 to 0.89. This is remarkably close to the values we have seen reported above. Overfitting is especially relevant when using wearable sensors, where hundreds of characteristics can be extracted from one assessment and combined in a bid to predict falls [66]. Validation of the prediction model in a non-training, or test dataset can help guard against overfitting. If the model performs poorly in the test dataset, it is unlikely to generalize well. There are different methods of performing this validation. The strongest form of validation is where the model is tested on an independently collected dataset by an external group. So far, these validation methods have been under-utilized in fall risk literature but increasing awareness and availability of data are likely to lead to improvements in generalizability of fall risk models.

Conclusions

Technology holds great promise for fall detection and fall risk assessment. Technological advances now allow for automatic detection of falls and remote monitoring of fall risk in daily life. However, despite encouraging results in controlled settings, these technologies are not yet ready for clinical use. Automatic fall detection suffers from high false positive rates and while some wearable-based fall risk assessments are finding their way into clinical settings, current validation and standardization is insufficient. It is likely that open science approaches of data and code sharing, together with further advances in sensors and algorithms, will result in the ongoing improvement of available tools. This combined with technology acceptance and current social changes will likely lead to the widespread uptake of new technology for falls management in clinical cohorts.

Finally, it is anticipated that bridging fall risk assessment with fall detection, and eventually real-time feedback, can assist in the clinical utility of these technologies. Current approaches tend to predict falls over months or years, but fall risk is dynamic process that may change over minutes or seconds. The reasons people fall may be broadly categorized at the macro level, for example, as a slip or a trip. However, at the micro level, each fall may be slightly different, defined by a unique series of unexpected events for the individual. The next challenge will be to implement these conceptual models into computational risk profiles, so that we can truly demonstrate the potential of technology to quantify falls and fall risk in real time in the natural environment at the individual level.

REFERENCES

1. Fleming J, Brayne C. Inability to get up after falling, subsequent time on floor, and summoning help: prospective cohort study in people over 90. *Br Med J.* 2008;337:a2227.
2. Tinetti ME, Liu WL, Claus EB. Predictors and prognosis of inability to get up after falls among elderly persons. *J Am Med Assoc.* 1993;269:65–70.
3. Nevitt MC, Cummings SR, Hudes ES. Risk factors for injurious falls: a prospective study. *J Gerontol.* 1991;46:M164–70.
4. Heinbüchner B, Hautzinger M, Becker C et al. Satisfaction and use of personal emergency response systems. *Z Gerontol Geriatr.* 2010;43:219–23.
5. Noury N, Rumeau P, Bourke AK et al. A proposal for the classification and evaluation of fall detectors. *Irbm.* 2008;29:340–9.
6. Becker C, Schwickert L, Mellone S et al. Proposal for a multiphase fall model based on real-world fall recordings with body-fixed sensors. *Z Gerontol Geriatr.* 2012;45:707–15.
7. Wu G. Distinguishing fall activities from normal activities by velocity characteristics. *J Biomech.* 2000;33:1497–500.
8. O'Connor JJ, Phillips LJ, Folarinde B et al. Assessment of fall characteristics from depth sensor videos. *J Gerontol Nurs.* 2017;43:13–19.
9. Litvak D, Zigel Y, Gannot I, (Eds.) Fall detection of elderly through floor vibrations and sound. In: *2008 30th Annual International Conference of the IEEE Engineering in Medicine and Biology Society.* Vancouver, BC: IEEE; 2008.
10. Minvielle L, Atiq M, Serra R, Mougeot M, Vayatis N. Fall detection using smart floor sensor and supervised learning. In: *2017 39th Annual International Conference of the IEEE Engineering in Medicine and Biology Society (EMBC).* Seogwipo, South Korea: IEEE; 2017.
11. Lord CJ, Colvin DP, (Eds.) Falls in the elderly: detection and assessment. In: *Annual International Conference of the IEEE Engineering in Medical and Biology Society.* Orlando, FL, USA: IEEE;1991.
12. Williams G, Doughty K, Cameron K, Bradley D, (Eds). A smart fall & activity monitor for telecare applications. In: *Proceedings of the 20th Annual International Conference of the IEEE Engineering in Medicine and Biology Society.* Hong Kong: IEEE; 1998.
13. Bianchi F, Redmond SJ, Narayanan MR et al. Barometric pressure and triaxial accelerometry-based falls event detection. *IEEE Trans Neural Syst Rehabilitation Eng.* 2010;18:619–27.

14. Bagala F, Becker C, Cappello A et al. Evaluation of accelerometer-based fall detection algorithms on real-world falls. *PloS One*. 2012;7:e37062.

15. Wu G, Xue S, (Eds.) Automatic fall detection based on kinematic characteristics during the pre-impact phase of falls. In: *6th World Congress of Biomechanics*. Singapore: WCB; 2010.

16. Bourke AK, van de Ven PJW, Chaya AE OLaighin GM, Nelson J. Testing of a long-term fall detection system incorporated into a custom vest for the elderly. In: *30th Annual International Conference of the IEEE Engineering in Medicine and Biology Society*. Vancouver, BC: IEEE; 2008.

17. Zhang T, Wang J, Liu P et al. Fall detection by embedding an accelerometer in cellphone and using KFD algorithm. *Int J Comput Sci Netw Secur*. 2006;6:277–84.

18. Kerdegari H, Samsudin K, Rahman Ramli A et al. Development of wearable human fall detection system using multilayer perceptron neural network. *Int J Comput Intell Syst*. 2013;6:127–36.

19. Palmerini L, Bagalà F, Zanetti A et al. A wavelet-based approach to fall detection. *Sensors*. 2015;15:11575–86.

20. Aziz O, Klenk J, Schwickert L et al. Validation of accuracy of SVM-based fall detection system using real-world fall and non-fall datasets. *PloS One*. 2017;12:e0180318.

21. Lipsitz LA, Tchalla AE, Iloputaife I et al. Evaluation of an automated falls detection device in nursing home residents. *J Am Geriatr Soc*. 2016;64:365–8.

22. Klenk J, Schwickert L, Palmerini L et al. The FARSEEING real-world fall repository: a large-scale collaborative database to collect and share sensor signals from real-world falls. *Eur Rev Aging Phys Act*. 2016;13:8.

23. Gates S, Smith LA, Fisher JD et al. Systematic review of accuracy of screening instruments for predicting fall risk among independently living older adults. *J Rehabil Res Dev*. 2008;45:1105–16.

24. Scott V, Votova K, Scanlan A et al. Multifactorial and functional mobility assessment tools for fall risk among older adults in community, home-support, long-term and acute care settings. *Age Ageing*. 2007;36:130–9.

25. Lee J, Geller AI, Strasser DC. Analytical review: focus on fall screening assessments. *PM R*. 2013;5:609–21.

26. Ejupi A, Brodie M, Gschwind YJ et al. Kinect-based five-times-Sit-to-Stand Test for clinical and in-home assessment of fall risk in older people. *Gerontology*. 2015;62:118–24.

27. Mehdizadeh S, Dolatabadi E, Ng K-D et al. Vision-based assessment of gait features associated with falls in people with dementia. *J Gerontol A Biol Sci Med Sci*. 2020;75:1148–53.

28. Kwok B-C, Clark RA, Pua Y-H. Novel use of the Wii Balance Board to prospectively predict falls in community-dwelling older adults. *Clin Biomech*. 2015;30:481–4.

29. Aicha AN, Englebienne G, Kröse B. Continuous measuring of the indoor walking speed of older adults living alone. *J Ambient Intell Humaniz Comput*. 2018;9:589–99.

30. Montero-Odasso M, Schapira M, Soriano ER et al. Gait velocity as a single predictor of adverse events in healthy seniors aged 75 years and older. *J Gerontol A Biol Sci Med Sci*. 2005;60:1304–9.

31. Quach L, Galica AM, Jones RN et al. The nonlinear relationship between gait speed and falls: the maintenance of balance, independent living, intellect, and zest in the elderly of Boston study. *J Am Geriatr Soc*. 2011;59:1069–73.

32. Moe-Nilssen R. A new method for evaluating motor control in gait under real-life environmental conditions. Part 1: the instrument. *Clin Biomech*. 1998;13:320–7.

33. Moe-Nilssen R. A new method for evaluating motor control in gait under real-life environmental conditions. Part 2: gait analysis. *Clin Biomech*. 1998;13:328–35.

34. Weiss A, Brozgol M, Dorfman M et al. Does the evaluation of gait quality during daily life provide insight into fall risk? A novel approach using 3-day accelerometer recordings. *Neurorehabil Neural Repair*. 2013;27:742–52.

35. Rispens SM, van Schooten KS, Pijnappels M et al. Identification of fall risk predictors in daily life measurements: gait characteristics' reliability and association with self-reported fall history. *Neurorehabil Neural Repair*. 2015;29:54–61.

36. Brodie MA, Lord SR, Coppens MJ et al. Eight-week remote monitoring using a freely worn device reveals unstable gait patterns in older fallers. *IEEE Trans Biomed Eng*. 2015;62:2588–94.

37. Brodie MA, Coppens MJ, Lord SR et al. Wearable pendant device monitoring using new wavelet-based methods shows daily life and laboratory gaits are different. *Med Biol Eng Comput*. 2016;54:663–74.

38. Brodie MA, Coppens MJ, Ejupi A et al. Comparison between clinical gait and daily-life gait assessments of fall risk in older people. *Geriatr Gerontol Int*. 2017;17:2274–82.

39. Howcroft J, Kofman J, Lemaire ED. Review of fall risk assessment in geriatric populations using inertial sensors. *J Neuroeng Rehabil*. 2013;10:91.

40. van Schooten KS, Pijnappels M, Rispens SM et al. Ambulatory fall-risk assessment: amount and quality of daily-life gait predict falls in older adults. *J Gerontol A Biol Sci Med Sci*. 2015;70:608–15.

41. Brodie MA, Okubo Y, Annegarn J et al. Disentangling the health benefits of walking from increased exposure to falls in older people using remote gait monitoring and multi-dimensional analysis. *Physiol Meas*. 2016;38:45–62.

42. van Schooten KS, Pijnappels M, Rispens SM et al. Daily-life gait quality as predictor of falls in older people: a 1-year prospective cohort study. *PloS One*. 2016;11:e0158623.

43. Kikkert LH, De Groot MH, van Campen JP et al. Gait dynamics to optimize fall risk assessment in geriatric patients admitted to an outpatient diagnostic clinic. *PloS One*. 2017;12:e0178615.

44. Del Din S, Galna B, Godfrey A et al. Analysis of free-living gait in older adults with and without Parkinson's disease and with and without a history of falls: identifying generic and disease-specific characteristics. *J Gerontol A Biol Sci Med Sci*. 2017;74:500–6.

45. Punt M, Bruijn SM, van Schooten KS et al. Characteristics of daily life gait in fall and non fall-prone stroke survivors and controls. *J Neuroeng Rehabil*. 2016;13:67.

46. Mancini M, Schlueter H, El-Gohary M et al. Continuous monitoring of turning mobility and its association to falls and cognitive function: a pilot study. *J Gerontol A Biol Sci Med Sci*. 2016;71:1102–8.

47. Pozaic T, Lindemann U, Grebe A-K et al. Sit-to-stand transition reveals acute fall risk in activities of daily living. *IEEE J Transl Eng Health Med*. 2016;4:1–11.

48. Bergmann J, Chandaria V, McGregor A. Wearable and implantable sensors: the patient's perspective. *Sensors*. 2012;12:16695–709.

49. Helbostad JL, Leirfall S, Moe-Nilssen R et al. Physical fatigue affects gait characteristics in older persons. *J Gerontol A Biol Sci Med Sci.* 2007;62:1010–15.

50. Manor B, Wolenski P, Guevaro A et al. Differential effects of plantar desensitization on locomotion dynamics. *J Electromyogr Kinesiol.* 2009;19:e320–8.

51. Hamacher D, Hamacher D, Rehfeld K et al. Motor-cognitive dual-task training improves local dynamic stability of normal walking in older individuals. *Clin Biomech.* 2016;32:138–41.

52. Henderson EJ, Lord SR, Brodie MA et al. Rivastigmine for gait stability in patients with Parkinson's disease (ReSPonD): a randomised, double-blind, placebo-controlled, phase 2 trial. *Lancet Neurol.* 2016;15:249–58.

53. van Schooten KS, Sloot LH, Bruijn SM et al. Sensitivity of trunk variability and stability measures to balance impairments induced by galvanic vestibular stimulation during gait. *Gait Posture.* 2011;33:656–60.

54. Varghese JP, McIlroy RE, Barnett-Cowan M. Perturbation-evoked potentials: significance and application in balance control research. *Neurosci Biobehav Rev.* 2017;83:267–80.

55. Fechir M, Schlereth T, Purat T et al. Patterns of sympathetic responses induced by different stress tasks. *Open Neurol J.* 2008;2:25–31.

56. Wang W, Adamczyk PG. Analyzing gait in the real world using wearable movement sensors and frequently repeated movement paths. *Sensors.* 2019;19:1925.

57. Bennett T, Jafari R, Gans N, (Eds.) An extended Kalman filter to estimate human gait parameters and walking distance. In: *2013 American Control Conference.* Washington, DC: Proc Am Control Conf; 2013.

58. Ihlen EA, Van Schooten KS, Bruijn SM et al. Improved prediction of falls in community-dwelling older adults through phase-dependent entropy of daily-life walking. *Front Aging Neurosci.* 2018;10:44.

59. Browne MG, Franz JR. More push from your push-off: joint-level modifications to modulate propulsive forces in old age. *PloS One.* 2018;13:e0201407.

60. Klenk J, Becker C, Palumbo P et al. Conceptualizing a dynamic fall risk model including intrinsic risks and exposures. *J Am Med Dir Assoc.* 2017;18:921–7.

61. Pang I, Okubo Y, Sturnieks D et al. Detection of near falls using wearable devices: a systematic review. *J Geriatr Phys Ther.* 2019;42:48–56.

62. Weiss A, Shimkin I, Giladi N et al. Automated detection of near falls: algorithm development and preliminary results. *BMC Res Notes.* 2010;3:62.

63. Bachlin M, Plotnik M, Roggen D et al. Wearable assistant for Parkinson's disease patients with the freezing of gait symptom. *IEEE Trans Inf Technol Biomed.* 2009;14:436–46.

64. Jovanov E, Wang E, Verhagen L Fredrickson M, Fratangelo R. deFOG – a real time system for detection and unfreezing of gait of Parkinson's patients. In: *31st Annual International Conference of the IEEE Engineering in Medicine and Biology Society.* Minneapolis, MN: EMBS; 2009.

65. Palumbo P, Palmerini L, Chiari L. A probabilistic model to investigate the properties of prognostic tools for falls. *Methods Inf Med.* 2015;54:189–97.

66. Shany T, Wang K, Liu Y et al. Review: are we stumbling in our quest to find the best predictor? Over-optimism in sensor-based models for predicting falls in older adults. *Healthc Technol Lett.* 2015;2:79–88.

14

Fall Risk Screening and Assessment

Anne Tiedemann and Stephen R. Lord

As outlined in previous chapters, falls are not random events and are associated with multiple risk factors. Fall risk increases in line with the cumulative effect of impairments, making a multi-factorial risk assessment important. A risk assessment should include tests with proven validity and reliability in the relevant setting and population, and linked to appropriate, evidence-based interventions to reduce fall risk. This chapter discusses the relevance and role of fall risk screening and assessment and provides information about validated tools that can be used to measure fall risk in the community, hospitals, and residential aged care.

Screening

Fall risk screening provides a quick means of identifying individuals at increased risk of falling who need greater surveillance or who require subsequent fall risk assessments. Fall risk screening usually involves consideration of a few brief items. Several studies have identified previous falls as one of the strongest predictors for falling again in the following year. Thus, the inclusion of this question is used in most fall risk screens, along with simple assessments of balance and mobility [1].

Assessment

Assessment tools aim to elucidate underlying factors contributing to falls. Assessing fall risk typically involves either the use of multi-factorial assessment tools that cover a wide range of fall risk factors, or functional assessments that focus on cognition, vision, strength, co-ordination, balance, and gait. Several multi-factorial assessment tools have been developed for use in a range of settings and some examples are provided below. The choice of tool depends on the time and equipment available and the level of functional ability of the individuals being assessed.

Screening and Assessment in Community-Dwellers

The United Kingdom National Institute for Health and Care Excellence (NICE) Guidelines recommend that older people in contact with health care professionals should be routinely asked about the frequency, context, and characteristics of any falls in the past year [2]. In addition, the American Geriatrics Society/British Geriatrics Society/American Academy of Orthopaedic Surgeons Guidelines [3] and NICE guidelines [2] recommend the Timed Up and Go Test (TUGT) as a simple screening tool to identify people warranting an assessment of balance and gait [4]. It involves measuring the time taken for a person to rise from a chair, walk three metres at normal pace and with usual assistive devices, turn, return to the chair, and sit down. However, a systematic review involving 25 studies found the predictive value of the TUGT for falls in community-dwelling older adults was limited and no cut point for impaired performance could be recommended [5]. Alternatives to the TUGT that are simple to administer and have good predictive accuracy for falls include the Alternate Step Test [6], Sit to Stand Test [6], and the Short Physical Performance Battery [7] – see Table 14.1.

The NICE guidelines [2] also recommend that older people who seek fall-related medical attention, or who report more than one fall in the past year, or demonstrate abnormalities of gait and/or balance should be offered a multi-factorial fall risk assessment. This assessment should be performed by a trained and experienced health care professional as part of an individualized, multi-factorial intervention. Such multi-factorial fall risk assessments may evaluate the following factors: fall history, gait, balance, mobility, muscle weakness, self-reported functional ability, fear of falling, visual impairment, osteoporosis risk, cognitive impairment, neurological issues, urinary incontinence, cardiovascular conditions, medication use, and home hazards. Examples of assessments for many of these fall risk domains are outlined in Table 14.1.

Physiological System Risk Assessments

As indicated in Chapter 10, several studies have identified many medical conditions which contribute to fall risk, including chronic and degenerative diseases such as stroke, Parkinson's disease, arthritis, foot problems, cognitive impairment, diabetes, cataracts, and dizziness. However, attribution of a degree of fall risk to a medical diagnosis is problematic because the severity of such conditions varies across individuals and co-morbidity is common in older age. Furthermore, sensory and motor impairments associated with increased age, inactivity, medication use, or minor pathology are highly prevalent in older people without documented medical conditions.

Table 14.1 Fall risk factors and validated assessment tools

Risk factor	Assessment tool
Balance and gait	The Berg Balance Scale is a 14-item scale with a maximum total score of 56 points [21]. It is most suited to lower-functioning groups
	The Mini Balance Evaluation Systems Test includes 14 balance tests including a test of reactive balance control [22]
	The Alternate Step Test measures the ability of patients to alternatively place their left and right feet as fast as possible onto an 18 cm high step. A test time >10 s to complete eight alternating steps indicates an impaired performance [6]
	The Sit to Stand Test measures the ability of patients to complete five chair rises as fast as possible. A test time >12 s to complete the test indicates an impaired performance [6]
	The Short Physical Performance Battery comprises simple assessments of standing balance, chair rise ability, and gait [7]. Each test is graded from 0 to 4 with a total test score of 12
Vision	Vision screening should include asking older people about their vision and checking for signs of visual deterioration. Visual acuity can be assessed using standard or low-contrast letter charts [10] and contrast sensitivity can be assessed with the Melbourne Edge Test [23].
Muscle strength	Lower limb muscle strength is best assessed using simple rigs that isolate specific muscle groups [8, 24]. The Sit to Stand Test provides a measure of functional strength [6]
Cognitive impairment	The Montreal Cognitive Assessment (MOCA) is a 10-minute cognitive screening tool for mild cognitive impairment [25]. The MOCA tests seven cognitive function domains: short term memory, visuospatial abilities, executive functioning, attention, concentration, working memory, and language. The maximum score is 30 with a score ≤25 indicating mild cognitive impairment
	The Confusion Assessment Method (CAM) is a comprehensive assessment instrument that screens for four clinical features of delirium (i.e. onset of mental status changes or a fluctuating course, inattention, disorganized thinking, and an altered level of consciousness). An older person is diagnosed as delirious if they have both of the first two features, and either the third or fourth feature [26]
Syncope/dizziness	Assessments for syncope and dizziness may include an electrocardiogram, echocardiography, Holter monitoring, tilt-table testing, and carotid sinus massage or insertion of an implantable loop recorder. Key risk factors for dizziness handicap in middle-aged and older people have recently been elucidated in a large prospective study [27]. Key assessments include the Dix–Hallpike test for diagnosing benign paroxysmal positional vertigo, the Halmagyi head-thrust test for assessing peripheral vestibular function as well as assessments of cardiovascular medication use, anxiety, and postural sway
Medications	A medication review should focus on appropriate prescribing (i.e. ensuring that medications are used safely and effectively)

Table 14.1 (*cont.*)

Risk factor	Assessment tool
Fear of falling	Falls Efficacy Scale International (FES-I) assesses fear of falling across a wide range of activities of daily living (such as cleaning the house, shopping, walking on uneven surfaces). The higher the score, the greater the concern about falling [28] Iconographical Falls Efficacy Scale (Icon-FES) assesses fear of falling using 30 pictures to describe a range of activities and situations (FES-I items with additional risk-taking activities). The items are scored on a four-point scale with 1 = not at all concerned to 4 = very concerned, along with facial expression icons to assess the level of concern about falling [29]
Feet and footwear	An assessment of footwear and foot problems involves assessing foot pain and other foot problems as well as using a safe shoe checklist [30]
Home hazards	Several home hazard checklists have been developed and are often culturally dependent. The Home Falls and Accidents Screening Tool (HOME FAST) [31] is a 25-item assessment of hazards in the physical environment, and assessment of functioning and personal behavioural factors. An alternative is the Westmead Home Safety Assessment [32]

To address this issue, Lord et al. [8, 9] devised an 'impairment profiling' rather than a 'disease-based/medical' approach. Termed the physiological profile assessment (PPA), it involves quantitative assessment of sensorimotor abilities critical for the control of balance and safe mobility. The short form takes 15–20 minutes to administer and comprises tests of visual contrast sensitivity, lower-limb proprioception, knee extension strength, reaction time, and postural sway. A marked deficit in any one system may be sufficient to predispose an older person to fall, but a combination of mild or moderate impairments across physiological systems is also likely to increase fall risk. Based on extensive normative data, this assessment provides a graph indicating the patient's fall risk score, a profile of individual test performance results, a table indicting individual test performances in relation to age-matched norms, and a written report outlining tailored interventions. Physiological profiling can therefore complement the disease-based/medical approach to fall risk assessment by quantifying the degree of fall risk, irrespective of co-morbidities, and inform tailored interventions to address identified physiological impairments.

The PPA requires equipment items and test-administrator training and is most suited to falls clinics, physiotherapy outpatient clinics, and other specialist settings. To widen the reach of the physiological approach to fall risk assessment, Tiedemann et al. [10] devised *QuickScreen* – a simplified assessment designed for home assessments and use in primary care. *QuickScreen* takes less than 10 minutes to administer and assesses previous falls, medication usage, vision, peripheral sensation, lower-limb strength, balance, and mobility. The cut points indicating increased fall risk for the five vision and physical performance tests (illustrated in Figure 14.1) were determined from prospective cohort studies of community-dwelling older people [11]. Figure 14.2 shows the *QuickScreen* form that provides suggested interventions based on the assessment results and a fall risk probability score derived from the number of identified risk factors [12].

Fall Risk Assessment in Hospitals

The UK NICE guidelines recommend that patients aged 65 years and over or those aged 50 to 64 years who have an underlying condition that places them at risk, such as recent stroke, should be assumed to be at risk and automatically undergo multifactorial assessments and interventions [13]. Such assessments should have good predictive accuracy, validation across multiple hospitals, and evaluate risk factors for falls that can be addressed or managed during the inpatient stay, such as, for example, postural instability, cognitive impairment, visual impairment, continence issues, and medication use. This information should then form the basis for an individualized fall prevention plan. Oliver has also argued against using fall risk screening in hospitals, particularly without an action plan for fall prevention, and instead suggest that high-quality care of all older adults should prevent falls [14].

The Peninsula Health Falls Risk Assessment Tool [15] is one validated assessment for the subacute hospital setting. It comprises three sections that cover: (i) fall risk status, (ii) a risk factor checklist, and (iii) an action plan. Such action plans have been incorporated into daily care plans to address patient (medications, vision, blood pressure, mobility) and environmental (appropriate bed height, nurse call bell accessibility) risk factors and used as part of a successful fall prevention intervention in the hospital setting [16]. Patients, and their family members and carers, if appropriate, should also be provided with oral and written information to explain the patient's risk factors for falling and appropriate prevention strategies while in hospital [17]. However, as it has yet to be demonstrated that fall risk assessment and intervention trials can prevent falls in acute hospitals, there remains some uncertainty about how best to keep older people safe in this setting. This is discussed in Chapter 26.

Fall Risk Assessment in Residential Care

Fall prevention guidelines from the Australian Commission on Safety and Quality in Healthcare [18] recommend that all older people who are admitted to

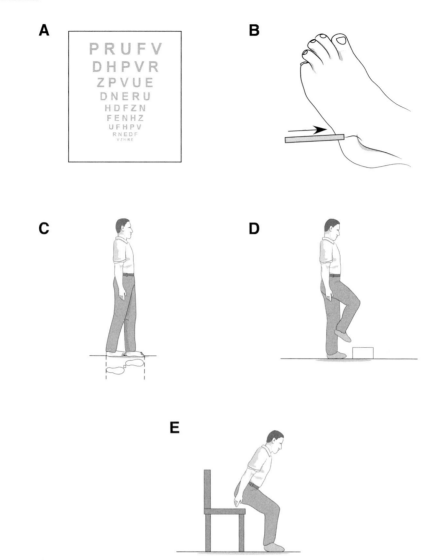

Figure 14.1   The 5 tests making up *QuickScreen.* A = low contrast visual acuity, B = tactile sensitivity, C = near tandem stand, D = alternate step test, E = sit to stand.

residential care facilities should undergo a fall screen as soon as practicable after they are admitted. This fall screen should also be undertaken every six months and when a change in functional status is evident. Formal fall risk screening, such as a question of whether the resident has fallen in the previous 12 months, for all residents has the advantage of forming part of routine clinical management and should prompt further assessment and fall prevention strategies for all residents.

The Australian Commission on Safety and Quality in Healthcare Guidelines also recommend that residents who score at risk on a screening tool should

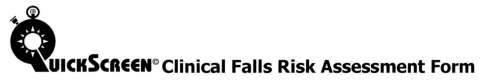

QUICKSCREEN© Clinical Falls Risk Assessment Form

CLIENT NAME   *DATE*

For the following risk factors score 'YES' if risk factor is present, score 'NO' if risk factor is not present

MEASURE	RISK FACTOR PRESENT? (please circle)	ACTION
Previous Falls		
One/more in previous year	Yes/No	
Medications		
Four or more (excluding vitamins)	Yes/No	
Any psychotropic	Yes/No	

Recommendation: Review current medications.

Vision

Low contrast visual acuity test Unable to see all of line 16	Yes/No	

Recommendation: Give vision information sheet. Examine for glaucoma, cataracts and suitability of spectacles. Refer if necessary.

Peripheral Sensation

Tactile sensitivity test Unable to feel 2 out of 3 trials	Yes/No	

Recommendation: Give sensation loss information sheet. Check for diabetes.

Strength/ Reaction Time/ Balance

Near tandem stand test Unable to stand for 10 secs	Yes/No	
Alternate step test Unable to complete in 10 secs	Yes/No	
Sit to stand test Unable to complete in 12 secs	Yes/No	

Recommendation: Give strength/balance information sheet. Refer to community exercise class or home exercise program if appropriate to individual level of functioning.

Number of risk factors	0-1	2-3	4-5	6+

Figure 14.2   The *QuickScreen* assessment form.

undergo a comprehensive fall risk assessment, as well as residents who experience a fall, or who move to or reside in a setting where most people are considered to have a high risk of falls (e.g. high-care facilities, dementia units) [18]. In many residential care settings, however, most residents are at an increased risk of falls so it may be pragmatic to omit the screening process and implement regular fall risk assessments of all residents.

The Care Home Falls Screen [19], uses easily collectable measures to identify older people living in residential care facilities at high risk of falls. It was developed in seven residential care homes involving 240 residents in the United Kingdom, using information that could be obtained from care records, medical notes, and by questioning carers, and thus did not require any active involvement of the residents. Logistic regression identified cognitive impairment, impulsivity, poor standing balance, requiring a walking frame, falling in the previous year, and use of anti-depressants and hypnotics/anxiolytics as independent and significant predictors of falls over a six-month follow-up period. The area under the receiver operating curve (ROC) for this model was 0.79 (95% CI: 0.73,0.84), and the absolute risk of falling ranged from zero in those with no risk factors to 100% in those with six or more risk factors. While labelled a screen, this tool assists in identifying important explanatory risk factors for falls that may be amenable to targeted interventions. This may assist in optimizing fall prevention strategies, as to date many intervention trials have not been effective in this population and those that have been effective have used approaches that involved identification of risk factors with ensuing interventions [20]. Finally, fall risk assessments should be supported by education for staff and regular reviews to ensure its appropriate and consistent use.

Conclusions

Fall risk screening provides a quick means of identifying individuals at increased risk of falling who need greater surveillance or who require subsequent fall risk assessments. Fall risk assessment is more detailed and can identify fall risk factors amenable to interventions. A range of simple through to more comprehensive assessments that have good predictive accuracy have been devised for community, hospital, and residential aged care facility settings. Physiological profiling can complement the disease-based/medical approach to fall risk assessment by quantifying the degree of fall risk, irrespective of co-morbidities, and inform tailored interventions to address identified physiological impairments. Older people in sub-acute hospitals and residential aged care facilities should be assumed to be at increased risk of falling and undergo multi-factorial assessments and interventions. This may assist in optimizing the prevention of falls, as to date the most effective interventions in these settings have based their interventions on such assessment protocols.

REFERENCES

1. Panel on Prevention of Falls in Older Persons, American Geriatrics Society, and British Geriatrics Society. Summary of the Updated American Geriatrics Society/British Geriatrics Society clinical practice guideline for prevention of falls in older persons. *J Am Geriatr Soc.* 2011;59:148–57.

2. National Collaborating Centre for Nursing and Supportive Care. *Clinical Practice Guideline for the Assessment and Prevention of Falls in Older People.* London, UK: Royal College of Nursing (NICE); 2004.

3. American Geriatrics Society, British Geriatrics Society, and American Academy of Orthopedic Surgeons Panel on Falls Prevention. Guideline for the prevention of falls in older persons. *J Am Geriatr Soc.* 2001;49:664–72.

4. Podsialdo D, Richardson S. The timed "Up & Go": a test of basic functional mobility for frail elderly persons. *J Am Geriatr Soc.* 1991;39:142–8.

5. Schoene D, Wu SM, Mikolaizak AS et al. Discriminative ability and predictive validity of the timed up and go test in identifying older people who fall: systematic review and meta-analysis. *J Am Geriatr Soc.* 2013;61:202–8.

6. Tiedemann A, Shimada H, Sherrington C et al. The comparative ability of eight functional mobility tests for predicting falls in community-dwelling older people. *Age Ageing.* 2008;37:430–5.

7. Guralnik JM, Simonsick EM, Ferrucci L et al. A short physical performance battery assessing lower extremity function: association with self-reported disability and prediction of mortality and nursing home admission. *J Gerontol.* 1994;49:M85–94.

8. Lord SR, Menz HB, Tiedemann A. A physiological profile approach to falls risk assessment and prevention. *Phys Ther.* 2003;83:237–52.

9. Lord SR, Delbaere K, Gandevia SC. Use of a physiological profile to document motor impairment in ageing and in clinical groups. *J Physiol.* 2016;594:4513–23.

10. Tiedemann A, Lord SR, Sherrington C. The development and validation of a brief performance-based fall risk assessment tool for use in primary care. *J Gerontol A Biol Sci Med Sci.* 2010;65A:896–903.

11. Lord SR, Ward JA, Williams P et al. Physiological factors associated with falls in older community-dwelling women. *J Am Geriatr Soc.* 1994;42:1110–17.

12. Lord SR, Tiedemann A, Chapman K et al. The effect of an individualized fall prevention program on fall risk and falls in older people: a randomized controlled trial. *J Am Geriatr Soc.* 2005;53:1296–304.

13. National Institute for Health and Care Excellence. *Falls in Older People: Assessing Risk and Prevention.* London, England: NICE; 2013.

14. Oliver D. Falls risk-prediction tools for hospital inpatients: time to put them to bed?*Age Ageing.* 2008;37:248–50.

15. Haines TP, Bennell KL, Osborne RH et al. A new instrument for targeting falls prevention interventions was accurate and clinically applicable in a hospital setting. *J Clin Epidemiol.* 2006;59:168–75.

16. Healey F, Monro A, Cockram A et al. Using targeted risk factor reduction to prevent falls in older in-patients: a randomised controlled trial. *Age Ageing*. 2004;33:390–5.

17. Hill AM, McPhail SM, Waldron N et al. Fall rates in hospital rehabilitation units after individualised patient and staff education programmes: a pragmatic, stepped-wedge, cluster-randomised controlled trial. *Lancet*. 2015;385:2592–9.

18. Australian Commission on Safety and Quality in Health Care. *Preventing Falls and Harm from Falls in Older People. Best Practice Guidelines for Australian Community Care.* Sydney, NSW: ACSQHC; 2009.

19. Whitney J, Close JC, Lord SR et al. Identification of high risk fallers among older people living in residential care facilities: a simple screen based on easily collectable measures. *Arch Gerontol Geriatr*. 2012;55:690–5.

20. Becker C, Kron M, Lindemann U et al. Effectiveness of a multifaceted intervention on falls in nursing home residents. *J Am Geriatr Soc*. 2003;51:306–13.

21. Berg KO, Wood-Dauphinee SL, Williams JI et al. Measuring balance in the elderly: validation of an instrument. *Can J Public Health*. 1992;83:S7–11.

22. Franchignoni F, Horak F, Godi M et al. Using psychometric techniques to improve the Balance Evaluation Systems Test: the mini-BESTest. *J Rehabil Med*. 2010;42:323–31.

23. Verbaken JH, Johnston AW. Clinical contrast sensitivity testing: the current status. *Clin Exp Optom*. 1986;69:204–12.

24. Sherrington C, Lord SR. Reliability of simple portable tests of physical performance in older people after hip fracture. *Clin Rehabil*. 2005;19:496–504.

25. Nasreddine ZS, Phillips NA, Bédirian V et al. The Montreal Cognitive Assessment, MoCA: a brief screening tool for mild cognitive impairment. *J Am Geriatr Soc*. 2005;53:695–9.

26. Inouye SK, van Dyck CH, Alessi CA et al. Clarifying confusion: the confusion assessment method. A new method for detection of delirium. *Ann Intern Med*. 1990;113:941–8.

27. Menant JC, Meinrath D, Sturnieks DL et al. Identifying key risk factors for dizziness handicap in middle-aged and older people. *J Am Med Dir Assoc*. 2020;21:344–50.e2.

28. Yardley L, Beyer N, Hauer K et al. Development and initial validation of the Falls Efficacy Scale-International (FES-I). *Age Ageing*. 2005;34:614–19.

29. Delbaere K, Smith ST, Lord SR. Development and initial validation of the Iconographical Falls Efficacy Scale. *J Gerontol A Biol Sci Med Sci*. 2011;66:674–80.

30. Menz HB, Sherrington C. The Footwear Assessment Form: a reliable clinical tool to assess footwear characteristics of relevance to postural stability in older adults. *Clin Rehabil*. 2000;14:657–64.

31. Mackenzie L, Byles J, Higginbotham N. Designing the Home Falls and Accidents Screening Tool (HOME FAST): selecting the items. *Br J Occup Ther*. 2000;63:260–9.

32. Clemson L, Fitzgerald MH, Heard R. Content validity of an assessment tool to identify home fall hazards: The Westmead Home Safety Assessment. *Br J Occup Ther*. 1999;62:171–9.

15

The Relative Importance of Fall Risk Factors: Analysis and Summary

Stephen R. Lord, Catherine Sherrington, and Vasi Naganathan

In this chapter, we have brought together the findings from published studies cited in Chapters 1 to 14 that have addressed fall risk in older people. We have rated the major socio-demographic, physiological, psychological, health, and environmental factors that have been posited as important fall risk factors according to the strength of the published evidence associating that factor with falls, using the following four-level rating system:

*** strong evidence of association (consistently found in good studies/systematic review evidence),

** moderate evidence of association (usually but not always found),

* weak evidence of association (occasionally but not usually found) and

– little or no evidence of association (not found in published studies despite research to examine the issue).

The factors have been classified as: socio-demographic factors, balance and mobility factors, sensory and neuromuscular factors, psychological factors, medical factors, medication factors, and environmental factors.

Socio-Demographic Factors

Table 15.1 shows that a range of socio-demographic aspects have been systematically studied as potential fall risk factors.

As falls are generally considered to be a marker of frailty and decreased mobility it is not surprising that falls are associated with advanced age and impairments in activities of daily living. The finding that a history of falling is strongly associated with future falls is also not surprising. Most studies undertaken in community settings have shown a higher incidence of falls in women. This may be due to reduced strength, slower reaction time (most notably for choice reaction time variability [1]) and increased visual field dependence in women [2]. It has also been reported that older women are slower than older men in executing fast and accurate steps in a choice reaction stepping time task that required whole body

Table 15.1 Socio-demographic factors associated with falls

Factor	Strength of association
Advanced age	***
ADL/mobility limitations	***
History of falls	***
Female gender	**
Race	***
Living alone	**
Sleep disturbances	**
Inactivity	**
Walking aid use	**
Alcohol consumption	–

movement [3]. However, in hospitals and institutions, where inpatient populations have high prevalences of acute and chronic disease, frailty, impaired mobility, etc., the reported incidence of falling in men is similar to or higher than in women. The finding that living alone is a risk factor for falls may be confounded by age and sex, in that older women comprise most of this group, but may also reflect the need to undertake challenging daily activities without assistance. The differences in fall rates among racial groups may reflect different behavioural characteristics related to amount and type of habitual physical activity as well as genetic differences.

As is described in Chapter 16, exercise can improve strength, balance, and functional abilities in older people [4] and can prevent falls [5]. However, being more physically active does not necessarily prevent falls [6]. This is probably because the more physically active older person takes part in activities which increase exposure to fall risk situations. Clearly, this risk should be balanced against the benefits of increased physical functioning and independence that exercise brings.

Too little, too much, or poor sleep quality have been found to be independently associated with increased odds of falls in both community and residential aged care settings [7, 8]. Further studies are required to elucidate mechanisms for these associations.

The most surprising finding regarding associations between socio-demographic factors and falls is that alcohol consumption has not been shown to be a fall risk factor. Despite examining the issue, several early prospective studies found no significant associations between alcohol use and falls in older people [9–14]. In fact, most of these studies have found that those who are current drinkers have fewer falls than those who abstain [9, 10, 12, 14]. Campbell et al. [14]

have suggested that this unexpected protective association may be due to alcohol use being lower in those with poor physical health or those taking psychoactive drugs; however, this was not the case in a community study by Lord et al. [10]. It may also be the case that the lack of a positive association between alcohol use and falls is due to response and selection biases, in that heavy alcohol consumers may under-report their drinking levels or simply decline participation in research studies. However, despite the lack of an association between current alcohol use and falls in cohort studies, national health survey data indicates people who drink above low-risk drinking guidelines have elevated rates of non-fatal fall injuries [15], and there is strong evidence that long-term high alcohol intake can lead to multiple medical problems, including osteoporosis, cerebellar atrophy, and peripheral neuropathy [16].

Postural Instability

Table 15.2 summarizes the results of the many investigations that have been performed to evaluate whether various measures of balance, gait, and mobility are associated with increased fall risk. Challenging stability tasks are stronger risk factors for falls than less challenging tasks. For example, while impaired stability when standing and walking on level surfaces are moderate risk factors, measures of leaning balance, transfers, and standing from a sitting position are consistently reported as strong risk factors in well-designed studies. On the other hand, the more global or non-specific measures provide less information about the underlying mechanisms predisposing older people to falls.

A recent systematic review and meta-analysis of 61 studies involving more than 9000 participants demonstrated that stepping impairment is a significant risk factor for falls among older adults. Both volitional and reactive step tests were found to significantly distinguish fallers from non-fallers, and with respect to reactive stepping, the quality of the step (i.e. the speed, size, and direction), rather

Table 15.2 Balance and mobility factors associated with falls

Factor	Strength of association
Impaired stability when standing	**
Impaired stability when leaning and reaching	**
Slow voluntary stepping	***
Poor reactive stepping responses	***
Impaired sit-to-stand/transfer ability	***
Reduced gait velocity/cadence/step length	***
Increased gait variability	***

than the ability to withstand a perturbation appears more important for fall avoidance [17]. Finally, measures of gait variability and other indices of gait quality when assessed either in the laboratory or remotely have been found to be associated with falls in older people.

Sensory and Neuromuscular Factors

As outlined in Chapter 2, postural control is a complex process involving many body systems. Table 15.3 shows that reduced functioning in peripheral sensation, strength, and reaction time – major contributors to postural control – are strongly associated with falls. Impaired vision is also a strong falls risk factor, and the fact that it is only moderately associated with falls in some studies appears to be due to the use of a sub-optimal test, i.e. Snellen letter charts. These charts measure discrimination of fine detail, whereas the ability to accurately perceive depth and detect larger visual stimuli under low-contrast conditions are more pertinent visual measures for avoiding hazards and thus falls [18]. There is also evidence that, if measured rigorously, vestibular impairments [19], reduced muscle power [20], and endurance [21] are also important fall risk factors in older people.

Table 15.3 Sensory and neuromuscular factors associated with falls

Factor	Strength of association
Vision	
Poor visual contrast sensitivity	***
Decreased depth perception	***
Poor visual acuity	**
Visual field loss	*
Increased visual field dependence	*
Poor hearing	*
Reduced vestibular function	*
Peripheral sensation	
Reduced vibration sense	***
Reduced tactile sensitivity	***
Reduced proprioception	**
Muscle strength	
Reduced muscle strength	***
Reduced muscle power	*
Reduced muscle endurance	*
Reaction time	
Poor simple reaction time	***
Poor choice reaction time	***

Finally, there are inconsistent reports that hearing impairment contributes to falls in older people [22, 23].

Studies by Lord et al. have found that measurements of vision, peripheral sensation, strength, reaction time, and balance significantly and independently contribute to the discrimination between fallers and non-fallers in multi-variate analyses [24, 25]. This suggests that poor functioning in any of these physiological domains predisposes older people to falls and that multiple impairments greatly increase fall risk. However, when the standardized weightings of each measure are compared, it is apparent that they do not contribute equally to the prediction of falls. Slow reaction time and increased sway (particularly when challenged by having participants close their eyes or stand on a compliant surface) appear to be particularly strong physiological risk factors for falls [24, 25].

Psychological Risk Factors

Table 15.4 outlines the psychological factors that have been implicated in falls in older people. Neuropsychological measures identified as fall risk factors include slow processing speed, reduced executive functioning, and poor selective attention. Several studies have shown that with increasing age, balance tasks become more attentionally demanding and frail older people require even more attentional resources for postural control, to the extent that even simple tasks like answering a question may interfere with standing, stepping, and walking [26]. In these situations, older people with attentional limitations are at increased risk of falls [27], although systematic review evidence indicates adding secondary tasks to tests of gait speed does not improve their ability to predict falls in older people [28].

Fear of falling is prevalent in older people. In many cases, this fear may be excessive and lead to unnecessary restrictions in physical and social activity. Fear of falling is strongly associated with falls [29], but most studies have not demonstrated fear of falling to be a risk factor for falls after adjusting for physical risk

Table 15.4 Psychological factors associated with falls

Factor	Strength of association
Increased fear of falling	***
Anxiety	**
Impaired executive functioning	***
Reduced processing speed	***
Impaired selective attention	**
Risk taking	*

factors. However, it has been shown many older people under- or overestimate their risk of falling, and that undue perceived risk is primarily associated with psychological measures such as anxiety, depression, and reduced executive functioning [30]. There is preliminary evidence that risk-taking behaviours increase fall risk in older people [31].

Medical Factors

Many studies have identified a range of medical factors that are associated with an increased risk of falls [10–12, 14, 32–34]. As illustrated in Table 15.5, these include the presence of stroke or Parkinson's disease, acute illness, arthritis, foot problems, depression, incontinence, impaired cognition, cerebral white matter lesions, and abnormal neurological signs. These conditions/problems have been shown to be risk factors for falls in both community and institutional settings, although the importance of some of these, such as incontinence and impaired cognition may be most important in institutions. The distinction between strong and moderate evidence for these factors relates to some extent to the difficulty in rigorously measuring some of these conditions/problems. This has meant that fewer studies have addressed these factors or that crude measures (with resultant imprecision) have been used as substitutes. This is particularly the case for neurological conditions, arthritis, and foot problems.

However, as also shown in Table 15.5, certain conditions commonly perceived to be strong risk factors for falls, such as vestibular disorders and orthostatic

Table 15.5 Medical factors associated with falls

Factor	Strength of association
Dementia / impaired cognition	***
Stroke	***
Parkinson's disease	***
White matter lesions	**
Abnormal neurological signs	**
Depression	***
Dizziness	**
Acute illness	**
Incontinence	**
Arthritis	**
Foot problems	**
Orthostatic hypotension	*
Vestibular disorders	–
Number of chronic conditions	***

hypotension, have not been found to be important risk factors at a population level in research studies. The lack of reported associations between either vestibular disorders or dizziness and falls appears paradoxical, as such disorders have marked effects on balance. Three factors could account for the lack of association. Firstly, increased age results in a *loss* of vestibular functioning, not an increase in *aberrant* vestibular information, as is the case with vestibular disease. Older people with adequate peripheral sensation and/or vision may be able to compensate for reduced vestibular functioning. Secondly, vestibular disorders (as opposed to diminished vestibular function) have such a marked effect on balance in older people that sufferers take steps to avoid falling – quite often by lying down. The final factor may relate to study limitations in that assessment measures used in prospective studies on falls have not taken into account the transient nature of certain vestibular disorders.

As indicated in Chapter 10, orthostatic hypotension, whether idiopathic or iatrogenic, has not been found to increase the risk of falling in older people in prospective cohort studies. This indicates that in comparison with impairments of sensorimotor function, balance, and gait, orthostatic hypotension is a relatively unimportant or rare cause of falls at a population level. As is the case with vestibular disorders, the lack of a demonstrated link between orthostatic hypotension and falls may be due to study limitations. Most studies have tested for orthostatic hypotension on a single occasion, usually when the older subject visits a clinic or laboratory. These subjects are then followed up in prospective studies to determine falling rates. It is possible that as orthostatic hypotension can be of an intermittent nature, patients may test negatively on the baseline testing day, but suffer postural blood pressure drops and falls on one or more occasions in the follow-up period. Further research is therefore required to determine the timing and frequency of orthostatic blood pressure measurement that is most predictive of falls [35]. It has also been reported that carotid sinus hypersensitivity, often cited as a cause of drop attacks and syncope, may be responsible for a proportion of unexplained falls [36], but is probably too rare to be detected in representative community samples of older people.

Medication Use

Table 15.6 outlines medications that have been implicated in falls in older people. Studies undertaken in both community and institutional settings have consistently reported significant associations between psychoactive medication (sedatives, antianxiety agents, antipsychotics, and antidepressants) use and falls [37]. In contrast, the association between antihypertensives and falls is inconsistent [38]. For these medications, the risk of falling appears to be highest on initiation or

Table 15.6 Medication factors associated with falls

Factor	Strength of association
Use of multiple medications	***
Benzodiazepines	***
Antidepressants	***
Antipsychotics	***
Psychoactive medications	***
Opioids	**
Antiarrhythmics	*
Antihypertensives	*
Analgesics	-
Anti-inflammatory drugs	-

within the first 24 hours of a dosage adjustment, then decreases to non-significant levels afterward. Regarding other cardiovascular drug classes, digoxin and type IA antiarrhythmic drugs may increase fall risk, and beta blockers may reduce it. Finally, there is consistent evidence indicating that opiates and antiepileptics increase fall risk and that non-steroidal anti-inflammatory drugs are not a risk factor for falls once confounding variables are taken into account [39].

The use of multiple medications (usually 4+) has been shown to be a predictor of fall risk in several studies. However, multiple medication use may be primarily a marker for underlying chronic diseases, and with the rising number of pharmacological treatments available from which older people have potential to benefit both in terms of morbidity and mortality, the priority is to ensure that older people are able to access treatments from which they stand to benefit, while ensuring harmful drug interactions and unnecessary medications are avoided.

Environmental Factors

In contrast to socio-demographic, medical, and physiological factors, there is less evidence that environmental factors are strongly associated with falls (see Table 15.7). There is no conclusive data to indicate that the households of older people who fall are more 'hazardous' than those who do not fall. The lack of associations may reflect, at least in part, the difficulty of studying transient or intermittent risk factors. However, as many falls undoubtedly involve environmental factors, it seems that the interaction between the older person's functional abilities and the environment is a crucial factor in determining whether a fall will occur. Further, as reported in Chapter 23, home hazard reduction is effective if targeted to older people with a history of falls and mobility limitations, and combined with strategies for improving transfer abilities and other behavioural changes.

Table 15.7 Environmental factors associated with falls

Factor	Strength of association
Poor footwear	*
Inappropriate spectacles	*
Home hazards	-
External hazards	-

There is now preliminary evidence that poor footwear [40] and inappropriate spectacles [41] are risk factors for falls. Both factors have also been found to affect important physiological fall risk factors. For example, high-heeled shoes impair balance [42] and bifocal and multi-focal spectacles impair depth perception and contrast sensitivity at critical distances required for detecting obstacles in the environment [41].

Conclusions

Large epidemiological studies have identified many risk factors for falling in older people. Many socio-demographic factors, medical conditions, and impairments of sensorimotor function, balance, and gait have been shown to be strongly associated with falls. The lack of significant associations for other posited risk factors might indicate that these are relatively unimportant causes of falls or that these issues have not been subject to appropriate study. The risk factors that are of an intermittent nature are especially difficult to study.

The above summaries have listed risk factors in isolation and have used a simple classification scheme. Many of the risk factors are inter-related, as indicated by path analytic models [43, 44]. Furthermore, the commonly used intrinsic/extrinsic distinction is an oversimplification, and a better understanding of falls is usually obtained when taking an ecological perspective, that is, examining the person and their behaviour in association with environmental factors [45]. Finally, the above summaries, by definition, are based on findings from population studies. Clearly, in clinical practice many medical conditions and rare disorders in addition to those listed above as important risk factors may well be the cause of falls in individual patients and require investigation.

REFERENCES

1. Der G, Deary IJ. Age and sex differences in reaction time in adulthood: results from the United Kingdom Health and Lifestyle Survey. *Psychol Aging.* 2006;21:62–73.

2. Lord SR, Sambrook PN, Gilbert C et al. Postural stability, falls and fractures in the elderly: results from the Dubbo Osteoporosis Epidemiology Study. *Med J Aust*. 1994;160:684–5, 8–91.

3. Lord SR, Fitzpatrick RC. Choice stepping reaction time: a composite measure of falls risk in older people. *J Gerontol A Biol Sci Med Sci*. 2001;56:M627–32.

4. Buchner DM, Beresford SA, Larson EB et al. Effects of physical activity on health status in older adults. II. Intervention studies. *Annu Rev Public Health*. 1992;13:469–88.

5. Province MA, Hadley EC, Hornbrook MC et al. The effects of exercise on falls in elderly patients. A preplanned meta-analysis of the FICSIT Trials. Frailty and Injuries: Cooperative Studies of Intervention Techniques. *J Am Med Assoc*. 1995;273:1341–7.

6. Studenski S, Duncan PW, Chandler J et al. Predicting falls: the role of mobility and nonphysical factors. *J Am Geriatr Soc*. 1994;42:297–302.

7. Cauley JA, Hovey KM, Stone KL et al. Characteristics of self-reported sleep and the risk of falls and fractures: the Women's Health Initiative (WHI). *J Bone Miner Res*. 2019;34:464–74.

8. St George RJ, Delbaere K, Williams P et al. Sleep quality and falls in older people living in self- and assisted-care villages. *Gerontology*. 2009;55:162–8.

9. Nelson DE, Sattin RW, Langlois JA et al. Alcohol as a risk factor for fall injury events among elderly persons living in the community. *J Am Geriatr Soc*. 1992;40:658–61.

10. Lord SR, Ward JA, Williams P et al. An epidemiological study of falls in older community-dwelling women: the Randwick falls and fractures study. *Aust J Public Health*. 2010;17:240–5.

11. Sheahan SL, Coons SJ, Robbins CA et al. Psychoactive medication, alcohol use, and falls among older adults. *J Behav Med*. 1995;18:127–40.

12. Tinetti ME, Speechley M, Ginter SF. Risk factors for falls among elderly persons living in the community. *N Engl J Med*. 1988;319:1701–7.

13. Nevitt MC. Risk factors for recurrent nonsyncopal falls. *J Am Med Assoc*. 1989;261:2663.

14. Campbell AJ, Borrie MJ, Spears GF. Risk factors for falls in a community-based prospective study of people 70 years and older. *J Gerontol*. 1989;44:M112–17.

15. Chen CM, Yoon YH. Usual alcohol consumption and risks for nonfatal fall injuries in the United States: results from the 2004–2013 National Health Interview Survey. *Subst Use Misuse*. 2017;52:1120–32.

16. Carlson JE. Alcohol use and falls. *J Am Geriatr Soc*. 1993;41:346–7.

17. Okubo Y, Schoene D, Caetano MJ et al. Stepping impairment and falls in older adults: a systematic review and meta-analysis of volitional and reactive step tests. *Ageing Res Rev*. 2021;66:101238.

18. Lord SR, Clark RD, Webster IW. Visual acuity and contrast sensitivity in relation to falls in an elderly population. *Age Ageing*. 1991;20:175–81.

19. Di Fabio RP, Greany JF, Emasithi A et al. Eye-head coordination during postural perturbation as a predictor of falls in community-dwelling elderly women. *Arch Phys Med Rehab*. 2002;83:942–51.

20. Skelton DA. Explosive power and asymmetry in leg muscle function in frequent fallers and non-fallers aged over 65. *Age Ageing*. 2002;31:119–25.

21. Schwendner KI, Mikesky AE, Holt WS et al. Differences in muscle endurance and recovery between fallers and nonfallers, and between young and older women. *J Gerontol A Biol Sci Med Sci.* 1997;52A:M155–60.

22. Lin FR, Ferrucci L. Hearing loss and falls among older adults in the United States. *Arch Intern Med.* 2012,172.369 71.

23. Purchase-Helzner EL, Cauley JA, Faulkner KA et al. Hearing sensitivity and the risk of incident falls and fracture in older women: the study of osteoporotic fractures. *Ann Epidemiol.* 2004;14:311–18.

24. Lord SR, Clark RD, Webster IW. Physiological factors associated with falls in an elderly population. *J Am Geriatr Soc.* 1991;39:1194–200.

25. Lord SR, Ward JA, Williams P et al. Physiological factors associated with falls in older community-dwelling women. *J Am Geriatr Soc.* 1994;42:1110–17.

26. Woollacott M, Shumway-Cook A. Attention and the control of posture and gait: a review of an emerging area of research. *Gait Posture.* 2002;16:1–14.

27. Lundin-Olsson L, Nyberg L, Gustafson Y. "Stops walking when talking" as a predictor of falls in elderly people. *Lancet.* 1997;349:617.

28. Menant JC, Schoene D, Sarofim M et al. Single and dual task tests of gait speed are equivalent in the prediction of falls in older people: a systematic review and meta-analysis. *Ageing Res Rev.* 2014;16:83–104.

29. Legters K. Fear of falling. *Phys Ther.* 2002;82:264–72.

30. Delbaere K, Close JC, Brodaty H et al. Determinants of disparities between perceived and physiological risk of falling among elderly people: cohort study. *BMJ Clin Res.* 2010;341: c4165.

31. Butler AA, Lord SR, Taylor JL et al. Ability versus hazard: risk-taking and falls in older people. *J Gerontol A Biol Sci Med Sci.* 2015;70:628–34.

32. Campbell AJ, Reinken J, Allan BC et al. Falls in old age: a study of frequency and related clinical factors. *Age Ageing.* 1981;10:264–70.

33. Prudham D, Evans JG. Factors associated with falls in the elderly: a community study. *Age Ageing.* 1981;10:141–6.

34. Robbins AS. Predictors of falls among elderly people: results of two population-based studies. *Arch Intern Med.* 1989;149:1628–33.

35. McDonald C, Pearce M, Kerr SR et al. A prospective study of the association between orthostatic hypotension and falls: definition matters. *Age Ageing.* 2017;46:439–45.

36. Parry SW, Kenny RA. Drop attacks in older adults: systematic assessment has a high diagnostic yield. *J Am Geriatr Soc.* 2005;53:74–8.

37. Seppala LJ, Wermelink A, de Vries M et al. Fall-risk-increasing drugs: a systematic review and meta-analysis. II. Psychotropics. *J Am Med Dir Assoc.* 2018;19:371.e11–17.

38. de Vries M, Seppala LJ, Daams JG et al. Fall-risk-increasing drugs: a systematic review and meta-analysis. I. Cardiovascular drugs. *J Am Med Dir Assoc.* 2018;19:371.e1–9.

39. Seppala LJ, van de Glind EMM, Daams JG et al. Fall-risk-increasing drugs: a systematic review and meta-analysis. III. Others. *J Am Med Dir Assoc.* 2018;19:372.e1–8.

40. Tencer AF, Koepsell TD, Wolf ME et al. Biomechanical properties of shoes and risk of falls in older adults. *J Am Geriatr Soc.* 2004;52:1840–6.

41. Lord SR, Dayhew J, Howland A. Multifocal glasses impair edge-contrast sensitivity and depth perception and increase the risk of falls in older people. *J Am Geriatr Soc.* 2002;50:1760–6.

42. Lord SR, Bashford GM. Shoe characteristics and balance in older women. *J Am Geriatr Soc.* 1996;44:429–33.

43. Lord SR, Anstey KJ, Williams P et al. Psychoactive medication use, sensori-motor function and falls in older women. *Br J Clin Pharmacol.* 1995;39:227–34.

44. Kvelde T, Pijnappels M, Delbaere K et al. Physiological and cognitive mediators for the association between self-reported depressed mood and impaired choice stepping reaction time in older people. *J Gerontol A Biol Sci Med Sci.* 2010;65:538–44.

45. Hogue CC. Falls and mobility in late life. *J Am Geriatr Soc.* 1984;32:858–61.

Part II

Strategies for Prevention

16

Exercise to Prevent Falls

Catherine Sherrington, Anne Tiedemann, and Nicola Fairhall

Daily life requires humans to undertake tasks in a range of environmental settings. Falls occur due to a mismatch between an individual's physiological function, environmental demands and the individual's behaviour. Many of the physiological impairments that increase the risk of falls (as outlined in Part 1 of this book) can be improved with structured exercise interventions. Poor balance control and impaired muscle strength particularly increase the risk of falling but are amenable to change with exercise [1, 2]. Exercise may also prevent falls by enabling practise of safe negotiation of the environment and a greater awareness of one's abilities in different situations.

The Evolution of Evidence about Exercise for the Prevention of Falls

There is now strong evidence for the effectiveness of exercise in the prevention of falls in community-dwelling older people [3, 4]. Exercise was the most frequently researched fall prevention intervention in the 2012 Cochrane review, which identified 59 randomized controlled trials of exercise as a fall prevention intervention [3]. The 2019 Cochrane review of exercise for fall prevention included 108 trials and confirmed that exercise can prevent falls in the community in terms of the rate of falls (number of falls experienced per person) and the number of people experiencing one or more falls per year (proportion of fallers in each group) [5]. This review categorized programmes as primarily involving different types of exercise according to criteria established by the European-Union-funded ProFaNE group [6]. Significantly different effects were found for different types of exercise through an overall test of sub-group difference. The impact of different types of exercise was then explored separately. This led to the conclusion that: (i) exercise that primarily targeted functional abilities or balance, (ii) exercise with multiple components (most commonly function/balance and strength), and (iii) Tai Chi were effective forms of exercise. Conversely, there was no current evidence that strength training alone, walking alone, or dance prevents falls.

A complementary 88-trial systematic review [7] also highlighted the importance of a focus on postural control/balance in exercise for fall prevention and used slightly different methods. This review pooled all exercise programmes together and used meta-regression to identify programme features that were associated with greater fall prevention effects [7] and built on the team's previous reviews in 2008 (45 trials) [8] and 2011 (54 trials) [4]. The meta-regression confirmed the previous finding that greater effects of exercise on falls are seen from programmes of a higher dose that include balance-challenging exercises. Interventions were classified as including a high challenge to balance if the exercise was undertaken while standing and aimed to: (i) narrow the base of support (by standing with the feet closer together or on one foot), (ii) include exercise performed without the use of the arms to support the body, and (iii) involve controlled movement of the body in space. These results differed from the previous version in that the cut off of three hours per week of total exercise distinguished between less effective and more effective programmes, whereas the previous review had used the median cut off of two hours per week [4]. Also, previous analyses found that the inclusion of walking programmes reduced intervention effects, but this was not the case in the most recent analysis. This was probably driven by a new trial that delivered a walking programme that did not increase falls. If not prescribed carefully, walking programmes may increase the exposure to environmental fall hazards as well as not focusing sufficiently on improving balance.

An Updated Review of Exercise to Prevent Falls

This chapter includes an update of the 108-trial 2019 Cochrane review [5] with additional trials to bring the total number of trials to 116. The characteristics of the 108 trials from the Cochrane review are summarized in the review itself [5] and in an additional paper [9]. Table 16.1 summarizes the newer trials not included in the Cochrane review. All studies were randomized controlled trials (RCTs) and involved a total of 25,160 participants. Most trials were individually randomized and ten were cluster randomized. The median number of participants randomized per trial was 131 (interquartile range (IQR) 66 to 249). The included trials were carried out in 25 countries, the most common being the USA (21 trials), Australia (20 trials), Japan (11 trials), and the UK (7 trials). Overall, 73% of included participants were women. All participants were women in 28 trials and all participants were men in one trial. The average participant age in the included trials was 76 years. Of the included studies, 62 (53%) specified a history of falling or evidence of one or more risk factors for falling in their inclusion criteria; 79 trials (68%) excluded participants with cognitive impairment, either defined as an

Table 16.1 Characteristics of new trials since the 2019 Cochrane review [5, 9]

First author, year	Sample size at randomization	Trial location	Age	Gender (% women)	Falls risk at enrolment[a]	Inclusion criteria related to falls	Good adherence[b]
Arkkukangas, 2019 [35]	175	Sweden	83	70	0		NR
Barclay, 2018 [36]	9	Canada	76	78	0		Y
Bernardelli, 2019 [37]	186	Italy	76	80	0		Y
Gallo, 2018 [38]	69	United States	79	46	0		NR
Li, 2018 [39]	670	United States	78	65	1	Fall history/ assessed risk of falls or reduced mobility	Y
Lipsitz, 2019 [40]	180	United States	75	67	0		Y
Liu-Ambrose, 2019 [41]	345	Canada	82	67	1	Previous fall	Y
Ma, 2019 [40]	33	Hong Kong	70	84	0		NR
Oliveira, 2019 [42]	131	Australia	72	71	0		NR

[a] Presence of a particular risk factor for falls was used as an inclusion criterion for the trial (0 = No specific risk; 1 = Previous falls, poor balance, recent hospitalization, reduced lower strength, poor mobility, use of mobility aids, frail, prolonged bed rest, recent rehabilitation, functional limitation, all participants greater than age 80) [b] Determined using numbers in each age group; N = No, Y = Yes, NR = not reported

exclusion criterion or implied by the stated requirement to be able to give informed consent.

The results of this updated review remain essentially unchanged from the 2019 Cochrane review. A key feature of recent Cochrane reviews is the rigorous application of the GRADE system to assess the strength of evidence/level of certainty associated with included results. Cochrane reviews now also require calculation of the absolute impact of interventions. Using the fall rate in the control group in the included studies we estimated that if exercise was delivered to 1000 people who were followed for one year there would be 195 (95% CI: 144, 246) fewer falls than the estimated 850 falls that would occur without exercise. The updated Summary of Findings table showing the strength of evidence and estimated impacts is shown in Table 16.2.

The key findings are that:

1. *Exercise reduces the rate of falls by 23% compared with control* (rate ratio (RaR): 0.77, 95% CI: 0.71, 0.83; 14,306 participants, 64 studies, I^2: 61%; high-certainty evidence).

2. Exercise can prevent falls in the general older population (aged 60+ years) as well as in people at an increased risk of falls and those aged 75+ years. Sub-group analysis by fall risk at baseline found there was probably little or no difference in the effect of exercise (all types) on the rate of falls in trials where all participants were at an increased risk of falling (RaR: 0.76, 95% CI: 0.69, 0.84; 7872 participants, 32 studies, I^2: 65%) compared with trials that did not use increased risk of falling as an entry criterion (RaR: 0.78, 95% CI: 0.68, 0.89; 6434 participants, 32 studies, I^2: 57%); test for sub-group differences: Chi^2: 0.1, df: 1, P: 0.75, I^2: 65%. Subgroup analysis by participant age found there was probably little or no difference in the effect of exercise (all types) on the rate of falls in trials where participants were aged 75 years or older (Ra:R 0.85, 95% CI: 0.73, 1.0; 3841 participants, 14 studies, I^2: 61%) compared with trials where participants were aged less than 75 years (RaR: 0.74, 95% CI: 0.68, 0.81; 10465 participants, 50 studies, I^2: 60%); test for sub-group differences: Chi^2: 2.29, df: 1, P: 0.13, I^2: 56%.

3. Fall prevention exercise can be effective when delivered in groups or individually by health professionals or trained exercise instructors. Sub-group analyses found there may be no difference in the effect of exercise (all types) in trials where interventions were delivered by a health professional (usually a physiotherapist, RaR: 0.73, 95% CI: 0.64, 0.82; 5099 participants, 28 studies, I^2: 53%) and in trials where the interventions were delivered by trained instructors who were not health professionals (RaR: 0.79, 95% CI: 0.72, 0.88; 9207 participants, 36 studies, I^2: 65%); test for sub-group differences: Chi^2: 1.2, df: 1, P: 0.27, I^2: 16%. Notably, both approaches resulted in reductions in the

Table 16.2 Summary of findings: rate of falls outcome (falls per person-years) for types of exercise

Type of exercise	Follow-up range	Illustrative comparative risks (95% CI)		Relative effect (95% CI)	No. of participants (studies)	Certainty of the evidence (GRADE)	Comments
		Assumed risk	Corresponding risk				
Exercise[a] (all types) versus control[b] (e.g. usual activities)	3 to 30 months	Control All studies population 850 per 1000[c] Not selected for high-risk population 605 per 1000[c] Selected for high-risk population 1290 per 1000[c]	Exercise (all types) 655 per 1000 (604 to 706) 466 per 1000 (430 to 503) 993 per 1000 (915 to 1071)	Rate ratio 0.77 (0.71 to 0.83)[d]	14,306 (64 RCTs)	High[e]	Overall, there is a reduction of 23% (95% CI: 17,29) in the number of falls Guide to the data: If 1000 people were followed over one year, the number of falls in the overall population would be 655 (95% CI: 604, 706) compared with 850 in the group receiving usual care or attention control. In the unselected population, the corresponding data are 466 (95% CI: 430, 503) compared with 605 in the group receiving usual care or attention control. In the selected higher-risk population, the corresponding data are 993 (95% CI: 915, 1071) compared with 1290 in the control group
Balance, and functional exercises[f] versus control[b] (e.g. usual activities)	3 to 30 months	Control All studies population 850 per 1000[g] Specific exercise population 865 per 1000[g]	Exercise (gait, balance, and functional training) 646 per 1000 (595 to 689) 657 per 1000 (606 to 709)	Rate ratio 0.76 (0.70 to 0.82)	7989 (39 RCTs)	High[h]	Overall, there is a reduction of 24% (95% CI: 18,30) in the number of falls Guide to the data based on the all-studies estimate If 1000 people were followed over one year, the number of falls would be 646 (95% CI: 595, 689) compared with 850 in the group receiving usual care or attention control
Resistance exercises[j] versus control[b] (e.g. usual activities)	4 to 12 months	Control All studies population	Exercise (resistance training)	Rate ratio 1.14 (0.67 to 1.97)	327 (5 RCTs)	Very low[k]	The evidence is of very low certainty, hence we are uncertain of the findings of an

Table 16.2 (cont.)

Type of exercise	Follow-up range	Illustrative comparative risks (95% CI)		Relative effect (95% CI)	No. of participants (studies)	Certainty of the evidence (GRADE)	Comments
		Assumed risk	Corresponding risk				
		850 per 1000[i] Specific exercise population 630 per 1000[j]	969 per 1000 (570 to 1675) 719 per 1000 (423 to 1242)				increase of 14% (95% CI: 33% reduction, 97% increase) in the number of falls Guide to the data based on the all-studies estimate: If 1000 people were followed over one year, the number of falls would be 969 (95% CI: 570, 1675) compared with 850 in the group receiving usual care or attention control
3D (Tai Chi) exercise[l] versus control[b] (e.g. usual activities)	6 to 17 months	Control All studies population 850 per 1000[m] Specific exercise population 1290 per 1000[m]	Exercise (3D (Tai Chi)) 655 per 1000 (519 to 825) 993 per 1000 (787 to 1251)	Rate ratio 0.77 (0.61 to 0.97)	3169 (9 RCTs)	Moderate[n]	Overall, there is probably be a reduction of 23% (95% CI: 3%, 39%) in the number of falls Guide to the data based on the all-studies estimate: If 1000 people were followed over one year, the number of falls is probably 655 (95% CI: 519, 825) compared with 850 in the group receiving usual care or attention control
3D (dance) exercise[o] versus control[b] (e.g. usual activities)	12 months	Control All studies population 850 per 1000[p] Specific exercise population 800 per 1000[p]	Exercise (3D (dance)) 1139 per 1000 (833 to 1556) 1072 per 1000 (784 to 1464)	Rate ratio 1.34 (0.98 to 1.83)	522 (1 RCT)	Very low[q]	The evidence is of very low certainty, hence we are uncertain of the findings of an increase of 34% (95% CI: 2% reduction, 83% increase) in the number of falls Guide to the data based on the all-studies estimate: If 1000 people were followed over one year, the number of falls may be 1139 (95% CI: 833, 1556) compared with 850 in the group receiving usual care or attention control

Intervention	Time	Comparison	Effect (95% CI)	No. of participants (studies)	Certainty	Plain language summary
General physical activity (including walking) training[r] versus control[b] (e.g. usual activities)	12 to 24 months	Control All studies population 850 per 1000[s] Specific exercise population 670 per 1000[s]	Exercise (general physical activity (including walking)) Rate ratio 1.14 (0.66 to 1.97) 969 per 1000 (561 to 1675) 764 per 1000 (443 to 1320)	441 (2 RCTs)	Very low[t]	The evidence is of very low certainty, hence we are uncertain of the findings of an increase of 14% (95% CI: 34% reduction, 97% increase) in the number of falls Guide to the data based on the all-studies estimate If 1000 people were followed over one year, the number of falls may be 969 (95% CI: 561, 1675) compared with 850 in the group receiving usual care or attention control
Multiple categories of exercise (often including, as primary interventions: gait, balance, and functional (task) training[u] plus resistance training[b] versus control[b] (e.g. usual activities)	2 to 25 months	Control All studies population 850 per 1000[v] Specific exercise population 1205 per 1000[v]	Exercise (multiple types (including, as primary interventions: gait, balance, and functional (task) training plus resistance training)) Rate ratio 0.72 (0.56 to 0.93)[r] 612 per 1000 (476 to 791) 868 per 1000 (675 to 791)	2283 (15 RCTs)	Moderate[w]	Overall, there is probably a reduction of 28% (95% CI: 7%, 44%) in the number of falls Guide to the data based on the all-studies estimate If 1000 people were followed over one year, the number of falls would probably be 612 (95% CI: 476,791) compared with 850 in the group receiving usual care or attention control

CI: confidence interval

GRADE Working Group grades of evidence: High certainty - We are very confident that the true effect lies close to that of the estimate of the effect; Moderate certainty - We are moderately confident in the effect estimate, the true effect is likely to be close to the estimate of the effect, but there is a possibility that it is substantially different; Low certainty - Our confidence in the effect estimate is limited, the true effect may be substantially different from the estimate of the effect; Very low certainty - We have very little confidence in the effect estimate, the true effect is likely to be substantially different from the estimate of effect.

[a] Exercise is a physical activity that is planned, structured, and repetitive and aims to improve or maintain physical fitness. There is a wide range of possible types of exercise, and exercise programmes often include one or more types of exercise. Exercise is categorized using the Prevention of Falls Network Europe (ProFaNE) taxonomy that classifies exercise type as: (i) gait, balance, and functional training, (ii) strength/resistance (including power), (iii) flexibility, (iv) three-dimensional (3D) exercise (e.g. Tai Chi, Qigong, dance), (v) general physical activity, (vi) endurance, and (vii) other kind of exercises.

[b] A control intervention is one that is not thought to reduce falls, such as general health education, social visits, very gentle exercise, or 'sham' exercise not expected to impact on falls.

[c] The all-studies population risk was based on the number of events and the number of participants in the control group for this outcome over the 64 RCTs. We calculated the risk in the control group using the median falls per person-year for the sub-groups of trials for which: (i) an increased risk of falls was not an inclusion criterion (32 RCTs, 6434 participants), or (ii) increased risk of falls was an inclusion criterion (32 RCTs, 7872 participants).

d Sub-group analysis found no difference based on whether risk of falls was an inclusion criterion or not (test for sub-group differences: Chi^2: 0.1, df: 1, P: 0.75, I^2: 0%).

e There was no downgrading, including for risk of bias, as results were essentially unchanged with removal of the trials with a high risk of bias on one or more items.

f Using Prevention of Falls Network Europe (ProFaNE) taxonomy, gait, balance, and functional training is: gait training = specific correction of walking technique, and changes of pace, level, and direction; balance training = transferring bodyweight from one part of the body to another or challenging specific aspects of the balance systems; functional training = functional activities, based on the concept of task specificity. Training is assessment-based, tailored, and progressed. Exercise programmes included in this analysis contained a single primary exercise category (gait, balance, and functional training); these exercise programmes may also include secondary categories of exercise.

g The all-studies population risk was based on the number of events and the number of participants in the control group for this outcome over the 64 all-exercise types RCTs. The specific exercise population risk was based on the number of events and the number of participants in the control group for this outcome over the 39 RCTs.

h We did not downgrade for risk of bias, as results were essentially unchanged with the removal of the trials with a high risk of bias in one or more items.

i Using Prevention of Falls Network Europe (ProFaNE) taxonomy, resistance training is any type of weight training (contraction of muscles against resistance to induce a training effect in the muscular system). Resistance is applied by body weight or external resistance. Training is assessment-based, tailored, and progressed. Exercise programmes included in this analysis had resistance training as the single primary exercise category; these exercise programmes may also include secondary categories of exercise.

j The all-studies population risk was based on the number of events and the number of participants in the control group for this outcome over the 64 all-exercise types RCTs. The specific exercise population risk was based on the number of events and the number of participants in the control group for this outcome over the 5 RCTs.

k Downgraded by three levels due to risk of inconsistency (there was substantial heterogeneity (I^2: 67%), imprecision (wide CI due to small sample size), and risk of bias (removing studies with high risk of bias in one or more items had a marked impact on results).

l Using Prevention of Falls Network Europe (ProFaNE) taxonomy, 3D (Tai Chi) training uses upright posture, specific weight transferences, and movements of the head and gaze, during constant movement in a fluid, repetitive, controlled manner through three spatial planes. Exercise programmes included in this analysis had 3D (Tai Chi) training as the single primary exercise category; these exercise programmes may also include secondary categories of exercise.

m The all-studies population risk was based on the number of events and the number of participants in the control group for this outcome over the 64 all-exercise types RCTs. The specific exercise population risk was based on the number of events and the number of participants in the control group for this outcome over the nine RCTs.

n Downgraded by one level due to inconsistency (there was substantial heterogeneity (I^2: 83%). There was no downgrading for risk of bias, as results were essentially unchanged with removal of the trials with a high risk of bias on one or more items.

o Using Prevention of Falls Network Europe (ProFaNE) taxonomy, 3D (dance) training uses dynamic movement qualities, patterns, and speeds while engaged in constant movement in a fluid, repetitive, controlled manner through three spatial planes. Exercise programmes included in this analysis had 3D (dance) training as the single primary exercise category; these exercise programmes may also include secondary categories of exercise.

p The all-studies population risk was based on the number of events and the number of participants in the control group for this outcome over the 64 all-exercise types RCTs. The specific exercise population risk was based on the number of events and the number of participants in the control group for this outcome in the sole RCT.

q Graded very low due to serious imprecision (only one cluster-RCT, with a wide CI due to small sample size).

r Using Prevention of Falls Network Europe (ProFaNE) taxonomy, physical activity is any movement of the body, produced by skeletal muscle, that causes energy expenditure to be substantially increased. Recommendations regarding intensity, frequency, and duration are required in order to increase performance. Exercise programmes included in this analysis had general physical activity (including walking) training as the single primary exercise category; these exercise programmes may also include secondary categories of exercise.

s   The all-studies population risk was based on the number of events and the number of participants in the control group for this outcome over the 64 all-exercise types RCTs. The specific exercise population risk was based on the number of events and the number of participants in the control group for this outcome in the two RCTs.

t   Downgraded by three levels due to inconsistency (there was substantial heterogeneity (I²: 67%), imprecision (wide CI), and risk of bias (removing studies with high risk of bias on one or more items had a marked impact on results).

u   Exercise programmes included in this analysis had more than one primary exercise category. We categorized exercise based on the Prevention of Falls Network Europe (ProFaNE) taxonomy that classifies exercise type as: (i) gait, balance, and functional (task) training, (ii) strength/resistance (including power), (iii) flexibility, (iv) three-dimensional (3D) exercise (e.g. Tai Chi, Qigong, dance), (v) general physical activity, (vi) endurance, and (vii) other kind of exercises. The programmes of ten included, as the primary intervention, gait, balance, and functional (task) training plus resistance training. The exercise programmes may also include secondary categories of exercise.

v   The all-studies population risk was based on the number of events and the number of participants in the control group for this outcome over the 64 all-exercise types RCTs. The specific exercise population risk was based on the number of events and the number of participants in the control group for this outcome over the 15 RCTs.

w   Downgraded by one level due to inconsistency (there was substantial heterogeneity (I²: 71%). We did not downgrade for risk of bias, as results were essentially unchanged with removal of the trials at a high risk of bias in one or more items rate of falls. Sub-group analyses found there may be no difference in the effect of exercise (all types) on the rate of falls where interventions were delivered in a group setting (RaR: 0.74, 95% CI: 0.67, 0.83; 8909 participants, 43 studies, I^2: 66%) compared with trials where interventions were delivered individually (RaR: 0.81, 95% CI: 0.72, 0.91; 5397 participants, 23 studies, I^2: 47%); test for sub-group differences: Chi^2: 1.3, df: 1, P: 0.31, I^2: 3%. However, it is likely that the provision of exercise to high-risk people can be more safely and effectively undertaken by health professionals.

4. *Exercises that target balance/function are particularly effective.* Sub-group analysis by exercise type showed a variation in the effects of the different types of exercise on rate of falls, the visual impression being confirmed by the statistically significant test for sub-group differences: Chi^2: 18.91, df: 6, P: 0.004, I^2: 68.3%. Exercise interventions that were classified as being primarily balance and functional reduce the rate of falls by 24% compared with control (RaR: 0.76, 95% CI: 0.70, 0.82; 7989 participants, 39 studies, I^2: 31%, high-certainty evidence). Exercise interventions that include multiple categories of the ProFaNE taxonomy (most commonly balance and functional exercises plus resistance exercises) probably reduce the rate of falls by 28% compared with controls (RaR: 0.72, 95% CI: 0.56, 0.93; 2283 participants, 15 studies; I^2: 65%; moderate-certainty evidence). Sensitivity analyses revealed little difference in the results when we pooled only trials that included the most common two components (balance and functional exercises plus resistance exercises) (RaR: 0.69, 95% CI: 0.48, 0.97; 1084 participants, 8 studies; I^2: 71%). Exercise interventions that were classified as 3D (Tai Chi or similar) probably reduce the rate of falls by 23% compared with control (RaR: 0.77, 95% CI: 0.61, 0.97; 3169 participants, 9 studies, I^2: 83%; moderate-certainty evidence). We are uncertain whether exercises, classified as being primarily 3D (dance) using the ProFaNE taxonomy, reduce the rate of falls compared with control (RaR: 1.34, 95% CI: 0.98, 1.83; 522 participants, 1 study; very low-certainty evidence). We are uncertain whether interventions, classified as being primarily walking programmes using the ProFaNE taxonomy, reduce the rate of falls compared with control (RaR: 1.14, 95% CI: 0.66, 1.97; 441 participants, 2 studies; I^2: 67%; very low-certainty evidence).

Programmes Found to Prevent Falls

The interventions used in many of the trials included in the reviews involved individualized exercise prescription based on assessment of an individual's abilities and limitations. As several exercise programmes that target balance/functional abilities or include multiple components have been found to prevent falls, current evidence supports the availability of a range of programmes and exercise prescription according to an individual's physical functioning and interests. Several of the trials have published manuals to guide the implementation of the exercise programmes tested. For example, the Otago Exercise Programme is a home-based programme that has been found in a meta-analysis of several trials to reduce the rate of falls by 35% in community-dwelling older people recruited via general practice [10]. An interesting approach to exercise prescription that has recently been found to be effective in the prevention of falls [11] is the Lifestyle-Integrated Functional Exercise (LiFE) programme, where participants are taught how to integrate the balance and leg-strengthening exercises into their daily routines. For example, participants are taught to practise standing on one leg while waiting for the kettle to boil or while cleaning their teeth and are encouraged to perform squats while bending to pick up washing from the washing basket. Table 16.3 outlines the categories of exercise intervention and other characteristics of the additional studies published since the 2019 Cochrane review [5, 9].

Exercise to Prevent Falls in Different Populations

The role of exercise as a single fall prevention intervention in people who are at a very high risk of falls is less clear than in the general older population. It is often assumed that people at greater risk of falls will obtain greater benefits from interventions but this is not supported by the current evidence [4]. However, an intervention of similar relative effectiveness will prevent more falls in absolute terms in high-risk populations who experience a greater number of falls.

There is mounting evidence that exercise can prevent falls in people with dementia and in people with Parkinson's disease but there is no evidence as yet that falls can be prevented with exercise as a single intervention in people after stroke, or in people who have recently been in hospital [7].

The role of exercise as a single intervention in populations defined by a particular fall risk factor not amenable to change by exercise is less clear. The Otago Exercise Programme is clearly effective in the prevention of falls in general community-dwelling older people [10] yet, in factorial studies by its developers, did not have the same impact in people with visual impairments [12] or in people taking psychoactive medications [13]. Whereas the other non-exercise arms of these studies – a home safety intervention for people with visual impairment and gradual reduction of psychoactive medications for those taking these medications – were effective. It may be certain risk factors are 'dominant' in certain populations and falls can only be prevented in such a population by addressing this particular risk factor.

Table 16.3 Components of new trials since our Cochrane review [5, 9] in categories of exercise found to prevent falls

First author, year, and interventions	Type of exercise according to ProFaNE classification [6]ᵃ							Duration of intervention (weeks)	Hours of intervention	Delivery modeᵇ	Participants per instructorᶜ	Tailored to the individual initially	Progressed based on individual assessment	Tailored in intensity or type
	Balance or functional training	Strength or resistance training	Flexibility training	3D exercise	General physical activity	Endurance exercise	Other exercise							
Gait/Balance/functional training														
Arkkukangas 2019 Individual Otago Exercise Programme [35]	P	S	-	-	S	-	-	52	84	3	None	Y	Y	Y
Multiple primary exercise categories														
Arkkukangas 2019 Individual Otago Exercise Programme + motivational interviewing [35]	P	S	-	-	S	-	P	52	84	3	None	Y	Y	Y
Barclay 2018 [36]	P	-	-	-	P	-	-	9	18	1	3	Y	Y	Y
Li 2018 Group-based balance, gait, resistance and flexibility training [39]	P	P	P	-	-	-	-	24	48	1	9–21	Y	Y	Y
Liu-Ambrose 2019 Individualised Otago Exercise Programme [41]	P	P	-	-	P	-	-	52	130	3	None	Y	Y	Y

ᵃ Classification (P = Primary; S = Secondary); ᵇ Delivery mode (1 = Group; 2 = Individual supervised; 3 = Individual unsupervised; 4 = Group + Home exercise); ᶜ 1 if delivery mode was individual supervised, None if delivery mode was individual unsupervised

Exercise for Fall Prevention in Residential Care

Although it is clear that exercise as a single intervention can prevent falls in community dwellers, this is not as clearly the case in residential aged care [14]. A recent Australian trial [15] did find a significant impact of an exercise-based Intervention on falls in residential care, so warrants replication.

Successful multi-factorial fall prevention interventions in residential care have included exercise. A particularly successful intervention for residential care was developed and tested by Becker et al. [16] in Germany. This programme involved staff and resident education on fall prevention, advice on environmental adaptations, progressive balance and resistance training, and hip protectors. This programme also appeared to prevent femoral fractures when disseminated across the state of Bavaria [17]. A group in New Zealand attempted to replicate this programme without increasing staff levels and did not find it to be effective. In fact, they found an increase in falls in the intervention group and concluded that a low-intensity programme may actually be worse than usual care [18]. This suggests that real investment is required to prevent falls and fractures in residential aged care.

Impact of Exercise on Fractures

Falls that lead to fractures and other serious injuries are usually of greater concern to individuals and health systems than non-injurious falls. Low bone mineral density has been identified as a risk factor for fracture and there is evidence that fractures can be prevented by medications that enhance bone mineral density. As most fractures result from falls it is also likely that interventions that prevent falls can also prevent fractures. There is evidence from meta-analyses that exercise interventions can prevent fractures. A meta-analysis of the Otago Exercise Programme trials [10] found a similar impact on injurious falls (IRR: 0.65, 95% CI: 0.53, 0.81) as on all falls (IRR: 0.65, 95% CI: 0.57, 0.75). Our Cochrane review [5] also gives a promising indication that exercise may prevent fractures (RR: 0.73, 95% CI: 0.56, 0.95) and falls that require medical care (RR: 0.61, 95% CI: 0.47, 0.79) although there is much less certainty around the conclusions for these rarer outcomes.

Two recent very large trials have tested the impact of fall prevention interventions including exercise on fractures [19] and serious fall injuries [20]. Both reported disappointing findings for the primary outcomes but give some indication of effects on secondary falls outcomes. Both trials were undertaken in general practice settings and sought to implement interventions within existing services primarily using existing resources. These studies raise interesting questions about the challenge of funding and implementing fall prevention interventions as well as the ability of investigators to support and even measure uptake of appropriate exercise interventions in very large trials, especially when delivered in addition to other fall prevention strategies.

Implications for Practice

Box 16.1 below summarizes the implications for practice from our work, as well as associated work by others. Key aspects are the importance of exercise for fall prevention, greater benefits from balance training/functional exercises and from

---

Box 16.1 Recommendations for Exercise to Prevent Falls among Community-Dwelling Older People

1. Exercise must provide a moderate or high challenge to balance – exercises should aim to challenge balance in three ways:
   a. reducing the base of support
   b. movement of the centre of gravity
   c. reducing the need for upper limb support
2. Exercise must be of a sufficient dose to have an effect – exercise should be undertaken for at least two hours per week
3. Ongoing exercise is necessary – the benefits are rapidly lost when exercise is ceased
4. Fall prevention exercise should be targeted at the general community as well as those at high risk for falls – there is a larger relative effect from programmes offered to the general community than programmes offered to high-risk groups, yet high-risk groups actually have more falls so a greater number of falls can be prevented in this population
5. Fall prevention exercise may be undertaken in a group or home-based setting – group sessions should be supplemented with additional home-based exercise in order to obtain the recommended exercise dose
6. Walking training may be included in addition to balance training but high-risk individuals should not be prescribed brisk walking programmes – walking training may be included in a programme as long as it is not at the expense of balance training
7. Strength training may be included in addition to balance training – effective strength training overloads the muscles by providing an amount of resistance that ensures that an exercise can only be done 10–15 times before muscles fatigue
8. Exercise providers should make referrals for other risk factors to be addressed – older people who have fall risk factors not amenable to change with exercise (such as visual problems and certain medications) should receive a full assessment at a falls clinic or ask their general practitioner for appropriate referrals

---

Adapted from Sherrington et al. [4]

a higher dose of exercise. Walking may be included in addition to balance training if the person is safe to walk outdoors. Resistance training may also be included but should not be the focus of intervention if the aim is fall prevention.

Taken together with the findings on the effectiveness of other interventions [3, 21] current evidence indicates: (i) group exercise, home safety, and multi-factorial interventions prevent falls in community-dwelling people at an increased risk of falls, and (ii) group and home-based exercise and multi-factorial interventions also prevent falls in unscreened groups. Therefore, fall assessment tools can be used to predict who will fall and to tailor interventions but may not be needed to decide who should do group exercise or multi-factorial interventions since all older people are likely to obtain benefits from these interventions.

Unfortunately, community participation rates in the type of exercise shown to prevent falls are relatively low. Only 8–12% of older people in NSW, Australia regularly undertake the type of exercise/physical activities that challenge balance and so prevent falls [22]. There is therefore an urgent need to address this evidence–practice gap.

Health professional promotion of exercise for fall prevention to their patients and the broader community is a potentially useful strategy to address the evidence–practice gap on exercise for fall prevention. Health professionals can offer and support evidence-based interventions. This may involve one or more of: (i) individualized prescription of home-based programmes, (ii) referral to community group programmes known to be suitable, (iii) offering group programmes in one's practice or hospital department, and (iv) contributing to broader community awareness raising about the importance of exercise in the prevention of falls, e.g. talks to groups of older people or fellow health professionals, and articles for local newspapers.

As other interventions have also been found to prevent falls for people with particular risk factors, health professionals and exercise providers could also screen patients for these risk factors and refer for specialized intervention (i.e. medication management, podiatry, occupational therapist home visits for high-risk people, cataract removal, and assessment of suspected carotid sinus hypersensitivity).

More falls are prevented in high-risk people with interventions of the same relative effectiveness, but it is not necessarily the case that high-risk people will benefit more from interventions. This can be considered when prioritizing limited resources.

The Broader Context of Physical Activity for Healthy Ageing

As exercise is a type of physical activity, the promotion of exercise for fall prevention forms part of broader initiatives to promote physical activity for healthy ageing at a population level. The World Health Organization (WHO) life course approach to healthy ageing is outlined in the 2015 report *Ageing and Health*, [23] which explains that health systems have traditionally focused on individual diseases but the concept of 'intrinsic capacity' is crucial to healthy ageing regardless of concurrent disease status. WHO defines healthy ageing as 'the process of developing and maintaining the functional ability that enables wellbeing in older age'. Functional ability is affected by the environment and the person's physical and mental capacity. The WHO report calls for the development and testing of interventions to enhance physical and mental capacity across the lifespan. To date, there is yet to be a comprehensive approach taken to this endeavour. Enhancement of intrinsic capacity across the lifespan at a population level would also prevent many falls.

Physical activity [24] is an important enabler of healthy ageing due to its impact on physical and mental capacity. The loss of independence (defined as the need for help with daily tasks) is up to 15 years later in more active people [25]. Physical activity participation is also associated with a lower risk of functional limitations, with greater benefits from more vigorous activities. Figure 16.1, from a systematic review of cohort studies, [26] shows the dose–response relationship between physical activity participation and difficulty with activities of daily living in people aged 65 to 80 after adjusting for other factors likely to be associated with functional limitations [26]. Health and economic benefits of physical activity have been demonstrated in terms of reduced mortality and disease incidence [27] and

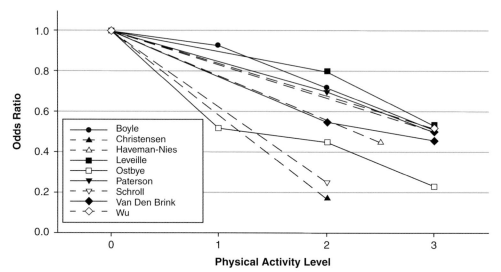

Figure 16.1   Odds of functional limitations by physical activity level for adults aged 65+ (1 = light activities, 2 = moderate activity 3–5 days/week, 30 min/day, 3 = vigorous activities). Reproduced with permission from Paterson DH, Warburton DE. Physical activity and functional limitations in older adults: a systematic review related to Canada's Physical Activity Guidelines. Int J Behav Nutr Phys Act. 2010;7:38 [26].

health care costs saved from hospital admissions [28]. Less is known about the impact on health care costs from improvements in functional capacity and quality of life. As falls are predicted by functional limitations, interventions that focus on maintaining functional capacity at a population level will also prevent many falls.

Physical activity is defined as any bodily movement produced by skeletal muscles that results in energy expenditure [29]. Exercise is considered a sub-set of physical activity that is planned, structured, and repetitive, and aims to improve or maintain physical fitness [29]. Exercise enhances mobility through improved aerobic capacity, muscle strength, balance, and co-ordination [30]. More demanding mobility tasks such as stair-climbing and walking longer distances require greater levels of physical functioning. If a person's physical functioning is lower than that required for independent performance of a particular activity, i.e. below the 'disability threshold', they will require assistance or aids. Greater physical functioning provides 'reserve capacity', which acts as a buffer to ensure that functioning remains above the disability threshold, even in the face of deterioration from factors such as physiological ageing, illness, or injury. Much of the deterioration in physical fitness and mobility commonly thought to be due to ageing/health conditions is actually due to inactivity and thus partially treatable and preventable [31, 32]. Trials have confirmed that certain forms of physical activity can improve walking abilities and prevent the onset of disability [33]. For example, the onset of mobility disability was prevented (HR: 0.82, 95% CI: 0.69, 0.98 p: 0.03) by a structured physical activity programme in people aged 70–89 who had some physical limitation at baseline [34]. As falls are predicted by functional limitations, interventions that focus on maintaining functional capacity at a population level also have the potential to prevent many falls.

Conclusions

Current evidence points to the role of carefully designed exercise programmes in the prevention of falls in community-dwelling older adults. There remain unanswered questions, especially with regard to the prevention of falls in higher-risk populations and the prevention of fractures. The broader context of healthy ageing can help us understand the importance of implementation and scale-up of exercise interventions known to prevent falls at a population level.

REFERENCES

1. Howe TE, Rochester L, Neil F, Skelton DA, Ballinger C. Exercise for improving balance in older people. *Cochrane Database Syst Rev.* 2011;9:CD004963.

2. Liu C-J, Latham NK. Progressive resistance strength training for improving physical function in older adults. *Cochrane Database Syst Rev.* 2009;2009:CD002759.

3. Gillespie LD, Robertson MC, Gillespie WJ et al. Interventions for preventing falls in older people living in the community. *Cochrane Database Syst Rev.* 2012;CD007146.

4. Sherrington C, Tiedemann A, Fairhall N et al. Exercise to prevent falls in older adults: an updated meta-analysis and best practice recommendations. NSW Public Health Bull. 2011;22:78–83.

5. Sherrington C, Fairhall NJ, Wallbank GK et al. Exercise for preventing falls in older people living in the community. *Cochrane Database Syst Rev.* 2019;1:CD012424.

6. Lamb SE, Jørstad EC, Hauer K et al. Development of a common outcome data set for fall injury prevention trials: the Prevention of Falls Network Europe consensus. *J Am Geriatr Soc.* 2005;53:1618–22.

7. Sherrington C, Michaleff ZA, Fairhall N et al. Exercise to prevent falls in older adults: an updated systematic review and meta-analysis. *Br J Sports Med.* 2017;51:1750–8.

8. Sherrington C, Whitney JC, Lord SR et al. Effective exercise for the prevention of falls: a systematic review and meta-analysis. *J Am Geriatr Soc.* 2008;56:2234–43.

9. Ng C, Fairhall N, Wallbank G et al. Exercise for falls prevention in community-dwelling older adults: trial and participant characteristics, interventions and bias in clinical trials from a systematic review. *BMJ Open Sport Exerc Med.* 2019;5:e000663.

10. Robertson MC, Campbell AJ, Gardner MM et al. Preventing injuries in older people by preventing falls: a meta-analysis of individual-level data. *J Am Geriatr Soc.* 2002;50:905–11.

11. Clemson L, Singh MAF, Bundy A et al. Integration of balance and strength training into daily life activity to reduce rate of falls in older people (the LiFE study): randomised parallel trial. *Br Med J.* 2012;345:e4547.

12. Campbell AJ, Robertson MC, La Grow SJ et al. Randomised controlled trial of prevention of falls in people aged > or =75 with severe visual impairment: the VIP trial. *Br Med J.* 2005;331:817.

13. Campbell AJ, Robertson MC, Gardner MM et al. Psychotropic medication withdrawal and a home based exercise programme to prevent falls: results of a randomised controlled trial. *J Am Geriatr Soc.* 1999;47:850–3.

14. Cameron ID, Dyer SM, Panagoda CE et al. Interventions for preventing falls in older people in care facilities and hospitals. *Cochrane Database Syst Rev.* 2018;9:CD005465.

15. Hewitt J, Goodall S, Clemson L et al. Progressive resistance and balance training for falls prevention in long-term residential aged care: a cluster randomized trial of the Sunbeam Program. *J Am Med Dir Assoc.* 2018;19:361–9.

16. Becker C, Kron M, Lindemann U et al. Effectiveness of a multifaceted intervention on falls in nursing home residents. *J Am Geriatr Soc.* 2003;51:306–13.

17. Becker C, Cameron ID, Klenk J et al. Reduction of femoral fractures in long-term care facilities: the Bavarian fracture prevention study. *PloS One.* 2011;6:e24311.

18. Kerse N, Butler M, Robinson E et al. Fall prevention in residential care: a cluster, randomized, controlled trial. *J Am Geriatr Soc.* 2004;52:524–31.

19. Lamb SE, Bruce J, Hossain A et al. Screening and intervention to prevent falls and fractures in older people. *N Engl J Med.* 2020;383:1848–59.

20. Bhasin S, Gill TM, Reuben DB et al. A randomized trial of a multifactorial strategy to prevent serious fall injuries. *N Engl J Med.* 2020;383:129–40.

21. Hopewell S, Adedire O, Copsey BJ et al. Multifactorial and multiple component interventions for preventing falls in older people living in the community. *Cochrane Database Syst Rev.* 2018;7:CD012221.

22. Merom D, Pye V, Macniven R et al. Prevalence and correlates of participation in fall prevention exercise/physical activity by older adults. *Prev Med.* 2012;55:613–17.

23. WHO. *World Report on Ageing and Health.* Switzerland: World Health Organisation; 2015.

24. Caspersen CJ, Powell KE, Christenson GM. Physical activity, exercise, and physical fitness: definitions and distinctions for health-related research. *Public Health Rep.* 1985;100:126–31.

25. Lee C, Dobson AJ, Brown WJ et al. Cohort profile: the Australian Longitudinal Study on women's health. *Int J Epidemiol.* 2005;34:987–91.

26. Paterson DH, Warburton DE. Physical activity and functional limitations in older adults: a systematic review related to Canada's Physical Activity Guidelines. *Int J Behav Nutr Phys Act.* 2010;7:38.

27. Ding D, Lawson KD, Kolbe-Alexander TL et al. The economic burden of physical inactivity: a global analysis of major non-communicable diseases. *Lancet.* 2016;388:1311–24.

28. Farag I, Howard K, Ferreira ML et al. Economic modelling of a public health programme for fall prevention. *Age Ageing.* 2015;44:409–14.

29. Caspersen CJ, Powell KE, Christenson GM. Physical activity, exercise, and physical fitness: definitions and distinctions for health-related research. *Public Health Rep.* 1985;100:126–31.

30. Garber CE, Blissmer B, Deschenes MR et al. American College of Sports Medicine position stand. Quantity and quality of exercise for developing and maintaining cardiorespiratory, musculoskeletal, and neuromotor fitness in apparently healthy adults: guidance for prescribing exercise. *Med Sci Sports Exerc.* 2011;43:1334–59.

31. Chodzko-Zajko WJ, Proctor DN, Fiatarone Singh MA, American College of Sports Medicine position stand: exercise and physical activity for older adults. *Med Sci Sports Exerc.* 2009;41:1510–30.

32. Pollock RD, Carter S, Velloso CP et al. An investigation into the relationship between age and physiological function in highly active older adults. *J Physiol.* 2015;593:657–80.

33. Durstine JL, Moore G, Painter P et al. *ACSM's Exercise Management for Persons with Chronic Diseases and Disabilities, 3rd Edn.* United States: Human Kinetics; 2009.

34. Pahor M, Guralnik JM, Ambrosius WT et al. Effect of structured physical activity on prevention of major mobility disability in older adults: the LIFE study randomized clinical trial. *J Am Med Assoc.* 2014;311:2387–96.

35. Arkkukangas M, Johnson ST, Hellstrom K et al. Fall prevention exercises with or without behavior change support for community-dwelling older adults: a two-year follow-up of a randomized controlled trial. *J Aging Phys Act.* 2019:1–26.

36. Barclay R, Webber S, Ripat J et al. Safety and feasibility of an interactive workshop and facilitated outdoor walking group compared to a workshop alone in increasing outdoor walking activity among older adults: a pilot randomized controlled trial. *Pilot Feasibility Stud.* 2018;4:179.

37. Bernardelli G, Roncaglione C, Damanti S et al. Adapted physical activity to promote active and healthy ageing: the PoliFIT pilot randomized waiting list-controlled trial. *Aging Clin Exp Res*. 2019;31:511–18.

38. Gallo E, Stelmach M, Frigeri F et al. Determining whether a dosage-specific and individualized home exercise program with consults reduces fall risk and falls in community-dwelling older adults with difficulty walking: a randomized control trial. *J Geriatr Phys Ther*. 2018;41:161–72.

39. Li F, Harmer P, Fitzgerald K et al. Effectiveness of a therapeutic Tai Ji Quan intervention vs a multimodal exercise intervention to prevent falls among older adults at high risk of falling. *JAMA Intern Med*. 2018;178:1301–10.

40. Lipsitz LA, Macklin EA, Travison TG et al. A cluster randomized trial of Tai Chi vs health education in subsidized housing: the MI-WiSH Study. *J Am Geriatr Soc*. 2019;67:1812–19.

41. Liu-Ambrose T, Davis JC, Best JR et al. Effect of a home-based exercise program on subsequent falls among community-dwelling high-risk older adults after a fall: a randomized clinical trial. *J Am Med Assoc*. 2019;321:2092–100.

42. Oliveira JS, Sherrington C, Paul SS et al. A combined physical activity and fall prevention intervention improved mobility-related goal attainment but not physical activity in older adults: a randomised trial. *J Physiother*. 2019;65:16–22.

43. Buchner DM, Cress ME, de Lateur BJ et al. The effect of strength and endurance training on gait, balance, fall risk, and health services use in community-living older adults. *J Gerontol A Biol Sci Med Sci*. 1997;52:M218–24.

17

Volitional and Reactive Step Training

Yoshiro Okubo and Daina L. Sturnieks

Step Training

Step training can be defined as training of single or multiple volitional or reactive steps in an upright (standing or walking) position in response to an environmental challenge. For example, stepping onto a target, avoiding an obstacle, or responding to a postural perturbation large enough to require reconfiguration of the base of support [1]. Volitional step training uses stepping targets or distractors (no-go zones), whereas reactive step training exposes participants to repeated mechanical perturbations that displace body segments and induce unplanned stepping responses. Reactive step training is also referred to as 'perturbation training' [2], 'reactive balance training' [3], or 'perturbation-based balance training' [4].

Effects of Step Training on Preventing Falls

A systematic review and meta-analysis by Okubo et al. [1], synthesized the effects of step training on falls and fall risk factors. Meta-analyses of seven RCTs (n = 660) showed that stepping interventions significantly reduced the rate of falls (rate ratio: 0.48, 95% CI: 0.36, 0.65; p<0.0001) and the proportion of fallers (risk ratio: 0.51, 95% CI: 0.38, 0.68; p<0.0001) [2, 4–9]. Subgroup analyses stratified by reactive and volitional stepping interventions revealed a similar efficacy for rate of falls and proportion of fallers for both training modalities.

Although the evidence is based on preliminary RCTs, the effects of step training for fall prevention is encouraging. The 50% reduction of falls following step training appears to be superior to that found for traditional exercise training, shown to be a 21–39% reduction [10]. Step training may be more effective than other forms of exercise due to greater task specificity. Step training involves directly training or shaping the neuropsychological and sensorimotor skills required for avoiding falls [1]. During trips, slips, and lateral loss of balance, quick stepping in forward, backward, and sideways directions are required, respectively [11]. The repetitive task-relevant stepping exercises delivered in the studies included in meta-analyses may generate stored motor programmes that can be promptly accessed when anticipatory or reactive postural threats are detected. Interestingly, significantly increased lower-extremity muscle strength following 14 to 16 weeks of traditional resistance training did not transfer to improved responses to laboratory-induced trips [12] and slips [13], suggesting other mechanisms at play. Regardless of the mechanisms, according to the principle of task specificity, step training may directly train the ability to avoid falls.

Volitional Step Training Programmes

Volitional step training programmes involve planned stepping movements in response to presented stimuli or a planned sequence, and often utilize equipment including stepping targets, such as mats partitioned into squares [6], exergame dance mats [14], or coloured tiles [9]. The volitional step training interventions conducted to date have involved regular sessions (one to three per week) of 6–55 minutes, conducted over two to six months, leading to total step training doses of 4.8–32 hours [6–8, 14–19], with some stepping exercises incorporated into broader multi-component exercise programmes [7–9, 15]. Volitional step training is associated with improved performances in tests of gait and mobility, simple reaction time, and choice stepping reaction time [1], indicating improvements in central processing speed, and initiation and velocity of movement execution. Some volitional step training programmes also incorporate specific cognitive tasks, such as divided attention, inhibition of irrelevant stimuli, switching between tasks, rotating objects, and making rapid decisions [20], or stepping pattern memorization [19]. One advantage of volitional step training is the relatively high clinical feasibility in terms of safety, enjoyment, required equipment, and skills. Commonly the intensity of volitional step training is also easily progressed, for example by increasing the pace and/or the complexity of stepping patterns.

Volitional Step Training Using Targets While Walking

Several studies have examined the use of step training interventions involving mats and targets. The Square Stepping Exercise [15] challenges participants to memorize

Multi-Target Stepping Test

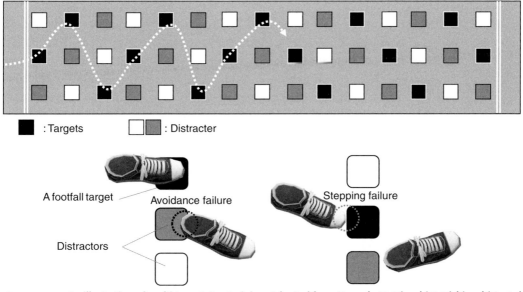

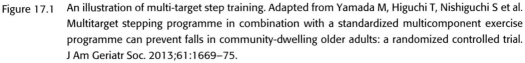

Figure 17.1   An illustration of multi-target step training. Adapted from Yamada M, Higuchi T, Nishiguchi S et al. Multitarget stepping programme in combination with a standardized multicomponent exercise programme can prevent falls in community-dwelling older adults: a randomized controlled trial. J Am Geriatr Soc. 2013;61:1669–75.

and perform stepping patterns on a low-profile mat (2.5 × 1 m) partitioned into 40 squares. This stepping intervention has been shown to improve agility, leg power, gait speed, and single leg balance [15], and reduce the rate of falls per trip [7]. A second trial evaluated the efficacy of a 24-week Multi-Target Stepping Programme incorporating inhibition (Figure 17.1) in preventing falls over 12 months in 264 people aged 65+ years [9]. Both intervention and control groups performed a strength and balance programme. In addition, the intervention participants were required to step on target squares (e.g. blue), avoiding distractor squares (e.g. red, yellow, and green), while walking along a 10 m mat. Over the 12-month follow-up, the intervention group experienced 65% fewer falls and 78% fewer fall-related fractures compared to the control group [9]. Finally, Fung et al. [18] conducted a Progressive Stepping Programme that involved walking and stepping on targets, onto cushions and over obstacles for 3–6 minutes, three times per week for 10 weeks. The main findings were that at the end of the trial, intervention participants had significantly shorter Timed Up and Go Test times compared to controls but that the two groups performed similarly in a single leg stance test [18]. Taken together, these findings show simple step training programmes are feasible and can improve mobility and prevent falls in older people.

Volitional Step Training Using Exergames While Standing

Interactive stepping mats interfaced with computer systems have recently been used for volitional step training interventions [14, 16, 20]. In contrast to the abovementioned programmes using stepping targets that are suitable for group settings, the interactive systems are designed to be used by one person at a time and may be used by an older person at home [14]. Step training using such technologies is explained in detail in Chapter 18. Briefly, exergames and virtual reality systems deliver interactive cognitive-motor training that may enhance uptake and adherence to exercise due to features such as goal-setting, feedback, positive reinforcement, challenges, and the ability to monitor performance and progression. These systems have been shown to be enjoyable, safe, and can elicit improvements in physical and cognitive outcomes. Furthermore, exergames and virtual reality training have been shown to be effective in improving stepping, balance, mobility, and preventing falls in some RCTs.

Recently, Morat et al. [21] developed a volitional stepping exergame incorporating an unstable platform supported by springs. In their eight-week RCT involving 51 healthy older adults, step training in both unstable and stable conditions improved functional balance, mobility, and calf strength endurance. However, the unstable step training induced greater improvements in leg extension strength compared the stable condition [21]. A further study is required to examine its effect on preventing falls.

Reactive Step Training

Reactive step training is an emerging paradigm that utilizes repeated exposure to sudden external perturbations, aimed at inducing locomotor adaptations and training balance recovery responses for fall avoidance [1, 22–24]. Reactive step training is founded on the principle of task specificity and the basis that a loss of balance is necessary for learning the optimal balance recovery responses based on error-feedback to directly train the skills required to avoid a fall. Repeated exposure to postural perturbations exploits the central nervous system's tendency to continuously adjust the peripheral output to correct posture and avoid falling. There is good evidence that both young and older adults can substantially reduce laboratory falls following a few repeated perturbation trials by proactively adapting gait and improving reactive balance responses [22, 25–31]. Hence, the total dose of reactive step training is considerably lower than the 50 hours recommended for traditional exercise training for fall prevention [32]. Of the seven reactive step training RCTs included in the systematic review by Okubo et al. [1], a total training dose of 4–10 hours was reported in three trials over 6–24 weeks [4,

5, 8], with the remaining four reporting only one or two 30–90 minute training sessions [2, 28, 33, 34].

The mechanisms for the effects of reactive step training on preventing falls are likely to be largely within the central nervous system. Theoretically, exposure to postural perturbations during reactive step training will reduce the risk of falling in the advent of unexpected slips and trips experienced in everyday life by shaping the motor programmes required for effective balance recovery in such situations. These motor adaptations may be predictive as well as reactive in their nature [35–37].

Predictive adaptation utilizes prior experience and knowledge of a potential perturbation in a feedforward manner to proactively adjust gait and balance (e.g. modifications of the base of support and/or centre of mass position). Such predictive adaptations can diminish the intensity of the perturbation by changing the mechanical response of the body to the perturbation, reducing the magnitude of the required balance recovery response [38]. Predictive adaptation can be observed as changes in gait and balance parameters before the perturbation onset or when the perturbation is removed (i.e. aftereffect) and likely involves a rapid update of one's existing internal model to improve its feedforward control [22, 37]. Studies have shown that repeated exposure to slips consistently induces an anterior shift of the body centre of mass (CoM) in a forward leaning posture, a decreased ankle angle (flat foot) at foot strike, and shorter step lengths while walking (Figure 17.2A) [27, 29, 31]. In contrast, repeated exposure to trips induces a posterior shift of the body CoM in a backward leaning posture, increased toe clearance, and shorter step lengths while walking (Figure 17.2B) [29, 39, 40]. These predictive gait alterations are adjusted by the central nervous system to minimize the impact of the upcoming perturbations, i.e. reduced slip severity [41]. Such predictive adaptations likely play a major role in the positively reported

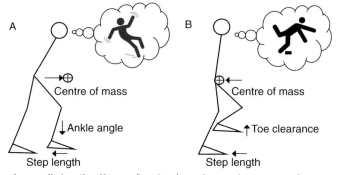

Figure 17.2   The predictive (feedforward) gait adaptation against repeated exposure to (A) a slip or (B) a trip hazard.

effects of very low dose reactive step training [2, 22, 28, 33, 34]. In addition, a balance-threatening experience in the laboratory might help the individual to become more aware of his or her own ability (i.e. reducing the gap between perceived and actual abilities) and of the consequences of daily life hazards.

Reactive adaptation is a change of balance recovery responses that are initiated at the onset of an unexpected perturbation (e.g. faster response initiation). Reactive adaptation can be achieved by: (i) early detection of the perturbation and recovery initiation [28, 42], (ii) optimization of motor programmes for balance recovery, including facilitation and suppression of functionally relevant and irrelevant reflexes, respectively [43–45], and (iii) increased force production capacity in skeletal (especially weight-bearing) muscles for rapid motor actions [12, 22, 46, 47]. However, an assessment of pure reactive adaptation is challenging as it requires true unpredictability of the perturbation, via sufficient washout or regulation of the predictive adaptation, and/or novelty of perturbation type, magnitude, and timing [25, 40]. In a systematic review by Bohm et al. [48], only one of 18 included studies was found to have a sufficient washout phase to eliminate predictive adjustments when examining reactive adaptation. Moreover, the distinction between predictive and reactive adaptations is not always clear, as feedforward modification of the sensitivity of the central nervous system (e.g. corticospinal excitability) prior to a perturbation can determine the magnitude of the evoked responses [49, 50]. Studies have shown that knowledge of a possible upcoming hazard (e.g. timing [51], magnitude [52, 53], or direction [54]) can enhance the reflexive muscle activation through increased corticospinal excitability [49, 55] to assist with balance recovery.

Reactive Step Training Using Treadmill Perturbation Systems

Methods for inducing perturbations vary but often involve walking on a treadmill and the use of ankle-cable pulls (to obstruct the swing limb) [56], treadmill belt accelerations (to induce a trip-like response), decelerations (similar to forward slipping) [8], and lateral shifts [57]. In the first RCT of treadmill perturbation training, which involved a total of 600 minutes of training over six months in 32 long-term care facility residents and outpatients, a significant improvement in balance and reaction time, and a non-significant reduction in falls (odds ratio: 0.42, 95% CI: 0.08, 2.07) was reported [8]. In another study, Wang et al. [58] reported a programme of only 40 slip-like perturbations on a treadmill in a single session reduced slips on an overground walkway. In a double-blind RCT with 53 community-dwelling older adults, 24 training sessions over three months with perturbations induced by a treadmill translating longitudinally, laterally, or in combination resulted in significant improvements in voluntary step execution times and standing balance [59]. Further studies are required to determine whether these improvements in balance and stepping performance following treadmill perturbation protocols transfer to fewer falls in daily life.

Simulated trips achieved via treadmill belt accelerations lack the physical obstruction of the swing foot that is a primary feature of a trip. To address this issue, ankle cable pulls have been used. Using ankle cable pulls, Konig et al. [60] reported at least eight repetitions were needed to see retention of the training effect for 14 weeks. Epro et al. [61] showed that the gait adaptation obtained from the eight trip-like perturbation exposures in two sessions (at baseline and 14 weeks) was significantly retained for 1.5 years with only minor decay. However, an additional 14-week resistance training programme targeting triceps surae had no effects on gait stability following the trip-like perturbations [61]. King et al. [62] developed a stumble perturbation system that incorporates a tripping obstruction; i.e. physical obstacles are released on the treadmill belt at precise times to induce trips that require either an elevating or lowering strategy to recover balance [47]. However, no intervention studies to date have been undertaken using physical obstacles on a treadmill.

Reactive Step Training Using Overground Perturbation Systems

Perturbations during overground gait include trips induced by hidden obstacles [3, 29, 46, 63] and soft floor surfaces [64], and slips induced by low-friction movable plates [27, 28] and floor-mounted rollers [65]. Overground perturbation systems probably have the highest ecological validity (i.e. similarity to real-life hazards), but the perturbation usually occurs at a fixed location and may result in a loss of 'unpredictability' in repeated trials [25, 66].

Pai et al. [26] found that exposing 38 older participants to 24 slips with a movable plate during walking in 37 trials significantly reduced laboratory falls from 48% in the first slip trial to <5% in the fifth and later slip trials. This rapid learning was found to be primarily due to predictive/feedforward adaptation to shift the CoM forward when approaching the visible movable plate, which could be unlocked to slide forward upon foot contact [27]. This forward CoM shift (lean) reduces the shear forces of the step on the movable plate, enabling a 'skateover' or 'walkover' (for slip distances <5 cm) response to avoid backward loss of balance [27]. This predictive adaptation was found to be retained for six months when participants were re-exposed to a slip in the same laboratory [33], and transferred to similar conditions, i.e. from a movable platform to a slippery floor [67], from short to long slips [68], and from one leg to the other [30]. Importantly, in a large RCT involving 212 community-dwelling older adults, a single training session of 24 slip exposures was found to significantly reduce daily-life falls by 50% over the subsequent year [2]. However encouraging, further studies are required to confirm this finding.

An issue with predictive adaptation emerges when the knowledge used in the feedforward model is inaccurate or inappropriate. The forward shift of the body CoM following slip perturbations is protective against slipping but might increase the risk of falling against an opposing perturbation (i.e. trip). For example, Bhatt et al. [29] found that when 16 young adults were unexpectedly exposed to a trip after exposure to eight slip trials, they had significantly greater forward instability and trunk sway following the trip compared to 16 participants who did not have such prior slip experience. These findings suggest the need for a mixed training to avoid any adverse transfer of training effects.

Okubo et al. developed a protocol involving both trips and slips with increasing unpredictability to specifically induce reactive adaptation while preventing predictive adaptation (Figure 17.3) [3, 40, 69]. Using this setup in a blinded RCT, 44 older adults were randomized to undergo either three 40 minutes sessions that exposed them to (i) 20 trips, (ii) 20 slips, and (iii) 10 trips and 10 slips in mixed order over two days, or a sham training control. Relative to the control group, the intervention group experienced fewer laboratory falls (rate ratio: 0.40, 95% CI:

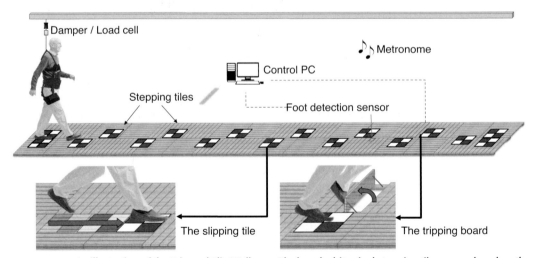

Figure 17.3   An illustration of the Trip and Slip Walkway. Black and white vinyl stepping tiles were placed on the walkway to regulate step length and a metronome was set to regulate cadence. A slip is induced by a movable tile on two hidden low-friction rails with linear bearings that could slide up to 70 cm upon foot contact. A trip is induced using a 14 cm high tripping board that could spring up from the walkway. The tripping board is triggered 50 ms before the foot arrives by an automatic foot detection sensor. The trip and slip tiles are hidden and can be positioned in the near, middle, and far left and right sides of the walkway.

0.22, 0.76) following induced trips and slips with no significant predictive gait adaptations [3].

While most reactive step training requires sophisticated perturbation systems, Allin et al. [70] devised a low-tech, slip training system using a visible slip hazard (i.e. nylon fabric on a lubricated polycarbonate sheet). This predictable slip training involving in a protocol of 100 slip trials was compared with unpredictable slip training involving 20 slips interspersed within 120+ regular walk trials in a pilot study involving 36 young adults [70]. Both the predictable and unpredictable slip training groups showed significantly improved balance recovery. Surprisingly, participants allocated to the low-tech predictable slip training primarily showed improved reactive balance control while those allocated to the unpredictable training programme showed greater predictive gait adaptations to reduce slip severity (e.g. flat foot landing). These findings suggest that sufficient training dosage may be more important than strictly maintaining perturbation unpredictability during the motor learning process.

Reactive Step Training Using Standing Perturbation Systems

Perturbations applied during standing include surface translations [4], waist-pulls [71], tether release [72], and manual pulls and pushes to the torso [73, 74]. In one RCT, repeated trials of standing on a perturbation platform that could move suddenly in one of four directions reduced multi-step reactions and foot collisions following the surface translations [4]. Similarly, voluntary or waist-pull-induced lateral step training has been shown to improve step initiation time [75]. Grabiner et al. [47] specifically trained an 'elevating stepping strategy' by suddenly starting a treadmill while a participant stood in front of a 5 cm foam block in four one-hour sessions over two weeks. At the completion of the training session, participants who received the intervention experienced fewer laboratory falls induced by an overground trip compared with controls [76], as well as fewer trip-related falls in the following year (incident rate ratio: 0.54, 95% CI: 0.30, 0.97) [77].

Mansfield et al. [73] developed a perturbation-based balance training programme using manually applied perturbations that comprises voluntary stepping tasks and torso push/pulls conducted one on one with a physiotherapist. They then conducted an RCT involving an initial six-week training period completed twice a week, followed by booster sessions at three and nine months in 88 long-term stroke survivors. Those in the intervention group had a non-significant 15% reduced rate of falls over 12 months (rate ratio: 0.85, 95% CI: 0.42, 1.69), compared to a control group who received usual balance training. A three-month RCT of balance training that included some time devoted to perturbations applied by an instructor or a partner to evoke reactive stepping responses has also been conducted. This trial involving 66 community-dwelling older adults showed significantly improved voluntary step execution times although effects were lost at the six-month follow-up [78]. While manual perturbations are simple, inexpensive, and likely have good clinical feasibility, more research is required to confirm their efficacy and whether such benefits transfer to daily-life fall prevention.

Reactive Training Programme Characteristics

Community-dwelling older adults comprise the group most likely to benefit from reactive step training, since trips and slips are the most common types of falls in this group [79]. In clinical practice, training of reactive balance and stepping using perturbations can be added as a challenging component to existing balance training programmes. In contrast, reactive training may be less appropriate for older people living in aged care facilities, as most falls experienced by this population do not involve external mechanical perturbations [80]. It appears that people with Parkinson's disease can benefit from reactive step training protocols with high frequency (three times/week) for long periods (eight weeks). It is unclear whether these protocols are effective in people with chronic stroke [73] or multiple sclerosis [81, 82].

The optimal dose of reactive step training is unclear but likely depends on the type of motor adaptation targeted. Many recent trials have included only a few or even single training sessions to examine acute training effects [2, 3, 26, 28, 29, 34, 83]. Lee et al. [84] found no significant difference in practice dosage (40 versus 24 slip-like perturbations on a treadmill) on an overground slip outcome. Feedforward adaptation has commonly been observed after only a few perturbation repetitions [26, 33, 39]. Indeed, Bhatt and Pai reported that watching a video of feedforward adaptation to slips was somewhat effective in achieving a change in slip response, though actual motor training was superior [85]. Despite this, the broader evidence suggests that reactive adaptation to improve balance recovery from unpredictable perturbations generally requires a training dose of multiple sessions [3, 40] over weeks or months [8, 86].

McCrum et al. [83] recently reported that rapid adaptations to only eight trip-like perturbations (sudden treadmill belt accelerations) were retained for a month and showed faster re-adaptation on re-exposure to the same perturbation. Training effects primarily due to feedforward adaptation can be retained for six months [33] to 1.5 years [61], and there is evidence that a booster session can assist in maintaining the effect [33]. Generally, a greater perturbation magnitude (e.g. slip distance and belt acceleration) is associated with a greater training effect [68, 87], and magnitude should be gradually increased [87].

Perturbation modalities vary greatly. Manual perturbations applied by push/ pull, lean-and-release, a foot trip during walking [73], water turbulence [88], catching a ball [89], or sudden start of a treadmill [70, 76] are inexpensive options, although their effectiveness for fall prevention is yet to be confirmed. Specialized perturbation treadmills have been commercialized and can be installed in a clinic with costs of USD $50,000 to $400,000. In contrast, overground walkways, ankle-cable-pulls, and tether-release systems are custom-made and not usually readily available. Finally, some step training programmes have been conducted in water [74] or while seated on a chair [90, 91]. While these can be an alternative or initial approach for individuals with contraindications to step training on the ground, their effects on balance control and preventing falls are unknown.

Conclusions

Emerging evidence suggests that both volitional and reactive step training can effectively prevent falls in older adults. Volitional step training likely contributes to stable gait and balance, improving the ability to proactively avoid hazards, whereas reactive step training likely contributes to an improved ability to recover balance in the event of an unexpected perturbation such as a trip or a slip. Despite these differences, cross-over effects are possible, but the extent and exact mechanisms are yet to be determined. The promising findings published regarding the effects of step training in reducing falls should encourage clinicians to incorporate both volitional and reactive step training as part of their balance training practice for older people and clinical populations. Rapid effects from very low-dose reactive step training are likely attributable to predictive/feedforward adaptation specific to the induced perturbations. Their generalization to fall prevention in daily life as well as training effect retention requires further study.

REFERENCES

1. Okubo Y, Schoene D, Lord SR. Step training improves reaction time, gait and balance and reduces falls in older people: a systematic review and meta-analysis. *Br J Sports Med.* 2017;51:586–93.
2. Pai Y-C, Bhatt T, Yang F et al. Perturbation training can reduce community-dwelling older adults' annual fall risk: a randomized controlled trial. *J Gerontol A Biol Sci Med Sci.* 2014;69:1586–94.
3. Okubo Y, Sturnieks DL, Brodie MA et al. Effect of reactive balance training involving repeated slips and trips on balance recovery among older adults: a blinded randomized controlled trial. *J Gerontol A Biol Sci Med Sci.* 2019;74:1489–96.

4. Mansfield A, Peters AL, Liu BA et al. Effect of a perturbation-based balance training program on compensatory stepping and grasping reactions in older adults: a randomized controlled trial. *Phys Ther.* 2010;90:476–91.

5. Lurie JD, Zagaria AB, Pidgeon DM et al. Pilot comparative effectiveness study of surface perturbation treadmill training to prevent falls in older adults. *BMC Geriatr.* 2013;13:49.

6. Shigematsu R, Okura T, Nakagaichi M et al. Square-stepping exercise and fall risk factors in older adults: a single-blind, randomized controlled trial. *J Gerontol A Biol Sci Med Sci.* 2008;63:76–82.

7. Shigematsu R, Okura T, Sakai T et al. Square-stepping exercise versus strength and balance training for fall risk factors. *Aging Clin Exp Res.* 2008;20:19–24.

8. Shimada H, Obuchi S, Furuna T et al. New intervention program for preventing falls among frail elderly people: the effects of perturbed walking exercise using a bilateral separated treadmill. *Am J Phys Med Rehabil.* 2004;83:493–9.

9. Yamada M, Higuchi T, Nishiguchi S et al. Multitarget stepping program in combination with a standardized multicomponent exercise program can prevent falls in community-dwelling older adults: a randomized controlled trial. *J Am Geriatr Soc.* 2013;61:1669–75.

10. Sherrington C, Michaleff ZA, Fairhall N et al. Exercise to prevent falls in older adults: an updated systematic review and meta-analysis. *Br J Sports Med.* 2017;51:1750–8.

11. Grabiner MD, Crenshaw JR, Hurt CP et al. Exercise-based fall prevention: can you be a bit more specific? *Exerc Sport Sci Rev.* 2014;42:161–8.

12. Pijnappels M, Reeves ND, Maganaris CN et al. Tripping without falling; lower limb strength, a limitation for balance recovery and a target for training in the elderly. *J Electromyogr Kinesiol.* 2008;18:188–96.

13. Kim S, Lockhart T. Effects of 8 weeks of balance or weight training for the independently living elderly on the outcomes of induced slips. *Int J Rehabil Res.* 2010;33:49–55.

14. Schoene D, Lord SR, Delbaere K et al. A randomized controlled pilot study of home-based step training in older people using videogame technology. *PloS One.* 2013;8:e57734.

15. Shigematsu R, Okura T. A novel exercise for improving lower-extremity functional fitness in the elderly. *Aging Clin Exp Res.* 2006;18:242–8.

16. Pichierri G, Murer K, de Bruin ED. A cognitive-motor intervention using a dance video game to enhance foot placement accuracy and gait under dual task conditions in older adults: a randomized controlled trial. *BMC Geriatr.* 2012;12:74.

17. Teixeira CV, Gobbi S, Pereira JR et al. Effect of square-stepping exercise and basic exercises on functional fitness of older adults. *Geriatr Gerontol Int.* 2013;13:842–8.

18. Fung L, Lam M. Effectiveness of a progressive stepping program on lower limb function in community dwelling older adults. *J Exerc Sci Fit.* 2012;10:8–11.

19. Teixeira CVL, Gobbi S, Pereira JR et al. Effects of square-stepping exercise on cognitive functions of older people. *Psychogeriatrics.* 2013;13:148–56.

20. Schoene D, Valenzuela T, Toson B et al. Interactive cognitive-motor step training improves cognitive risk factors of falling in older adults: a randomized controlled trial. *PloS One.* 2015;10:e0145161.

21. Morat M, Bakker J, Hammes V et al. Effects of stepping exergames under stable versus unstable conditions on balance and strength in healthy community-dwelling older adults: a three-armed randomized controlled trial. *Exp Gerontol.* 2019;127:110719.

22. Pai YC, Bhatt TS. Repeated-slip training: an emerging paradigm for prevention of slip-related falls among older adults. *Phys Ther.* 2007;87:1478–91.

23. Mansfield A, Wong JS, Bryce J et al. Does perturbation-based balance training prevent falls? Systematic review and meta-analysis of preliminary randomized controlled trials. *Phys Ther.* 2015;95:700–9.

24. Horak FB, Henry SM, Shumway-Cook A. Postural perturbations: new insights for treatment of balance disorders. *Phys Ther.* 1997;77:517–33.

25. Bohm S, Mademli L, Mersmann F et al. Predictive and reactive locomotor adaptability in healthy elderly: a systematic review and meta-analysis. *Sports Med.* 2015;45: 1759–77.

26. Pai YC, Bhatt T, Wang E et al. Inoculation against falls: rapid adaptation by young and older adults to slips during daily activities. *Arch Phys Med Rehabil.* 2010;91:452–9.

27. Bhatt T, Wening JD, Pai YC. Adaptive control of gait stability in reducing slip-related backward loss of balance. *Exp Brain Res.* 2006;170:61–73.

28. Parijat P, Lockhart TE. Effects of moveable platform training in preventing slip-induced falls in older adults. *Ann Biomed Eng.* 2012;40:1111–21.

29. Bhatt T, Wang TY, Yang F et al. Adaptation and generalization to opposing perturbations in walking. *Neuroscience.* 2013;246:435–50.

30. Bhatt T, Pai YC. Immediate and latent interlimb transfer of gait stability adaptation following repeated exposure to slips. *J Mot Behav.* 2008;40:380–90.

31. Pavol MJ, Runtz EF, Pai YC. Young and older adults exhibit proactive and reactive adaptations to repeated slip exposure. *J Gerontol A Biol Sci Med Sci.* 2004;59:494– 502.

32. Sherrington C, Tiedemann A, Fairhall N et al. Exercise to prevent falls in older adults: an updated meta-analysis and best practice recommendations. *NSW Public Health Bull.* 2011;22:78–83.

33. Bhatt T, Yang F, Pai CY. Learning to resist gait-slip falls: long-term retention in community-dwelling older adults. *Arch Phys Med Rehabil.* 2012;93:557–64.

34. Bieryla KA, Madigan ML, Nussbaum MA. Practicing recovery from a simulated trip improves recovery kinematics after an actual trip. *Gait Posture.* 2007;26:208–13.

35. Patla AE. Strategies for dynamic stability during adaptive human locomotion. *IEEE Eng Med Biol.* 2003;22:48–52.

36. Wolpert DM, Miall RC. Forward models for physiological motor control. *Neural Netw.* 1996;9:1265–79.

37. Shadmehr R, Smith MA, Krakauer JW. Error correction, sensory prediction, and adaptation in motor control. *Annu Rev Neurosci.* 2010;33:89–108.

38. Ting LH, van Antwerp KW, Scrivens JE et al. Neuromechanical tuning of nonlinear postural control dynamics. *Chaos.* 2009;19:026111.

39. Wang TY, Bhatt T, Yang F et al. Adaptive control reduces trip-induced forward gait instability among young adults. *J Biomech.* 2012;45:1169–75.

40. Okubo Y, Brodie MA, Sturnieks DL et al. Exposure to trips and slips with increasing unpredictability while walking improves balance recovery responses with minimal predictive gait alterations. *PloS One*. 2018;13:e0202913.

41. Moyer BE, Chambers AJ, Redfern MS et al. Gait parameters as predictors of slip severity in younger and older adults. *Ergonomics*. 2006;49:329–43.

42. Nashner LM. Balance adjustments of humans perturbed while walking. *J Neurophysiol*. 1980;44:650–64.

43. Nashner LM. Adapting reflexes controlling the human posture. *Exp Brain Res*. 1976;26:59–72.

44. Dietz V, Quintern J, Sillem M. Stumbling reactions in man: significance of proprioceptive and pre-programmed mechanisms. *J Physiol*. 1987;386:149–63.

45. Haridas C, Zehr EP, Misiaszek JE. Adaptation of cutaneous stumble correction when tripping is part of the locomotor environment. *J Neurophysiol*. 2008;99:2789–97.

46. Pijnappels M, Bobbert MF, van Dieen JH. Contribution of the support limb in control of angular momentum after tripping. *J Biomech*. 2004;37:1811–18.

47. Eng JJ, Winter DA, Patla AE. Strategies for recovery from a trip in early and late swing during human walking. *Exp Brain Res*. 1994;102:339–49.

48. Bierbaum S, Peper A, Karamanidis K et al. Adaptive feedback potential in dynamic stability during disturbed walking in the elderly. *J Biomech*. 2011;44:1921–6.

49. Fujio K, Obata H, Kitamura T et al. Corticospinal excitability is modulated as a function of postural perturbation predictability. *Front Hum Neurosci*. 2018;12:68.

50. Welch TD, Ting LH. Mechanisms of motor adaptation in reactive balance control. *PloS One*. 2014;9:e96440.

51. Fujio K, Obata H, Kawashima N et al. The effects of temporal and spatial predictions on stretch reflexes of ankle flexor and extensor muscles while standing. *PloS One*. 2016;11: e0158721.

52. Horak FB, Diener HC, Nashner LM. Influence of central set on human postural responses. *J Neurophysiol*. 1989;62:841–53.

53. Beckley DJ, Bloem BR, Remler MP et al. Long latency postural responses are functionally modified by cognitive set. *Electroencephalogr Clin Neurophysiol*. 1991;81:353–8.

54. Diener HC, Horak F, Stelmach G et al. Direction and amplitude precuing has no effect on automatic posture responses. *Exp Brain Res*. 1991;84:219–23.

55. Fujio K, Obata H, Kawashima N et al. Presetting of the corticospinal excitability in the tibialis anterior muscle in relation to prediction of the magnitude and direction of postural perturbations. *Front Hum Neurosci*. 2019;13:4.

56. Karamanidis K, Süptitz F, Catalá MM et al. *Reactive Response and Adaptive Modifications in Dynamic Stability to Changes in Lower Limb Dynamics in the Elderly while Walking.* Berlin, Heidelberg: Springer; 2011.

57. Shapiro A, Melzer I. Balance perturbation system to improve balance compensatory responses during walking in old persons. *J Neuroeng Rehabil*. 2010;7:32.

58. Wang Y, Bhatt T, Liu X et al. Can treadmill-slip perturbation training reduce immediate risk of over-ground-slip induced fall among community-dwelling older adults? *J Biomech*. 2019;84:58–66.

59. Kurz I, Gimmon Y, Shapiro A et al. Unexpected perturbations training improves balance control and voluntary stepping times in older adults: a double blind randomized control trial. *BMC Geriatr.* 2016;16:58.

60. Konig M, Epro G, Seeley J et al. Retention of improvement in gait stability over 14 weeks due to trip-perturbation training is dependent on perturbation dose. *J Biomech.* 2019;84:243–6.

61. Epro G, Mierau A, McCrum C et al. Retention of gait stability improvements over 1.5 years in older adults: effects of perturbation exposure and triceps surae neuromuscular exercise. *J Neurophysiol.* 2018;119:2229–40.

62. King ST, Eveld ME, Martinez A et al. A novel system for introducing precisely-controlled, unanticipated gait perturbations for the study of stumble recovery. *J Neuroeng Rehabil.* 2019;16:69.

63. Pavol MJ, Owings TM, Foley KT et al. The sex and age of older adults influence the outcome of induced trips. *J Gerontol A Biol Sci Med Sci.* 1999;54:M103–8.

64. Bierbaum S, Peper A, Karamanidis K et al. Adaptational responses in dynamic stability during disturbed walking in the elderly. *J Biomech.* 2010;43:2362–8.

65. Marigold DS, Patla AE. Strategies for dynamic stability during locomotion on a slippery surface: effects of prior experience and knowledge. *J Neurophysiol.* 2002;88:339–53.

66. McCrum C, Gerards MHG, Karamanidis K et al. A systematic review of gait perturbation paradigms for improving reactive stepping responses and falls risk among healthy older adults. *Eur Rev Aging Phys Act.* 2017;14:3.

67. Bhatt T, Pai YC. Generalization of gait adaptation for fall prevention: from moveable platform to slippery floor. *J Neurophysiol.* 2009;101:948–57.

68. Yang F, Wang TY, Pai YC. Reduced intensity in gait-slip training can still improve stability. *J Biomech.* 2014;47:2330–8.

69. Okubo Y, Brodie M, Sturnieks D et al. A pilot study of reactive balance training using trips and slips with increasing unpredictability in young and older adults: biomechanical mechanisms, falls and clinical feasibility. *Clin Biomech.* 2019;67:171–9.

70. Allin LJ, Nussbaum MA, Madigan ML. Two novel slip training methods improve the likelihood of recovering balance after a laboratory-induced slip. *J Appl Biomech.* 2018:1–31.

71. Mille ML, Johnson-Hilliard M, Martinez KM et al. One step, two steps, three steps more . . . directional vulnerability to falls in community-dwelling older people. *J Gerontol A Biol Sci Med Sci.* 2013;68:1540–8.

72. Carty CP, Cronin NJ, Lichtwark GA et al. Mechanisms of adaptation from a multiple to a single step recovery strategy following repeated exposure to forward loss of balance in older adults. *PloS One.* 2012;7:e33591.

73. Mansfield A, Aqui A, Danells CJ et al. Does perturbation-based balance training prevent falls among individuals with chronic stroke? A randomised controlled trial. *BMJ Open.* 2018;8:e021510.

74. Elbar O, Tzedek I, Vered E et al. A water-based training program that includes perturbation exercises improves speed of voluntary stepping in older adults: a randomized controlled cross-over trial. *Arch Gerontol Geriatr.* 2013;56:134–40.

75. Rogers MW, Johnson ME, Martinez KM et al. Step training improves the speed of voluntary step initiation in aging. *J Gerontol A Biol Sci Med Sci.* 2003;58:46–51.

76. Grabiner MD, Bareither ML, Gatts S et al. Task-specific training reduces trip-related fall risk in women. *Med Sci Sports Exerc.* 2012;44:2410–14.

77. Rosenblatt NJ, Marone J, Grabiner MD. Preventing trip-related falls by community-dwelling adults: a prospective study. *J Am Geriatr Soc.* 2013;61:1629–31.

78. Melzer I, Oddsson L. Improving balance control and self-reported lower extremity function in community-dwelling older adults: a randomized control trial. *Clin Rehabil.* 2013;27:195–206.

79. Berg WP, Alessio HM, Mills EM et al. Circumstances and consequences of falls in independent community-dwelling older adults. *Age Ageing.* 1997;26:261–8.

80. Robinovitch SN, Feldman F, Yang Y et al. Video capture of the circumstances of falls in elderly people residing in long-term care: an observational study. *Lancet.* 2013;381:47–54.

81. Gera G, Fling BW, Van Ooteghem K et al. Postural motor learning deficits in people with MS in spatial but not temporal control of center of mass. *Neurorehabil Neural Repair.* 2016;30:722–30.

82. Van Liew C, Dibble LE, Hunt GR et al. Protective stepping in multiple sclerosis: impacts of a single session of in-place perturbation practice. *Mult Scler Relat Disord.* 2019;30:17–24.

83. McCrum C, Karamanidis K, Willems P et al. Retention, savings and interlimb transfer of reactive gait adaptations in humans following unexpected perturbations. *Commun Biol.* 2018;1:230.

84. Lee A, Bhatt T, Liu X et al. Can higher training practice dosage with treadmill slip-perturbation necessarily reduce risk of falls following overground slip? *Gait Posture.* 2018;61:387–92.

85. Bhatt T, Pai YC. Can observational training substitute motor training in preventing backward balance loss after an unexpected slip during walking? *J Neurophysiol.* 2008;99: 843–52.

86. Protas EJ, Mitchell K, Williams A et al. Gait and step training to reduce falls in Parkinson's disease. *NeuroRehabilitation.* 2005;20:183–90.

87. Liu X, Bhatt T, Pai YC. Intensity and generalization of treadmill slip training: high or low, progressive increase or decrease? *J Biomech.* 2016;49:135–40.

88. Melzer I, Elbar O, Tsedek I et al. A water-based training program that include perturbation exercises to improve stepping responses in older adults: study protocol for a randomized controlled cross-over trial. *BMC Geriatr.* 2008;8:19.

89. Oddsson LIE, Boissy P, Melzer I. How to improve gait and balance function in elderly individuals: compliance with principles of training. *Eur Rev Aging Phys Act.* 2007;4:15–23.

90. Yamada M, Aoyama T, Hikita Y et al. Effects of a DVD-based seated dual-task stepping exercise on the fall risk factors among community-dwelling elderly adults. *Telemed J E-Health.* 2011;17:768–72.

91. Yamada M, Aoyama T, Tanaka B et al. Seated stepping exercise in a dual-task condition improves ambulatory function with a secondary task: a randomized controlled trial. *Aging Clin Exp Res.* 2011;23:386–92.

18

Cognitive-Motor Interventions and Their Effects on Fall Risk in Older People

Daniel S. Schoene and Daina L. Sturnieks

Many studies have now shown that both physical and cognitive factors are important in fall risk. In accordance with the common-cause theory of cognitive ageing, which states that age-related declines in cognitive, sensory, and motor functioning are attributed to a common neurobiological mechanism, there is evidence of shared variance between sensorimotor and cognitive age-related changes. Indeed, cognitive, sensory, and motor inter-relationships strengthen with age [1]. It is, therefore, of little surprise that parameters of the postural control system are influenced by the cognitive demand of a task, particularly in older people. Undertaking daily tasks, such as maintaining upright posture and safely navigating complex environments, requires adequate sensory perception, cognitive integration, and subsequent motor adjustments [2], with increased cognitive processing required with aging [3]. Furthermore, many daily activities require the handling of two or more simultaneous tasks, such as walking while talking, carrying a basket with laundry while navigating the stairs, or crossing a busy road safely [4]. Older people appear not to be able to process multiple tasks as quickly and/or as well as younger adults and such impairments have been linked to falls in older people [5]. Figure 18.1 displays a hypothetical model of how the sensory, cognitive, and motor domains are inter-linked and how these factors and interactions might contribute to falls.

As indicated in Chapter 16, interventions for fall prevention in the general (community-dwelling) older population commonly prescribe strength and balance exercises [6], which are usually considered physical training. However, it has become clear that physical exercise can influence cognitive functions such as attention, memory, and executive functions in both healthy and cognitively impaired older people [7]. In turn, there is some evidence that (seated) cognitive training (e.g. playing computer games) transfers to improvements in parameters of balance and mobility [8]. Given the significant and independent contributions of physical and cognitive factors to fall risk, interventions that purposely combine cognitive, motor, and/or sensory domains have good face validity, with promising complementary benefits for physical and cognitive health.

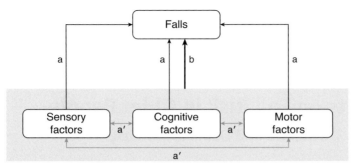

Figure 18.1   Inter-relationships between sensory, cognitive, and motor factors and fall-risk in older people. a: single-domain deficits, such as impaired vision (sensory domain) may cause a fall by the person overlooking an obstacle; a′: within and across domain, (partial) compensation by other domains help to avoid falling, e.g. increased attention and proactive avoidance of a balance threat (cognitive domain) and fast reaction (motor domain) compensate for vision-related increase in fall risk; b: the complex interplay between individual domains contributes to falls (in addition to external task and environmental factors)

Classification of Cognitive-Motor Training

There is no consensus definition for cognitive-motor or motor-cognitive interventions; however, they involve a combination of physical and cognitive tasks that might occur either serially (e.g. thinking then moving) or simultaneously (dual- or multi-tasking) [9]. This chapter will focus on cognitive-motor training interventions that have cognitive and motor components combined in the same exercise/s. This is a narrower definition than found in some areas of this growing body of literature, yet reflects the multi-tasking required during daily activities and has been recommended as the most promising approach to enhance cognitive reserve [10]. Body-mind exercises (e.g. tai chi, yoga) are not included here.

Figure 18.2 shows a classification scheme of cognitive-motor interventions for fall prevention based on current published studies. Except for some studies administering dual- or multi-task interventions, such as walking with additional secondary tasks (handling objects, counting, word recall, etc.), the majority of interventions are classified as combined programmes, having both serial and simultaneous cognitive-motor training components. In the combined programmes, participants have completed tasks serially (e.g. solving a cognitive task immediately before a motor action) or simultaneously (e.g. dual-tasking) as well as combinations of these, while the motor components often comprised walking, stepping, and balancing in place. The combined training interventions can be subdivided into modalities that include traditional physical activities, such as

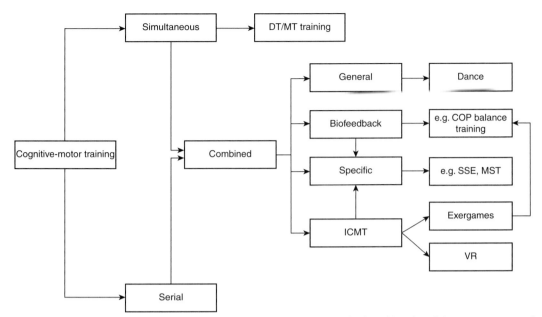

Figure 18.2   Classification of cognitive-motor interventions. DT/MT: dual/multi-task training; COP: centre of pressure; SSE: square stepping exercise; MST: multi-target step training; ICMT: interactive cognitive-motor training; VR: virtual reality.

dancing, and those specifically developed to target fall risk factors, such as prescribed step training (see Chapter 17). Over the past two decades, the use of computerized interventions has enabled the development of specific cognitive-motor training technologies. These include balance training under real-time feedback of one's centre of pressure (i.e. biofeedback) and interactive cognitive-motor training (ICMT) [9]. ICMT is an exercise modality that requires participants to interact with a computer interface via gross motor movements, such as stepping, while receiving immediate (visual and/or auditory) feedback. ICMT includes virtual reality (VR) training, such as navigating simulated street scenes using VR goggles as well as exergames (exercise while playing video games), such as the Nintendo Wii, Microsoft Kinect, or custom-built systems that vary greatly in cost and complexity [11]. It should be noted that balance biofeedback training can be incorporated into ICMT.

Efficacy of Cognitive-Motor Interventions on Fall Risk

Numerous studies have examined the effects of cognitive-motor training interventions on falls and fall risk factors in older people. While too many to provide an extensive review, some are worthy of specific mention, as they provide insight into the efficacy of this type of intervention. The following overview of the literature includes studies that administered any form of cognitive-motor intervention in cohorts of people aged 65 years and older for improving fall risk factors or fall outcomes. Studies not covered include those that did not require the participant to be in an upright position, and robot-assisted or exoskeleton interventions. Studies conducted in clinical populations, such as people with stroke and Parkinson's disease, are also not included in this chapter.

The findings of 13 prospective studies [12–26] examining the effects of motor-cognitive training on prospectively ascertained falls in older people are summarized in Table 18.1. These studies are diverse in terms of sample populations (frail nursing home residents versus higher-functioning community-dwellers) and intervention modalities (dancing, off-the-shelf exergames, and balance and stepping exercises).

Several high-quality studies (i.e. randomized controlled trial (RCT) designs, blinded assessments, prospective falls ascertainment of at least six months) have demonstrated lower fall rates in participants undertaking cognitive-motor interventions, compared to control groups. However, only a few studies have had appropriate sample sizes for the study of falls [20, 24, 25]. Physical components of the successful studies include functional dynamic balance challenges under cognitive load and sensory changes, including stepping, walking, and controlled centre of mass movements. Cognitive components have included the detection of relevant stimuli in complex environments, objects to be hit or avoided, distracters, no-go stimuli to be supressed, among others. Interventions were also often accompanied by music. It is important to note that several other trials with similar interventions did not show significant effects in terms of preventing falls [14, 17, 19, 21]. More high-quality studies of sufficient size with appropriate control groups are needed to determine whether cognitive-motor training programmes are superior to other forms of exercise.

Overall, it appears that research-facility-based cognitive-motor training interventions prevent falls, whereas interventions delivered more widely [19], or unsupervised at home [21] have no or smaller effects. These reduced effects may be due to lower adherence to the intervention or lack of appropriate exercise progression. Future studies should consider the intervention suitability for the population, feasibility, uptake, and adherence. Research-facility-based studies should be tested in implementation studies to ensure they can be effective in the community and thus have an impact on public health.

To date, no studies have investigated the effects of serial cognitive-motor training (e.g. solving cognitive task first and before a motor action) alone on fall risk or related factors in older people. However, serial tasks have been included in combined training along with simultaneous cognitive-motor tasks (e.g. dual-tasking).

Table 18.1 RCTs of cognitive-motor interventions examining effects on falls in older people

Study	Sample size	Population and setting	Intervention category	Interventions	Control	Findings
Simultaneous training						
Trombetti 2011 [24]/ Hars 2014 [27]	106/52 (4 y)	65+ years, mean 75.5 (6.9); high fall risk; no neurological or orthopaedic condition affecting gait and balance; community	DT/MT	Various multitask exercises involving wide range of movements and challenging balance to music. Supervised, group. 6 mo, 1/wk, 60 min. 4 y maintained exercise participation (n = 23). Jaques Dalcroze Eurhythmics	None. 4 y discontinued participation (n = 29)	6 mo IRR 0.49 (0.27–0.91) RR 0.69 (0.44–1.07), p=0.06, RR mF 0.21 (0.06–0.99) Falls past 12 mo IRR 0.39 (0.14–1.08), p = 0.07 RR 0.45 (0.19–1.07), p = 0.07 Falls over 4 y IRR 0.78 (0.47–1.28), p = 0.32, RR 0.69 (0.53–0.91)
Combined serial and simultaneous training						
Merom 2016 [19]	522	Mean 78 y, 39% >80; able to walk 50 m; MMSE>23; self-care retirement villages	General – Dance	Folk or Ballroom Dancing 12 mo, 2/wk, 60 min (80 h total) Supervised, group. Folk = 5 villages Ballroom = 7 villages	None	12 mo All IRR 1.19 (0.83–1.71) Folk dance IRR 1.68 (1.03–2.73) Ballroom IRR 0.92 (0.65–1.29) Ballroom high attendance IRR 0.71 (0.48–1.05)
da Silva Borges 2014 [12]	59	Mean 67.5 (8.0) years; no ADL impairment, no regular exercise; no cognitive impairment; long-stay institution	General – Dance	Ballroom dancing 12 wk, 3/wk, 50 min Supervised, group. Foxtrot, Waltz, Rumba, Samba, Swing, Bolero, Salsa, Merengue, Square Dancing, Forro, Pagode, Baiao, Cirandas	None	Fewer falls (p <0.001)

Table 18.1 (*cont.*)

Study	Sample size	Population and setting	Intervention category	Interventions	Control	Findings
Yamada 2013 [25]	230	65+ years, mean 76.7 (8.0); able to walk independent w/o cane; RDST >4; community	Specific – DT/MT, Serial	Specific; multi-target stepping + multi-component standard Supervised, group 24 wk, 2/wk, 35 min (2 min multi-target stepping)	Indoor walking 50 m + multi-component standard Supervised, group 24 wk, 2/wk, 35 min (2 min walking)	12 mo IRR 0.35 (0.19–0.66), Fractures RR 0.22 (0.06–0.80)
Shigematsu 2008 [22]	68	65–74, mean 69.1 (2.7); no mobility-limiting orthopaedic conditions; community	Specific – DT/MT, Serial	Memorized step patterns; 12 wk, 2/wk, 70 min (40 min SSE) Supervised, group	Walking 12 wk, 1/wk, 70 min (40 min walking) Supervised, group	8 mo RR 0.64 ns* HR walking 2.32 (0.59–9.04)
Shigematsu 2008 [23]	39	65–74, mean 69.0 (2.8); no mobility-limiting orthopaedic conditions; community	Specific – DT/MT, Serial	Memorized step patterns; 12 wk, 2/wk, 70 min (40 min SSE) Supervised, group	Strength and balance (S&B) 12 wk, 2/wk, 70 min (40 min strength and balance) Supervised, group	14 mo trip-related falls SSE 30% versus S&B 58%, p = 0.08 falls per trip SSE 17% versus S&B 50%, p = 0.04
Mirelman 2016 [20]	282	60–90 years, mean 73.8 (6.7); high fall risk; able to walk unassisted 5min; MMSE >20; including MCI, PD; community	ICMT	Motion capture camera (Kinect) with computer-generated simulation with obstacles, distracters, path-walking; real-time projection feet VR treadmill Supervised, single 6 wk, 3/wk, 45 min	Treadmill Supervised, single 6 wk, 3/wk, 45 min	6 mo IRR 0.58 (0.36–0.96)

Study	N	Design	Population	Intervention	Intervention details	Comparison	Outcome
Schoene 2015 [21]	86	ICMT	70+ years, 81.5 (7.0); able to walk w/o walking aid; able to step unassisted; Mini-Cog >2; retirement villages and community	Stepping exergames Unsupervised at home 16 wk, 3/wk, 20 min recommended	Stepping tasks focusing on precise, rapid stepping, including go/no-go tasks, spatial orientation and task-switching	Evidence-based recommendations on health topics, including fall prevention	6 months IRR 0.78 ns*
Kwok and Pua 2016 [17]	80	ICMT	60+ years, mean 70.2 (7.1); SPPB 5-9; mFES <10; AMT 8.9 (1.2); community	Exergames + standard multi-component 12 wk, 1/wk, 60 min (20 min cog-mot) + home exercise (20 min S&B) Supervised, group	WiiActive exercises with balance board	Standard multi-component 12 wk, 1/wk, 60 min + home exercise (20 min S&B) Supervised, group	12 mo IRR 0.95 (0.37–2.43) (EX reference)
Eggenberger 2015 [14]	66	1. ICMT 2. DT	70+ years, mean 78.9 (5.4); able to walk 20 m w/o walking aid; MMSE >21; community or residence facilities (only need for little care)	1. Dance exergame 2. Treadmill + verbal memory + S&B Supervised, group 26 wk, 2/wk, 60 min (20 min cog-mot)	1. Modified Dance Dance Revolution 2. DT, memorizing word lists	Treadmill + S&B Supervised, group 26 wk, 2/wk, 60 min (20 min walking)	12 mo no differences
Fu 2015 [15]	60	ICMT	65+ years, mean 82.4 (4.1); history of falls; frail; compromised mobility; able to follow instructions; nursing home	Balance exergame 6 wk, 3/wk, 60 min Supervised, group	Wii Fit Balance Board (three games)	Otago Exercise Programme, 6 wk, 3/wk, 60 min Supervised, group	12 mo IRR 0.35 (0.20–0.64)

Table 18.1 *(cont.)*

Study	Sample size	Population and setting	Intervention category	Interventions	Control	Findings
Duque 2013 [13]	60	65+, history of falls; impaired balance; able to walk w/o walking aid; MMSE >21; community	ICMT	VR balance games + general recommendation on fall prevention and evidence-based care plan Supervised, alone 6 wk, 2/wk, 20 min	Postural control in VR under different sensory conditions	General recommendation on fall prevention andevidence-based care plan	9 mo significantly lower number of falls (1.1 (0.7) versus 2.0 (0.2), p<0.01)
Lauze 2017 [18]	31	65+ years, mean 81.2 (7.2); able to stand w/o assistance 1 min; MoCA 22.9 (4.5); assisted living community	ICMT	Exergame 12 wk, 2/wk, 45 min Partially supervised, alone	Kinect, Jintronix; seven aerobic and eight resistance/ balance exercises	None	Change in number of falls previous 3 mo from baseline to 24 weeks EX –0.1 (0.6) versus CG 0.3 (0.5), p = 0.03

* Calculated based on data in publication

DT/MT = Dual-task/multi-task; ICMT = Interactive cognitive-motor training; MMSE = Mini Mental Status Examination; MoCA = Montreal Cognitive Assessment; IRR = Incident rate ratio; RR = Relative risk; VR = Virtual reality; MCI = Mild cognitive impairment; PD = Parkinson's disease; EX = Exercise; CG = Control Group; SPPB = Short Physical Performance Battery; AMT = Abbreviated Mental Test; mFES = Modified Falls Efficacy Scale; w/o = without

Simultaneous (Dual- and Multi-Task) Training

Simultaneous interventions include dual- or multi-task exercises, such as walking with an additional physical (e.g. handling objects) or cognitive task (e.g. counting, word recall). One music-based multi-task training programme conducted for one hour per week for six months reduced the rate of falls by >50% and fall risk by 39%, compared to a delayed intervention control group [24]. The movements involved multi-directional weight-shifting, walking and turning, and exaggerated upper body movements, thus challenging balance in line with systematic review recommendations [6]. In parallel, participants were required to react to changes in the music as well as to handle objects. Improvements were also observed in outcomes of balance, gait, and physical functioning that partially persisted for six months beyond training [24], in addition to improved executive functioning and reduced anxiety levels [27]. A sub-set of people (n = 52) was followed up at four years, with outcomes compared between those who kept training and those that stopped after the initial trial [26]. Gait speed, standing balance, mobility, functional strength of the lower extremities, and hand grip strength were all better in the group that maintained training, and this group tended to have fewer falls, compared to those who did not keep training.

In healthy older people, dual-task training intervention studies have demonstrated improvements in both cognitive and motor components of dual tasks, more so than single-task training [28]. While meta-analytic evidence has demonstrated the efficacy of balance training on improving outcomes of postural stability in older people [29], little or limited effect has been shown under dual-task conditions. To measure this effect properly, it is important to assess both the motor task and the cognitive task, but relatively few studies have done this. In one small study, participants were assigned to three sessions of no training, single-task training (quiet standing on a compliant surface and counting backwards in threes, separately) or dual-task training (same tasks simultaneously) [30]. Sway under dual-task conditions increased in the no training and single-task training groups but not in the dual-task group. In another three-arm study, Azadian et al. [31] found an eight-week programme of 24 sessions of dual-task training to be beneficial for some temporal-spatial parameters of single-task gait and walking symmetry compared to a control group. Training combined cognitive tasks with different standing and walking tasks that included multi-directional stepping and controlled weight shifts. However, seated cognitive training focusing on executive functions has also shown beneficial effects on gait. For instance, gait speed increased by 8% in the dual-tasking group but by 21% in the cognitive training group, while other gait parameters only improved in the cognitive training group.

Interestingly, this included walking symmetry under dual-task gait conditions, confirming findings linking gait to different cognitive domains, including executive networks [32]. Similarly, Wongcharoen et al. [33] demonstrated home-based cognitive-motor dual-task training was superior to single task (i.e. balance) training, as was seated cognitive training, in improving gait under single and dual-task conditions. No transfer from practiced to novel dual tasks was observed in this study, in contrast to earlier findings by Silsupadol et al. [34].

Some considerations of the findings of dual-task training studies should be borne in mind. Falbo et al. [35] compared two co-ordination training programmes that both involved dual-tasking, one with a motor dual-task focus (e.g. combining walking and balance exercises with other body movements or handling objects, changing walking patterns in response to stimuli) and one with a cognitive-motor dual-task focus specific to executive functions (e.g. according to equipment features, stimulus-response patterns changed). The programmes comprised 12 weekly 30-minute sessions and were administered to healthy older people. Both groups improved in gait performance (speed, stride time variability) during level walking, but the cognitive-motor training group also demonstrated improved inhibition after the intervention in line with corresponding improvements in gait performance.

Task prioritization during training appears to influence the outcomes of dual-task intervention studies. In older people, including those with balance impairments, balance improved under alternating priority conditions (half the time prioritizing the postural control task and the other half the cognitive task), compared to fixed priority conditions (equally prioritizing both components during all exercises), indicating improved co-ordination between tasks can be learned [36]. For instance, Silsupadol et al. [37] compared a four-week balance training programme under single-task, fixed priority dual-task, and alternating priority dual-task conditions. While all three groups improved their balance (Berg Balance Scale), and gait speed after four weeks, only the alternating priority group improved gait speed under dual-task conditions following the training phase and at 12 weeks follow-up [37], indicating relevance of transfer effects to daily-life performance. Overall, the results on dual-task training show the efficacy of incorporating cognitive demands into physical training. However, more studies, especially in balance-impaired and frailer older people are warranted.

Combined Training

Dancing

Dancing, without automatisms (i.e. actions without conscious volition) can be considered cognitive-motor training. It involves challenging dynamic balance exercises and requires serial as well as simultaneous cognitive processing. Dancing is popular in many cultures and communities and has been shown to lead to improvements in balance, gait, mobility, strength, and proprioception in older people [38–40]. In healthy older adults, a twice weekly six-month intervention of training novel dances from different genres led to improved dual-task gait performance and cognition compared to a health-enhancing multi-component exercise programme that had the same frequency, duration, and intensity [41]. Gait speed increased in both groups [41], but no difference between groups was observed for gait variability. However, the dance group increased their local dynamic stability during walking and thus the postural system's sensitivity to small perturbations [42]. Two other small RCTs have been conducted in relatively young and well-functioning older adults without major cognitive impairments [43, 44]. One administered an eight-week Salsa dancing programme (twice weekly for 60 minutes) and found a tendency towards an improvement in static postural control in the antero-posterior direction as well as changes in gait (increased stride velocity and stride length and decreased stride time) but not gait variability or lower extremity power [43]. The other administered traditional Greek folk dances, which involved self-imposed perturbations that substantially challenged the postural control system [44]. At the end of the ten-week trial, participants assigned to the intervention (20 sessions of moderate intensity (50–60% maximum heart rate) dancing, demonstrated improved one-legged stance and upper body range of motion compared to the controls. These findings suggest that in mobile and well-functioning seniors, dancing leads to task-specific adaptations in static and dynamic balance important for postural stability in daily life.

Three small studies conducted by the same team have administered ballroom dancing (foxtrot, waltz, rumba, swing, samba, and bolero) over 12 weeks for three 50-minute sessions a week (30 minutes dancing) [12, 45, 46]. Included participants were relatively young (mean age <70 years), sedentary residents of long-stay institutions who were mobile and independent in ADLs, and in one of these studies, a large proportion of participants were cognitively impaired [46]. Consistent findings demonstrated better performance in balance (stabilometer balance platform) and performance-based functional performance (gait speed, chair rise, standing up from prone position, standing up from a chair and moving about the room, putting on/taking off a shirt) compared to non-active control groups. Moreover, in one study, fewer falls over a six-month follow-up were reported [12].

The evidence for dancing effects on cognition in older people is inconsistent, reflecting the diversity of dances across cultures and the difficulty in administering interventions with standardized doses and cognitive stimuli. A recently published systematic review and meta-analysis, including 13 studies of ballroom, folk, or contemporary dances, found a large effect for improved global cognition, very limited evidence for a beneficial effect on memory and no effect on executive functioning [47]. After controlling for age, education, IQ, lifestyle, health, and fitness, it appears there is no added benefit of social dancing on cognitive functioning and grey matter volume in older long-term dancers compared to non-dancers [48], potentially indicating a lack of cognitive stimulation and progression in habitual dancers. Dancing may be therefore a cognitive-motor intervention only in novices, meaning that the inclusion of additional stimuli or the learning of new dances is required for maximising beneficial cognitive and motor abilities.

The one adequately powered RCT of twice weekly one-hour social dancing classes (folk or ballroom dancing) did not show significant benefits for fall prevention over 12 months [19]. Furthermore, physical and cognitive fall-related measures were also unchanged. Exploratory post-hoc sub-group analysis showed the rate of falls was higher for the folk-dance group, compared to ballroom dance group, and people at increased risk at baseline appeared not to benefit from the programme. The authors argue that besides the lack of sufficient balance intensity, low adherence (median attendance 56%) may help to explain these results, which is in line with other studies [6, 49]. Therefore, despite improvements in fall-related factors, there is currently insufficient evidence to recommend dancing, especially folk dancing, for fall prevention in older people, particularly those at increased risk. Further studies comparing different styles and doses of dancing may be warranted.

Cognitive Stepping (Low Tech)

The Square Stepping Exercise programme [22] requires participants to step precisely (full foot, toe, or heel) on a grid-marked carpet, following up to 196 different stepping patterns of increasing complexity. This low-cost cognitive-motor intervention involves serial and simultaneous processing. Compared to a strength and balance training programme of equal dose, the Square Stepping participants reported a reduced number of trip-related falls over 14 months following 12 weeks of training with 24 group sessions and otherwise similar improvements in functional tests, including leg strength (chair rise, leg power), balance (one leg stance), stepping, and gait speed [23]. Comparing the same programme to supervised and home-based walking, Square Stepping Exercise was associated with greater improvements in leg power, balance, agility, and reaction time [22].

Another example of a cognitive-motor step intervention is Yamada et al.'s multi-target stepping programme that combines square stepping and colour-based go/no-go tasks for deciding where to step [25]. In a 24-week randomized controlled trial involving people reporting fear of falling, Yamada et al. [25]

compared this multi-target stepping programme with a dose-matched multi-component exercise programme. They found that two 30-minute sessions a week of the multi-component exercise plus only two minutes of precise stepping under cognitive load improved stepping accuracy, mobility, and gait, compared to the multi-component exercise control group. Moreover, the multi-target stepping training reduced the proportion of fallers and the fall rate by 60% over one year.

Technology-Enriched Interactive Cognitive-Motor Training

Interactive cognitive-motor training (ICMT) involves exercising while interacting with a computer. Sometimes called 'serious games' or 'exergames', most ICMT systems include features such as point scoring, rankings, achievements, badges, and feedback. Also, a stepwise progression for binding the 'player' to the task is often incorporated, meaning a slight increase in difficulty that provides a challenging task, which is important for maintaining motivation. ICMT can provide enriched environments and require complex sensory, cognitive, and motor integration for undertaking a task [50], making it a suitable technology to deliver cognitive-motor interventions.

Fall-related studies using ICMT have involved a range of technologies and exercise modalities. Technologies include pressure-sensing boards, virtual reality (VR) environments, inertial sensors, instrumented stepping mats, and motion capture systems to facilitate balance, stepping, strength, and aerobic training (as outlined in Figure 18.3). For instance, balance-board programmes incorporate exergames with underfoot pressure sensors, upon which the participant undertakes feet-in-place balance exercises. Step training programmes incorporate exergames with step pads that require the participant to take well-timed steps in multiple directions for game play. On the other hand, VR walking interventions involve treadmill walking through screen-displayed environments and may include distractors. Multi-component programmes have used sport simulations, such as tennis or golf that require the player to mimic sport-specific movements and thus train specific fitness components at lower intensity compared to the real-world sporting activities. Lastly, some studies have used balance-board training for mostly aerobic exercises, such as step aerobics or walking in place.

It is important to consider the acceptability and usability of ICMT in older adults and other specific populations. Laver et al. [51] reported that in aged rehabilitation, only a small proportion of patients were able and willing to participate in therapist-led exergames. There may also be a trade-off between commercially available games developed for younger people and the few specifically developed for older users to improve fall-related outcomes. While the first

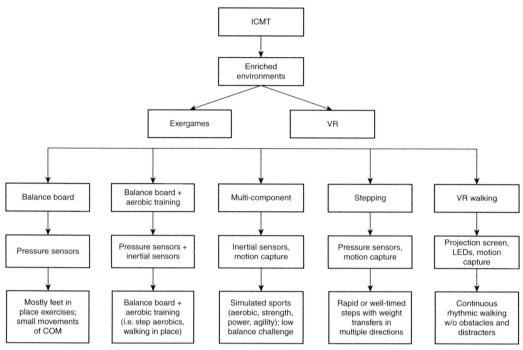

Figure 18.3   ICMT training components with respect to fall-risk interventions.

category (Nintendo Wii, Microsoft Kinect) has received considerable investment by large companies dedicated to usability and user interface, the latter often lacks these resources and may function less well. In trials by Schoene et al. [21, 52], adherence and usability were partially diminished by functionality issues that prevented older people playing the exergames unsupervised at home.

ICMT interventions, including both custom-made as well as off-the-shelf VR/exergame applications have been shown to improve balance, gait, and mobility measures, as shown in studies of within-group effects and comparisons between active and passive control groups [53, 54]. Meta-analytic evidence now shows the efficacy of exergaming for balance test batteries (e.g. Berg Balance Scale, Performance-Oriented Mobility Assessment), chair rise ability, dynamic balance (e.g. Timed-Up and Go Test), and perceived balance, with data lacking for reactive balance measures [55].

Regarding fall prevention, several trials have examined the potential benefits of ICMT. A sufficiently powered VR training intervention reported a significant fall prevention effect in a mixed cohort, i.e. people identified at high fall risk or with mild cognitive impairment or Parkinson's disease [20]. During thrice weekly 45 min sessions over six weeks, participants walked on a treadmill with (VR intervention) or without (control) a screen ahead displaying an avatar's feet walking through a virtual, life-like environment. This system enabled the VR intervention participants' feet to be projected in real-time within the VR scenes that included walking on paths, stepping over obstacles, and distractors. The VR group reported a >40% decline in falls relative to the treadmill-only control group over six months [20]. These findings suggest that enriched environments, such as VR or exergames that include a realistic and complex integration of sensory, cognitive, and motor processing, may provide a powerful tool for enabling exercise training for fall prevention. The VR training group also improved their obstacle negotiation ability, static balance, and 4-metre gait speed compared to the treadmill-only training group [20].

As for most cognitive-motor interventions, only a few ICMT studies have been undertaken in frailer or functionally impaired older adults. One VR training programme in a sample who experienced falls applied balance exercises under changing somatosensory, visual, and vestibular conditions for 12 sessions within six weeks and found improved balance, fewer falls, and reduced levels of fear of falling [13]. Similarly, Fu et al. [15] found that a three times per week, one-hour exergame (Wii Fit) balance training for six weeks, improved leg strength, body sway on a compliant surface and reaction time and reduced the incidence of falls over 12 months by 65% in frail nursing-home residents. Finally, a small study using the Microsoft Kinect and Jintronix software to administer multi-component exercise to residents of assisted living residences, found fewer falls, reduced frailty, increased physical performance scores as well as improved mobility and gait speed following up to 24 sessions within a 12-week period [18]. These encouraging findings suggest that with appropriate supervision, off-the-shelf games that have been developed for different target groups might be suitable for older adults, including those living in care facilities.

ICMT interventions have also demonstrated improvements in cognition. In a 12-week exergame study (n = 32) using the Nintendo Wii twice weekly, participants improved in tasks of executive functioning (e.g. Trail-Making Test, Stroop Test) and processing speed but not in visuo-spatial ability [56]. In an exergame stepping study delivered unsupervised at home using a step mat interfaced with the home television, individuals (n = 81) played four games targeting different cognitive functions with a recommended dose of three sessions per week over a 16-week period. Playing on average 32 sessions of 27 minutes, improvements were observed in measures of processing speed, visuo-spatial abilities, and concern about falling [21]. People with poorer baseline performance also improved in inhibition and cognitive-motor dual-tasking. Low adherers were lower-functioning individuals and tended to improve more in processing-speed-related tasks, while high adherers were already higher-functioning individuals at baseline and benefited more in executive functions, thus demonstrating adherence to exercise interventions being an important factor for further cognitive changes. The enriched environments of ICMT seem to help improving complex cognitive functions, such as gait speed under conditions of divided attention and executive functions [53]. In addition, fear of falling and balance confidence have been shown to improve after training in ICMT studies with durations of more than four weeks [53]. These findings corroborate those showing neuropsychological benefits from physical and cognitive training studies in older people without cognitive impairments [57–60] and since some of these cognitive functions are known risk factors for falls, suggest that ICMT is a promising intervention for fall prevention.

Cognitive-Motor Interventions versus Traditional Exercise

Several of the discussed studies included an active control group, comparing motor-cognitive training to traditional physical exercise, and evidence from some of the higher-quality studies suggest cognitive-motor interventions may be superior to traditional physical exercise regimens in older people. A recently published systematic review and meta-analysis of 41 studies found that physical exercise programmes combined with cognitive training components were better than exercise alone for improving cognition, and that training interventions with simultaneous designs tended to yield better effects on cognitive function that those with sequentially ordered cognitive and motor training components [61].

Regarding physical outcomes, several studies have shown beneficial effects of cognitive-motor training outcomes assessed under dual-task conditions. This is in line with the construct of task-specificity; however, transfer seems limited with no clear benefits for balance and walking outcomes [62]. When comparing traditional strength and balance training to the same exercises performed with additional cognitive load, such as calculation, visual search, and verbal fluency tasks, no differences were observed between groups after three months of training in tests of physical function performance [63], although, the intervention group performed significantly better in a cognitive task while maintaining balance [63]. In a trial of aerobic group-based exercise incorporating square stepping exercises, the group that received additional cognitive activities during square stepping showed improved gait speed, step length, and stride time variability under dual-task but not single-task conditions, demonstrating the task-specific benefit of added dual-task training [64].

The effects of cognitive-motor training on fall outcomes, compared to traditional exercise, have been shown in several studies of ICMT. When comparing ICMT interventions to motor-only interventions in older people, studies consistently demonstrated equal or improved effects (no negative findings) [54]. The previously described study comparing VR treadmill versus treadmill-only training [20] found only six weeks of training to show differences in several fall-related domains and fall rates between groups. Similarly, the study by Fu et al. [15] found a large effect on falls in nursing home residents after just a few weeks of Nintendo Wii balance board training, when compared to the Otago Exercise Programme, which has previously been shown in numerous studies to be effective in reducing falls and fall-related injuries [65].

Low-tech stepping cognitive-motor interventions have also shown beneficial effects on fall outcomes, compared to traditional exercise. A remarkable result warranting replication was the finding that two minutes of multi-target stepping added to a multi-component exercise programme achieved a large fall-reducing effect and improved several measures related to mobility [25]. Square stepping exercise has also been compared to traditional exercise programmes in two studies [22, 23]. Firstly, compared to strength and balance training (training that is often recommended for fall prevention) square stepping training led to fewer trip-related falls, perhaps highlighting the importance of task specificity in training paradigms [23]. This was despite no observed differences in performance-based tests of physical functioning. Secondly, when compared to walking (training that is often recommended for improving health), square stepping exercise showed superior outcomes on functional measures relevant to daily mobility, such as power, balance, and the ability to react quickly [22].

With relatively short intervention durations, these studies found lower fall rates and/or demonstrated significantly greater improvements for balance, gait, and other physical performance measures, and cognition compared to active control groups that received gold standard fall-preventive exercises or the same exercise as the intervention group without the cognitive component. This indicates that in older people, training in enriched environments improves transfer of acquired skills to daily life and therefore has good potential for improving gait, balance, cognition, and fall prevention. However, more research with equivalent-dose exercise programmes, including studies in clinical populations, long-term follow-up, and falls as the outcome is needed before definitive conclusions can be drawn [53, 54].

Mode of Action

The promising findings from cognitive-motor interventions suggest the two components trained together may exceed the sum of the effects of separate training. This means that cognitive-motor training is not just another mode of delivery of traditional exercise, but is in fact a distinct training modality with potentially enhanced benefits. Maintaining balance is an attention-demanding task and people with higher fall risk appear to have greater interference on balance control with cognitive load [66]. Cognitive-motor interventions improve both motor and cognitive performance as well as their inter-relationship and may reduce the level of interference (or the dual-task cost).

As it has been shown that locomotion in daily life is more closely related to dual- than single-task walking [4], cognitive-motor interventions reflect the interplay of sensory, cognitive, and motor factors in real-life better than traditional physical exercise that focus on strength and balance, but exclude aspects of cognitive processing. Situational awareness, i.e. understanding factors that contribute to optimal task performance in expected and unexpected conditions is important to facilitate protective postural responses and depends on correct coordination based on precise feedback from multiple sensory systems. For instance, non-fallers perform better in complex stepping tasks, suggesting that the quick and accurate appraisal of the individual–environment interaction is relevant [67]. Training in enriched environments can be considered a better reflection of these situational demands, which is supported by the findings of Mirelman et al. [20] showing that treadmill walking in virtual environments, including decision-making and obstacle avoidance is better than treadmill walking for balance, gait, and fall prevention.

Poor executive functioning is an independent risk factor for falls in older people [68] and preserved or improved executive functioning can compensate partially for reduced balance ability [69]. While physical exercise training is associated with increased oxygen and glucose metabolism and elevated levels of neuroprotective factors in the brain, these biochemical changes only translate to enhanced cognitive performance under cognitive-challenging conditions [70]. Anderson-Hanley et al. [71] found increased levels of brain-derived neurotrophic factor following ICMT cyber-cycling but not following normal cycling, suggesting enhanced neuroplasticity following ICMT. ICMT interventions have also been shown to induce changes in prefrontal cortical activity that is associated with executive functioning [72, 73]. Even simple exergames without explicit cognitive demands inherently require cognitive processing [50]. Applying cognitive-motor interventions that require those central processes, in addition to and in conjunction with motor execution, likely improve neural networks more so than traditional exercise training.

As adherence to conventional fall-prevention programmes is often low [74, 75], technology-based fall-prevention interventions, including ICMT, have been proposed as one possible solution to overcome issues of uptake and adherence [76]. ICMT interventions often include several features to promote uptake and adherence, such as realistic goal-setting, positive reinforcement, feedback, and the

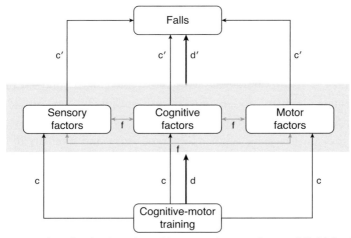

Figure 18.4   Proposed mode of action of cognitive-motor interventions on fall-risk in older people.
c: task-specific improvements in single domains due to cognitive-motor training, e.g. enhanced spatial attention following ICMT that focus on this skill; c': improvements in domain-specific functioning lead to reduced fall-risk, e.g. improved spatial attention affects daily life spatial attention, such as obstacle avoidance; d: cognitive-motor training has positive effects on the interplay between domains; d': this improved interplay transfers to real-life reduced fall risk; f: improvements in single domains also affect (partial) compensation positively and help to reduce fall risk.

ability to self-monitor performance [53]. For example, immediate feedback enables rapid adjustments to improve motor and/or cognitive performance for rapid skill development. Further, it has been suggested that through gamification in ICMT, perceived pain and exhaustion levels are lower [11]. These factors lead to increased levels of motivation and higher training doses, positively affecting efficacy. ICMT systems may also address barriers to participation by enabling home-based training, saving costs and reaching people in remote areas. However, few studies have been conducted in the home setting and issues of safety and technological usability must first be overcome. Thus, cognitive-motor interventions seem to be efficacious on both the single-domain level, e.g. by improving balance, executive functions, and reducing concerns about falling, and the multiple-domain level, e.g. improving the task-specific inter-play of different domains in situations when falls occur (see Figure 18.4).

Conclusion

Physical and cognitive factors contribute to the risk of falls in older people. While there is good evidence that physical exercise training can prevent falls in older people, evidence is only emerging for cognitive-motor training. Cognitive-motor training programmes appear to be promising strategies for improving fall-related factors and preventing falls in older people. In particular, the use of technology in ICMT, such as exergaming appears to be valuable, providing task-specific functional cognitive and physical stimuli and addressing the issue of low exercise adherence by providing an enjoyable and engaging method of training. Training programmes that simultaneously target cognitive and motor functions that involve balance control and maximize task specificity may provide enhanced value for fall prevention. However, most studies conducted to date have been small in size, and few have reported the type, dose, and intensity of balance and cognitive training. Moreover, most of the studies have been conducted in relatively well-functioning people and it remains unclear how feasible and effective cognitive-motor interventions are in people at high risk of falling. Thus, adequately powered studies are required, comparing cognitive-motor training to adequate controls to establish definitive evidence for the effects of cognitive-motor interventions for preventing falls in different populations of older people.

REFERENCES

1. Schäfer S, Huxhold O, Lindenberger U. Healthy mind in healthy body? A review of sensori-motor–cognitive interdependencies in old age. *Eur Rev Aging Phys Act*. 2006;3:45–54.
2. Amboni M, Barone P, Hausdorff JM. Cognitive contributions to gait and falls: evidence and implications. *Mov Disord*. 2013;28:1520–33.
3. Boisgontier MP, Beets IA, Duysens J et al. Age-related differences in attentional cost associated with postural dual tasks: increased recruitment of generic cognitive resources in older adults. *Neurosci Biobehav Rev*. 2013;37:1824–37.
4. Hillel I, Gazit E, Nieuwboer A et al. Is every-day walking in older adults more analogous to dual-task walking or to usual walking? Elucidating the gaps between gait performance in the lab and during 24/7 monitoring. *Eur Rev Aging Phys Act*. 2019;16:6.
5. Lundin-Olsson L, Nyberg L, Gustafson Y. "Stops walking when talking" as a predictor of falls in elderly people. *Lancet*. 1997;349:617.
6. Sherrington C, Michaleff ZA, Fairhall N et al. Exercise to prevent falls in older adults: an updated systematic review and meta-analysis. *Br J Sports Med*. 2017;51:1750–8.
7. Sanders LMJ, Hortobagyi T, la Bastide-van Gemert S et al. Dose-response relationship between exercise and cognitive function in older adults with and without cognitive impairment: a systematic review and meta-analysis. *PLos One*. 2019;14:e0210036.
8. Verghese J, Mahoney J, Ambrose AF et al. Effect of cognitive remediation on gait in sedentary seniors. *J Gerontol A Biol Sci Med Sci*. 2010;65:1338–43.
9. Pichierri G, Wolf P, Murer K et al. Cognitive and cognitive-motor interventions affecting physical functioning: a systematic review. *BMC Geriatr*. 2011;11:29.
10. Herold F, Hamacher D, Schega L et al. Thinking while moving or moving while thinking: concepts of motor-cognitive training for cognitive performance enhancement. *Front Aging Neurosci*. 2018;10:228.

11. de Bruin ED, Schoene D, Pichierri G et al. Use of virtual reality technique for the training of motor control in the elderly. Some theoretical considerations. *Z Gerontol Geriatr.* 2010;43:229–34.

12. da Silva Borges EG, de Souza Vale RG, Cader SA et al. Postural balance and falls in elderly nursing home residents enrolled in a ballroom dancing program. *Arch Gerontol Geriatr.* 2014;59:312–16.

13. Duque G, Boersma D, Loza-Diaz G et al. Effects of balance training using a virtual-reality system in older fallers. *Clin Interv Aging.* 2013;8:257–63.

14. Eggenberger P, Theill N, Holenstein S et al. Multicomponent physical exercise with simultaneous cognitive training to enhance dual-task walking of older adults: a secondary analysis of a 6-month randomized controlled trial with 1-year follow-up. *Clin Interv Aging.* 2015;10:1711–32.

15. Fu AS, Gao KL, Tung AK et al. Effectiveness of exergaming training in reducing risk and incidence of falls in frail older adults with a history of falls. *Arch Phys Med Rehabil.* 2015;96:2096–102.

16. Hars M, Herrmann FR, Fielding RA et al. Long-term exercise in older adults: 4-year outcomes of music-based multitask training. *Calcif Tissue Int.* 2014;95:393–404.

17. Kwok BC, Pua YH. Effects of WiiActive exercises on fear of falling and functional outcomes in community-dwelling older adults: a randomised control trial. *Age Ageing.* 2016;45:621–7.

18. Lauze M, Martel DD, Aubertin-Leheudre M. Feasibility and effects of a physical activity program using gerontechnology in assisted living communities for older adults. *J Am Med Dir Assoc.* 2017;18:1069–75.

19. Merom D, Mathieu E, Cerin E et al. Social dancing and incidence of falls in older adults: a cluster randomised controlled trial. *PLoS Med.* 2016;13:e1002112.

20. Mirelman A, Rochester L, Maidan I et al. Addition of a non-immersive virtual reality component to treadmill training to reduce fall risk in older adults (V-TIME): a randomised controlled trial. *Lancet.* 2016;388:1170–82.

21. Schoene D, Valenzuela T, Toson B et al. Interactive cognitive-motor step training improves cognitive risk factors of falling in older adults: a randomized controlled trial. *PLos One.* 2015;10:e0145161.

22. Shigematsu R, Okura T, Nakagaichi M et al. Square-stepping exercise and fall risk factors in older adults: a single-blind, randomized controlled trial. *J Gerontol A Biol Sci Med Sci.* 2008;63:76–82.

23. Shigematsu R, Okura T, Sakai T et al. Square-stepping exercise versus strength and balance training for fall risk factors. *Aging Clin Exp Res.* 2008;20:19–24.

24. Trombetti A, Hars M, Herrmann FR et al. Effect of music-based multitask training on gait, balance, and fall risk in elderly people: a randomized controlled trial. *Arch Phys Med Rehabil.* 2011;171:525–33.

25. Yamada M, Higuchi T, Nishiguchi S et al. Multitarget stepping program in combination with a standardized multicomponent exercise program can prevent falls in community-dwelling older adults: a randomized, controlled trial. *J Am Geriatr Soc.* 2013;61:1669–75.

26. Hars M, Herrmann FR, Fielding RA et al. Long-term exercise in older adults: 4-year outcomes of music-based multitask training. *Calcif Tissue Int.* 2014;95:393–404.

27. Hars M, Herrmann FR, Gold G et al. Effect of music-based multitask training on cognition and mood in older adults. *Age Ageing*. 2014;43:196–200.

28. Wollesen B, Voelcker-Rehage C. Training effects on motor–cognitive dual-task performance in older adults. *Eur Rev Aging Phys Act*. 2014;11:5–24.

29. Lesinski M, Hortobagyi T, Muehlbauer T et al. Effects of balance training on balance performance in healthy older adults: a systematic review and meta-analysis. *Sports Med*. 2015;45:1721–38.

30. Pellecchia GL. Dual-task training reduces impact of cognitive task on postural sway. *J Mot Behav*. 2005;37:239–46.

31. Azadian E, Torbati HR, Kakhki AR et al. The effect of dual task and executive training on pattern of gait in older adults with balance impairment: a randomized controlled trial. *Arch Gerontol Geriatr*. 2016;62:83–9.

32. Morris R, Lord S, Bunce J et al. Gait and cognition: mapping the global and discrete relationships in ageing and neurodegenerative disease. *Neurosci Biobehav Rev*. 2016;64:326–45.

33. Wongcharoen S, Sungkarat S, Munkhetvit P et al. Home-based interventions improve trained, but not novel, dual-task balance performance in older adults: a randomized controlled trial. *Gait Posture*. 2017;52:147–52.

34. Silsupadol P, Lugade V, Shumway-Cook A et al. Training-related changes in dual-task walking performance of elderly persons with balance impairment: a double-blind, randomized controlled trial. *Gait Posture*. 2009;29:634–9.

35. Falbo S, Condello G, Capranica L et al. Effects of physical-cognitive dual task training on executive function and gait performance in older adults: a randomized controlled trial. *Biomed Res Int*. 2016;2016:5812092.

36. Ghai S, Ghai I, Effenberg AO. Effects of dual tasks and dual-task training on postural stability: a systematic review and meta-analysis. *Clin Interv Aging*. 2017;12:557–77.

37. Silsupadol P, Shumway-Cook A, Lugade V et al. Effects of single-task versus dual-task training on balance performance in older adults: a double-blind, randomized controlled trial. *Arch Phys Med Rehabil*. 2009;90:381–7.

38. Fernandez-Arguelles EL, Rodriguez-Mansilla J, Antunez LE et al. Effects of dancing on the risk of falling related factors of healthy older adults: a systematic review. *Arch Gerontol Geriatr*. 2015;60:1–8.

39. Hwang PW, Braun KL. The effectiveness of dance interventions to improve older adults' health: a systematic literature review. *Altern Ther Health Med*. 2015;21:64–70.

40. Marmeleira JF, Pereira C, Cruz-Ferreira A et al. Creative dance can enhance proprioception in older adults. *J Sports Med Phys Fitness*. 2009;49:480–5.

41. Hamacher D, Hamacher D, Rehfeld K et al. The effect of a six-month dancing program on motor-cognitive dual-task performance in older adults. *J Aging Phys Act*. 2015;23:647–52.

42. Hamacher D, Hamacher D, Rehfeld K et al. Motor-cognitive dual-task training improves local dynamic stability of normal walking in older individuals. *Clin Biomech*. 2016;32:138–41.

43. Granacher U, Muehlbauer T, Bridenbaugh SA et al. Effects of a salsa dance training on balance and strength performance in older adults. *Gerontology*. 2012;58:305–12.

44. Sofianidis G, Hatzitaki V, Douka S et al. Effect of a 10-week traditional dance program on static and dynamic balance control in elderly adults. *J Aging Phys Act.* 2009;17:167–80.

45. Borges EG, Cader SA, Vale RG et al. The effect of ballroom dance on balance and functional autonomy among the isolated elderly. *Arch Gerontol Geriatr.* 2012;55:192 6.

46. Borges E, Vale RGS, Pernambuco CS et al. Effects of dance on the postural balance, cognition and functional autonomy of older adults. *Rev Bras Enferm.* 2018;71:2302–9.

47. Meng X, Li G, Jia Y et al. Effects of dance intervention on global cognition, executive function and memory of older adults: a meta-analysis and systematic review. *Aging Clin Exp Res.* 2020;32:7–19.

48. Niemann C, Godde B, Voelcker-Rehage C. Senior dance experience, cognitive performance, and brain volume in older women. *Neural Plast.* 2016;2016:9837321.

49. Chin APMJ, van Poppel MN, Twisk JW et al. Once a week not enough, twice a week not feasible? A randomised controlled exercise trial in long-term care facilities. *Patient Educ Couns.* 2006;63:205–14.

50. Anders P, Lehmann T, Muller H et al. Exergames inherently contain cognitive elements as indicated by cortical processing. *Front Behav Neurosci.* 2018;12:102.

51. Laver K, George S, Ratcliffe J et al. Use of an interactive video gaming program compared with conventional physiotherapy for hospitalised older adults: a feasibility trial. *Disabil Rehabil.* 2012;34:1802–8.

52. Schoene D, Lord SR, Delbaere K et al. A randomized controlled pilot study of home-based step training in older people using videogame technology. *PLos One.* 2013;8:e57734.

53. Schoene D, Valenzuela T, Lord SR et al. The effect of interactive cognitive-motor training in reducing fall risk in older people: a systematic review. *BMC Geriatr.* 2014;14:107.

54. Skjaeret N, Nawaz A, Morat T et al. Exercise and rehabilitation delivered through exergames in older adults: an integrative review of technologies, safety and efficacy. *Int J Med Inform.* 2016;85:1–16.

55. Fang Q, Ghanouni P, Anderson SE et al. Effects of exergaming on balance of healthy older adults: a systematic review and meta-analysis of randomized controlled trials. *Games Health J.* 2020;9:11–23.

56. Maillot P, Perrot A, Hartley A. Effects of interactive physical-activity video-game training on physical and cognitive function in older adults. *Psychol Aging.* 2012;27:589–600.

57. Tyndall AV, Clark CM, Anderson TJ et al. Protective effects of exercise on cognition and brain health in older adults. *Exerc Sport Sci Rev.* 2018;46:215–23.

58. Saez de Asteasu ML, Martinez-Velilla N, Zambom-Ferraresi F et al. Role of physical exercise on cognitive function in healthy older adults: a systematic review of randomized clinical trials. *Ageing Res Rev.* 2017;37:117–34.

59. Lampit A, Hallock H, Valenzuela M. Computerized cognitive training in cognitively healthy older adults: a systematic review and meta-analysis of effect modifiers. *PLoS Med.* 2014;11:e1001756.

60. Mowszowski L, Lampit A, Walton CC et al. Strategy-based cognitive training for improving executive functions in older adults: a systematic review. *Neuropsychol Rev.* 2016;26:252–70.

61. Gheysen F, Poppe L, DeSmet A et al. Physical activity to improve cognition in older adults: can physical activity programs enriched with cognitive challenges enhance the effects? A systematic review and meta-analysis. *Int J Behav Nutr Phys Act.* 2018;15:63.

62. Konak HE, Kibar S, Ergin ES. The effect of single-task and dual-task balance exercise programs on balance performance in adults with osteoporosis: a randomized controlled preliminary trial. *Osteoporos Int.* 2016;27:3271–8.

63. Hiyamizu M, Morioka S, Shomoto K et al. Effects of dual task balance training on dual task performance in elderly people: a randomized controlled trial. *Clin Rehabil.* 2012;26:58–67.

64. Gregory MA, Gill DP, Zou G et al. Group-based exercise combined with dual-task training improves gait but not vascular health in active older adults without dementia. *Arch Gerontol Geriatr.* 2016;63:18–27.

65. Thomas S, Mackintosh S, Halbert J. Does the 'Otago exercise programme' reduce mortality and falls in older adults? A systematic review and meta-analysis. *Age Ageing.* 2010;39:681–7.

66. Lacour M, Bernard-Demanze L, Dumitrescu M. Posture control, aging, and attention resources: models and posture-analysis methods. *Neurophysiol Clin.* 2008;38:411–21.

67. Schoene D, Delbaere K, Lord SR. Impaired response selection during stepping predicts falls in older people-a cohort study. *J Am Med Dir Assoc.* 2017;18:719–25.

68. Mirelman A, Herman T, Brozgol M et al. Executive function and falls in older adults: new findings from a five-year prospective study link fall risk to cognition. *PLos One.* 2012;7: e40297.

69. Pieruccini-Faria F, Lord SR, Toson B et al. Mental flexibility influences the association between poor balance and falls in older people: a secondary analysis. *Front Aging Neurosci.* 2019;11:133.

70. Lauenroth A, Ioannidis AE, Teichmann B. Influence of combined physical and cognitive training on cognition: a systematic review. *BMC Geriatr.* 2016;16:141.

71. Anderson-Hanley C, Arciero PJ, Brickman AM et al. Exergaming and older adult cognition: a cluster randomized clinical trial. *Am J Prev Med.* 2012;42:109–19.

72. Eggenberger P, Wolf M, Schumann M et al. Exergame and balance training modulate prefrontal brain activity during walking and enhance executive function in older adults. *Front Aging Neurosci.* 2016;8.

73. Schättin A, Arner R, Gennaro F et al. Adaptations of prefrontal brain activity, executive functions, and gait in healthy elderly following exergame and balance training: a randomized-controlled study. *Front Aging Neurosci.* 2016;8:278.

74. Nyman SR, Victor CR. Older people's recruitment, sustained participation, and adherence to falls prevention interventions in institutional settings: a supplement to the Cochrane systematic review. *Age Ageing.* 2011;40:430–6.

75. Nyman SR, Victor CR. Older people's participation in and engagement with falls prevention interventions in community settings: an augment to the Cochrane systematic review. *Age Ageing.* 2012;41:16–23.

76. Valenzuela T, Okubo Y, Woodbury A et al. Adherence to technology-based exercise programs in older adults: a systematic review. *J Geriatr Phys Ther.* 2018;41:49–61.

19

Cognitive Behavioural Interventions for Addressing Fear of Falling and Fall Risk

G.A. Rixt Zijlstra and Kim Delbaere

Fear of falling refers to ongoing concerns about falls which can compromise an individual's quality of life. 'Fear of falling' is often used as an umbrella term to include both cognitive constructs, like balance confidence and fall-related self-efficacy, and affect-based constructs, like concern or worry about falling [1]. Fear of falling can be an adaptive and justified response for people who are frail, preventing them from taking part in risky activities [2]. However, approximately one-third of community-dwelling older people experience high levels of fear of falling, which has been associated with restriction in physical and social activities with consequent negative impacts on quality of life [3]. Fear of falling is multi-dimensional in nature. Physical (poor balance and muscle weakness), psychological (unrealistic appraisals of one's ability to avoid falls), and behavioural factors (reduced outdoor and social activities) can interact and contribute to a vicious cycle of fear of falling and activity avoidance [2].

Cognitive behavioural interventions have been used to address both fear of falling and falls themselves [4, 5]. Cognitive behavioural interventions aim to identify, evaluate, and change maladaptive beliefs regarding fear of falling and the risk of falling, as well as related avoidance behaviour [4, 6]. These interventions often consist of multiple components, combining cognitive restructuring and goal setting with physical exercises and/or activities exposing the older person to situations in which fear of falling is experienced. The 'A Matter of Balance' programme is the most studied and implemented cognitive behavioural intervention for community-dwelling older people in this area and applies a range of principles derived from cognitive behavioural therapy [7] (see Table 19.1). The programme is designed to: (i) challenge misconceptions about falls to promote the view that fall risk and fear of falling are controllable, (ii) set realistic goals to increase activity level, (iii) create a risk-free home environment, and (iv) promote physical exercises aimed at increasing strength and balance.

Table 19.1 Cognitive behavioural therapy principles, relevant to fear of falling in older people and applied within the "A Matter of Balance" programme

Principle	Example
Phenomenology	The older person's experiences with fear of falling
Collaboration	With the facilitator or group participants to share knowledge, empathy and resources
Activity	Practical skills training like physical exercises, getting up from the floor after a fall, assessing a home environment
Empiricism	Education based on empirical data that falls can be prevented
Generalization	During and after the programme, logging situations that invoke fear, applying cognitive restructuring techniques in these situations and evaluating the results, and identifying problems and applying problem-solving to a variety of situations
Use of behavioural assessment	Regarding safe and unsafe behaviour, the home environment
Individualization of treatment strategies and treatment aimed at specific behaviours or components of behaviours	Action planners and goal setting are used to specify one's behavioural goals in order to prevent falls and to match activities to a person's situation, including one's physical abilities

Effect of Cognitive Behavioural Interventions on Fear of Falling

Original and Adapted 'A Matter of Balance' Interventions

The original version of A Matter of Balance (AMB) consisted of eight two-hour group sessions over four weeks and was led by trained, professional facilitators [6]. The programme focused on instilling adaptive beliefs on falls, strength exercises, fall risk and safety, problem solving, and action planning. In a randomized controlled trial with older people reporting activity restriction due to fear of falling, AMB showed an immediate effect on increasing the level of intended activities and mobility control compared to a control group receiving a single two-hour group session on falls [6]. In post-hoc analysis, in the sub-group who were more compliant with the interventions, benefits were also seen in falls efficacy (confidence in performing activities without falling), directly following the programme and at 12 months.

Following this original trial, the programme has been adapted. While still focusing on instilling adaptive beliefs on falls, strength exercises, fall risk and safety, problem solving, and action planning, the programme is delivered over eight weekly sessions by registered nurses and includes a booster session after six months [4]. It utilizes a variety of techniques and materials such as lectures, videos, group discussions, problem-solving sessions, and assertiveness training. This adapted programme was evaluated in a randomized controlled trial in the Netherlands with community-dwelling older people who reported some concerns about falling and some activity avoidance due to these concerns [4]. Compared to the usual-care control group, the intervention group showed significant short-term and long-term reductions in concerns about falling. To further facilitate participation and retention, a home-based version of AMB was developed for frail older people [8]. The same content (i.e. instilling realistic view of fall risk, restructuring misconceptions about falls and fall risk, setting realistic goals for increasing physical activity and safe behaviour) was delivered via seven one-on-one sessions with therapists, i.e. three home visits and four telephone contacts, to encourage independence [8]. The primary findings from a randomized controlled trial indicated the programme significantly reduced fear of falling at 5 and 12 months follow up time-points [8].

'A Matter of Balance' as Part of a Combined Intervention Programme with Exercise

The effect of AMB has also been evaluated in combination with exercise, showing similar positive effects on fear of falling in older people. These include studies by Huang et al. and Liu et al., who both combined AMB programmes with exercise training [5, 9–11]. Huang et al. [9] developed a fear of falling management model, which focuses on restructuring misconceptions to promote a view of fall, risk and fear of falling as controllable, strategies to manage fear of falling and family support during daily life activities, and problem-solving (during a fall learning how to fall, stand up, and call for help). Huang et al. [5, 9] combined their AMB programme with either Tai Chi or strength and endurance training in two separate randomized controlled trials, showing positive effects on fear of falling in both. Liu et al. [11] compared a combined AMB–Tai Chi programme with Tai Chi alone and found no difference in fear of falling. In a second trial, Liu et al. [10] combined AMB[1] with Task-Oriented Balance Training (TOBT), i.e. five progressive exercises for strength and balance. They found that this combined programme had a positive effect on balance confidence compared with a combined health education–TOBT programme [10].

---

[1] Omitting the cognitive and behavioural factors known to generate and aggravate impaired subjective balance confidence and fear-avoidance behaviour component.

Other Cognitive Behavioural Interventions

In a randomized controlled trial involving 230 older people living in senior centres, Reinsch et al. [12] compared three programmes, i.e. strength and balance group exercises, a cognitive behavioural programme for falls and injuries, and a combination of both, with group discussions. The cognitive behavioural programme addressed health and safety, relaxation, and reaction time. At the completion of the 12-month trial, none of the interventions showed effects on fear of falling. Parry et al. [13] took a slightly different approach by examining factors that predisposed the patient to the problem, triggered the current problem and factors that might be perpetuating the problem in terms of cognitive, behavioural, emotional, physical, and social factors. In a randomized controlled trial involving 415 community-dwelling older people with excessive concern about falls, this cognitive behavioural programme had a positive effect on fear of falling after 12 months. More recently, Wetherell et al. [14, 15] investigated the effect of an at-home CBT programme combined with exercise to target fear of falling in older people with high levels of fear of falling. Their Activity, Balance, Learning, and Exposure (ABLE) programme employed physical therapists to conduct an eight-session at-home intervention which included a fall prevention exercise programme, home safety evaluation, and exposure-based CBT (psycho-education, creation of a fear hierarchy, exposure practice, cognitive restructuring, and problem solving). Participants in the intervention group showed a significant decrease in fear of falling directly after the intervention. However, contrary to some other cognitive behavioural interventions, there were no significant long-term benefits at the three-month and six-month follow-up time-points [15].

Table 19.2 displays an overview of the characteristics of cognitive behavioural interventions and their effect on fear of falling in older people. Overall, the evidence suggests that a two-month CBT programme can reduce fear of falling. Booster CBT sessions at six months and CBT programmes in combination with exercise programmes appear to provide additional long-term benefits.

Effect of Cognitive Behavioural Interventions on Falls and Other Outcomes

In addition to its positive effect on fear of falling, cognitive behavioural therapy is an effective treatment for depression and generalized anxiety in older people [16, 17], with evidence indicating it can also reduce falls in people with fear of falling. For decision-making regarding the implementation of evidence-based interventions for fear of falling, it is important to also consider other outcomes, including falls, feasibility, and costs.

Table 19.2 Characteristics and outcomes of randomized controlled trials evaluating the effect of cognitive behavioural interventions on fear of falling in older people[a]

Study, sample size and primary aim	Study sample description	Intervention [dose]	Follow-up	Outcomes on FoF[b]	Outcomes on falls
Original and adapted 'A Matter of Balance' interventions					
Dorresteijn, 2016, [8] Netherlands, n = 389 *Concerns about falling*	• Community-living • ≥70 years • Fair/poor health, concerns about falling	IG: home-based AMB [dose: three home visits of 1 h, four telephone contacts of 35 min] CG: usual care (no programme)	5 months 12 months	+ +	+
Tennstedt, 1998 [6], United States, n = 432 *Fear of falling and related activity restriction*	• Living in senior housing sites • ≥60 years • Concerns about falling and activity restriction	IG: CBT group programme, AMB [dose: four weeks, twice weekly sessions, two h] CG: community-based, one attention-control session, two h	1.5 months 6 months 12 months	+ + +	–
Zijlstra, 2009 [4], The Netherlands, n=540 *Concerns about falling and activity avoidance*	• Community-living • ≥70 years • Concerns about falling and activity avoidance	IG: adapted AMB [dose: eight weekly sessions, 2 h, and one booster session after six months] CG: usual care (no programme)	2 months 8 months 14 months	+ + +	+
'A Matter of Balance' as part of a combined intervention programme with exercise					
Huang, 2011 [9], Taiwan, n = 186 *Fear of falling and falls*	• Community-living • ≥60 years	IG1: adapted AMB, including Huang FoF management model [dose: eight weekly sessions of 1–1.5 h] and Tai Chi group programme [dose: eight weeks, five sessions/wk, 1 h] IG2: adapted AMB [dose: eight weekly sessions of 1–1.5 h] CG: usual care (no programme)	2 months 5 months	IG1-CG: + IG1-CG: + IG1-IG2: +	–
Huang, 2016 [5],	• Nursing home residents		2 months	IG1-CG: +	+

Table 19.2 (cont.)

'A Matter of Balance' as part of a combined intervention programme with exercise

Study, n, outcome	Inclusion criteria	Interventions	Follow-up	Result	
Taiwan, n = 80 *Fear of falling and falls*	• ≥65 years • MMSE >13	IG1: adapted AMB, including Huang FoF management model, [dose: eight weekly sessions of 20–25 min], and supervised group exercise programme for strength and endurance [dose: eight twice weekly sessions, 30 min] IG2: adapted AMB [dose: eight weekly sessions of 20–25 min] CG: usual care (no programme)	5 months	IG1-IG2: + IG1-CG: +	na
Liu, 2014 [11], Hong Kong, n = 122 *Concerns about falling*	• Living in community centres • ≥1 fall in the last year, concerns about falling	IG: adapted AMB [dose: eight weekly sessions of 1–1.5 h], and a Tai Chi group programme [dose: eight weekly sessions of 1 h] CG: Tai Chi group programme [dose: eight weekly sessions of 1 h]	2 months 4 months	– –	na
Liu, 2018 [10], Hong Kong, n = 89 *Concerns about falling*	• 1–6 years post-stroke • 55–85 years • Cognitively intact, low balance confidence	IG: adapted AMB as small-group programme and TOBT (task-oriented balance training) [dose: eight twice weekly sessions, 45 min AMB and 45 min TOBT] CG: general health education (GHE) as small-group programme and TOBT programme [dose: eight twice weekly sessions, 45 min GHE and 45 min TOBT]	2 months 5 months 14 months	+ + +	

Other cognitive behavioural interventions

Study	Population	Intervention / Control	Follow-up	Outcome
Parry, 2016 [13], United Kingdom, n = 415 *Concerns about falling*	• Community-living • ≥60 years • Excessive concerns about falling	IG: CBT programme, home- or community-based [dose: eight weekly sessions, 45 minutes, and one booster session after six months] CG: usual care	12 months	−
Reinsch, 1992 [12], United States, n = 230 *Falls and fear of falling*	• Living in senior centres • >60 years	IG1: group exercises for strength and balance [dose: one year, three weekly sessions, 1 h] IG2: CBT group programme [dose: one year, weekly sessions, 1 h] IG3: combination of IG1 and IG2 [dose: one year, weekly CBT of 1 h and twice-weekly exercise sessions of 1 h] CG: group discussions, topics not fall related [dose: one year, weekly sessions, 1 h]	12 months	−
Wetherell, 2018 [15], United States, n = 42 *Time to first fall*	• Community-living • ≥65 years • High concerns about falling	IG: home-based, Activity, Balance, Learning and Exposure programme (ABLE) [dose: eight weekly sessions, 1 h] CG: home-based, fall prevention education, eight weekly sessions, 1 h	2 months 3 months 6 months	+ −

Effect on Falls

The outcomes of studies that evaluated AMB or adapted versions indicate that cognitive behavioural interventions can reduce falls [5, 8] or recurrent falls [4], and increase older people's fall management [6]. The studies by Huang et al. [5] and Zijlstra et al. [4] included exercise, i.e. strength and endurance training, and basic exercise training, respectively, and provided evidence that using cognitive behavioural therapy with exercise is successful in reducing fear of falling and fall risk. Other cognitive behavioural interventions have not prevented falls [12–14], raising the question that cognitive behavioural therapy alone might not be sufficient to reduce falls in people with fear of falling. However, the addition of cognitive behavioural therapy principles to multi-factorial fall prevention interventions, especially in combination with exercise programmes, may be more effective in reducing fall risk in people with fear of falling compared to exercise alone. Future research should evaluate different combinations of interventional components addressing the multi-dimensional nature of fear of falling in older people, over a period of 12 months or longer.

Effect on Fall Risk Factors

Evaluations of adapted AMB interventions and trials have reported improvements in mental health through decreased symptoms of depression [13], reduced activity avoidance [14], and improved psychological and social outcomes relating to mastery, general self-efficacy, physical self-efficacy, perceived control over falling, social support satisfaction and interactions, and community integration [4–6, 8–10]. AMB also showed improved physical and behavioural outcomes, relating to daily activity, mobility, gait, balance, and disability in some studies [4–6, 8–10], but not others [13, 14]. Cognitive behavioural interventions have shown consistent improvement in mental-health-related risk factors of falling in older people. This confirms its value as a fall prevention strategy in older people with fear of falling, and co-morbid symptoms of depression.

Cost-Effectiveness

The studies by Zijlstra et al. [4] and Dorresteijn et al. [8] included extensive process and cost evaluations and these indicated the cognitive behavioural interventions are feasible and likely more cost-effective than usual care [18–21]; the interventions by Parry et al. and Wetherell et al. were not considered cost-effective [13, 14]. However, it should be noted that in both AMB trials, drop-out from the intervention was substantial, suggesting adherence to parts of the intervention could be improved, particularly in relation to the uptake of home work and the performance of a feared activity under supervision of a facilitator. In an implementation study, it was found that the inclusion of a personal intake interview instead of a written intake procedure [4, 22], and more attention to the homework reduced the drop-out rate from 42% (observed in the RCT) to 7% [18] and increased adherence to homework from 75% (in the RCT) to 82% [18].

Conclusions

Several reviews and meta-analyses suggest that fear of falling, multi-dimensional in nature, can be reduced through multi-factorial interventions including exercise (balance and strength exercises, or Tai Chi) and principles of cognitive behavioural therapy [23, 24]. Fear of falling has been linked to a reduction in overall activity levels which can result in physical decline and in turn increase the risk of falls. In the context of fear of falling research, exercise is a healthy way of exposing people to situations inside and outside their home that may lead to enhanced feelings of confidence while improving physical health, and in consequence reduced fall risk. However, the effects of exercise interventions are mostly apparent immediately post-intervention with limited long-term effects [25]. The addition of cognitive behavioural therapy principles to multi-factorial fall prevention interventions, especially in combination with exercise programmes, may be more effective in reducing fall risk in people with fear of falling compared to exercise alone. More research is required to understand impacts on falls and which specific components of interventions are associated with longer-term effects and whether adding specific components leads to increased effect sizes [26].

REFERENCES

1. Zijlstra GA, Van Haastregt JCM, Van Rossum E et al. Interventions to reduce fear of falling in community-living older people: a systematic review. *J Am Geriatr Soc.* 2007;55:603–15.
2. Delbaere K, Close JC, Brodaty H et al. Determinants of disparities between perceived and physiological risk of falling among elderly people: cohort study. *Br Med J.* 2010;341:c4165.
3. Delbaere K, Crombez G, Vanderstraeten G et al. Fear-related avoidance of activities, falls and physical frailty: a prospective community-based cohort study. *Age Ageing.* 2004;33:368–73.
4. Zijlstra GA, Van Haastregt JCM, Ambergen T et al. Effects of a multicomponent cognitive behavioral group intervention on fear of falling and activity avoidance in community-dwelling older adults: results of a randomized controlled trial. *J Am Geriatr Soc.* 2009;57:2020–8.
5. Huang TT, Chung ML, Chen FR et al. Evaluation of a combined cognitive-behavioural and exercise intervention to manage fear of falling among elderly residents in nursing homes. *Aging Ment Health.* 2016;20:2–12.

6. Tennstedt S, Howland J, Lachman M et al. A randomized, controlled trial of a group intervention to reduce fear of falling and associated activity restriction in older adults. *J Gerontol B Psychol Sci Soc Sci*. 1998;53B:P384–92.

7. Peterson EW. Using cognitive behavioral strategies to reduce fear of falling: a matter of balance. *Generations*. 2003;26:53–9.

8. Dorresteijn TAC, Zijlstra GAR, Ambergen AW et al. Effectiveness of a home-based cognitive behavioral program to manage concerns about falls in community-dwelling, frail older people: results of a randomized controlled trial. *BMC Geriatr*. 2016;16:2.

9. Huang T-T, Yang L-H, Liu C-Y. Reducing the fear of falling among community-dwelling elderly adults through cognitive-behavioural strategies and intense Tai Chi exercise: a randomized controlled trial. *J Adv Nurs*. 2011;67:961–71.

10. Liu TW, Ng GYF, Chung RCK et al. Decreasing fear of falling in chronic stroke survivors through cognitive behavior therapy and task-oriented training. *Stroke*. 2018: Strokeaha118022406.

11. Liu YW, Tsui CM. A randomized trial comparing Tai Chi with and without cognitive-behavioral intervention (CBI) to reduce fear of falling in community-dwelling elderly people. *Arch Gerontol Geriatr*. 2014;59:317–25.

12. Reinsch S, MacRae P, Lachenbruch PA et al. Attempts to prevent falls and injury: a prospective community study. *Gerontologist*. 1992;32:450–6.

13. Parry SW, Bamford C, Deary V et al. Cognitive-behavioural therapy-based intervention to reduce fear of falling in older people: therapy development and randomised controlled trial. The Strategies for Increasing Independence, Confidence and Energy (STRIDE) study. *Health Technol Assess*. 2016;20:1–206.

14. Wetherell JL, Johnson K, Chang D et al. Activity, balance, learning, and exposure (ABLE): a new intervention for fear of falling. *Int J Geriatr Psychiatry*. 2016;31:791–8.

15. Wetherell JL, Bower ES, Johnson K et al. Integrated exposure therapy and exercise reduces fear of falling and avoidance in older adults: a randomized pilot study. *Am J Geriatr Psychiatry*. 2018;26:849–59.

16. Proudfoot J, Clarke J, Birch MR et al. Impact of a mobile phone and web program on symptom and functional outcomes for people with mild-to-moderate depression, anxiety and stress: a randomised controlled trial. *BMC Psychiatry*. 2013;13:312.

17. Cockayne NL, Glozier N, Naismith SL et al. Internet-based treatment for older adults with depression and co-morbid cardiovascular disease: protocol for a randomised, double-blind, placebo controlled trial. *BMC Psychiatry*. 2011;11.

18. van Haastregt JC, Zijlstra GA, van Rossum E et al. Feasibility of a cognitive behavioural group intervention to reduce fear of falling and associated avoidance of activity in community-living older people: a process evaluation. *BMC Health Serv Res*. 2007;7:156.

19. Evers S, Dorresteijn TAC, Wijnen BFM et al. Economic evaluation of a home-based programme to reduce concerns about falls in frail, independently-living older people. *Expert Rev Pharmacoecon Outcomes Res*. 2020:20;641–51.

20. Dorresteijn TA, Rixt Zijlstra GA, Van Haastregt JC et al. Feasibility of a nurse-led in-home cognitive behavioral program to manage concerns about falls in frail older people: a process evaluation. *Res Nurs Health*. 2013;36:257–70.

21. van Haastregt JC, Zijlstra GA, Hendriks MR et al. Cost-effectiveness of an intervention to reduce fear of falling. *Int J Technol Assess Health Care*. 2013;29:219–26.

22. Zijlstra GA, van Haastregt JC, van Eijk JT et al. Mediating effects of psychosocial factors on concerns about falling and daily activity in a multicomponent cognitive behavioral group intervention. *Aging Ment Health*. 2011;15:68–77.

23. Rand D, Miller WC, Yiu J et al. Interventions for addressing low balance confidence in older adults: a systematic review and meta-analysis. *Age Ageing*. 2011;40:297–306.

24. Whipple MO, Hamel AV, Talley KMC. Fear of falling among community-dwelling older adults: a scoping review to identify effective evidence-based interventions. *Geriatr Nurs*. 2018;39:170–7.

25. Kendrick D, Kumar A, Carpenter H et al. Exercise for reducing fear of falling in older people living in the community. *Cochrane Database Syst Rev*. 2014:Cd009848.

26. Vestjens L, Kempen GI, Crutzen R et al. Promising behavior change techniques in a multicomponent intervention to reduce concerns about falls in old age: a Delphi study. *Health Educ Res*. 2015;30:309–22.

20

The Medical Management of Older People at Risk of Falls

Mark D. Latt and Vasi Naganathan

The vast majority (75%) of falls among community-dwelling older persons are not reported to a health care professional [1]. When falls are reported, 68% are to general practitioners (GPs) and 16% to emergency department clinicians. Older people may present with falls, risk factors for falling, or complications of a fall. Risk factors for falls include a history of a fall [2], dementia [3], stroke [4] and Parkinson's disease [5], and use of fall-risk-increasing drugs (FRIDs) [6–12]. Complications of falls may present as fractures, soft tissue injury, fear of falling and loss of independence [13, 14].

Medical practitioners are responsible for assessing conditions that predispose to falls, recommending appropriate treatment and co-ordinating multi-disciplinary healthcare. Multi-factorial strategies that include assessment and appropriate intervention have been shown in meta-analyses to reduce the rate of falls significantly and may also reduce fall-related injury [15, 16].

Identification of At-Risk Populations

Although 22% of persons aged ≥65 years fall in any given year, only 31% of female and 24% of male fallers will mention the fall to a health care professional [17]. As a fall in the preceding year is a highly significant predictor of falling in the subsequent year [2], clinical practice guidelines recommend that all persons aged ≥65 years be asked about falls, fall-related injuries, and mobility difficulties at least annually [18], and ideally whenever they present to a health care professional [19].

Older persons living in institutional care or presenting to the Emergency Department are high fall-risk populations [20, 21]. Diseases which are significant predictors of falls include dementia [3], stroke [4], and Parkinson's disease [5]. A significantly increased risk of falling is associated with several classes of medication (FRIDs), including antipsychotic, sedative, anxiolytic, antidepressant [6, 8, 11], and antihypertensive drugs [7, 9, 12], and with medication regimes involving four or more drugs of any type per day [22] (see Table 12.1).

A proactive approach to documenting falls and identifying risk of falling is important, as primary prevention strategies, such as interventions to improve exercise, mobility, and nutrition, reduce medication side effects and modify environmental hazards in the home and may reduce the incidence of falls [23–25].

Clinical Assessment of the Older Faller

Most falls occur from an interaction between environmental, behavioural, and physiological factors, when the location and type of activity exceeds the individual's postural stability. Many diseases prevalent among older persons can contribute to falls (see Chapter 6). Unlike older definitions of a fall [26], current definitions do not exclude incidents resulting from seizure, syncope, stroke, or external perturbations [27, 28].

Information should be obtained regarding the environment, activity, and symptoms associated with the fall. It is also important to determine cognitive performance at an early stage in the consultation and obtain collateral information from witnesses, carers, and health care practitioners, as there is a significant association between falling and many conditions that cause transient self-limited loss of consciousness (TLOC) [29, 30] or memory impairment [3].

Questions to ask older people include:

(i)   Did you lose consciousness or is it difficult to remember how you fell?
Impaired recall may be due to TLOC, delirium, or dementia. TLOC may result from syncope and non-syncopal conditions, such as stroke, seizure, intoxication, or hypoglycaemia. Many individuals will be unaware that they lost consciousness prior to the fall. Up to 42% of older people who experience TLOC due to vasovagal (neurocardiogenic) syncope, for example, will be unaware that they lost consciousness [31].

(ii)   Where did you fall?
Environmental hazards include slippery or uneven flooring, stairs, obstacles, and sub-optimal lighting [32]. Individuals who fall in their homes are more likely to be frail, while those who fall outdoors may be more physically active and independent [33, 34].

(iii)   What were you doing just before the fall?
Intoxication or medication ingestion may be complicated by hypotension, drowsiness, disequilibrium, or hypoglycaemia. After meals, falls may occur due to post-prandial hypotension [35]. Falls at night may occur in the setting of nocturia [36] or sedative use. Alcohol consumption appears to be associated with falls when it is greater than four standard drinks for men and three standard drinks for women per day [37].

Rising from lying or seated positions may result in postural hypotension and syncope. Syncope may be situational, resulting from coughing, urinating, defaecating, pain or intense emotion, suggesting neurocardiogenic or vasovagal disorders [38]. Turning, bending, or reaching may exacerbate vestibular deficits and cause dizziness or disequilibrium [39]. Individuals who fall during routine daily activities, such as rising from a bed or walking to the toilet, after minimal exertion may be more frail than those engaging in outdoor activities [34].

Risk-taking behaviour is associated with falls, independent of physical ability, indicating some older persons who fall may be unaware of their reduced physical ability and may fail to adjust their activities accordingly [40].

(iv) Did you have lightheadedness, dizziness, palpitations or weakness?
Lightheadedness may indicate conditions causing hypotension (postural hypotension, dehydration, antihypertensive medication use, or structural heart disease). Palpitations can occur in the setting of cardiac arrhythmias, while weakness of sudden onset may suggest a stroke.

(v) Were you able to pick yourself up after the fall?
Inability to rise after a fall may indicate of frailty, injury, loss of alertness, weakness, or impaired balance. It may also suggest a need for harm minimization strategies such as personal alarms and increased levels of supervision and assistance [41].

(vi) What injuries did you have?
Low-trauma fractures necessitate treatment of osteoporosis. Falls resulting in major injuries, such as hip, facial, or skull fractures, or intracranial haemorrhage, may be more likely to occur in frail older individuals [42]. Facial and intra-cranial injury may also suggest an inability to break the fall, possibly due to TLOC, impaired postural reflexes or bradykinesia [43].

(vii) Have you been diagnosed with any of the following diseases?
An increased background risk of falling can occur in the setting of a history of a fall [2], dementia [3], stroke [4], Parkinson's disease [5], syncope [38], cardiac arrhythmia, ventricular or valvular heart disease [44], orthostatic hypotension [45], musculoskeletal gait disorders [46], impaired vision [47], and vestibular disease [38].

(viii) What medications do you take (including non-prescribed, over-the-counter and herbal ones)?
Drugs commonly associated with an increased risk of falling (FRIDs) include sedatives, antidepressants, antipsychotics [6, 11] (see Chapter 11), and antihypertensives [7–9, 12]. Polypharmacy (four or more

regularly prescribed medications) has been consistently associated with falls [48, 49].

(ix)   How much do you move around during the day? What do you do? How much help do you need? What do you eat each day?

Reduced physical activity in older people increases the number of falls per hour or distance mobilized, probably due to muscle weakness [50]. Frail older people, with malnutrition, sarcopenia, and reduced independence, [51] are also more likely to fall.

Examination

Table 20.1 highlights the more common and important examination findings that may provide insight into the cause of an individual's fall.

The examination should include an assessment of level of alertness, attention and concentration, and signs of delirium. An increased risk of falling has been significantly associated with worse performance in tests of executive function, such as the Trails B Test [52] or Frontal Assessment Battery [5], and Mini Mental State Exam [53]. Postural blood pressure and pulse measurements may reveal hypotension, orthostatic hypotension, arrhythmia, and autonomic instability. Cardiovascular examinations may detect signs of valvular heart disease and heart failure.

Assessment of Mobility, Gait, and Postural Stability

Mobility examinations attempt to determine the contributions of neurological and musculoskeletal conditions to the risk of falling. A gait examination may demonstrate reduced armswing, shuffling, or small steps (reflecting extrapyramidal disorders such as Parkinson's disease), Trendelenburg gait (osteoarthritis), leg scissoring or circumduction (upper motor neurone leg weakness), antalgic gait (pain in the lower limbs), waddling gait (proximal weakness), high stepping gait (peroneal nerve palsy), or ataxia (cerebellar disease). Tremor, bradykinesia (reduced amplitude or speed of movements) suggest an extrapyramidal disorder. Neurological examinations include tests of central and peripheral nerves (tone, power, reflexes, sensation, and coordination), vestibular and cerebellar pathways (dysmetria, dysdiadochokinesis, nystagmus, and diplopia), and vision (visual fields and acuity). Bedside tests of postural stability include the Modified Romberg, Unterberger-Fukuda stepping, Head Impulse (vestibular disease) and Hallpike Tests (positional vertigo). Deformity, reduced range of motion and stability in the knees, hips and spine may be seen in arthritis.

The Timed Up and Go Test (TUGT) has been recommended as a simple screening tool to identify people warranting more detailed assessment of gait and balance [54]. It involves measuring the time taken for a person to rise from a chair, walk three metres at normal pace and with usual assistive devices, turn, return to the

Table 20.1 Suggestions for management of medical risk factors in general practice

Risk factor	GP management	Referral/liaison
Impaired vision (inc. refractive errors, macular degeneration, cataracts, glaucoma, and retinopathies)	Simple visual acuity test (preferably low contrast) and fundoscopy	Optician/optometrist, ophthalmologist, occupational therapist
Orthostatic hypotension Supine blood pressure measured after minimum of five minutes lying down and then postural pressures checked at one, three and five minutes after standing	Review any potential culprit medications, hydration status and consider possibility of autonomic problem. Increase fluid intake, offer compression hosiery, stop culprit medications	If symptoms fail to settle – consider referral to geriatrician or cardiologist
Foot disorders (inc. corns and calluses, bunions, nail problems, ulceration)	Scalpel reduction of calluses, orthotic devices/insoles, footwear and home footcare advice and education	Podiatrist, orthopaedic surgeon, orthotist, boot-maker
Musculoskeletal disorders (inc. osteoarthritis, rheumatoid arthritis, acute soft-tissue injuries)	Appropriate diagnostic evaluation, appropriate medications, mobility aids (frames, walking sticks), education and advice on exercise and weight loss if appropriate	Physiotherapist, orthopaedic surgeon, prosthetist, orthotist, rheumatologist, occupational therapist
Peripheral neuropathy	Check for evidence of B12 deficiency, diabetes, alcohol misuse, or other causes of a peripheral neuropathy	If cause uncertain – refer to neurologist. If diabetic, ensure regular diabetic foot review, including podiatry
Use of medications	Avoid all centrally acting medications where possible. Withdrawal of benzodiazepines if possible. Review need for all medications and prescribe lowest effective dose	Geriatrician or pharmacist
Vestibular dysfunction Consider Meniere's disease, benign paroxysmal positional vertigo	Avoidance of drugs with vestibular effects. Undertake Epley manoeuvre.	Consider referral to ENT surgeon, neurologist or vestibular rehabilitation program
Neurological disorders (inc. stroke, cerebellar disorders, Parkinson's disease)	Appropriate diagnostic evaluation, disease modifying medications	Geriatrician, neurologist, physiotherapist, occupational therapist
Psychological factors (inc. dementia, depression, anxiety)	Exclude acute delirium. Detect reversible causes of dementia or depression	Geriatrician, psychiatrist, neurologist, psychologist
Incontinence	Determine nature of incontinence and review any medications precipitating incontinence	Refer for formal urodynamics and further assessment/ intervention
Unexplained falls, dizziness and syncope	12-lead ECG	Refer for further specialist evaluation, geriatrician, cardiologist, neurologist

chair and sit down. However, a systematic review involving 25 studies found the predictive value of the TUGT for falls in community-dwelling older adults was limited and no cut-point for impaired performance could be recommended [55]. Quick, multi-factorial fall risk screens should be considered to provide additional information for identifying older people at risk of falls.

QuickScreen

QuickScreen is a brief risk assessment suitable for use in primary care. It is based on the sensorimotor functional model for falls prediction. The multi-factorial aetiology of falls lends itself well to a sensorimotor model as it allows the clinician not only to predict which older patients are likely to fall, but also to determine which sensori-motor systems are impaired. This gives greater insight into the causes of instability and falls and provides guidance for the tailoring of appropriate intervention strategies. The fall risk assessment requires minimal equipment: a low-contrast eye chart, an aesthesiometer filament for measuring touch sensation, and a small step. The assessment takes less than 10 minutes to complete and includes information which can be given to the patient to educate them about their fall risk and assist them to reduce or compensate for any identified risk factors. It is also portable so that an assessment can be performed in the home, a GP surgery, hospital ward, or residential care setting. *QuickScreen* is described in greater detail in Chapter 14.

Investigations

Further laboratory investigation of older persons who fall should be guided by the clinician's impressions of possible background and precipitating factors, as the yield for routine testing in clinical practice is low. Laboratory investigation guided by history and examination may include serum tests of renal function (urea and creatinine), hepatic enzymes, electrolyte balance (sodium, potassium, magnesium, and calcium), nutritional status (albumin, iron, vitamin B12, and folate), endocrine function (glucose, vitamin D, and thyroid function) and drug levels (e.g. for digoxin and anticonvulsants), and haematological tests for anaemia (haemoglobin). Where TLOC and syncope are suspected, investigations such as electrocardiogram, echocardiography, ambulatory cardiac telemetry, or tilt-table tests, with or without carotid sinus massage, may be rarely indicated [56, 57]. Stroke and other intra-cerebral disease may be assessed by cerebral computer tomography or magnetic resonance imaging.

Treatment

Gait and Balance Problems

Where gait and balance problems are identified, it may be possible to reduce fall risk through exercise interventions that aim to improve strength and balance.

Specific exercise interventions are discussed in detail in Chapter 16. Choice is often limited by service constraints, with group exercise or one to one physiotherapy being the more common means of delivery. Exercise programs can provide cost-effective strength and balance training to reduce falls in the community [58, 59].

Vision Problems

Interventions to improve visual acuity in older people may reduce the incidence of falls. Examinations by an optometrist should be performed annually to identify treatable deficits in vision. Visual acuity is often assessed using a traditional high-contrast Snellen chart. However, low contrast visual acuity tests may be better predictors of falls in community and residential home populations [60–62]. Patients are asked to read the smallest letters that they can see on a low contrast Snellen chart from a set distance (usually three metres). A Snellen fraction score of greater than 6/20 indicates severely impaired low-contrast visual acuity.

Where spectacles are necessary to improve visual acuity, older people benefit from wearing unifocal, rather than bifocal or multi-focal, lenses, particularly when negotiating stairs and unfamiliar environments [47]. Multi-focal lenses impair depth perception and edge-contrast sensitivity at critical distances for detecting obstacles in the environment and are not recommended for older people at risk of falling. If visual acuity is impaired by cataracts, removal of the cataract in the first affected eye may reduce the incidence of falls [63, 64]. There is evidence that expediting cataract extraction (surgery within one month) may reduce incidence of falls and fractures when compared to a routine 12-month wait [64]. Cataract removal in the second eye may also provide some incremental benefit in reducing falls. In frail older people, however, interventions to improve vision may not reduce, and may actually increase, the incidence of falls [65]. Even in this population, these interventions may still be necessary to maintain independence and quality of life, and should be recommended in conjunction with other strategies to reduce falls.

'Drop Attacks' and Transient Loss of Consciousness

'Drop attacks' and TLOC may be due to a number of diseases causing seizure, stroke, or syncope. Causes of syncope include reflex syncope (neurally medicated syncope), a category which includes vasovagal syncope, situational syncope (micturition, defecation, cough, laugh, and swallow) and carotid sinus syndrome, orthostatic hypotension, cardiac arrhythmia, and structural heart disease (including valvular heart disease and cardiomyopathy). A low index of suspicion is required for these conditions, older people may be unaware of having lost of consciousness prior to a fall [66].

When 'drop attacks' are recurrent and not clearly attributable to any of the above conditions or acute inter-current illness, such as myocardial infarction, infection, malignancy, electrolyte disturbance, or gastrointestinal haemorrhage, a diagnosis may still be obtained in almost 90% of patients [56]. Twelve-lead electrocardiogram and 24-hour cardiac telemetry may be indicated in specific older people, but have a low diagnostic yield and need to be complemented by other assessments such as 24-hour ambulatory blood pressure monitoring, orthostatic blood pressure measurements, electroencephalogram, and tilt-table testing, which may include bilateral supine and erect carotid sinus massage.

The European Society of Cardiology [57] and the American College of Cardiology [67] have produced guidelines for the assessment and management of syncope.

Reflex (Neurally Medicated) Syncope

Vasovagal syncope represents the most common form of reflex syncope and is characterized by a failure of the autonomic nervous system to maintain a pulse and blood pressure sufficient to ensure adequate cerebral perfusion [68, 69]. The low blood pressure is due to reduced peripheral vascular resistance and venous return, and a slow heart rate, due to paradoxical reflex bradycardia [70, 71]. Vasovagal syncope can be orthostatic (usually from prolonged standing) or provoked by emotion such as fear, pain, instrumentation, or blood phobia.

Although the diagnosis may be made through bedside history and examination, tilt-table testing may be required to investigate reflex syncope [57] . Treatment usually involves counselling about the relatively benign prognosis, avoidance of possible precipitating factors, instructions about assuming safe supported, seated, or lying postures when an episode is imminent and counterpressure manoeuvres, such as isometric arm, fist, or lower limb tensing [57, 72]. There are rare individuals with reflex syncope who have recurrent episodes of collapse and no associated warning symptoms and may warrant further intervention. However, the strength of evidence for treatment [67] is only moderate – for midodrine [73, 74] – or weak – for fludrocortisone, beta-blockers [75], selective serotonin reuptake inhibitors [76], and dual chamber pacemakers [77–79].

Orthostatic Hypotension

People who demonstrate orthostatic hypotension, defined as a 20 mmHg decrease in systolic blood pressure or a 10 mmHg decrease in diastolic blood pressure within three minutes of standing compared with blood pressure in the supine position, are at a significantly higher risk of falling [45]. Orthostatic hypotension was found to account for 14% of all causes of syncope referred to a dedicated syncope unit [80]. It may be associated with post-prandial hypotension (drops in blood pressure following meals), postural tachycardia syndrome or reflex syncope, and can be caused or exacerbated by vasodilator medications, diuretics, autonomic failure associated with diabetes and Parkinson's disease, and, less commonly, adrenal insufficiency and valvular or structural heart disease.

Formal testing involves the patient lying initially in the supine position for a minimum of five minutes before lying blood pressure is recorded. Subsequent readings are taken on assuming the upright position at one, three and five minutes using a standard sphygmomanometer, although continuous beat-to-beat monitoring is more accurate.

Treatment of symptomatic orthostatic hypotension firstly involves removal or avoidance of contributing medications, alcohol, and large, carbohydrate-rich meals. Other measures include regular fluid and salt intake, graded compression stockings, exercises to increase venous return from the legs (such as leg tensing or crossing exercises) prior to standing, education regarding awareness of symptoms and rising carefully from seated or lying positions, and, rarely, head-up/toe-down tilt of the bed. Pharmacological treatments may be infrequently required when falls persist despite other interventions, although the evidence of benefit is weak (fludrocortisone and pyridostigmine) to moderate (midodrine), and the drugs have potential prohibitive side effects (fluid retention and supine hypertension) [67, 81–84].

Carotid Sinus Syndrome

Carotid sinus syndrome is a rarer form of reflex syncope. There are three sub-types of the carotid sinus syndrome (CSS) – cardioinhibitory, vasodepressor, and mixed. The *cardioinhibitory* response is characterized by a period of more than three seconds of asystole following carotid sinus massage. This is usually seen within a few seconds of onset of massage and tends to be self-limiting, although atropine and full resuscitation facilities should be readily accessible. The *vasodepressor* response is identified by a fall in systolic blood pressure of greater than 50 mmHg in the absence of a significant bradycardia. The *mixed* type is a combination of both responses. The drop in blood pressure is seen within seconds of massage and as such is difficult to detect without the use of continuous non-invasive blood pressure monitoring.

The Newcastle protocol is useful to investigate carotid sinus syndrome [85]. A history of a stroke, transient ischaemic attack, or myocardial infarction within the last three months is a contraindication to undertaking carotid sinus massage. Those with carotid artery bruits should undergo carotid Dopplers before undertaking the study to exclude significant carotid artery disease, and if proceeding in the presence of carotid artery disease, the risks and benefits need to be discussed with the individual.

Surface ECG monitoring, non-invasive beat-to-beat monitoring of blood pressure and immediate access to resuscitation facilities should be available.

Patients are initially tested in the supine position with the neck slightly extended. Massage is applied over the point of maximal carotid impulse, medial to the sternomastoid muscle at the level of the upper border of the thyroid cartilage. Firm longitudinal massage is applied for 5 seconds, initially on the right, and after a 60 second interval repeated on the left. The procedure is then repeated with the patient tilted upright to 70°.

Carotid sinus studies are not without risk of complications, including both transient and permanent neurological damage [86–88]. Of the four series published, the highest reported rate of any neurological complication was 0.9% and this corresponded with 0.1% of all cases having persistent neurological deficits. It is possible that the difference in complication rates documented at different sites relates more to methodological issues and possibly case mix rather than any true difference as differences in definition are apparent in the existing literature.

With regard to treatment, symptomatic cardioinhibitory CSS can be treated with dual-chamber pacing [89]. Atrial pacing is contraindicated in view of the high incidence of atrioventricular block during baroreflex stimulation, while ventricular pacing fails to control symptoms in many patients due to either aggravation of co-existing vasodepression or the development of the pacemaker syndrome. However, the level of evidence for these interventions remains moderate to weak [67].

People with vasodepressor CSS have an impaired responsiveness to vasoconstrictive stimuli [90]. A review of prescribed medications is the first step, particularly looking for drugs with vasodilator or vagal activity. One small case series reported an improvement in symptoms with the alpha agonist midodrine [91].

Cardiac Syncope

Both brady and tachy arrhythmias have the potential to cause a fall in older people. A 12-lead ECG may assist diagnosis in less than 11% of syncopal patients [92] and is only useful if symptoms and signs are present at the time of the recording or if there are persisting abnormalities in rhythm and morphology between episodes.

The 24-h ECG has been the mainstay clinical investigation for people with intermittent palpitations, dizziness, and syncope occurring at least daily, but has a low diagnostic yield when used routinely. Patient-activated recorders and implantable loop recorders are preferred when an intermittent cardiac arrhythmia is suspected. Implantable loop recorders are small devices inserted subcutaneously under local anaesthetic that can store retrospective ECG recording when triggered by the individual. The device can remain in situ for a few years with reported diagnostic yields of up to 40% [93] and are useful if symptoms occur at least a few times each year. Diagnostic utility can be improved further by implantable monitors that monitor heart rhythm and record irregularities continuously, rather than relying on patient triggering [94].

Cardiac ischaemia-related syncope is confirmed when syncope presents with evidence of acute myocardial ischaemia with or without myocardial infarction [57]. Syncope can also occur due to structural cardiopulmonary disorders such as severe aortic stenosis, acute aortic dissection, and pulmonary embolus.

Medication Review

The risk of falls increases proportionally with the number of medications taken [48]. In older people, the risk may also increase, irrespective of number of medications, with higher defined daily doses of certain drugs, such as antidepressants [95] and antihypertensives [96, 97], cumulative exposure to a drug with sedative and anticholinergic properties (drug burden index) [98], or commencement of antihypertensives [12].

Routine assessment of medications, including commencement of a drug, duration of use, and change in dose, should be undertaken at least six monthly (for those with four or more medications, higher defined daily doses, or drug burden) to yearly (for those on one to three drugs) [99].

Appropriate medication use involves regular assessment of indications, identification of possible side effects (due to drug pharmacokinetics, pharmacodynamics, and interactions), discussion of risks and benefits with older persons and their carers, and prescription or deprescription of medications in appropriate doses, frequencies, and combinations to achieve desired outcomes. Although its incremental benefit is unclear, medication assessment and rationalization have been important adjuncts in several randomized controlled trials [21, 100–105] which have used a multi-faceted approach to fall prevention. In the PROFET study [21], 10.5% of the intervention group were referred to their GP for a further review of medication and the majority of these referrals related to benzodiazepine use. Tinetti et al. [101] reduced the number of prescribed medications in a group of community-dwelling older people and also saw a reduction in sedative/hypnotic use during the one year follow-up.

Centrally Acting Medications

Centrally acting medications have consistently been shown to increase fall risk [7, 8]. Campbell et al. [106] assessed the benefits of withdrawing centrally acting medications as part of a 2×2 factorial randomized controlled trial. Subjects were recruited through their local GP practice. A 14-week structured withdrawal programme and a follow-up period of 44 weeks showed a 66% reduction in falls in the medication withdrawal group when compared to those remaining on medication. Of those in the medication withdrawal arm, 67% were on a benzodiazepine, 33% on an antidepressant, and 17% were prescribed a major tranquillizer. Within one month of study termination, however, 47% of subjects had restarted centrally acting medications. A more recent systematic review involving 1309 participants in clinical trials found fall-risk-inducing drugs withdrawal strategy (mostly targeting centrally acting medications) did not significantly reduce fall rates (RaR: 0.98, 95% CI: 0.63, 1.51) in older people over a 6–12 month follow-up period [107]. This suggests strategies to prevent the initial uptake of centrally acting medications are warranted. Furthermore, the prescription of benzodiazepines, Z-drugs, or other psychotropic medication for the management of insomnia in older persons should be avoided, unless there is a clear pattern of addiction or inability to complete a withdrawal program. Non-pharmacological approaches to the management of insomnia should be considered.

Vitamin D Supplementation

Vitamin D insufficiency is common in older people, particularly those who are housebound or who reside in nursing homes [108, 109]. In addition to increasing the risk of osteoporosis [110], there is also evidence that inadequate vitamin D impairs psychomotor function and exacerbates muscle weakness [105]. Vitamin D supplementation may improve postural stability [111] and muscle strength [112]. Calcium and vitamin D supplementation (in doses of 700–1000 IU/day) may also reduce the risk of falls [113] and fractures [114]. Therefore, in the absence of individual contraindications (such as conditions predisposing to hypercalcaemia), vitamin D and calcium supplementation should be recommended to older persons to reduce rate of falls, particularly in residential care facilities [115]. The one proviso is that monthly or yearly doses of vitamin D should be avoided as such high doses appear to increase fall risk [116, 117].

Conclusions

The multi-factorial aetiology of falls is such that input and expertise from disciplines including medicine is often required to prevent falls. Identification of at-risk populations needs to be considered and those at high risk often present via the general practice route. Basic clinical assessments include medication review and simple tests of cognition, postural stability, gait, balance, and vision. Centrally acting medications should be avoided or actively withdrawn where possible and alternate non-pharmacological approaches considered in high-risk individuals. Strength and balance training programmes are beneficial in reducing falls. An additional environmental assessment may be required. Individuals with unexplained falls, 'drop attacks', syncope, or dizziness may require specialist assessment, investigations, and interventions.

REFERENCES

1. Graham HJ, Firth J. Home accidents in older people: role of primary health care team *Br Med J*. 1992;305:30–2.

2. Close JC, Hooper R, Glucksman E et al. Predictors of falls in a high risk population: results from the prevention of falls in the elderly trial (PROFET). *Emerg Med J*. 2003;20:421–5.

3. Fernando E, Fraser M, Hendriksen J et al. Risk factors associated with falls in older adults with dementia: a systematic review. *Physiother Can*. 2017;69:161–70.

4. Kerse N, Parag V, Feigin VL et al. Falls after stroke: results from the Auckland Regional Community Stroke (ARCOS) Study, 2002 to 2003. *Stroke*. 2008;39:1890–3.

5. Latt MD, Lord SR, Morris JG et al. Clinical and physiological assessments for elucidating falls risk in Parkinson's disease. *Mov Disord*. 2009;24:1280–9.

6. Leipzig RM, Cumming RG, Tinetti ME. Drugs and falls in older people: a systematic review and meta-analysis. I. Psychotropic drugs. *J Am Geriatr Soc*. 1999;47:30–9.

7. Leipzig RM, Cumming RG, Tinetti ME. Drugs and falls in older people: a systematic review and meta-analysis. II. Cardiac and analgesic drugs. *J Am Geriatr Soc*. 1999;47:40–50.

8. Woolcott JC, Richardson KJ, Wiens MO et al. Meta-analysis of the impact of 9 medication classes on falls in elderly persons. *Arch Intern Med*. 2009;169:1952–60.

9. de Vries M, Seppala LJ, Daams JG et al. Fall-risk-increasing drugs: a systematic review and meta-analysis. I. Cardiovascular Drugs. *J Am Med Dir Assoc*. 2018;19:371.e1–9.

10. Seppala LJ, van de Glind EMM, Daams JG et al. Fall-risk-increasing drugs: a systematic review and meta-analysis. III. Others. *J Am Med Dir Assoc*. 2018;19:372.e1–8.

11. Seppala LJ, Wermelink A, de Vries M et al. Fall-risk-increasing drugs: a systematic review and meta-analysis. II. Psychotropics. *J Am Med Dir Assoc*. 2018;19:371.e11–17.

12. Kahlaee HR, Latt MD, Schneider CR. Association between chronic or acute use of antihypertensive class of medications and falls in older adults: a systematic review and meta-analysis. *Am J Hypertens*. 2018;31:467–79.

13. Tinetti ME, Doucette J, Claus E et al. Risk factors for serious injury during falls by older persons in the community. *J Am Geriatr Soc*. 1995;43:1214–21.

14. Vellas BJ, Wayne SJ, Romero LJ et al. Fear of falling and restriction of mobility in elderly fallers. *Age Ageing*. 1997;26:189–93.

15. Gillespie LD, Robertson MC, Gillespie WJ et al. Interventions for preventing falls in older people living in the community. *Cochrane Database Syst Rev*. 2012:CD007146.

16. Hopewell S, Adedire O, Copsey BJ et al. Multifactorial and multiple component interventions for preventing falls in older people living in the community. *Cochrane Database Syst Rev*. 2018;7:CD012221.

17. Stevens JA, Ballesteros MF, Mack KA et al. Gender differences in seeking care for falls in the aged Medicare population. *Am J Prev Med.* 2012;43:59–62.

18. Panel on Prevention of Falls in Older Persons, American Geriatrics Society and British Geriatrics Society. Summary of the updated American Geriatrics Society/British Geriatrics Society clinical practice guideline for prevention of falls in older persons. *J Am Geriatr Soc.* 2011;59:148–57.

19. Quality statement 1: Identifying people at risk of falling. National Institute for Clinical Excellence; 2015, updated 31 January 2017. www.nice.org.uk/guidance/qs86/chapter/quality-statement-1-identifying-people-at-risk-of-falling#quality-statement-1-identifying-people-at-risk-of-falling (accessed April 2021).

20. Rubenstein LZ, Josephson KR, Robbins AS. Falls in the nursing home. *Ann Intern Med.* 1994;121:442–51.

21. Close J, Ellis M, Hooper R et al. Prevention of falls in the elderly trial (PROFET): a randomised controlled trial. *Lancet.* 1999;353:93–7.

22. Buatois S, Perret-Guillaume C, Gueguen R et al. A simple clinical scale to stratify risk of recurrent falls in community-dwelling adults aged 65 years and older. *Phys Ther.* 2010;90:550–60.

23. Albert SM, King J, Boudreau R et al. Primary prevention of falls: effectiveness of a statewide program. *Am J Public Health.* 2014;104:e77–84.

24. Gawler S, Skelton DA, Dinan-Young S et al. Reducing falls among older people in general practice: the ProAct65+ exercise intervention trial. *Arch Gerontol Geriatr.* 2016;67:46–54.

25. McClure R, Turner C, Peel N et al. Population-based interventions for the prevention of fall-related injuries in older people. *Cochrane Database Syst Rev.* 2005;CD004441.

26. The prevention of falls in later life: a report of the Kellogg International Work Group on the prevention of falls by the elderly. *Dan Med Bull.* 1987;34(4):1–24.

27. Stark A, Kaduszkiewicz H, Stein J et al. A qualitative study on older primary care patients' perspectives on depression and its treatments: potential barriers to and opportunities for managing depression. *BMC Fam Pract.* 2018;19:2.

28. Lamb SE, Jørstad-Stein EC, Hauer K et al. Development of a common outcome data set for fall injury prevention trials: the Prevention of Falls Network Europe consensus. *J Am Geriatr Soc.* 2005;53:1618–22.

29. Dey AB, Stout NR, Kenny RA. Cardiovascular syncope is the most common cause of drop attacks in the elderly. *Pacing Clin Electrophysiol.* 1997;20:818–19.

30. Kenny RA, Traynor G. Carotid sinus syndrome: clinical characteristics in elderly patients. *Age Ageing.* 1991;20:449–54.

31. O'Dwyer C, Bennett K, Langan Y et al. Amnesia for loss of consciousness is common in vasovagal syncope. *Europace.* 2011;13:1040–5.

32. Cumming RG, Thomas M, Szonyi G et al. Home visits by an occupational therapist for assessment and modification of environmental hazards: a randomized trial of falls prevention. *J Am Geriatr Soc.* 1999;47:1397–402.

33. Bergland A, Jarnlo GB, Laake K. Predictors of falls in the elderly by location. *Aging Clin Exp Res.* 2003;15:43–50.

34. Kelsey JL, Berry SD, Procter-Gray E et al. Indoor and outdoor falls in older adults are different: the maintenance of balance, independent living, intellect, and Zest in the Elderly of Boston Study. *J Am Geriatr Soc*. 2010;58:2135–41.

35. Aronow WS, Ahn C. Association of postprandial hypotension with incidence of falls, syncope, coronary events, stroke, and total mortality at 29-month follow-up in 499 older nursing home residents. *J Am Geriatr Soc*. 1997;45:1051–3.

36. Vaughan CP, Brown CJ, Goode PS et al. The association of nocturia with incident falls in an elderly community-dwelling cohort. *Int J Clin Pract*. 2010;64:577–83.

37. Chen CM, Yoon YH. Usual alcohol consumption and risks for nonfatal fall injuries in the united states: results from the 2004–2013 National Health Interview Survey. *Subst Use Misuse*. 2017;52:1120–32.

38. Brignole M. Distinguishing syncopal from non-syncopal causes of fall in older people. *Age Ageing*. 2006;35(2):ii46–ii50.

39. Schlick C, Schniepp R, Loidl V et al. Falls and fear of falling in vertigo and balance disorders: a controlled cross-sectional study. *J Vestib Res*. 2016;25:241–51.

40. Butler AA, Lord SR, Taylor JL et al. Ability versus hazard: risk-taking and falls in older people. *J Gerontol A Biol Sci Med Sci*. 2014;70:628–34.

41. Fleming J, Brayne C. Inability to get up after falling, subsequent time on floor, and summoning help: prospective cohort study in people over 90. *Br Med J*. 2008;337:a2227.

42. Koski K, Luukinen H, Laippala P et al. Risk factors for major injurious falls among the home-dwelling elderly by functional abilities: a prospective population-based study. *Gerontology*. 1998;44:232–8.

43. Owings JT, Wisner DH, Battistella FD et al. Isolated transient loss of consciousness is an indicator of significant injury. *Arch Surg*. 1998;133:941–6.

44. Tan MP, Kenny RA. Cardiovascular assessment of falls in older people. *Clin Interv Aging*. 2006;1:57–66.

45. McDonald C, Pearce M, Kerr SR et al. A prospective study of the association between orthostatic hypotension and falls: definition matters. *Age Ageing*. 2017;46:439–45.

46. Campbell AJ, Borrie MJ, Spears GF. Risk factors for falls in a community-based prospective study of people 70 years and older. *J Gerontol*. 1989;44:M112–17.

47. Lord SR, Dayhew J, Howland A. Multifocal glasses impair edge-contrast sensitivity and depth perception and increase the risk of falls in older people. *J Am Geriatr Soc*. 2002;50:1760–6.

48. Dhalwani NN, Fahami R, Sathanapally H et al. Association between polypharmacy and falls in older adults: a longitudinal study from England. *BMJ Open*. 2017;7:e016358.

49. Morin L, Calderon Larrañaga A, Welmer AK et al. Polypharmacy and injurious falls in older adults: a nationwide nested case-control study. *Clin Epidemiol*. 2019;11:483–93.

50. Klenk J, Kerse N, Rapp K et al. Physical activity and different concepts of fall risk estimation in older people: results of the ActiFE-Ulm study. *PLoS One*. 2015;10:e0129098-e.

51. Speechley M, Tinetti M. Falls and injuries in frail and vigorous community elderly persons. *J Am Geriatr Soc*. 1991;39:46–52.

52. Holtzer R, Friedman R, Lipton RB et al. The relationship between specific cognitive functions and falls in aging. *Neuropsychology.* 2007;21:540–8.

53. Gleason CE, Gangnon RE, Fischer BL et al. Increased risk for falling associated with subtle cognitive impairment: secondary analysis of a randomized clinical trial. *Dement Geriatr Cogn Disord.* 2009;27:557–63.

54. Podsialdo D, Richardson S. The timed "up & go": a test of basic functional mobility for frail elderly persons. *J Am Geriatr Soc.* 1991;39:142–8.

55. Schoene D, Wu SM, Mikolaizak AS et al. Discriminative ability and predictive validity of the timed up and go test in identifying older people who fall: systematic review and meta-analysis. *J Am Geriatr Soc.* 2013;61:202–8.

56. Parry SW, Kenny RA. Drop attacks in older adults: systematic assessment has a high diagnostic yield. *J Am Geriatr Soc.* 2005;53:74–8.

57. Brignole M, Moya A, de Lange FJ et al. 2018 ESC Guidelines for the diagnosis and management of syncope. *Eur Heart J.* 2018;39:1883–948.

58. Campbell AJ, Robertson MC, Gardner MM et al. Randomised controlled trial of a general practice programme of home based exercise to prevent falls in elderly women. *Br Med J.* 1997;315:1065–69.

59. Robertson MC, Gardner MM, Devlin N et al. Effectiveness and economic evaluation of a nurse delivered home exercise programme to prevent falls. 2 Controlled trial in multiple centres. *Br Med J.* 2001;322:701–4.

60. Lord SR, Ward JA, Williams P et al. Physiological factors associated with falls in older community-dwelling women. *J Am Geriatr Soc.* 1994;42:1110–17.

61. Lord SR, Clark RD, Webster IW. Visual acuity and contrast sensitivity in relation to falls in an elderly population. *Age Ageing.* 1991;20:175–81.

62. Verbaken JH, Johnston AW. Clinical contrast sensitivity testing: the current status. *Clin Exp Optom.* 1986;69:204–12.

63. Brannan S, Dewar C, Sen J et al. A prospective study of the rate of falls before and after cataract surgery. *Br J Ophthalmol.* 2003;87:560–2.

64. Harwood RH, Foss AJ, Osborn F et al. Falls and health status in elderly women following first eye cataract surgery: a randomised controlled trial. *Br J Ophthalmol.* 2005;89:53–9.

65. Cumming RG, Ivers R, Clemson L et al. Improving vision to prevent falls in frail older people: a randomized trial. *J Am Geriatr Soc.* 2007;1:175–81.

66. Davies AJ, Kenny RA. Falls presenting to the accident and emergency department: types of presentation and risk factor profile. *Age Ageing.* 1996;25:362–6.

67. Shen WK, Sheldon RS, Benditt DG et al. 2017 ACC/AHA/HRS guideline for the evaluation and management of patients with syncope: executive summary: a Report of the American College of Cardiology/American Heart Association Task Force on Clinical Practice Guidelines and the Heart Rhythm Society. *J Am Coll Cardiol.* 2017;70:620–63.

68. Shepherd RFJ, Shepherd JT. Control of the blood pressure and circulation in man. In: Mathias CJ, Bannister R, (Eds.) *Autonomic Failure: a Textbook of Clinical Disorders of the Autonomic Nervous System.* 4th Edn. Oxford: Oxford University Press; 1999.

69. Grubb BP, Karas B. Clinical disorders of the autonomic nervous system associated with orthostatic intolerance: an overview of classification, clinical evaluation, and management. *Pacing Clin Electrophysiol.* 1999;22:798–810.

70. Lurie K, Benditt D. Syncope and the autonomic nervous system. *J Cardiovasc Electrophysiol.* 1996;7:760–76.

71. Kosinski D, Grubb BP. Pathophysiological aspects of neurocardiogenic syncope: current concepts and new perspectives. *Pacing Clin Electrophysiol.* 1995;18:716–24.

72. Krediet CT, van Dijk N, Linzer M et al. Management of vasovagal syncope: controlling or aborting faints by leg crossing and muscle tensing. *Circulation.* 2002;106:1684–9.

73. Kaufmann H, Saadia D, Voustianiouk A. Midodrine in neurally mediated syncope: a double-blind, randomised, crossover study. *Ann Neurol.* 2002;52:342–5.

74. Perez-Lugones A, Schweikert R, Pavia S et al. Usefulness of midodrine in patients with severely symptomatic neurocardiogenic syncope: a randomized control study. *J Cardiovasc Electrophysiol.* 2001;12:935–8.

75. Sheldon R, Connolly S, Rose S et al. Prevention of Syncope Trial (POST): a randomized, placebo-controlled study of metoprolol in the prevention of vasovagal syncope. *Circulation.* 2006;113:1164–70.

76. Di Girolamo E, Di Iorio C, Sabatini P et al. Effects of paroxetine hydrochloride, a selective serotonin reuptake inhibitor, on refractory vasovagal syncope: a randomized, double-blind, placebo-controlled study. *J Am Coll Cardiol.* 1999;33: 1227–30.

77. Sutton R, Brignole M, Menozzi C et al. Dual-chamber pacing in treatment of neurally mediated tilt-positive cardioinhibitory syncope: pacemaker versus no therapy: a multicenter randomized study. *Circulation.* 2000;102:294–9.

78. Connolly SJ, Sheldon R, Thorpe KE et al. Pacemaker therapy for prevention of syncope in patients with recurrent severe vasovagal syncope. Second Vasovagal Pacemaker Study (VPS II): a randomized trial. *J Am Med Assoc.* 2003;289:2224–9.

79. Raviele A, Giada F, Menozzi C et al. A randomized, double-blind, placebo-controlled study of permanent cardiac pacing for the treatment of recurrent tilt-induced vasovagal syncope: the Vasovagal Syncope and Pacing trial (synpace). *Eur Heart J.* 2004;25:1741–8.

80. McIntosh S, Da Costa D, Kenny RA. Outcome of an integrated approach to the investigation of dizziness, falls and syncope in elderly patients referred to a 'syncope' clinic. *Age Ageing.* 1993;22:53–8.

81. Jankovic J, Gilden JL, Hiner BC et al. Neurogenic orthostatic hypotension: a double-blind, placebo-controlled study with midodrine. *Am J Med.* 1993;95:38–48.

82. Grijalva CG, Biaggioni I, Griffin MR et al. Fludrocortisone is associated with a higher risk of all-cause hospitalizations compared with midodrine in patients with orthostatic hypotension. *J Am Heart Assoc.* 2017;6(10).

83. Byun JI, Moon J, Kim DY et al. Efficacy of single or combined midodrine and pyridostigmine in orthostatic hypotension. *Neurology.* 2017;89:1078–86.

84. Izcovich A, González Malla C, Manzotti M et al. Midodrine for orthostatic hypotension and recurrent reflex syncope: a systematic review. *Neurology.* 2014;83:1170–7.

85. Kenny RA, O'Shea D, Parry SW. The Newcastle protocols for head-up tilt table testing in the diagnosis of vasovagal syncope, carotid sinus hypersensitivity, and related disorders. *Heart*. 2000;83:564–9.

86. Davies AJ, Kenny RA. Frequency of neurologic complications following carotid sinus massage. *Am J Cardiol*. 1998;81:1256–7.

87. Munro N, McIntosh S, Lawson J et al. Incidence of complications after carotid sinus massage in older patients with syncope. *J Am Geriatr Soc*. 1994;42:1248–51.

88. Puggioni E, Guiducci V, Brignole M et al. Results and complications of the carotid sinus massage performed according to the "method of symptoms". *Am J Cardiol*. 2002;89:599–601.

89. Kenny RA. Syncope in the elderly: diagnosis, evaluation, and treatment. *J Cardiovasc Electrophysiol*. 2003;14:S74–S7.

90. Mangoni AA, Ouldred E, Allain TJ et al. Paradoxical vasodilation during lower body negative pressure in patients with vasodepressor carotid sinus syndrome. *J Am Geriatr Soc*. 2003;51:853–7.

91. Moore A, Watts M, Sheehy T et al. Treatment of vasodepressor carotid sinus syndrome with midodrine: a randomized, controlled pilot study. *J Am Geriatr Soc*. 2005;53:114–18.

92. Kapoor WN. Diagnostic evaluation of syncope. *Am J Med*. 1991;90:91–106.

93. Fitzpatrick AP. Ambulatory electrocardiographic (AECG) monitoring for evaluation of syncope. In: Benditt DG, Blanc J-J, Brignole M, Sutton R, (Eds.) *The Evaluation and Treatment of Syncope: a Handbook for Clinical Practice*. New York: Futura Publishing; 2003:63–70.

94. Burkowitz J, Merzenich C, Grassme K et al. Insertable cardiac monitors in the diagnosis of syncope and the detection of atrial fibrillation: a systematic review and meta-analysis. *Eur J Prev Cardiol*. 2016;23:1261–72.

95. Sterke CS, Ziere G, van Beeck EF et al. Dose-response relationship between selective serotonin re-uptake inhibitors and injurious falls: a study in nursing home residents with dementia. *Br J Clin Pharmacol*. 2012;73:812–20.

96. Tinetti ME, Han L, Lee DSH et al. Antihypertensive medications and serious fall injuries in a nationally representative sample of older adults. *JAMA Intern Med*. 2014;174:588–95.

97. Callisaya ML, Sharman JE, Close J et al. Greater daily defined dose of antihypertensive medication increases the risk of falls in older people: a population-based study. *J Am Geriatr Soc*. 2014;62:1527–33.

98. Nishtala PS, Narayan SW, Wang T et al. Associations of drug burden index with falls, general practitioner visits, and mortality in older people. *Pharmacoepidemiol Drug Saf*. 2014;23:753–8.

99. Department of Health and Social Care. *National Service Framework for Older People*. London: DoHaSC; 2001.

100. Davison J, Bond J, Dawson P et al. Patients with recurrent falls attending Accident & Emergency benefit from multifactorial intervention: a randomised controlled trial. *Age Ageing*. 2005;34:162–8.

101. Tinetti ME, Baker DI, McAvay G et al. A multifactorial intervention to reduce the risk of falling among elderly people living in the community. *N Engl J Med*. 1994;331:821–7.

102. Rubenstein LZ, Robbins AS, Josephson KR et al. The value of assessing falls in an elderly population: randomized clinical trial. *Ann Intern Med.* 1990;113:308–16.

103. Ray WA, Taylor JA, Meador KG et al. A randomized trial of a consultation service to reduce falls in nursing homes *J Am Med Assoc.* 1997;278:557–62.

104. Shaw FE, Bond J, Richardson DA et al. Multifactorial intervention after a fall in older people with cognitive impairment and dementia presenting to the accident and emergency department: a randomised controlled trial. *Br Med J.* 2003;326:73.

105. Boonen S, Lysens R, Verbeke G et al. Relationship between age-associated endocrine deficiencies and muscle function in elderly women: a cross-sectional study. *Age Ageing.* 1998;27:449–54.

106. Campbell AJ, Robertson MC, Gardner MM et al. Psychotropic medication withdrawal and a home-based exercise program to prevent falls: a randomized, controlled trial. *J Am Geriatr Soc.* 1999;47:850–3.

107. Lee J, Negm A, Wong E et al. Does deprescribing fall-associated drugs reduce falls and its complications? A systematic review. *Innov Aging.* 2017;1:268.

108. Gloth FM, 3rd. Osteoporosis in long term care. Part 1 of 2: recognizing bone and beyond. *Director.* 2004;12:175–6, 179–80.

109. Sambrook PN, Cameron ID, Cumming RG et al. Vitamin D deficiency is common in frail institutionalised older people in northern Sydney. *Med J Aust.* 2002;176:560.

110. Peacock M, Liu G, Carey M et al. Bone mass and structure at the hip in men and women over the age of 60 years. *Osteoporos Int.* 1998;8:231–9.

111. Pfeifer M, Begerow B, Minne HW et al. Effects of a short-term vitamin D and calcium supplementation on body sway and secondary hyperparathyroidism in elderly women. *J Bone Miner Res.* 2000;15:1113–18.

112. Dhesi JK, Bearne LM, Monitz C et al. Neuromuscular and psychomotor function in elderly subjects who fall and the relationship with vitamin D status. *J Bone Miner Res.* 2002;17:891–7.

113. Bischoff HA, Stahelin HB, Dick W et al. Effects of vitamin D and calcium supplementation on falls: a randomized controlled trial. *J Bone Miner Res.* 2003;18:343–51.

114. Chapuy MC, Arlot ME, Duboeuf F et al. Vitamin D3 and calcium to prevent hip fractures in the elderly women. *N Engl J Med.* 1992;327:1637–42.

115. Cameron ID, Dyer SM, Panagoda CE et al. Interventions for preventing falls in older people in care facilities and hospitals. *Cochrane Database Syst Rev.* 2018;9:CD005465.

116. Bischoff-Ferrari HA, Dawson-Hughes B, Orav EJ et al. Monthly high-dose vitamin D treatment for the prevention of functional decline: a randomized clinical trial. *JAMA Intern Med.* 2016;176:175–83.

117. Sanders KM, Stuart AL, Williamson EJ et al. Annual high-dose oral vitamin D and falls and fractures in older women: a randomized controlled trial. *J Am Med Assoc.* 2010;303:1815–22.

21

Fall Prevention Interventions for People with Visual Impairment

Stephen R. Lord

As indicated in Chapter 4, there is good evidence that important visual functions including poor contrast sensitivity, deficient depth perception, and visual field loss increase the risk of falls and fall-related fractures in older people. Some visual impairments are amenable to intervention by surgery or refractive correction, and accordingly several randomized controlled trials have investigated visual interventions as a fall prevention strategy. This chapter provides summaries of these trial findings as well as a complementary study that evaluated the roles of exercise and home safety programmes for older people with visual impairment.

Cataract Surgery

Two randomized controlled trials have investigated the effect of cataract surgery on fall incidence. The first, involving 306 women aged 70 years and over, examined cataract surgery for one eye [1]. Participants were randomly allocated to receive either expedited (approximately four weeks' wait) or routine (12 months' wait) surgery. Vision, visual disability, physical activity levels, anxiety, depression, and balance confidence improved significantly in the operated group at the six-month retest and over the 12 months of follow-up, the fall rate in the operated group was reduced by 34% compared with the controls (IRR: 0.66, 95% CI: 0.45, 0.96).

A follow-on study by the same authors evaluated whether surgery on the second eye led to further reductions in falls, with the rationale that improving vision in both eyes would lead to better depth perception and subsequently fewer falls [2]. Again, participants (239 women aged over 70) were randomized to either expedited (approximately four weeks' wait) or routine (12 months' wait) surgery. Visual function (especially stereopsis), confidence, visual disability, and handicap all improved in the operated compared with the control group. Over the one-year trial period, the fall rate in the intervention group was reduced, although not significantly, by 32% (IRR: 0.68, 95% CI: 0.39, 1.19). This study planned for a larger sample size, whereby a reduction of this magnitude would have been significant. Ironically, the success of the first trial triggered policy changes whereby waiting times for cataract surgery fell from more than one year to less than six months in the period the study was carried out, making recruitment of the proposed sample numbers impossible. Therefore, it can be concluded that second eye cataract surgery improves depth perception, visual disability, and general health status, but the effect on rate of falling is uncertain.

Complementary research has also been conducted using data from over 1 million US Medicare beneficiaries aged 65 years and older with a diagnosis of cataract between 2002 and 2009. This showed that those who had cataract surgery within a year of diagnosis (36.9% of the sample) had a 16% lower incidence of hip fracture compared to those who did not have cataract surgery in this one-year period (adjusted OR: 0.84, 95% CI: 0.81, 0.87) [3].

Provision of New Glasses

Many older people who wear glasses with outdated prescriptions or no glasses at all may benefit from wearing new glasses with correct prescriptions. For example, an Australian survey involving 1695 older people showed that 39% had not visited an eye specialist in the past year [4]. Similarly, a USA study found 47% of 2433 had not had their vision examined in the past year and 37% of those who wore protective glasses could benefit from a visual intervention [5]. To address this issue, two RCTs have evaluated the efficacy of visual assessment and provision of new glasses as an intervention to prevent falls. Day et al. [6] used a factorial design to assess the separate and combined effects of interventions aimed at vision improvement, home hazard reduction, and group exercise among 1090 participants aged 70 years and over. In the visual improvement intervention, participants with impaired vision were provided a referral to their usual eye-care provider (if they exhibited poor visual acuity, decreased stereopsis, and/or reduced field of view and were not already being treated for the impairment). There was a non-significant reduction in prospective falls over 12 months in the visual intervention group (rate ratio for time to first fall: 0.89, 95% CI: 0.75, 1.04). It is worth noting, however, that of the 547 participants randomly assigned to receive the vision intervention, only 26 received a treatment they would not otherwise have had.

In the second study [7], 616 older people aged 70 years and over, were randomized to either an intervention group (n = 309) or a control group (n = 307). Of the intervention group, 44% (n = 92) received vision-related treatments (most often a new pair of glasses). During the follow-up period, participants from the intervention group reported significantly more falls than those from the control group (RR: 1.57, 95% CI: 1.20, 2.95). There was also a trend for more fall-related fractures in the intervention group (RR: 1.74, 95% CI: 0.97, 3.11). The authors suggested two factors may have accounted for these unexpected findings: (i) since the participants in the intervention group often received large changes to prescriptions, they might need considerable time to adapt to their new glasses, while being at greater risk of falling during this period [8] and (ii) with the improvement in vision, the intervention group may have changed their behaviour, becoming overconfident and adopting more risk-taking activities (thus increasing the exposure to falls). As evidence of the former, the authors observed that fall rates were higher among those who had a larger change in prescription, than for those who had a smaller change. Thus, time for adaptation to new glasses is recommended and optometrists are advised to gradually change prescriptions and to counsel clients as to the likely short-term risks of a new prescription [9].

Neither of the above interventions involving updating glasses aimed to restrict the use of multi-focal glasses and, in not doing so, may have left a significant risk factor unaltered. Multi-focal glasses are worn by over 50% of older adults who have visual acuity deficits and have benefits for tasks that require changes in focal length, including everyday tasks of driving, shopping, and cooking. However, the lower lenses of all types of multi-focal glasses (bifocals, trifocals, and progressive lens glasses) blur objects in the lower visual field and impair distant depth perception and contrast sensitivity [10]. For example, three studies in older people have found that multi-focal glasses impair step negotiation and accuracy of foot placement when stepping onto a raised surface [10–12] or negotiating an obstacle course [13]. Other studies have reported that wearing multi-focal glasses increases the risk of trips [14, 15] and falls in older people [10]. In particular, older multi-focal glasses wearers have an elevated risk of falls when outside their homes, and when walking up or down stairs [10].

To explicitly intervene with respect to multi-focal glasses as a fall risk factor, Haren et al. [16] conducted an RCT involving 606 older people and 13 months follow-up to determine whether fall rates among habitual multi-focal users could be reduced by assisting participants to wear single-vision correction when active outdoors or in unfamiliar indoor settings. The intervention targeted older habitual multi-focal wearers at increased risk of falls (i.e. suffered one or more falls in the past year or had a Timed Up and Go Test completion time>15 s).

Participants were provided with an additional pair of single-vision glasses and counselled to wear these for walking and activities out of the home and to restrict their use of multi-focal glasses to seated activities that require changes in focal length, such as driving, and minimal-risk walking activities such as shopping and cooking. An optometrist/counsellor also demonstrated how multi-focal glasses can impair the visual abilities required for detecting obstacles and judging depth [17]. This was achieved by administering the tests of distance edge contrast

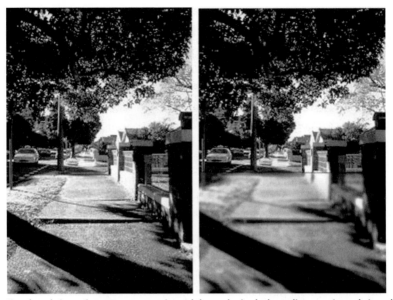

Figure 21.1   Simulated view of street scene as viewed through single-lens distance (panel a) and bifocal glasses (panel b). The footpath misalignment (a commonly reported environmental factor involved in outdoor falls) is clearly seen in panel a, but blurred in panel b. Reproduced with permission from Haran MJ, Cameron ID, Ivers RQ et al. Preventing falls in older multifocal glasses wearers by providing single-lens distance glasses: the protocol for the VISIBLE randomised controlled trial. BMC Geriatrics 2009, 9:10.

sensitivity and depth perception with participants viewing the visual stimuli through the upper and lower portion of their multi-focal lenses and distance lenses [10]. The difference in upper and lower visual performance was shown to the participant and the rationale for performing these tests was explained. Participants were also shown photographs of steps and streetscapes with and without simulated lower field blur to further reinforce how multi-focal glasses may increase the risk of falls. Figure 21.1 shows the photographs of a simulated view of a street scene as viewed through single-lens distance (panel a) and bifocal glasses (panel b). The counselling session was considered crucial to convince older wearers of multi-focal glasses that they are personally at risk of fall-related injuries and that the benefits of wearing single lens glasses may outweigh the inconvenience of dealing with two pairs of glasses.

The intervention produced a non-significant overall 8% reduction in falls (IRR: 0.92, 95% CI: 0.73, 1.16). The intervention was effective in preventing falls in the sub-group of people who more regularly undertook outside activities. In this group there were significant reductions in all falls (IRR: 0.60, 95% CI: 0.4, 0.85), falls outside the home (IRR: 0.61, 95% CI: 0.42, 0.87) and injurious falls (IRR: 0.62,

95% CI: 0.42, 0.92). However, there was a significant increase in outside falls in people who undertook little outside activity in the intervention group (IRR: 1.56, 95% CI: 1.11,2.19). These findings suggest that, with appropriate counselling, compliance with the intervention was acceptable and that the provision of single-lens glasses for older multi-focal wearers who take part in regular outdoor activities is an effective fall prevention strategy. The intervention may be harmful, however, in multi-focal wearers with low levels of outdoor activity.

Exercise and Home Safety Programmes for Visually Impaired Older People

In contrast to the above trials that have attempted to improve vision, Campbell et al. [18, 19] conducted a study evaluating the efficacy of a home safety programme and home-based exercise programme in older adults with low vision. Three hundred and ninety-one visually impaired people aged 75 years and over living in the community were randomized to either a home safety programme (n = 100), an exercise programme with vitamin D supplementation (n = 97), both interventions (n = 98), or a social visit control group (n = 96). Falls were reduced by 41% across groups receiving the home safety programme [18]. The possible mechanisms attributed to the success of this intervention were: (i) the removal of hazards around the home; (ii) the participants increased awareness and ability to negotiate hazards, and (iii) a reduction in activity due to a heightened fear of falling and therefore reduced exposure to risk [19]. In contrast, there was no reduction in falls in participants randomized to exercise and a subsequent systematic review that included three trials with a total of 539 participants with visual impairment revealed no impact of exercise on falls (RR: 1.05, 95%CI: 0.73, 1.50, p: 0.81) [20]. A fourth large trial that is examining whether falls can be prevented in older people with vision loss through a home-based exercise programme that embeds balance and strength training within everyday activities is currently underway [21].

Summary

In summary, randomized controlled trial evidence indicates cataract surgery for the first eye and maximizing vision through restricting multi-focal glasses use in active older people are effective fall prevention strategies. Occupational therapy interventions involving home hazard reductions are also effective in preventing falls in severely visually impaired older people. Although interventions involving vision assessment and provision of new spectacles undoubtedly improve performance in visual tests in community-dwelling older people, such interventions have not yet shown they can reduce the risk of falls. In fact, it is recommended that optometrists counsel their clients about their likely short-term increased fall risk when dispensing new prescription glasses.

REFERENCES

1. Harwood RH, Foss JE, Osborn F et al. Falls and health status in elderly women following first eye cataract surgery: a randomised controlled trial. *Brit J Ophthalmol.* 2005;89:53–9.

2. Foss AJE, Harwood RH, Osborn F et al. Falls and health status in elderly women following second eye cataract surgery: a randomised controlled trial. *Age Ageing.* 2006;35:66–71.

3. Tseng VL, Yu F, Lum F et al. Risk of fractures following cataract surgery in Medicare beneficiaries. *J Am Med Assoc.* 2012;308:493–501.

4. Müller A, Keeffe JE, Taylor HR. Changes in eye care utilization following an eye health promotion campaign. *Clin Exp Optom.* 2007;35:305–9.

5. Puent BD, Klein BE, Klein R et al. Factors related to vision care in an older adult cohort. *Optom Vis Sci.* 2005;82:612–16.

6. Day L, Fildes B, Gordon I et al. Randomised factorial trial of falls prevention among older people living in their own homes. *Br Med J.* 2002;325:128–31.

7. Cumming RG, Ivers R, Clemson L et al. Improving vision to prevent falls in frail older people: a randomized trial. *J Am Geriatr Soc.* 2007;55:175–81.

8. Elliott DB, Chapman GJ. Adaptive gait changes due to spectacle magnification and dioptric blur in older people. *Invest Ophth Vis Sci.* 2010;51:718–22.

9. Elliott DB. The Glenn A. Fry Award Lecture 2013: blurred vision, spectacle correction, and falls in older adults. *Optom Vis Sci.* 2014;91:593–601.

10. Lord SR, Dayhew J, Sc BA et al. Multifocal glasses impair edge-contrast sensitivity and depth perception and increase the risk of falls in older people. *J Am Geriatr Soc.* 2002;50:1760–6.

11. Johnson L, Buckley JG, Harley C et al. Use of single-vision eyeglasses improves stepping precision and safety when elderly habitual multifocal wearers negotiate a raised surface. *J Am Geriatr Soc.* 2008;56:178–80.

12. Johnson L, Buckley JG, Scally AJ et al. Multifocal spectacles increase variability in toe clearance and risk of tripping in the elderly. *Invest Ophth Vis Sci.* 2007;48:1466–71.

13. Menant JC, St. George RJ, Sandery B et al. Older people contact more obstacles when wearing multifocal glasses and performing a secondary visual task. *J Am Geriatr Soc.* 2009;57:1833–8.

14. Connell BR, Wolf SL, Group AF. Environmental and behavioral circumstances associated with falls at home among healthy elderly individuals. *Arch Phys Med Rehab.* 1997;78:179–86.

15. Davies J, Kemp G, Stevens G et al. Bifocal/varifocal spectacles, lighting and missed-step accidents. *Saf Sci.* 2001;38:211–26.

16. Haran MJ, Cameron ID, Ivers RQ et al. Effect on falls of providing single lens distance vision glasses to multifocal glasses wearers: VISIBLE randomised controlled trial. *Br Med J.* 2010;340:c2265.

17. Haran MJ, Lord SR, Cameron ID et al. Preventing falls in older multifocal glasses wearers by providing single-lens distance glasses: the protocol for the VISIBLE randomised controlled trial. *BMC Geriatr.* 2009;9:10.

18. Campbell AJ, Robertson MC, La Grow SJ et al. Randomised controlled trial of prevention of falls in people aged >= 75 with severe visual impairment: the VIP trial. *Br Med J.* 2005;331:817.

19. La Grow S, Robertson MC, Campbell AJ et al. Reducing hazard related falls in people 75 years and older with significant visual impairment: how did a successful program work? *Inj Prev.* 2006;12:296–301.

20. Dillon L, Clemson L, Ramulu P et al. A systematic review and meta-analysis of exercise-based falls prevention strategies in adults aged 50+ years with visual impairment. *Ophthalmic Physiol Opt.* 2018;38:456–67.

21. Keay L, Dillon L, Clemson L et al. PrevenTing Falls in a high-risk, vision-impaired population through specialist ORientation and Mobility services: protocol for the PlaTFORM randomised trial. *Inj Prev.* 2018;24:459–66.

22

Footwear, Orthoses, Walking Aids, Wearable Technology, and Restraint Devices for Fall Prevention

Hylton B. Menz

As discussed in Chapter 1, falls result from the interaction between intrinsic risk factors (i.e. those pertaining to the individual, such as poor vision and reduced strength) and extrinsic risk factors (i.e. those relating to environmental hazards). The interface between the individual and their environment is also important and can be modified by a range of physical assistive devices, which are used by approximately one in seven people aged over 65 years [1]. Devices to be addressed in this chapter include footwear, orthoses, walking aids, wearable technology, and physical restraints. The demonstrated and potential impact of each of these approaches on falls is discussed.

Footwear

As outlined in Chapter 6, many older people wear sub-optimal footwear, which may impair balance and increase the risk of falling. Specifically, shoes with elevated heels, excessive midsole cushioning, and inadequate slip resistance have been shown to be detrimental to balance [2], and the wearing of socks or slippers has been associated with incident falls [3–5] and fractures [6]. Optimizing footwear in older people, either by minimizing the use of potentially hazardous footwear or by encouraging use of footwear with balance-enhancing design features, therefore has some potential as a fall prevention strategy. Based on evidence from laboratory-based gait and balance studies and prospective fall risk factor studies, the ideal safe shoe for older people at risk of falling is considered to be a shoe with a low, broad, firm heel with 10° bevel to prevent slipping, fixation using laces, buckles, or Velcro straps, a supportive heel collar around the ankle, a 15° anterior rocker sole to prevent tripping, and a slip-resistant outer sole [2] (see Figure 22.1). Three randomized trials of multi-faceted podiatry interventions incorporating footwear advice and provision of more appropriate footwear based on these recommendations have demonstrated an overall 27% reduction in fall rate [7].

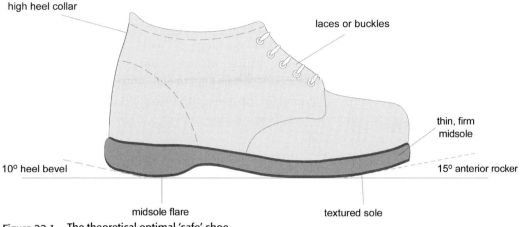

high heel collar

laces or buckles

thin, firm
midsole

10° heel bevel

15° anterior rocker

midsole flare

textured sole

Figure 22.1   The theoretical optimal 'safe' shoe.

However, whether footwear designed to enhance balance can prevent falls as a stand-alone intervention is unclear. Several prototype shoes have been developed, including shoes with very broad midsoles to improve lateral stability reactions [8], shoe outsole modifications to optimize slip resistance on icy surfaces [9, 10], shoes encompassing multiple design features known to be beneficial for balance [11], and even shoes which detect postural sway and automatically perform a corrective backwards step using an in-built motion device [12]. Although improvements in some aspects of balance (including prevention of slipping incidents [10]) have been reported with these footwear designs, it remains to be seen whether they are effective in preventing falls and whether older people are prepared to wear them, as many design features that are optimal for balance may not be aesthetically acceptable [13].

Indoor footwear poses a particular challenge in relation to fall prevention, as it tends to be less supportive than outdoor footwear, is infrequently replaced, and is selected primarily for comfort [14]. The most frequently worn indoor footwear is slippers, which often feature soft midsoles and smooth outsoles, and have been shown to increase the risk of falls [3–5]. However, not all slippers are equally hazardous, and there is some potential to improve the safety of slippers while maintaining the desired degree of comfort. Menz et al. [15] recently reported that slippers with a thin, firm sole, firm heel counter, and Velcro fastening improved gait and balance in older women compared to soft, backless slippers, and despite being perceived to be heavier, were more comfortable.

In older people who do not want to wear slippers, non-slip socks have been proposed as a safer alternative to standard socks or hosiery, and many inpatient settings have adopted non-slip socks as footwear to prevent falls [16]. However, whether non-slip socks are effective at increasing slip resistance and preventing falls is uncertain. Although non-slip socks appear to offer better slip resistance compared to standard socks and slippers, they may be no better than going barefoot or wearing compression stockings [17–19]. Furthermore, quality improvement studies in inpatient settings incorporating non-slip socks have not demonstrated consistent reductions in slipping incidents [16]. In one study, there was a 33% reduction in slipping on the floor with urine, but this was partly offset by increases in falls resulting from getting out of a chair (12%) or from an unknown cause (19%) [20].

These findings suggest that minimizing the use of potentially hazardous footwear or wearing appropriate footwear in combination with other interventions such as orthoses and foot exercises may have a role in preventing falls, but there is limited evidence for the effectiveness of specialized footwear or hosiery as a stand-alone intervention.

Orthoses

Orthoses are externally applied devices designed to correct or accommodate deformity, improve balance and gait patterns, and reduce pain. The most commonly used orthoses in relation to fall prevention are *foot orthoses* (insoles placed inside the shoe that alter the timing and magnitude of the ground reaction forces acting on the plantar aspect of the foot) and *ankle-foot orthoses* (braces which extend from the posterior aspect of the lower leg to the plantar surface of the foot) (see Figure 22.2). Orthoses vary considerably in relation to the underlying prescription principles, manufacturing methods, and materials used. However, in the context of fall prevention, the overall goal of orthoses is to improve balance, which may be achieved by improving mechanical stability and/or enhancing sensory feedback from the foot and ankle [21, 22].

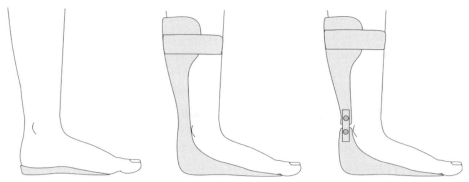

Figure 22.2   Types of orthoses. From left: foot orthosis, solid ankle-foot orthosis, hinged/articulated ankle-foot-orthosis.

Several studies have demonstrated improvements in a range of balance tests in older people using a variety of foot orthoses, including custom-moulded, contoured foot orthoses [23–26], flat insoles with a raised projection around the periphery of the heel [27, 28], textured insoles [29], and insoles which generate a vibratory stimulus to the plantar surface of the foot [30, 31]. No clinical trials with adequate follow-up have demonstrated that the use of foot orthoses in isolation is effective at reducing falls, although as mentioned previously, three randomized trials of multi-faceted podiatry interventions (which all incorporated pre-fabricated, contoured foot orthoses) have demonstrated an overall 27% reduction in fall rate [32]. Similarly, several laboratory-based studies have demonstrated improvements in balance and gait when wearing ankle-foot orthoses, particularly following stroke [32–35], but whether these improvements translate to a reduction in the incidence of falls is yet to be determined.

As with the evidence pertaining to footwear, these findings suggest that there may be a role for foot orthoses and ankle-foot orthoses in preventing falls when used in combination with other foot-related interventions. However, given that orthoses have also been shown to be detrimental to balance in some studies [36, 37], it is essential that such devices are appropriately prescribed by trained health professionals, taking into account individual variations in lower limb structure and function. Furthermore, the acceptability and practicality of ankle-foot orthoses needs to be carefully considered in frailer older people who may have difficulty securing them in the correct position and removing them when not required.

Walking Aids

A range of walking aids are commonly recommended to older people as a means of increasing their walking ability, including walking sticks (single or four-pronged), crutches (axillary or forearm), and frames (forearm support, rollator, and pick-up) [38, 39] (see Figure 22.3). The main indications for a walking aid are excessive pain on weight bearing, leg muscle weakness and/or control, instability, shortness of breath, poor vision, and poor distal lower limb proprioception. These deficits may either be associated with acute events such as surgery or major illness, or with chronic conditions leading to a more gradual decline in physical abilities. Many of these deficits increase an individual's risk of falling. Thus, walking with an appropriate walking aid may reduce the risk of falling by compensating for these risk factors and thus lessening their potential to contribute to a fall.

A walking aid is best prescribed by a health professional after an individualized assessment of gait, muscle strength, balance, and pain [40–43]. As different

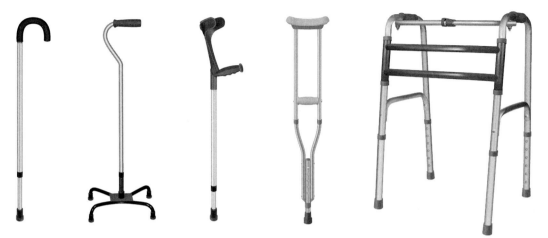

Figure 22.3   Commonly used walking aids in older people. From left: standard walking stick, four-pronged (or quad) stick, forearm support stick, axillary crutches, pick-up frame.

walking aids have different characteristics, the person's abilities and environment need to be considered when prescribing an aid. For example, a rollator frame may be difficult to manoeuvre in a small bathroom, a pick-up frame may be unsafe for someone who is unable to stand unsupported while moving the frame forwards, and the stability of a quad stick may encourage a person to bear excessive weight through their upper limb. A person may also need to use different aids when walking outdoors than when indoors [44]. The skill required to use an aid also should be considered. For example, attentional demands have been found to be greater with a pick-up frame than with a rollator frame [45].

The potential benefits of walking aids need to be considered in the context of several disadvantages, including social stigma [46], adverse effects on upper limbs due to additional load-bearing [47], and over-reliance on the aid. Once an older person has learnt to walk with a walking aid, it may be difficult for them to walk unaided [48], and they may be less safe when they attempt to stand or reach without support. This may interfere with their ability to carry out activities of daily living independently. The cost of walking aids may also be prohibitive for many older people, with studies demonstrating that low income and lack of health care insurance are barriers to their use [49]. Indeed, the World Health Organization estimates that only one in ten people have sufficient access to affordable assistive devices, and have developed the Global Cooperation on Assistive Technology initiative to address this need [50].

Although the available evidence suggests that walking aids enhance mobility, activity, and participation in older people [51], their effectiveness in preventing falls is less certain. Somewhat paradoxically, several studies have found that use of a walking aid is associated with a *higher* risk of falling [52, 53]. In most cases, it is likely that the use of a walking aid is merely a marker for a gait or balance impairment, i.e. the impairment causes the increased risk of falls, not the use of the walking aid *per se* [54]. However, there is also evidence that walking aids may directly cause falls due to tripping over the aid or catching the aid on furniture [55], or indirectly, by increasing the attentional demands of weightbearing activities or interfering with limb movement when responding to perturbations [56]. To date, no studies have found that walking aid prescription alone is effective in preventing falls, although some multi-factorial interventions that include the use of walking aids have demonstrated significant reductions in the rate of falls [57].

Wearable Technology

As outlined in Chapter 13, recent advances in electronic component miniaturization have given rise to a range of wearable technology devices based on inertial motion sensors that have practical applications to gait assessment and detection of falls [58]. When combined with biofeedback, such devices may also have a role in fall prevention by compensating for sensory and neuromuscular deficits associated with neurological conditions such as stroke, diabetic peripheral neuropathy, and Parkinson's disease.

Foot drop is a common consequence of stroke which results in insufficient foot clearance during walking, thereby increasing the risk of trip-related falls [59]. However, by electrically stimulating the common peroneal nerve at the head of the fibula with a surface electrode, the ankle dorsiflexor muscles can be activated to correct this abnormal walking pattern. Functional electrical stimulation devices for foot drop were first developed in the 1960s but were not widely adopted due to their cumbersome construction. In recent years, however, wireless systems which use either heel switches (Bioness™) or accelerometers (WalkAide™) to determine the appropriate timing of nerve stimulation have been made commercially available. Although no studies have specifically determined whether these devices can prevent falls, several studies have demonstrated improvements in gait speed and range of motion, and decreased spasticity [60]. Interestingly, comparative trials have found that functional electrical stimulation devices produce equivalent gait outcomes to ankle-foot orthoses [61]. However, acceptability is generally higher for functional electrical stimulation devices [62–64], possibly due to improved comfort, appearance, and ability to freely move the ankle.

Another recently developed wearable aid with possible applications to fall prevention in people with diabetic peripheral neuropathy is WalkJoy™. This device consists of an accelerometer and vibrotactile actuator contained in a small casing that is attached to the legs with an elastic strap. The underlying principle of this device is to replace the sensation of the foot striking the ground that is diminished or absent in people with neuropathy. To achieve this, the accelerometer detects the vertical acceleration generated at heel strike, and then immediately applies an equivalent vibration signal to the tibial tuberosity. This works because neuropathy has a distal to proximal pattern of progression, the sensory nerves around the knee retain their function in a large number of people with neuropathy and are therefore able to 'compensate' for plantar sensory loss. To date, however, no studies have been conducted to assess the effectiveness of the device in preventing falls.

Finally, a novel shoe-mounted device to prevent freezing of gait in people with Parkinson's disease has recently been developed. The device contains a laser which projects a thin line on the ground perpendicular to the direction of travel, thereby providing an external visual cue to assist step initiation [65]. Although visual cueing is a well-established intervention approach [66] and walking stick-mounted laser cues have shown modest benefits in relation to freezing episodes in people with Parkinson's disease [67, 68], evidence to support the shoe-mounted device is currently limited to case studies [65].

Although promising, the effectiveness of wearable technology for the prevention of falls is yet to be established, and much work still needs to be done to ensure that these devices are acceptable to older people from the perspective of comfort, practicality, and cost.

Physical Restraint

Physical restraint is defined as 'any action or procedure that prevents a person's free body movement to a position of choice and/or normal access to his/her body by the use of any method, attached or adjacent to a person's body that he/she cannot control or remove easily' [69]. Examples of physical restraints include wrist or leg cuffs, belts, vests, or jackets to stop a person sitting up in bed or getting out of a chair, bed rails, and use of low chairs or beds to prevent the person standing up [70]. Physical restraints are used in residential aged care facilities and acute care hospitals in some countries to control disruptive or potentially dangerous behaviours and prevent falls [71]. This practice sometimes arises out of concerns regarding legal liability in the case of injury.

The use of restraints is highly controversial and has declined since the 1990s because of legislative changes focused on the rights of older people in residential aged care [70, 72]. It is clear that the widespread use of restraints impinges on an older person's autonomy and personal freedom, with associated philosophical and legal ramifications [73]. Furthermore, the external pressure required to physically restrain an older person may directly cause injuries such as skin tears, pressure sores, and nerve damage [74], and several deaths have been specifically attributed to the use of restraints leading to mechanical asphyxia [75].

The effectiveness of physical restraint in the prevention of falls is questionable. A recent systematic review found nine studies evaluating the use of bed rails, belts, and wheelchairs in acute care hospitals and nursing homes, and concluded that these approaches were not effective at preventing falls [76]. In one study conducted in an acute care facility, fall-related injuries were more severe in those who were restrained compared to those who were not, which was attributed to patients falling more awkwardly, or in the case of bed rails, from a greater height [77]. Long-term restraint use is also likely to lead to deconditioning, thereby increasing the risk of falls during unrestrained periods [78]. Further confirmation of the ineffectiveness of physical restraints is provided by studies in which physical restraints are removed and no increase in falls or fall-related injuries is subsequently observed [79, 80].

Contemporary aged care practice guidelines recommend against the use of restraints where possible and advocate alternative strategies such as such as bed alarms, removal of hazardous furniture, and improved layout of aged care facilities [72]. The older person should also be given the opportunity to minimize their physiological risk of falling through appropriate medication use, management of medical risk factors, appropriate footwear, and effective exercise programmes to improve strength and balance. If these alternatives are not effective, restraint may need to be considered as a last resort; however, this needs to be preceded by a full documented assessment involving consultation with the resident and their legal representative. The least restrictive form of restraint to ensure the older person's safety should be implemented, and all restraint decisions need to be subjected to regular monitoring and review [72].

Conclusions

A range of physical assistive devices have been discussed in this chapter. These impact either positively or negatively on the physical abilities or safety of older people. However, for each type of assistive device discussed above, more research is required to clarify its potential contribution to fall prevention. Each of these assistive devices should be carefully prescribed following assessment of the person's abilities and needs.

REFERENCES

1. Kaye HS, Kang T, LaPlante MP. *Mobility Device Use in the United States. Disability Statistics Report 14.* Washington, DC: US Department of Education, National Institute on Disability and Rehabilitation Research; 2000.
2. Menant JC, Steele JR, Menz HB et al. Optimizing footwear for older people at risk of falls. *J Rehabil Res Dev.* 2008;45:1167–81.

3. Larsen ER, Mosekilde L, Foldspang A. Correlates of falling during 24 h among elderly Danish community residents. *Prev Med.* 2004;39:389–98.

4. Koepsell TD, Wolf ME, Buchner DM et al. Footwear style and risk of falls in older adults. *J Am Geriatr Soc.* 2004;52:1495–501.

5. Menz HB, Morris ME, Lord SR. Footwear characteristics and risk of indoor and outdoor falls in older people. *Gerontology.* 2006;52:174–80.

6. Kelsey JL, Procter-Gray E, Nguyen U-SDT et al. Footwear and falls in the home among older individuals in the MOBILIZE Boston Study. *Footwear Sci.* 2010;2:123–9.

7. Wylie G, Torrens C, Campbell P et al. Podiatry interventions to prevent falls in older people: a systematic review and meta-analysis. *Age Ageing.* 2019;48:327–36.

8. Yamaguchi T, Cheng KC, McKay SM et al. Footwear width and balance-recovery reactions: a new approach to improving lateral stability in older adults. *Gerontechnology.* 2015;13:359–67.

9. Yamaguchi T, Hsu J, Li Y et al. Efficacy of a rubber outsole with a hybrid surface pattern for preventing slips on icy surfaces. *Appl Ergon.* 2015;51:9–17.

10. McKiernan FE. A simple gait-stabilizing device reduces outdoor falls and nonserious injurious falls in fall-prone older people during the winter. *J Am Geriatr Soc.* 2005;53:943–7.

11. Menz HB, Auhl M, Munteanu SE. Preliminary evaluation of prototype footwear and insoles to optimise balance and gait in older people. *BMC Geriatr.* 2017;17:212.

12. Campbell AJ, Robertson MC, La Grow SJ et al. Randomised controlled trial of prevention of falls in people aged > or =75 with severe visual impairment: the VIP trial. *BMJ Clin Res.* 2005;331:817.

13. Davis A, Murphy A, Haines TP. "Good for older ladies, not me": how elderly women choose their shoes. *J Am Podiatr Med Assoc.* 2013;103:465–70.

14. Munro BJ, Steele JR. Household-shoe wearing and purchasing habits: a survey of people aged 65 years and older. *J Am Podiatr Med Assoc.* 1999;89:506–14.

15. Menz HB, Auhl M, Munteanu SE. Effects of indoor footwear on balance and gait patterns in community-dwelling older women. *Gerontology.* 2017;63:129–36.

16. Hartung B, Lalonde M. The use of non-slip socks to prevent falls among hospitalized older adults: a literature review. *Geriatr Nurs.* 2017;38:412–16.

17. Chari S, Haines T, Varghese P et al. Are non-slip socks really 'non-slip'? An analysis of slip resistance. *BMC Geriatr.* 2009;9:39.

18. Hatton AL, Sturnieks DL, Lord SR et al. Effects of non-slip socks on the gait patterns of older people when walking on a slippery surface. *J Am Podiatr Med Assoc.* 2013;103:471–9.

19. Hubscher M, Thiel C, Schmidt J et al. Slip resistance of non-slip socks: an accelerometer-based approach. *Gait Posture.* 2011;33:740–2.

20. Meddaugh DI, Friedenberg DL, Knisley R. Special socks for special people: falls in special care units. *Geriatr Nurs.* 1996;17:24–6.

21. Aboutorabi A, Bahramizadeh M, Arazpour M et al. A systematic review of the effect of foot orthoses and shoe characteristics on balance in healthy older subjects. *Prosthet Orthot Int.* 2016;40:170–81.

22. Hatton AL, Rome K, Dixon J, Martin DJ, McKeon PO. Footwear interventions: a review of their sensorimotor and mechanical effects on balance performance and gait in older adults. *J Am Podiatr Med Assoc.* 2013;103:516–33.

23. Gross MT, Mercer VS, Lin FC. Effects of foot orthoses on balance in older adults. *J Orthop Sports Phys Ther*. 2012;42:649–57.

24. de Morais Barbosa C, Barros Bertolo M, Marques Neto JF et al. The effect of foot orthoses on balance, foot pain and disability in elderly women with osteoporosis: a randomized clinical trial. *Rheumatology*. 2013;52:515–22.

25. Mulford D, Taggart HM, Nivens A et al. Arch support use for improving balance and reducing pain in older adults. *Appl Nurs Res*. 2008;21:153–8.

26. Chen TH, Chou LW, Tsai MW et al. Effectiveness of a heel cup with an arch support insole on the standing balance of the elderly. *Clin Interv Aging*. 2014;9:351–6.

27. Maki BE, Perry SD, Norrie RG et al. Effect of facilitation of sensation from plantar foot-surface boundaries on postural stabilization in young and older adults. *J Gerontol*. 1999;54A:M281–7.

28. Perry SD, Radtke A, McIlroy WE et al. Efficacy and effectiveness of a balance-enhancing insole. *J Gerontol A Biol Sci Med Sci*. 2008;63:595–602.

29. Palluel E, Nougier V, Olivier I. Do spike insoles enhance postural stability and plantar-surface cutaneous sensitivity in the elderly? *Age*. 2008;30:53–61.

30. Galica AM, Kang HG, Priplata AA et al. Subsensory vibrations to the feet reduce gait variability in elderly fallers. *Gait Posture*. 2009;30:383–7.

31. Stephen DG, Wilcox BJ, Niemi JB et al. Baseline-dependent effect of noise-enhanced insoles on gait variability in healthy elderly walkers. *Gait Posture*. 2012;36:537–40.

32. Yalla SV, Crews RT, Fleischer AE et al. An immediate effect of custom-made ankle foot orthoses on postural stability in older adults. *Clin Biomech*. 2014;29:1081–8.

33. Cikajlo I, Osrecki K, Burger H. The effects of different types of ankle-foot orthoses on postural responses in individuals with walking impairments. *Int J Rehabil Res*. 2016;39:313–19.

34. Rao N, Aruin AS. Role of ankle foot orthoses in functional stability of individuals with stroke. *Disabil Rehabil Assist Technol*. 2016;11:595–8.

35. Wang C, Goel R, Rahemi H et al. Effectiveness of daily use of bilateral custom-made ankle-foot orthoses on balance, fear of falling, and physical activity in older adults: a randomized controlled trial. *Gerontology*. 2018;65:1–9.

36. Hatton AL, Dixon J, Rome K et al. Altering gait by way of stimulation of the plantar surface of the foot: the immediate effect of wearing textured insoles in older fallers. *J Foot Ankle Res*. 2012;5:11.

37. Panwalkar N, Aruin AS. Role of ankle foot orthoses in the outcome of clinical tests of balance. *Disabil Rehabil Assist Technol*. 2013;8:314–20.

38. Ogle AA. Canes, crutches, walkers, and other ambulation aids. *Phys Med Rehabil*. 2000;14:485–92.

39. Bradley SM, Hernandez CR. Geriatric assistive devices. *Am Fam Physician*. 2011;84:405–11.

40. Breuer J. Assistive devices and adapted equipment for ambulation programs for geriatric patients. *Phys Occup Ther Geriatr*. 1981;1:51–77.

41. Hall J, Clarke A, Harrison R. Guide lines for prescription of walking frames. *Physiotherapy*. 1990;76:118–20.

42. Holliday P, Fernie G. Assistive devices: aids to independence. In: Pickles B, Compton A, Cott C et al. (Eds.) *Physiotherapy with Older People*. London: WB Saunders; 1995:360–81.

43. Prajapati C, Watkins C, Cullen H et al. The 'S' test: a preliminary study of an instrument for selecting the most appropriate mobility aid. *Clin Rehabil.* 1996;10:314–18.

44. York J. Mobility methods selected for use in home and community environments. *Phys Ther.* 1989;69:736–47.

45. Wright D, Kemp T. The dual-task methodology and assessing the attentional demands of ambulation with walking devices. *Phys Ther.* 1992;72:306–15.

46. Aminzadeh F, Edwards N. Exploring seniors' views on the use of assistive devices in fall prevention. *Public Health Nurs.* 1998;15:297–304.

47. Crosbie WJ, Nicol AC. Aided gait in rheumatoid arthritis following knee arthroplasty. *Arch Phys Med Rehabil.* 1990;71:299–303.

48. Carr J, Shepherd R. *Neurological Rehabilitation: Optimizing Motor Performance.* Oxford: Butterworth-Heinemann; 1998.

49. Mathieson KM, Kronenfeld JJ, Keith VM. Maintaining functional independence in elderly adults: the roles of health status and financial resources in predicting home modifications and use of mobility equipment. *Gerontologist.* 2002;42:24–31.

50. World Health Organization. Global Cooperation on Assistive Technology (GATE). 2014. www.who.int/disabilities/technology/gate/en/ (accessed April 2021).

51. Bertrand K, Raymond MH, Miller WC et al. Walking aids for enabling activity and participation: a systematic review. *Am J Phys Med Rehabil.* 2017;96:894–903.

52. West BA, Bhat G, Stevens J et al. Assistive device use and mobility-related factors among adults aged≥65years. *J Safety Res.* 2015;55:147–50.

53. Roman de Mettelinge T, Cambier D. Understanding the relationship between walking aids and falls in older adults: a prospective cohort study. *J Geriatr Phys Ther.* 2015;38:127–32.

54. Mahoney JE, Sager MA, Jalaluddin M. Use of an ambulation assistive device predicts functional decline associated with hospitalization. *J Gerontol A Biol Sci Med Sci.* 1999;54: M83–8.

55. Mann WC, Granger C, Hurren D et al. An analysis of problems with canes encountered by elderly persons. *Phys Occup Ther Geriatr.* 1995;13:25–49.

56. Bateni H, Maki BE. Assistive devices for balance and mobility: benefits, demands, and adverse consequences. *Arch Phys Med Rehabil.* 2005;86:134–45.

57. Hopewell S, Adedire O, Copsey BJ et al. Multifactorial and multiple component interventions for preventing falls in older people living in the community. *Cochrane Database Sys Rev.* 2018;7:CD012221.

58. Godfrey A. Wearables for independent living in older adults: gait and falls. *Maturitas.* 2017;100:16–26.

59. Weerdesteyn V, de Niet M, van Duijnhoven HJ et al. Falls in individuals with stroke. *J Rehabil Res Dev.* 2008;45:1195–213.

60. Bosch PR, Harris JE, Wing K. Review of therapeutic electrical stimulation for dorsiflexion assist and orthotic substitution from the American Congress of Rehabilitation Medicine Stroke Movement Interventions subcommittee. *Arch Phys Med Rehabil.* 2014;95:390–6.

61. Prenton S, Hollands KL, Kenney LPJ et al. Functional electrical stimulation and ankle foot orthoses provide equivalent therapeutic effects on foot drop: a meta-analysis providing direction for future research. *J Rehabil Med.* 2018;50:129–39.

62. Kluding PM, Dunning K, O'Dell MW et al. Foot drop stimulation versus ankle foot orthosis after stroke: 30-week outcomes. *Stroke.* 2013;44:1660–9.

63. Everaert DG, Stein RB, Abrams GM et al. Effect of a foot-drop stimulator and ankle-foot orthosis on walking performance after stroke: a multicenter randomized controlled trial. *Neurorehabil Neural Repair.* 2013;27:579–91.

64. Dunning K, O'Dell MW, Kluding P et al. Peroneal stimulation for foot drop after stroke: a systematic review. *Am J Phys Med Rehabil.* 2015;94:649–64.

65. Ferraye MU, Fraix V, Pollak P et al. The laser-shoe: a new form of continuous ambulatory cueing for patients with Parkinson's disease. *Parkinsonism Relat Disord.* 2016;29:127–8.

66. Ginis P, Nackaerts E, Nieuwboer A et al. Cueing for people with Parkinson's disease with freezing of gait: a narrative review of the state-of-the-art and novel perspectives. *Ann Phys Rehabil Med.* 2018;61:407–13.

67. McCandless PJ, Evans BJ, Janssen J et al. Effect of three cueing devices for people with Parkinson's disease with gait initiation difficulties. *Gait Posture.* 2016;44:7–11.

68. Donovan S, Lim C, Diaz N et al. Laserlight cues for gait freezing in Parkinson's disease: an open-label study. *Parkinsonism Relat Disord.* 2011;17:240–5.

69. Bleijlevens MH, Wagner LM, Capezuti E et al. Physical restraints: consensus of a research definition using a modified Delphi technique. *J Am Geriatr Soc.* 2016;64:2307–10.

70. Retsas AP. Survey findings describing the use of physical restraints in nursing homes in Victoria, Australia. *Int J Nurs Stud.* 1998;35:184–91.

71. Evans LK, Strumpf NE. Tying down the elderly. A review of the literature on physical restraint. *J Am Geriatr Soc.* 1989;37:65–74.

72. Commonwealth of Australia. *Decision-Making Tool: Supporting a Restraint Free Environment in Residential Aged Care.* Canberra: Commonwealth of Australia; 2012.

73. Griffith R. Restraint and the older patient: legal and professional considerations. *Br J Nurs.* 2014;23:132–3.

74. Evans D, Wood J, Lambert L. Patient injury and physical restraint devices: a systematic review. *J Adv Nurs.* 2003;41:274–82.

75. Bellenger EN, Ibrahim JE, Lovell JJ et al. The nature and extent of physical restraint-related deaths in nursing homes: a systematic review. *J Aging Health.* 2018;30:1042–61.

76. Sze TW, Leng CY, Lin SK. The effectiveness of physical restraints in reducing falls among adults in acute care hospitals and nursing homes: a systematic review. *JBI Libr Syst Rev.* 2012;10:307–51.

77. Tan KM, Austin B, Shaughnassy M et al. Falls in an acute hospital and their relationship to restraint use. *Ir J Med Sci.* 2005;174:28–31.

78. Tinetti ME, Liu WL, Ginter SF. Mechanical restraint use and fall-related injuries among residents of skilled nursing facilities. *Ann Intern Med.* 1992;116:369–74.

79. Capezuti E, Strumpf NE, Evans LK et al. The relationship between physical restraint removal and falls and injuries among nursing home residents. *J Gerontol A Biol Sci Med Sci.* 1998;53:M47–52.

80. Evans LK, Strumpf NE, Allen-Taylor SL et al. A clinical trial to reduce restraints in nursing homes. *J Am Geriatr Soc.* 1997;45:675–81.

23

Environmental Interventions to Prevent Falls at Home and in the Community

Lindy Clemson and Alison Pighills

As indicated in Chapter 12, the homes of many older people have environmental hazards [1–3] and the majority of these are amenable to modification. This chapter outlines environmental assessment, adaptations, and strategies to prevent falls and reviews the literature for interventions delivered individually or as part of multi-faceted programmes. It discusses the breadth and quality of assessments available; potential enablers and challenges to hazard removal and design strategies for minimizing older people's risk of falling at home and in public places. Fall prevention strategies involving the provision of new glasses and assistive devices are presented in Chapters 21 and 22 respectively.

Environmental Interventions to Reduce Fall Hazards

Environmental interventions can be characterized as programmes that remove fall hazards, provide assistive technologies and devices, or deliver information on environmental fall risk prevention [4–6]. Most fall hazard reduction research has been conducted in the home environment, as opposed to outdoor and public places. Assistive devices and technologies encompass personal mobility devices, body worn aids (e.g. anti-slip devices for shoes), aids to compensate for sensory loss (e.g. spectacles), protective technologies (monitoring systems), and self-care aids (e.g. grab bars) [5]. Information/education may cover environmental fall risks with examples of solutions or self-assessment home hazard check lists.

Fall hazard reduction encompasses environmental assessment, adaptation, and modification to reduce fall hazards in and around the home, outdoors, or both [6]. A successful home fall-hazard approach uses multiple strategies to raise the person's awareness of potential hazards and utilizes adaptations to the home along with behavioural safety strategies to prevent falls [7–9]. One home hazard reduction trial [10] also found falls reduced outside the home suggesting awareness of the environment may be generalizable. It is important to begin with the 'F' questions: (i) 'Tell me about your Fall/s?' and (ii) 'What do you think contributed to you Falling?'. Problem solving begins with engaging the person in the problem and the solution. Community safety interventions have not been tested in individual trials but have been included in multi-component programmes where strategies have been incorporated to manage crossing roads, negotiating uneven surfaces, and safe travel on public transport [11], or in community education programmes [12].

The quality, intensity, and consequent outcomes of environmental assessment and intervention have been framed in terms of person–environment fit models [9, 13]. For example, Law et al.'s [14] Person, Environment, Occupation (PEO) model posits that it is the interaction and fit between the person, environment, and occupation (task/activity) that is important, and that when one element is altered then this impacts on the others. Competence–environmental press models [15] further elaborate the connection between the person's competencies and the demand ('press') placed on the individual by the environment. Thus, the person's capacity and their task performance should be assessed and considered when determining environmental solutions.

Environmental interventions modify risk by enabling people to mobilize and engage in activities in a safer way, compensating for specific risk factors known to be predictive of falls (such as cognitive, visual, sensorimotor, balance, and gait impairments), modifying risky behaviours, or minimizing exposure to hazardous situations [6]. Some interventions, such as the provision of new glasses and non-slip shoes, might increase outdoor activity and exposure to risk, and increase falls. Conversely, activity avoidance to lessen fall risk may lead to physical deconditioning and increase fall risk. Importantly, one home fall-hazard reduction intervention [16] demonstrated that while activity avoidance was linked to higher fall rates, the intervention did not result in participants limiting activity to enhance their safety.

Profiling Risk to Environment and Activity

In a US study of indoor falls, Stevens et al. [17] found that most non-injurious falls (n = 528) occurred in living areas and bedrooms when the participants were undertaking everyday tasks. Injurious falls (n = 255) were more likely to occur in bathrooms, kitchens, and on stairs. In a Dutch study, Bleijlevens et al. [18] found frailer people sustained injurious falls mostly in the hall and bathroom, and predominately when visiting the toilet, whereas a more active group fell in other indoor locations and predominantly during activities of daily living. Hill et al. [19] found the bedroom was the location of most post-hospital injurious falls, reflecting the need to focus on bedroom activities and safety for this group with functional limitations.

Older people who fall outdoors are more often active, vigorous, walk quickly, and undertake many activities [20, 21]. Rushing is frequently mentioned as a cause, and falls are often attributed to unnoticed balance impairments or deteriorating vision. Bleiljevens et al. [18] found two categories of people who suffer outdoor injurious falls: those who fall near the home (garden, access paths, climbing ladders) and predominantly during instrumental activities of daily living, and a second group who experience injurious falls away from home, occurring predominately during walking, grocery shopping, or vigorous activity. In a US study, middle-aged men suffered the most injurious falls while using ladders and women suffered more trip-related injuries than men, the latter possibly due to gait or footwear differences [22].

A qualitative study [23] investigating reasons why older people recently discharged from hospital do not adopt fall-hazard recommendations has highlighted the need to not make assumptions about where risk prevention should be focused. For example, one older woman was provided with bathing aids, which she did not use as she was concerned her daughter would not be happy with them in her bathroom. Instead, an interview revealed that she was a very active woman preadmission who intended to return to previous activities, i.e. she was more concerned with how she might cope with stairs at train stations and how she might safely clean the gutters of her house. Ladder safety, home supports, and community mobility safety would have been a more appropriate fall prevention focus.

Environmental Adaptations as a Single Intervention

Systematic reviews have shown home fall-hazard reduction as a single intervention can significantly reduce falls [24, 25]. The most recent Cochrane review [25] found that home safety assessment and modification interventions were effective in reducing the rate of falls (RaR: 0.81, 95% CI: 0.68, 0.97; 6 trials, 4208 participants) and risk of falling (i.e. the number of people falling, RR: 0.88, 95% CI: 0.80, 0.96; 7 trials, 4051 participants). These interventions were more effective in people at higher risk of falls and for sub-groups of people, including those with vision impairment, those who had had a history of falling in the past year, those who had been hospitalized for a fall, and those with functional limitations [24, 25]. This suggests that this intervention should be primarily applied to people at higher risk rather than to the general population.

The interventions are also more effective when delivered by an occupational therapist [25], suggesting this approach is more sophisticated than the simple removal of hazards. Criteria have been developed as part of a meta-analysis [24] to determine the intensity or quality of home fall-hazard interventions. These include: a comprehensive process of hazard identification and priority setting, use of a validated assessment tool, formal observational evaluation of an older person's functional capacity within the context of their environment, provision of adequate follow-up for adaptations and modifications, and active involvement of the older person in the assessment and priority-setting. Interventions most effective in reducing falls [24, 25] include comprehensive assessments of the older person, the activity in which they are engaged, and the environment, with interventions consisting of person-, activity-, and environment-focused strategies [9].

To illustrate this notion of targeted intervention, the trial by Cumming et al. [10] with 530 community-dwelling older people recently discharged from hospital is useful as it included a sub-group of participants (n = 206) who had fallen in the year prior to the study. The intervention group received a home visit by an occupational therapist who assessed the home for environmental hazards using a validated assessment tool for fall hazards and facilitated any necessary home adaptations. There was a borderline significant reduction in falls in the intervention group as a whole (p = 0.05), and the sub-group analysis showed a significant reduction in the rate of falls among those who had fallen in the year prior to the study (36% reduction). These results were replicated by Pighills et al. [16] when the assessment was delivered by an occupational therapist using the Westmead content-valid assessment tool to identify hazards. It may be that a prior fall raises awareness of potential hazards and motivates older people to adopt environmental changes and implement protective behaviours.

Table 23.1 summarizes the evidence from eight trials that have included high-risk samples and sub-groups. The Chu et al. study [26] conducted in Hong Kong delivered their intervention to people admitted to the emergency department following a fall. They found a significant fall reduction at six months, but this was not maintained at 12 months. The non-significant difference at 12 months may result from insufficient power due to attrition and a low rate of falls in both groups [27]. The authors recommended a booster visit at six months.

The Falls-HIT trial [28] involved 361 people with mobility limitations who had recently been discharged from hospital. The intervention consisted of a home assessment and recommendations in addition to training in the use of mobility aids. It was implemented by an occupational therapist and, if indicated, also by a physiotherapist. At one-year follow-up, the intervention group had 31% fewer falls than the control group, with sub-group analysis revealing that the intervention was particularly effective in those with a history of multiple falls.

Campbell et al. [29] assessed the efficacy of a home safety programme on falls in people aged 75 years and over with severe visual impairment (visual acuity of 6/24 or worse). The intervention consisted of an occupational therapy home assessment and follow-up recommendation letter, along with facilitation of equipment purchase and installation. At the one-year follow-up, there were 41% fewer falls in those who received the home safety intervention compared to the control group.

Table 23.1 Summary of trials of home safety interventions in older people at risk of falls

Study	Participants	Intervention	Main Outcomes	Comments
Campbell 2005 New Zealand [29]	Severe vision impairment n = 391 Aged 75+, mean age: 83.6 (SD 4.8) Community living	Home safety assessment and recommendations delivered by OT Compliance 90% (with ≥1 recommendations)	41% fewer falls in home safety group versus control group IRR: 0.59 (95% CI: 0.42, 0.83)	No difference in reduction of falls at home compared with those away from home
Chu 2017 Hong Kong [26]	Emergency department following a fall n = 198 Aged 65 +	OT fall reduction home visit Compliance 76% environmental hazards; 39% education-fall reduction plans; 68% assistive devices	Non-significant RR: 0.66 (95% CI: 0.33, 1.14)	Effective at six months but not at 12 months Rates of falls reported in both groups were low so sample size not meeting expected power analysis
Cumming 1999 Australia [10]	Recently discharged from hospital n = 530 Aged 65+	Comprehensive home assessment by OT and supervision of home modifications Compliance: 19–75%	Not effective in full sample RR: 0.81 (95% CI: 0.66, 1.00)	Effective for the sub-group with a fall history: RR: 0.64 (95% CI: 0.50, 0.83) Falls reduced to a similar degree outside the home in previous fallers
Nikolaus 2003 [28]	Admitted from home to a geriatric hospital n = 360 Mean age: 81.5 (SD 6.4)	Home assessment by OT and physiotherapist, advice regarding modifications, training in use of mobility devices Compliance 33–83%	Effective in reducing falls in full sample IRR: 0.69 (95% CI: 0.51, 0.97)	More effective in subgroup who had two or more falls in previous 12 months. Effective in reducing proportion of frequent fallers IRR: 0.63 (95% CI: 0.43, 0.94)
Pardessus 2002 France [72]	Hospitalized after a fall n = 60 Aged 65+	Home assessment by OT, advice regarding modifications and how to live safely with fixed hazards Compliance: not described (average 3.6 recommendations)	Not effective in reducing falls RR: 0.87 (95% CI: 0.50, 1.49)	Small sample; underpowered for falls as an outcome measure
Pighills 2011 UK [16]	Fall in previous year n = 238 Aged 70+ Community living	Intervention administered by: (i) an OT (compliance: 88%), or (ii) non-OT trained assessors (compliance: 65%)	OT intervention effective in reducing falls: IRR: 0.54 (95% CI: 0.36, 0.83) Trained assessor intervention less effective in reducing falls: IRR: 0.78 (95% CI: 0.51,1.21)	The interventions had no effect on fear of falling

Notes: OT: occupational therapist, RR: relative risk, CI: confidence interval, IRR: incidence rate ratio

However, there was no difference in the reduction of falls at home compared to those outside the home. This suggests, as with the study by Cumming et al. [10], that the efficacy of the intervention was partly due to the changes made to the environment and partly due to the general fall prevention approach provided by the occupational therapist.

In contrast to the above, the trial by Day et al. [30] was not targeted towards an at-risk group but to a general sample of 1090 community-residing people aged 70 years and over. The home hazard reduction intervention comprised a home assessment by a trained assessor and advice, plus provision of materials and labour for modifications. A validated hazard assessment was not used, rather a pre-determined list of physical attributes for access was used that comprised minimal descriptors of known fall hazards (personal communication). As a single-mode intervention this did not result in a significant reduction in falls (RR: 0.92, 95% CI: 0.78, 1.08). A study by Stevens et al. [2] that was also conducted in a general community population sample was also not effective in reducing falls (RR: 1.11, 95% CI: 0.82, 1.50). The intervention in this study did not meet the intensity or quality criteria to be considered a comprehensive fall hazard assessment as it used a checklist of 11 hazards and advice provided to remediate just three hazards. The intervention resulted in only a small number of environmental changes – a reduction in unsafe steps by 16%, unsafe floor rugs and mats by 14%, rooms with trailing cords by 26%, and unsafe chairs by 12% [31].

Environmental Adaptations in Multi-Component and Multi-Factorial Interventions

Multiple component interventions involve administering two or more of the same interventions to all people in the treatment arm of a trial, whereas multi-factorial interventions involve the initial conduct of an assessment to guide the delivery of intervention components. A Cochrane systematic review concluded that multiple component interventions (17 trials) were likely to reduce falls (moderate level of evidence) [32]. Most of the included trials included exercise and either education or home hazard assessment. The review concluded that the multi-factorial interventions (43 trials) may be effective in reducing falls in older people, although the level of evidence was low. The most common intervention components included in these trials were exercise (37 trials) and environment/ assistive interventions (e.g. home hazard assessment and modifications, referral to occupational therapist) (34 trials), with medication reviews (28 trials) and cognitive behavioural (9 trials) interventions also common.

The design of multi-factorial studies does not allow assessment of the effects of individual strategies or their relative contributions to the success or otherwise of the interventions. In contrast, the factorial design used in the study by Day et al. [30] provides a means for contrasting the effectiveness of combining intervention strategies. They found that as a single intervention strategy, group-based exercise was effective in reducing falls (RR: 0.82, 95% CI: 0.70, 0.97) whereas home modifications (RR: 0.92, 95% CI: 0.78, 1.08) and vision improvement (RR: 0.89, 95% CI: 0.75, 1.04) interventions were not. However, the combined effect of the three interventions was greater than for exercise alone (RR: 0.67, 95% CI: 0.51, 0.88), as was the effect of home modifications in addition to exercise (RR: 0.76, 95% CI: 0.60, 0.95).

There is a great deal of diversity in the type of multi-factorial interventions and the mix of components as well as study designs and some have been effective (e.g. [11, 33–35]) while others have not (e.g. [36–38]). The following trials included an environmental aspect and demonstrated a significant reduction in the rate of falls. Tinetti et al. [34] assessed people for multiple fall risk factors, including home environmental hazards, and tailored the intervention accordingly. The Close et al. study [33] involved a medical assessment for risk factors and a home visit by an occupational therapist for environmental hazard assessment and intervention. The Logan et al. [35] study provided a multi-disciplinary fall prevention service, including balance training, muscle strengthening, and reduction of environmental hazards, education on how to get off the floor, and equipment provision. The Clemson et al. 2004 study [11] was a group-based multi-component programme which facilitated self-management of risks. They included both safe community mobility strategies as well as participants sharing home safety tips and solutions.

There is less evidence on the efficacy of multi-component interventions with injurious falls as an outcome measure. However, one systematic review has reported pooled results of combinations of different interventions on reducing injurious falls [39]. Their results included four different successful intervention combinations with one being exercise, vision assessment and treatment, and environmental assessment and modification (OR: 0.30, 95% CI: 0.13, 0.70).

Cost Effectiveness

Correction and/or removal of potential hazards is a one-off intervention that can be carried out relatively cheaply, over one or two home visits. The incremental cost-effectiveness ratios for home safety interventions have varied depending on the target group [40], but such interventions have been shown to be cost-effective when delivered to at-risk participants such as those with a previous fall [41]. Few studies have reported fall-related injuries or fractures, although one home safety trial has shown a significant reduction in injurious falls for people with vision impairment [29].

One economic modelling study conducted in New Zealand found that a low-cost home modification programme for recipients of community service benefits who lived in older housing stock [42] reduced injurious falls and was cost effective [43]. This intervention used a standard checklist and applied a specific set of home-safety modifications which included reducing the slipperiness of outside surfaces, and the provision of step edging, improved outdoor lighting, handrails for steps, grab rails in bathrooms, fixed edges of carpets and mats, and non-slip bathmats. This approach may be particularly relevant for developing countries where environmental fall risks are more common, widespread and context specific [44], i.e. narrow steps with poor lighting, a water source outside the home, earth floors, open street gutters, and hazardous walking areas.

Tailoring the Intervention

Building on the evidence for home fall-hazard reduction, the Westmead Schema – a conceptual framework for tailoring interventions – was developed and refined using an expert review process [45]. It has been used to develop an on-line home and community safety learning module and the schema can be downloaded from the website (https://fallspreventiononlineworkshops.com.au/). It consists of three key areas:

- 'Understanding the Person' and their risk related to their fall history, context and functional capacity. This highlights the importance of understanding the person's functional vision, mobility and cognition in order to tailor solutions.
- 'Moving through the Home Environment and Collaborative Problem-Solving' for risk reduction. This outlines five foundations forming the basis for clinical reasoning and a range of techniques and tools necessary for conducting the assessment and collaboratively problem solving.
- 'Prioritising and Planning' which involves constructing an action plan for change and adaptation.

Further, environmental and behavioural risks around the home should be assessed with consideration for safe mobility strategies outdoors and checking the need for referral for other interventions such as balance exercises or medication reviews.

Environmental Risk Screens and Assessments

Seventy seven assessments for measuring environmental fall risk have been published [46]. Individual 'in house' assessments have been used in 74% of studies, with 25% of the 77 assessments used in two or more studies and 6% in five or more studies. Blanchet and Edwards [46] have reviewed 42 of these checklists and found variability in the environmental hazards considered, whether the assessment was administered as part of a screening or assessment process, who carried out the hazard identification process, how comprehensive the components of the process were, and whether the tool targeted older people with specific health conditions that affect falls, such as visual impairment or dementia.

Key criteria for good quality interventions [24] are the inclusion of a comprehensive process of hazard identification and a validated assessment tool for a broad range of fall hazards. The available tools, however, vary considerably in the number of items they cover, which aspects of home are included, and the measurement objectivity of the criteria [46]. In addition, the studies have differed with respect to whether they used a screening or assessment process. Screening requires limited clinical reasoning and comprises a basic assessment involving a standardized process of information collection and interpretation, often supported by a template for collecting and scoring data for a small number of hazards. Studies using screening tools alone have not been effective in reducing falls (e.g. [2]).

In contrast, an assessment (as opposed to screening only) involves the collection, interpretation, and integration of information into clinical decision-making which informs subsequent care-planning decisions. Therefore, assessment, unlike with screening, is generally carried out by health professionals such as occupational therapists, who have an in-depth understanding of person–environment fit [47]. In Blanchet and Edwards' review [46], 37% of assessments were completed by occupational therapists, 32% by nurses, 16% by research assistants, 15% by the older person/family, 6% by physiotherapists, and 13% by other professionals. Unsurprisingly, health professionals identified more hazards than lay older adults. Blanchet and Edwards warn against adding the number of hazards to compute a composite risk score. In fact, assessments that have established strong content validity for the range and type of hazards still require clinical reasoning skills to establish priorities and solutions for the individual and benefit from assessing functional vision and mobility prior to a joint home tour [45].

Romli et al. [48] reviewed the psychometric properties of fall hazard assessments (36 tools) and recommended the Westmead Home Safety Assessment as a thorough assessment for occupational therapists. This tool is considered a gold standard and was developed specifically for falls. It contains 72 items (with a short version containing 44 items) for inside and outside items with each item having hazard descriptors. The tool has undergone expert review to determine the assessment criterion for tool development [49], and demonstrated content validity [45, 50] and inter-rater reliability [51]. The Home Safety Self-Assessment Tool (HSSAT) [52, 53] was recommended as a thorough self-administered environment assessment tool (64 items) with content validity determined by an expert panel. The Home Falls and Accidents Screening Tool (HOME FAST) [54] was recommended as a screening tool (25 items). It contains 18 environmental fall hazards plus seven items related to mobility and transfer difficulties. This tool has demonstrated predictive validity for falls but this may be due to the included mobility items. The tool has not been assessed to determine whether it has one or two dimensions and it is unlikely that hazards alone, or a small number of hazards are predictive of falls.

The Falls Behavioural (FaB) Scale for the Older Person [7] was designed to identify an older person's awareness of and practice of indoor and outdoor behaviours that could potentially protect against falling. The 30-item FaB includes day-to-day habitual and intentional behaviours that if not undertaken safely could place a person at risk of falling. It has established content validity and good inter-rater reliability. It has been used in practice by mailing it to the person prior to a home visit followed up with discussion on the visit. It can raise awareness as well as focus on behaviours that need attention. A shorter version has demonstrated validity for use as an outcome measure [55].

A new environmental assessment, the Outdoor Falls Questionnaire has been developed to assess fall risk in the wider community [56]. Content validity was established through qualitative interviews with older people, review of relevant studies and an expert review of the assessment. It consists of a range of background questions (e.g. physical activity, time spent outdoors) and questions on perceived outdoor fall risks and strategies used for outdoor fall prevention. Finally, environmental assessments have been developed specifically for people with health conditions including the Home Environment Assessment for the Visually Impaired [57] and the Home Environmental Assessment Protocol (HEAP) for individuals with dementia [58].

Solution Examples

Table 23.2 presents a list of environmental fall risk factors that have been suggested in the literature (see Chapter 12) with some examples of potential solutions. These solutions need to be tailored so they are relevant, acceptable, and target the behaviour for change. Resources such as handouts can be sourced from appropriate websites but should only be used when relevant for the person and not in place of problem-solving and tailoring. They provide suggestions for avoiding falls in public places, footwear safety, use of mobility aids, and coping with low vision (e.g. [59, 60]).

Adherence: Enablers and Challenges

Full or partial adherence to home fall-hazard recommendations when delivered by an occupational therapist has been reported to be between 53% and 88% [16,

Table 23.2 Suggested strategies to address environmental hazards

Area	Solution
Climbing and reaching	Have a secure, lightweight step ladder with a wide base and a high handrail
Flooring and mats	Use double sided tape to secure mats or replace with rubber backed non-slip mats
	Avoid thick-pile carpets that catch feet
	Avoid furniture with splayed legs
General	Avoid rushing to answer the phone, find out the number you can call to find out who was your last caller
	Use a fall detector if living alone
	Talk to neighbours about having a routine to show you are ok such as opening a front blind when getting up in the morning
	Keep pets confined during times of high activity and feed them in a corner away from where you walk.
	Mop up spills straight away. Use a cleaner if they are oil or butter spills
	Scan ahead when walking to observe hazards
	Use sensor lights at entrances
Steps and stairs	Use adhesive strips
	Avoid leaving things on the stairs and just carry things that you can with one hand when descending to hold on with the other
	Switch on stair lights when descending at night
	Remove loose rugs from the top of stairs
Lighting	Take care with sudden changes such as from brightly lit to more dimly lit rooms
	Use a night light or a plug in photosensitive light in a power point. These are soft enough not to 'awaken' you and automatically light up when dark so you don't have to remember
Clothes	Dressing gowns and loose long pants can be a trip hazard on the stairs
	Wear well-fitting shoes that allow a good grip and a feeling of the floor surface
	Make sure your shoe soles are not slippery
	Have bed socks with non-slip tread
Bathroom	Consider a rail in shower or toilet
	Use non-slippery bathroom mats
Public transport	Have money or ticket easily found and ready in advance
	Travel in off-peak times if you can
	Ask the driver to wait till you are seated
	Once off the bus, pause, get your balance, and maybe even walk first in the direction the bus is travelling
Outdoors	Allow extra time to get to places, particularly going somewhere new
	Have some strategies for crossing roads safely
	Avoid windy conditions
	Slow down your pace
	Wear some clothing that is easily seen
	Wear a rain hood rather than using an umbrella if you use a walking stick
Impaired vision to judge depth/distance	Take extra care when getting new prescriptions until adjust to changes, particularly at stairs and changes of level
	Consider having two pairs of spectacles instead of bifocals

61]. This is consistent with aggregated data showing adherence for home safety interventions to be 58–59%, and compares favourably to other fall prevention interventions [62], i.e. 52% for individually targeted exercise and 42% for the Otago Exercise Programme [63]. Given that good adherence is crucial for fall prevention, consideration of ways to support follow through is required. Strategies for promoting adherence include taking into account the persons' view of risk, joint determination of solutions, providing intervention options, and immediate and multiple home visit follow-ups to support the implementation of recommendations [27]. As part of a successful multi-faceted fall prevention intervention, Clemson et al. [11] used small group sessions using a self-efficacy enhancement approach and reported 70% of programme participants adhered to at least 50% of the home visit recommendations.

Few personal characteristics predict follow-through. However, available help from relatives and a belief that home modifications can prevent falls are associated with higher adherence [61]. Reasons for non-adherence include not seeing the need for the intervention or a belief that one is not at risk of falling. In some countries, community programmes which provide subsidized housing modifications to older people on low incomes, offer a means of addressing financial barriers. For example, the low intervention costs to participants is likely to have contributed to the high take-up of suggested modifications (90%) in the study by Thompson et al. [64]. Other barriers, particularly for assistive devices, are that older people may be concerned about the stigmatizing effects of such safety measures and feel that their view of their health and independence is being challenged [65]. Luz et al. [66] revealed a range of barriers regarding the use of walkers and mobility aids including a belief they were not needed or would not be easily reachable. They highlighted the importance of promoting personal relevance, proper fit, and training.

Public Places and Design Issues

Improvements in the design and maintenance of outdoor areas are likely to be an effective population-level fall prevention approach, as most falls in the wider community involve modifiable environmental risk factors [67]. The WHO Global Age-Friendly Cities Guide [68] provides checklists for features to consider for outdoor and city environments to be accessible, safe, and optimize participation for older people. Environments should be designed to safely provide for the needs of people with physical and sensory abilities across all weather conditions. Possible interventions in public places include programmes to provide more even and maintained pavements, timely removal of ice and snow, spilt liquids, and fallen leaves, better contrasting edges on curbs, stairs, and trip hazards, clear signage, adequate street lighting, traffic lights timing changes to allow longer pedestrian crossing times, and increased provision of resting places and grab rails.

One Australian fall prevention population level study conducted over four years targeted knowledge, attitudes, behaviours, medication use, footwear, home hazard reduction, and public environmental hazards in community-living people aged 60 years and over. It was delivered via a mix of community strategies utilizing brochures, posters, television and radio media, policy development (local and state government), home hazard reduction programmes, and engagement of local clinicians and other health professionals. This programme resulted in a significant 20% decrease in fall-related hospitalizations in the intervention area compared a comparison community [12].

Studies conducted in the US [56], UK, and Sweden [69] have highlighted the importance of involving older people in identifying hazards and generating solutions with respect to pedestrian experiences. Garner [70] proposed two checklists for public places, one for assessing the adequacy of footpaths, steps, stairs, ramps, and roadways, and a second for assessing safety in shopping centres, malls, and arcades. A Hong Kong study [71] used spatial mapping to identify high-risk locations or hot spots for falls. These approaches require coordinated efforts at multiple government levels to set and enforce design, construction, and maintenance standards and establish access and safety committees to oversee this. Standardized methods to assess outdoor environmental hazards and identify high-risk locations are required, along with ongoing monitoring and remediation of community fall hazards through falls surveillance and data-sharing. This will promote active and productive ageing among community-dwelling older people and reduce litigation and health-care costs associated with injurious falls.

Conclusions

Reducing hazards in the home is an effective fall prevention strategy, and particularly so in at-risk older people, for example, older people with a history of falls or mobility limitations. The effectiveness of home safety interventions may be enhanced by joint decision-making as well as by including interventions to ensure safe transfers, reaching and climbing strategies. Environmental assessment and modification by trained individuals appears to contribute to the success of multi-faceted fall prevention programmes. Solutions to potential barriers to an individual's adoption of home adaptations include engaging family, education, and financial assistance. Research is needed on assistive technologies, and public/community safety. Further implementation and evaluation of evidence-based monitoring and remediation systems, and building standards is required to improve safety in public places to reduce fall risk.

REFERENCES

1. Carter SE, Campbell EM, Sanson-Fisher RW et al. Environmental hazards in the homes of older people. *Age Ageing*. 1997;26:195–202.

2. Stevens M, Holman CD, Bennett N et al. Preventing falls in older people: outcome evaluation of a randomized controlled trial. *J Am Geriatr Soc*. 2001;49:1448–55.

3. Gill TM, Robison JT, Williams CS et al. Mismatches between the home environment and physical capabilities among community-living older persons. *J Am Geriatr Soc*. 1999;47:88–92.

4. Lamb SE, Jorstad-Stein EC, Hauer K et al. Development of a common outcome data set for fall injury prevention trials: the Prevention of Falls Network Europe consensus. *J Am Geriatr Soc*. 2005;53:1618–22.

5. Lamb SE, Hauer K, Becker C. Manual for the fall prevention classification system. Version 1. 2007. www.profane.eu.org/documents/Falls_Taxonomy.pdf (accessed April 2021).

6. Clemson L, Stark S, Pighills A et al. Environmental interventions for preventing falls in older people living in the community. *Cochrane Database Syst Rev*. 2019;2019:CD013258.

7. Clemson L, Cumming RG, Heard R. The development of an assessment to evaluate behavioral factors associated with falling. *Am J Occup Ther*. 2003;57:380–8.

8. Iwarsson S, Horstmann V, Carlsson G et al. Person-environment fit predicts falls in older adults better than the consideration of environmental hazards only. *Clin Rehabil*. 2009;23:558–67.

9. Pighills A, Ballinger C, Pickering R et al. A critical review of the effectiveness of environmental assessment and modification in the prevention of falls amongst community dwelling older people. *Br J Occup Ther*. 2016;79:133–43.

10. Cumming RG, Thomas M, Szonyi G et al. Home visits by an occupational therapist for assessment and modification of environmental hazards: a randomized trial of falls prevention. *J Am Geriatr Soc*. 1999;47:1397–402.

11. Clemson L, Cumming RG, Kendig H et al. The effectiveness of a community-based program for reducing the incidence of falls among the elderly: a randomized trial. *J Am Geriatr Soc*. 2004;52:1487–94.

12. Kempton A, van Beurden E, Sladden T et al. Older people can stay on their feet: final results of a community-based falls prevention programme. *Health Promotion International* 2000;15:27–33.

13. Gitlin L, Winter L, Corcoran M et al. Effects of the home environmental skill-building program on the caregiver-care recipient dyad: 6-month outcomes from the Philadelphia REACH Initiative. *Gerontologist*. 2003;43:532–46.

14. Law M, Cooper B, Strong S et al. The person environment occupation model: a transactive approach to occupational therapy. *Can J Occup Ther*. 1997;63:9–23.

15. Nahemow L. The ecological theory of aging: Powell Lawton's legacy. In: Rubinstein R, Moss M, Kieban M, Lawton M. (Eds.) *The Many Dimensions of Aging*. New York: Springer; 2000:22–40.

16. Pighills AC, Torgerson DJ, Sheldon TA et al. Environmental assessment and modification to prevent falls in older people. *J Am Geriatr Soc*. 2011;59:26–33.

17. Stevens JA, Mahoney JE, Ehrenreich H. Circumstances and outcomes of falls among high risk community-dwelling older adults. *Inj Epidemiol.* 2014;1:5.

18. Bleijlevens MHC, Diederiks JPM, Hendriks MRC et al. Relationship between location and activity in injurious falls: an exploratory study. *BMC Geriatr.* 2010;10.

19. Hill AM, Hoffmann T, Haines TP. Circumstances of falls and falls-related injuries in a cohort of older patients following hospital discharge. *Clin Interv Aging.* 2013;8:765–73.

20. O'Loughlin JL, Robitaille Y, Boivin JF et al. Incidence of and risk factors for falls and injurious falls among the community-dwelling elderly. *Am J Epidemiol.* 1993;137:342–54.

21. Nyman SR, Ballinger C, Phillips JE et al. Characteristics of outdoor falls among older people: a qualitative study. *BMC Geriatr.* 2013;13:125.

22. Timsina LR, Willetts JL, Brennan MJ et al. Circumstances of fall-related injuries by age and gender among community-dwelling adults in the United States. *PLoS One.* 2017;12.

23. Clemson L, Cusick A, Fozzard C. Managing risk and exerting control: determining follow through with falls prevention. *Disabil Rehabil.* 1999;13:531–41.

24. Clemson L, Mackenzie L, Ballinger C et al. Environmental interventions to prevent falls in community-dwelling older people: a meta-analysis of randomized trials. *J Aging Health.* 2008;20:954–71.

25. Gillespie LD, Robertson MC, Gillespie WJ et al. Interventions for preventing falls in older people living in the community. *Cochrane Database Syst Rev.* 2012:CD007146.

26. Chu MML, Fong KNK, Lit ACH et al. An occupational therapy fall reduction home visit program for community-dwelling older adults in Hong Kong after an emergency department visit for a fall. *J Am Geriatr Soc.* 2017;65:364–72.

27. Pighills A, Drummond A, Crossland S et al. What type of environmental assessment and modification prevents falls in community dwelling older people? *Br Med J.* 2019;364.

28. Nikolaus T, Bach M. Preventing falls in community-dwelling frail older people using a Home Intervention Team (HIT): results from the randomized Falls-HIT trial. *J Am Geriatr Soc.* 2003;51:300–5.

29. Campbell AJ, Robertson MC, La Grow SJ et al. Randomised controlled trial of prevention of falls in people aged >75 with severe visual impairment: the VIP trial. *Br Med J.* 2005;331:817–25.

30. Day L, Fildes B, Gordon I et al. Randomised factorial trial of falls prevention among older people living in their own homes. *Br Med J.* 2002;325:128.

31. Stevens M, Holman CD, Bennett N. Preventing falls in older people: impact of an intervention to reduce environmental hazards in the home. *J Am Geriatr Soc.* 2001;49:1442–7.

32. Hopewell S, Adedire O, Copsey BJ et al. Multifactorial and multiple component interventions for preventing falls in older people living in the community. *Cochrane Database Syst Rev.* 2018;7;CD012221.

33. Close J, Ellis M, Hooper R et al. Prevention of falls in the elderly trial (PROFET): a randomised controlled trial. *Lancet.* 1999;353:93–7.

34. Tinetti ME, Baker DI, McAvay G et al. A multifactorial intervention to reduce the risk of falling among elderly people living in the community. *N Engl J Med.* 1994;331:821–7.

35. Logan PA, Coupland CAC, Gladman JRF et al. Community falls prevention for people who call an emergency ambulance after a fall: a randomised controlled trial. *Br Med J.* 2010;340: c2102.

36. Fabacher D, Josephson K, Pietruszka F et al. An in-home preventative assessment program for independent older adults: a randomized controlled trial. *J Am Geriatr Soc.* 1994;42:630–8.

37. Rubenstein LZ, Robbins AS, Josephson KR et al. The value of assessing falls in an elderly population: a randomised clinical trial. *Ann Intern Med.* 1990;113:308–16.

38. Vetter NJ, Lewis PA, Ford D. Can health visitors prevent fractures in elderly people? *Br Med J.* 1992;304:888–90.

39. Tricco AC, Thomas SM, Veroniki AA et al. Comparisons of interventions for preventing falls in older adults: a systematic review and meta-analysis. *J Am Med Assoc.* 2017;318:1687–99.

40. Davis JC, Ashe MC, Liu-Ambrose T et al. Does a home based strength and balance programme in people aged ≥ 80 years provide the best value for money to prevent falls? A systematic review of economic evaluations of falls prevention interventions. *Br Med J.* 2009;44:80–9.

41. Salkeld G, Cumming RG, O'Neill R et al. The cost effectiveness of a home hazard reduction program to reduce falls among older persons. *Aust NZ J Public Health.* 2000;24:265–71.

42. Keall MD, Pierse N, Howden-Chapman P et al. Home modifications to reduce injuries from falls in the home injury prevention intervention (HIPI) study: a cluster-randomised controlled trial. *Lancet.* 2015;385:231–8.

43. Keall MD, Pierse N, Howden-Chapman P et al. Cost-benefit analysis of fall injuries prevented by a programme of home modifications: a cluster randomised controlled trial. *Inj Prev.* 2017;23:22–6.

44. Stewart Williams J, Kowal P, Hestekin H et al. Prevalence, risk factors and disability associated with fall-related injury in older adults in low- and middle-income countries: results from the WHO Study on global AGEing and adult health (SAGE). *BMC Med.* 2015;13:147.

45. Mandelbaum C, Clemson L, Glassman M et al. A scoping review of fall hazards in the homes of older adults and development of a framework for assessment and intervention. *Aust Occup Ther J.* 2019;67.

46. Blanchet R, Edwards N. A need to improve the assessment of environmental hazards for falls on stairs and in bathrooms: results of a scoping review. *BMC Geriatr.* 2018;18:272.

47. Peterson EW, Finlayson M, Elliott SJ et al. Unprecedented opportunities in fall prevention for occupational therapy practitioners. *Am J Occup Ther.* 2012;66:127–30.

48. Romli MH, Mackenzie L, Lovarini M et al. The clinimetric properties of instruments measuring home hazards for older people at risk of falling: a systematic review. *Eval Health Prof.* 2016:1–47.

49. Clemson L, Fitzgerald MH, Heard R. Content validity of an assessment tool to identify home fall hazards: the Westmead Home Safety Assessment. *Br J Occup Ther.* 1999;62:171–9.

50. Clemson L. Validity, usefulness, and reliability of an assessment tool to identify home fall hazards. Master of Applied Science Thesis: The University of Sydney (Lidcombe); 1997.

51. Clemson L, Fitzgerald MH, Heard R et al. Inter-rater reliability of a home fall hazards assessment tool. *OTJR.* 1999;19:83–98.

52. Horowitz BP, Nochajski SM, Schweitzer JA. Occupational therapy community practice and home assessments: use of the Home Safety Self-Assessment Tool (HSSAT) to support aging in place. *Occup Ther Health Care.* 2013;27:216–27.

53. Tomita M, Saharan S, Rajendran S et al. Development, psychometrics and use of Home Safety Self-Assessment Tool (HSSAT). *Am J Occup Ther.* 2014;68:711–18.

54. Mackenzie L, Byles J, Higganbotham N. Designing the Home Falls and Accidents Screening Tool (HOME FAST): selecting the items. *Br J Occup Ther.* 2000;63:261–9.

55. Clemson L, Bundy A, Cumming RG et al. Validating the Falls Behavioural (FaB) Scale for older people: a Rasch analysis. *Disabil Rehabil.* 2008;30:498–506.

56. Chippendale T, Boltz M. Perceived neighborhood fall risks and strategies used to prevent outdoor falls: does age matter? *J Am Geriatr Soc.* 2014;62:2210–12.

57. Swenor BK, Yonge AV, Goldhammer V et al. Evaluation of the Home Environment Assessment for the Visually Impaired (HEAVI): an instrument designed to quantify fall-related hazards in the visually impaired. *BMC Geriatr.* 2016;16:214.

58. Gitlin LN, Schinfeld S, Winter L et al. Evaluating home environments of persons with dementia: interrater reliability and validity of the Home Environmental Assessment Protocol (HEAP). *Disabil Rehabil.* 2002;24:59–71.

59. Clinical Excellence Commission. Patient safety information [Downloadable handouts on fall prevention]. Available from: https://www.cec.health.nsw.gov.au/keep-patients-safe/falls-prevention (accessed April 2021).

60. Clemson L, Swann M. Stepping On handouts 2016 https://ses.library.usyd.edu.au/handle/2123/14283 (accessed April 2021).

61. Cumming RG, Thomas M, Szonyi G et al. Adherence to occupational therapist recommendations for home modifications for falls prevention. *Am J Occup Ther.* 2001;55:641–8.

62. Nyman SR, Victor CR. Older people's participation in and engagement with falls prevention interventions in community settings: an augment to the Cochrane systematic review. *Age Ageing.* 2012;41:16–23.

63. Campbell AJ, Robertson MC, Gardner MM et al. Randomised controlled trial of a general practice programme of home based exercise to prevent falls in elderly women. *Br Med J.* 1997;315:1065–69.

64. Thompson PG. Preventing falls in the elderly at home: a community-based program. *Med J Aust.* 1996;164:530–2.

65. Connell B, Wolf S. Environmental and behavioural circumstances associated with falls at home among healthy elderly individuals. *Arch Phys Med Rehab.* 1997;78:179–86.

66. Luz C, Bush T, Shen X. Do canes or walkers make any difference? Nonuse and fall injuries. *Gerontologist.* 2017;57:211–18.

67. Li WJ, Keegan THM, Sternfeld B et al. Outdoor falls among middle-aged and older adults: a neglected public health problem. *Am J Public Health.* 2006;96:1192–200.

68. WHO. *Global Age-Friendly Cities: a Guide.* Geneva: World Health Organisation; 2007:80.

69. Wennberg H, Phillips J, Stahl A. How older people as pedestrians perceive the outdoor environment: methodological issues derived from studies in two European countries. *Ageing Soc.* 2018;38:2435–67.

70. Garner E. *Preventing Falls in Public Places. Challenge & Opportunity for Local Government. Report No: NCPHU 96–0026.* Lismore, NSW: North Coast Public Health Unit; 1996.

71. Lai PC, Wong WC, Low CT et al. A small-area study of environmental risk assessment of outdoor falls. *J Med Syst.* 2011;35:1543–52.

72. Pardessus V, Puisieux F, Di Pompeo C et al. Benefits of home visits for falls and autonomy in the elderly: a randomized trial study. *Am J Phys Med Rehabil.* 2002;81:247–52.

24

Fall Injury Prevention: Hip Protectors and Compliant Flooring

Susan Kurrle and Ian Cameron

This chapter reviews prevention from a different perspective. Instead of preventing the fall, this chapter examines fall injury prevention, a complementary approach that has a history of many decades. This approach has comprised two strategies. The first pertains to padding, or 'protecting' the hip or other body parts, including the head, while the second pertains to modifying the surface onto which the person falls to reduce fall impact. The main contrast between these approaches is that the use of body part protectors requires a commitment from the wearer or carers, whereas compliant flooring is a passive device requiring no such commitment or action.

Hip Protectors

The first patent for a hip protector was granted in the United States of America in 1959. The underlying principle of hip protectors is that a shield/pad/protector worn over the hip, and constructed with energy absorbing material or using an energy-shunting design, reduces the force transmitted to the greater trochanter and proximal components of the femur during a fall. As a result, the risk of fracturing the femur in a fall onto the lateral side of the thigh is reduced. This principle is valid because most hip fractures occur with a fall to the side and it is extremely rare for the femur to fracture spontaneously. Figure 24.1 shows an example of a hip protector.

Hip protectors are held in place over the greater trochanter of the femur by specially designed underwear that incorporates the hip protector in a pocket. The underwear is often elasticized to enable a close fit. Some designs of hip protector underwear allow the hip protector to be removed from the pocket to assist in laundering the underwear and limit that cost by having one pair of hip protectors and multiple underwear garments. Generally this system has been abandoned due to the hip protectors becoming misplaced or lost. Hip protectors can be directly applied to the skin with the use of an adhesive but this has not been widely used or accepted.

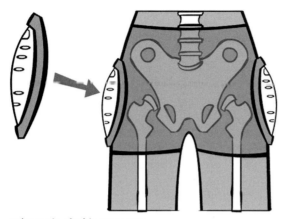

Figure 24.1   Schematic of a hip protector.

There are complex issues in modelling the biomechanics of hip fracture. Multiple testing systems have been devised for hip protectors, and while it is uncertain whether they address all in vivo issues relating to hip fractures, it is generally accepted that testing systems can accurately measure the force-attenuating properties of hip protectors [1]. Published studies have shown that the many commercially available hip protectors have differing biomechanical properties and not all are likely to be sufficiently effective in attenuating the force present in some falls to prevent a hip fracture [1].

Efficacy in Preventing Hip Fractures

The first randomized controlled trial of hip protectors was published in 1993 [2]. It was conducted in 701 nursing home residents and the hip protectors incorporated a firm outer shell and an inner foam section. The risk of fracture was significantly decreased in the intervention group (RR: 0.44). Although eight intervention group participants suffered hip fractures, none were wearing the hip protectors at the time of fracture. Another early study tested a different model of hip protector and also found a decreased fracture rate among residents of a randomly selected nursing home that was offered hip protectors compared with a control nursing home (RR: 0.33) [3].

Subsequent research into the efficacy and practicality of hip protector use has been less positive. The most recent Cochrane Collaboration review of 19 randomized trials concluded that for older people living in nursing care facilities, providing a hip protector probably decreases the risk of a hip fracture (RR: 0.82, 95% CI: 0.67, 1.00; 14 trials, 11,808 participants) [4]. For older people living in the community, the review concluded there is little or no evidence that hip protectors can prevent hip fractures (RR: 1.15, 95% CI; 0.84, 1.58; 5 trials, 5,614 participants). Hip protectors, even if worn correctly and at all times, do not prevent all hip fractures; the risk reduction is approximately 60 to 80% [5,6]. No new trials of hip protectors have been conducted since the 2014 Cochrane review. For the reasons outlined in the sections below, this may relate to the practical difficulties with this intervention strategy.

Potential Adverse Effects of Hip Protectors

The most recent Cochrane Collaboration review concluded that for older people living in nursing care facilities, hip protectors may slightly increase the chance of a pelvic fracture [4]. Hip protectors could also cause pressure injuries if not properly applied or if used at night, but this has not been scientifically substantiated. There have also been concerns about the use of hip protectors in people who have already had a hip fracture (or arthroplasty for other reasons), but again there is no evidence of adverse events in these circumstances. There are case reports of hip protectors causing people to fall when repositioning them for toileting. Finally, commercial laundering may damage hip protectors and their associated garments, which could render them ineffective or cause pressure injuries.

Adherence and 'Real Life' Issues

After the initial period of great enthusiasm for the use of hip protectors, practical issues with their use became evident. Markedly different levels of adherence with use of hip protectors have been reported in clinical trials, i.e. 30 to 75% [7,8], and the authors of the most recent Cochrane review concluded poor acceptance and adherence by older people offered hip protectors is a barrier to their effective use [4].

It has been reported that most older women at risk of hip fracture do not perceive themselves to be at risk and therefore are reluctant to consider their use [7]. Furthermore, hip protectors can be uncomfortable to wear and impede toileting. Hip protector cost has also been identified as a barrier to their use [8]. In a large randomized trial of hip protector use over two years in 600 community-dwelling older women who had fallen at least once, adherence with the use of hip protectors was approximately 53% during the two years of the study, and hip protectors were worn at the time of 51% of falls. The predictors for non-adherence were lower self-efficacy for hip protector use, higher number of perceived barriers to hip protector use, and lower self-rated health [9].

In residential care, adherence depends more on the attitudes of staff who supervise/assist with the wearing of hip protectors. In a randomized trial of 174 older people living in residential care who had fallen at least once, there was a mean adherence rate with their use of 57%, with hip protectors being worn for 54% of the recorded falls during the 18 months of the study [10]. In this early study of hip protector use in residential care, adherence was related to the assessed quality of care provided in each facility. Commitment of nursing and care staff, and the work practices of the aged care facility, also influenced adherence. Incontinence and dementia in participants, discomfort from hip protectors, and laundering difficulties negatively affected adherence. High staff turnover, reduced application of the interventions due to limited training, or staff prioritizing other aspects of daily care for residents have also been reported as factors limiting use of hip protectors in residential care [11].

Current Status of Hip Protectors

Despite the above issues, hip protectors are still recommended in guidelines [12], and as part of multi-factorial interventions aimed at preventing injury in residential care settings [13]. Indeed, hip protectors are in regular use in many aged care facilities where high levels of care are delivered, and where the older residents are at high risk of falls. Hip protector design continues to evolve with an emphasis on comfort, ease of use, and adequate energy attenuation. Recently, Korall et al. [14] investigated routine hip protector use in 14 residential aged care facilities in British Columbia, Canada, where there is a strong organizational and managerial commitment to hip protector use. Routine use of hip protectors was at an acceptable level as they were worn at the time of 60% of recorded falls. This finding builds on the authors' previous study that identified staff commitment as crucial for this injury prevention strategy [15].

Protectors for Other Body Regions

Head protectors are commercially available and used in some clinical settings, although no scientific studies of their efficacy have been undertaken. Wrist, hand, and lower leg protectors are also used to prevent skin lacerations and bruising.

Compliant Flooring

Controlled laboratory studies have shown that specific types of compliant flooring meaningfully reduce forces during impact to vulnerable locations, such as the hip and head, without impairing balance or mobility during daily activities, such as standing and walking [16]. The provision of compliant flooring for older people at high risk of fall injury therefore appears an attractive fall injury prevention strategy.

Effectiveness of Compliant Flooring in Preventing Fall-Related Injuries

Six non-controlled trials undertaken in hospitals and residential care facilities in Sweden, the United States, the United Kingdom, and New Zealand provided initial evidence that low-impact flooring can significantly reduce injuries and prevent fractures. In the most recent of these trials, Hanger compared fall and fall-related injury rates for low-impact flooring versus standard vinyl flooring in a prospective, non-randomized controlled study in 20 bedrooms within a sub-acute geriatrics ward [17]. He found the fall rate did not differ between the low impact floor and control floor bedrooms which indicates the compliant surface did not cause unstable gait for the older people walking on it. However, fall-related injuries were significantly less frequent when they occurred on low-impact floors (22% of falls versus 34% of falls on control flooring, p = 0 .02), and fewer fractures occurred from falls onto the low-impact floor compared with the control floor – 0.7% versus 2.3% respectively.

Following on from the above trial, a four-year, randomized superiority trial of compliant (low-stiffness) flooring (see Figure 24.2) has been conducted by Mackey et al. [18]. Residents in 150 single-occupancy resident rooms in a Canadian residential aged care facility were randomly allocated to rooms with 2.54 cm thick compliant (low-stiffness) rubber flooring or plywood flooring with identical overlying vinyl floor covering and over pre-existing concrete floors. Over the trial period, 1,907 falls were reported; 23 intervention residents experienced 38 serious injuries (from 29 falls in 22 rooms), while 23 control residents experienced 47 serious injuries (from 34 falls in 23 rooms). Compliant flooring did not affect the odds of ≥1 serious fall-related injury (12.5% intervention versus 13.3% control, OR: 0.98, 95% CI: 0.52, 1.84; p = 0.950) or ≥2 serious fall-related injuries (5.4% versus 7.5%, OR: 0.74, 95% CI: 0.31,1.75; p = 0.500). It is possible that the

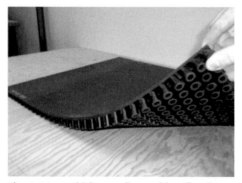

Figure 24.2   The 2.54 cm thick compliant rubber flooring used in Mackey et al. trial [18] (reproduced with permission from Simon Fraser University).

compliant flooring used was sub-optimal, and compliant flooring with greater impact attenuation may have prevented fall injuries. However, further trials are required to confirm this.

Additional Issues with Compliant Flooring

Soft surfaces can impair balance and gait in older people [19], but the compliant flooring used in the above trials was manufactured specifically to provide sufficient stiffness to have a negligible effect on these parameters [20]. The disadvantage of low-impact floors, however, is their rolling resistance when moving heavy equipment such as beds or hoists, and concerns have been raised about potential injuries to care staff as a result of pushing wheelchairs and other objects across compliant flooring due to increased forces on the hands [21]. These factors were considered a major issue for ward staff in the Hanger trial [17], and the low-impact flooring was removed from the study hospital at the completion of the trial. Finally, for routine use, additional factors that require consideration are the cost of installation and materials, and the durability of the flooring.

Conclusions

Hip protectors and compliant flooring have been assessed in clinical trials with reference to their efficacy in preventing fall-related injuries. These trials are complex because they involve interactions between human factors (the user and others who interact with the user) and environmental factors (the device or the flooring). Furthermore the threshold for injury (with reference to bone, muscle, and connective and brain tissue) varies from person to person. These are both intrinsic to the person (e.g. height and weight) and related to the type of fall, e.g. the direction and impact forces. For these reasons it is important to appreciate these devices and systems do not completely eliminate the risk of injury. Hip protectors can be viewed as a mature technology with established efficacy. However, their effectiveness in routine use is highly variable and complex, and requires considerable commitment from the older people and caregivers. Compliant flooring is attractive in theory as an intervention but it has practical difficulties. It can only be supported for use in carefully conducted research studies at this stage of its development.

REFERENCES

1. Robinovitch SN, Evans SL, Minns J et al. Hip protectors: recommendations for biomechanical testing-an international consensus statement (part I). *Osteoporos Int.* 2009;20:1977–88.

2. Lauritzen JB, Petersen MM, Lund B. Effect of external hip protectors on hip fractures. *Lancet*. 1993;341:11–13.

3. Ekman A, Mallmin H, Michaelsson K et al. External hip protectors to prevent osteoporotic hip fractures. *Lancet*. 1997;350:563–64.

4. Santesso N, Carrasco-Labra A, Brignardello-Petersen R. Hip protectors for preventing hip fractures in older people. *Cochrane Database Syst Rev*. 2014:CD001255.

5. Cameron ID, Cumming RG, Kurrle SE et al. randomised trial of hip protector use by frail older women living in their own homes. *Inj Prev*. 2003;9:138–41.

6. Cameron ID, Kurrle SE, Cumming RG et al. Proximal femoral fracture while wearing correctly applied hip protectors. *Age Ageing*. 2000;29:85–6.

7. Cameron ID, Quine S. External hip protectors: likely non-compliance among high risk elderly people living in the community. *Arch Gerontol Geriatr*. 1994;19:273–81.

8. Cameron ID, Kurrle SE, Quine S et al. Improving adherence with the use of hip protectors among older people living in nursing care facilities: a cluster randomized trial. *J Am Med Dir Assoc*. 2011;12:50–7.

9. Kurrle SE, Cameron ID, Quine S et al. Adherence with hip protectors: a proposal for standardised definitions. *Osteoporosis Int*. 2004;15:1–4.

10. Cameron ID, Venman J, Kurrle SE et al. Hip protectors in aged care facilities: a randomised trial of use by individual higher-risk residents. *Age Ageing*. 2001;30:477–81.

11. Roigk P, Becker C, Schulz C et al. Long-term evaluation of the implementation of a large fall and fracture prevention program in long-term care facilities. *BMC Geriatr*. 2018;18:233.

12. Australian Commission on Safety and Quality in Health Care. Preventing Falls and Harm from Falls in Older People: Best Practice Guidelines for Residential Aged Care Facilities. 2009. www.safetyandquality.gov.au/publications-and-resources/resource-library/preventing-falls-and-harm-falls-older-people-best-practice-guidelines-residential-aged-care-facilities (accessed April 2021).

13. Quigley P, Bulat T, Kurtzman E et al. Fall prevention and injury protection for nursing home residents. *J Am Med Dir Assoc*. 2010;11:284–93.

14. Korall AMB, Loughin TM, Feldman F et al. Determinants of staff commitment to hip protectors in long-term care: a cross-sectional survey. *Int J Nurs Stud*. 2018;82:139–48.

15. Korall AM, Feldman F, Scott VJ et al. Facilitators of and barriers to hip protector acceptance and adherence in long-term care facilities: a systematic review. *J Am Med Dir Assoc*. 2015;16:185–93.

16. Laing AC, Robinovitch SN. Low stiffness floors can attenuate fall-related femoral impact forces by up to 50% without substantially impairing balance in older women. *Accid Anal Prev*. 2009;41:642–50.

17. Hanger CH. Low-impact flooring: does it reduce fall-related injuries? *J Am Med Dir Assoc*. 2017;18:588–91.

18. Mackey DC, Lachance CC, Wang PT et al. The Flooring for Injury Prevention (FLIP) Study of compliant flooring for the prevention of fall-related injuries in long-term care: a randomized trial. *PLoS Med*. 2019;16(6):e1002843.

19. Redfern MS, Moore PL, Yarsky CM. The influence of flooring on standing balance among older persons. *Hum Factors*. 1997;39:445–55.

20. Sittichoke C, Buasord J, Boripuntakul S et al. Effects of compliant flooring on dynamic balance and gait characteristics of community-dwelling older persons. *J Nutr Health Aging.* 2019;23:665–8.

21. Lachance CC, Korall AM, Russell CM et al. External hand forces exerted by long-term care staff to push floor-based lifts: effects of flooring system and resident weight. *Hum Factors* 2016;58:927–43.

Multi-Factorial Fall Prevention Strategies: Where to Next?

Sarah E. Lamb and Hopin Lee

Introduction

There is compelling evidence that a range of risk factors contribute to falls in later life. A natural extension is to think that intervening on multiple risk factors as opposed to a single risk factor for falling might result in a greater reduction in falls. However, the evidence base suggests that interventions that target multiple risk factors are difficult to implement in practice and that the effect varies substantially across populations and practice settings. Multiple risk factor intervention is complex and requires greater commitment from participants and health care professionals than single-component interventions, and costs more to deliver.

In this chapter, we distinguish between single, multiple, and multi-factorial interventions (see Box) but focus on the multi-factorial fall prevention interventions (MFFP). We discuss the types of people who might benefit from MFFP and review the evidence base. We consider how multi-factorial interventions might be improved, whether they are likely to offer additional benefit over single intervention strategies and how research could help inform and improve prevention effectiveness.

Definition of Different Types Intervention According to the Prevention of Falls Network Europe Consensus Definitions [1]

• **Single-component interventions**: Only one intervention is provided.

Example:
  ◦ Supervised exercises.

• **Multiple-component interventions**: Interventions in which the same two or more interventions are given to every participant of the fall prevention programme.

(Cont.)

Examples:

- All participants of the fall prevention programme receive
    - Medication + supervised exercise
    - Geriatric assessment + environmental assessment in the patient's home.

- **Multi-factorial interventions (MFFP):** Two or more interventions in which each intervention is linked to an individual's risk profile (for example using the Physiological Performance Assessment [2] or the YALE FICSIT intervention [4]. Unlike multiple-component interventions, not all participants in a programme receive the same combination of sub-domains.

Examples:

- Each individual receives an assessment of known risk factors for falling (fall risk assessment) and receives an intervention matched to their risk factor profile
- Participation in any possible combination of intervention options according the participant's choice.

The Evidence for Multi-Factorial Interventions

It is over 30 years since the first well-designed prospective cohort studies identified risk factors for falls in older people [3]. Common risk factors identified include gait and balance disturbance, home and environmental hazards, vision impairment, culprit medications, polypharmacy, postural hypotension, poor footwear, and foot health. As these risk factors appear potentially modifiable through health care interventions, a new era of fall prevention ensued. MFFP requires the presence of at least two risk factors for falling, one of which might be a previous fall (not modifiable but a strong signature for future falls) and at least one other modifiable risk factor [1]. A typical risk factor assessment with linked interventions is shown in Figure 25.1 [5].

Summary of the Evidence Base

The evidence base of randomized controlled trials expanded rapidly in the 1990s with several highly influential trials [6–8]. The early trials were typically single-centre, small trials with interventions provided by specialist physicians. The early trials were promising and led to rapid implementation of falls clinics across many countries. National and international guidance

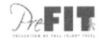

PreFIT Falls Risk Assessment Quick Reference Guide

EACH RISK FACTOR CHECKED	ASSESSMENT (TRAINED ASSESSOR) Q = Exploratory Questions	TREATMENT / ACTION
1. Falls history	**Q** Any falls in last year? Ask about context, consider potential causes & consequences.	Continue with full MFFP assessment.
2. Red flags	**Q** Refer to manual. Fainting / loss of consciousness? Any dizziness? Any tongue biting or facial injury?	Consider referral to consultant led-falls service or secondary care if red flags present.
3. Gait and balance	Conduct Timed Up and Go Test. Observe for balance problems whilst walking or turning. Observe gait: any shuffling or postural sway? Was TUGT completed within 14 seconds?	If problems with gait or balance, refer to physiotherapy for Otago strength & balance retraining programme.
4. Postural hypotension	**Q** Any dizziness on rising from bed? Check radial pulse rate & rhythm. Take lying & standing BP (within 3 minutes of standing). Conduct ECG if irregular pulse or brady/tachycardia.	Advice about postural change if symptomatic. Conduct medication review. GP to assess ECGs. Refer to other services if underlying disease suspected.
5. Medication review	**Q** Taking any meds to help you sleep or lift your mood? Check for any of the following: hypnotics, anxiolytics, anti-psychotics, anti-depressants. Also: BP, arrhythmia, angina, Parkinson's or prostate drugs.	Conduct full face-to-face medication review. Modify, reduce or stop culprit medications if indicated. Provide non-pharmaceutical advice for treatment of chronic conditions.
6. Vision	**Q** Explore last time eyes checked. Conduct Snellen chart test on all patients. Record acuity for both eyes.	Refer to optician for eye test if no test in last 12 months. If eye disease suspected, refer to optician or ophthalmology services.
7. Foot & footwear **Podiatry**	Visual inspection of feet on all patients. Check for corns, ingrowing toenails etc. **Q** Any problems with feet e.g. pain, numbness, any history of diabetes?	Conduct test for numbness & proprioception if indicated (numbness suspected). Refer to podiatry if indicated. Give AgeUK advice leaflet if not already received.
8. Environment hazards	**Q** Any use of furniture for support when walking? Difficulty getting out of a chair or using stairs/or steps at home? Any use of walking aids?	Give safety at home Tip Sheet. Raise awareness of potential home hazards (eg. rugs, wires etc.). Remind to use lights if rising in middle of night. Refer to OT if indicated.

Figure 25.1   A typical risk factor assessment with linked treatments [5]. Reproduced with permission from BMC Geriatrics

emerged for clinical care and developing fall prevention services but did not always include the details necessary for consistent clinical implementation. Health care teams adopted a wide variety of service delivery models and intervention strategies [9].

Since then, clinical trials of multi-factorial interventions have increased in size, with more centres and 'everyday' physicians and health care professionals being involved in treatment delivery. However, as the clinical trials became more pragmatic, the range of service delivery models has become more varied, along with trial quality. These pragmatic trials showed the first signals that MFFP might not be as effective as the early controlled trials suggested and that they may be difficult to implement. Figure 25.2 shows that over time, estimates of treatment effect for fall risk and rate (the risk of an individual being a faller or not) have declined.

In the most recent version of the Cochrane review, the evidence to support MFFP was weak, despite a large number of trials (44 trials, 15,778 participants). Overall, there was no reduction in the numbers of people who fall, but there was a modest difference in the rate of falling per person year. These findings were similar regardless of whether MFFP was compared to active or non-active controls [10, 11]. There was little evidence of reductions in fall-related injury, fracture rates, disability, and health-related quality of life. The findings indicate some falls can be prevented in people who fall several times a year, but interventions cannot change people from being a faller to a non-faller. On average, MFFP reduced the risk of being a faller by 4% and the rate of falls by 23%.

The findings of the Cochrane review broadly concur with the literature review published by Guirguis-Blake et al. [12] who report that exercise produces the most consistent effects and multi-factorial interventions have variable and more modest effects. Tricco et al. [13] pooled data across community, hospital, and long-term care settings and suggested exercise was the most robust intervention, but also recommended MF interventions alongside clinical quality-improvement interventions such as effective team working and audit processes. The main challenge with the Tricco et al. review is whether it is plausible to use evidence generated across diverse settings to apply to all, given the evidence in many settings is poor, and clinical experience tells us that the populations and targets for treatment may be very different [14].

This leaves us at an important crossroads in determining the value of MFFP interventions and ensuring that we deliver effective interventions to populations of older people. We need to consider a number of issues. These are the reliability of the research underpinning the evidence base, variations in the clinical approach used, that the premise of MFFP is wrong, and that we do not know which parts of the MFFP are effective.

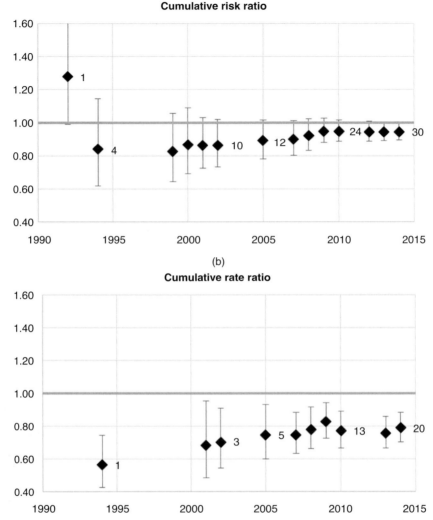

(a)

Cumulative risk ratio

(b)

Cumulative rate ratio

Figure 25.2   Estimates of the relative risk of being a faller (Panel I) and rate ratio (Panel 2) along with 95% confidence intervals in trials conducted over the last 30 years. Estimates are summarized at key points, and the numbers of trials contributing to the estimate are shown numerically.

Validity of the Evidence Base

Most systematic reviews include all randomized trials (and sometimes all quasi-randomized trials), regardless of quality of reporting or conduct of the trial. Randomization is the process by which allocation of treatment is determined by chance as opposed to clinician or patient preference. It is the cornerstone of a clinical trial design and helps to minimize many biases. Within the existing evidence base of trials, allocation concealment (which is a process used to ensure that clinicians, study personnel, and patients cannot anticipate or tamper with random allocation) was robust in only about 40% of trials [10]. Detection bias, whereby the person measuring outcomes (other than the patient) can work out the random allocation at some point later in the study, was also only robustly reported in 10 to 15% of trials [10]. Clearly, the standard of conduct and reporting of trials of fall prevention must improve if they are to be a reliable evidence base on which to base practice and policy decisions.

Small trials, particularly those from single centres of excellence, may overestimate the treatment effect in everyday settings and lead to biased statistical conclusions [15]. Poor-quality trials are also likely to overestimate the treatment effect. The trial base in MFFP suggests that small trial bias is a problem in this literature, and larger trials have often not been able to replicate the findings of promising smaller trials. In the future, research commissioners and ethics committees need to be vigilant to ensure that only the highest-quality trials are conducted and meaningfully add to the evidence base. Another indicator of usefulness of a trial is the duration of follow-up. Fortunately, the proportion of trials with greater than 12 months follow-up is increasing, and this substantially improves the utility of trials that are conducted. Over three-quarters of trials included in the Cochrane review of MFFP interventions had greater than 12 months follow-up and a quarter of trials had sample sizes of greater than 500 people [10].

Good reporting of trials is essential, not only to assess the quality of a trial, but also to improve their usefulness in implementation. The international fall prevention research community has agreed a core set of measures for fall prevention trials to encourage investigators to use at least some common outcome measures which are standardized in definition and method of measurement [16, 17]. In addition, a description system for fall prevention interventions has been devised to encourage investigators to report critical elements of their intervention so that other researchers and clinicians can replicate them [1].

Variations in Clinical Approach

Despite extensive analysis, it has been difficult to pinpoint a reason for variations in effectiveness of MFFP. In a review published in 2008, MFFP interventions which had a reliance on onward referral as opposed to the clinical team providing the intervention components, were less effective [18]. Other factors, such as the professional background of those providing the interventions or level of fall risk of participants, were not important [18]. Hopewell and colleagues recently repeated a similar analysis on newer evidence and did not found any determining factors [11].

Team changes (increasing the multi-disciplinarity of teams) may reduce the risk of injurious falls and a combination of case management, patient reminders, and staff education, as well as active case management may reduce the risk of falls [13]. Data from the Prevention of Fall Injury Trial demonstrated that despite extensive training, everyday clinicians find it very difficult to identify gait and balance impairments, and that timed tests may not provide an ideal solution to this problem [19].

Making Things More Complex May Not Make Them Better

The premise of multi-factorial interventions is that identifying multiple risk factors and intervening on these increases the precision and effectiveness of an intervention. There are also more steps in the intervention where errors may be introduced. Imprecision in determining the risk factors for treatment is likely to lead to redundancy in the intervention. For example, clinic-based measures of postural hypotension are unlikely to be accurate in everyday settings [20]. The mechanistic evidence of single interventions in the multi-factorial package have traditionally been ascertained from epidemiological evidence that has reported an association between a risk factor and subsequent falls. These relationships are not necessarily causal, and therefore intervening on the risk factor may not necessarily affect the outcome. A particular problem arises in epidemiological studies where analyses are not adjusted for fall history [21]. In many populations, being a faller is a recurring characteristic for at least some of the cohort.

For example, in the Women's Health and Aging Study [22], of the 279 participants who fell in the first year of the study, 147 (53%) had fallen in the year before. If we estimate the effect of urinary incontinence as a risk factor during the first year without adjusting for prior falls, we see that the relative risk of falling is significant at 1.34 (95% CI: 1.02, 1.77). If we adjust for prior falls the effect drops to 1.15 (95% CI: 0.86, 1.56) which is below the conventional levels of significance. The difference we see between the adjusted and unadjusted effects suggests that prior falling confounds the effect of incontinence on falls. The structure of this bias arises because prior falls is associated with incontinence and future falls. So, by not adjusting for prior falls, we observe a distorted effect that cannot be given a causal interpretation. Based on this observation, it would seem important to identify and adjust for all common causes of incontinence and falls if we were to identify the real causes of falling. Applying modern advanced epidemiological methods in causal modelling would help to improve our knowledge of causes of falls, and if applied within clinical trials would improve the understanding of treatment mechanisms [23, 24]. Similar methods of analysis are being applied with good effect in other fields and we would encourage their expanded use in this field.

Knowing Which Bits of a Multi-Factorial Treatment Are Effective Is Not so Clear

The most common treatments used in clinical trials of multi-factorial treatments are home safety programmes, exercise, medication reviews, and interventions to improve vision. While the evidence that exercise reduces falls is now robust [25], evidence of the effectiveness of other individual-level components being significant or independent contributors to the treatment effect is less strong and this makes refining interventions difficult. If we had robust evidence for all individual components, we could prioritize the most promising components to build tailored multi-factorial interventions for fall prevention. It would also be important to understand how the promising components interact with one another. It is possible that by combining some components, we produce super-additive effects that go beyond the sum of the effects of combined components. It would be important to explore these effects in factorial or adaptive trials. One problem with implementing multi-factorial interventions is that the clinician may be distracted from recommending and delivering an effective treatment (such as exercise), by focusing on addressing other risk factors which might have less therapeutic potential for the particular person they are seeing. A structured and prioritized approach to building multi-factorial interventions seems a more promising approach than simply combining individual components without guidance on their relative effects and interactions.

Why Not Deliver All Treatments at Once i.e., Use Multiple Interventions?

A handful of trials have investigated the effect of delivering two or more interventions, most commonly exercise and home-hazard modification. These types of combined treatments are expensive to deliver, and there are very few trials to inform decisions about which combination of interventions to focus on. More evidence is needed before this can be recommended as an approach.

Impact of Multi-Factorial Interventions on Fall-Related Fractures

Two recent very large trials have tested the impact of multi-factorial fall prevention interventions on fractures and serious fall injuries, respectively [26, 27]. Both were undertaken in general practice settings and sought to implement interventions within existing services, primarily using existing resources. Both studies found that the interventions did not significantly reduce falls or factures. These studies raise interesting questions about the challenge of funding and implementing fall prevention interventions as well as the ability of investigators to support and even measure uptake of intervention components in very large trials.

Conclusions

Multi-factorial interventions are complicated to deliver. With many differing risk factors for falls, and a poor understanding of how the risk factors interact, it is unsurprising that multi-factorial interventions are not consistent in effect. These issues are compounded in routine practice where standardization of clinical protocols, training, and quality assurance are less tightly monitored than in clinical trials. Further research aimed at elucidating effective treatment combinations and risk factor assessments, should be carefully structured to allow estimation of the effects of different treatment combinations in a sequential manner. At present, best practice guidelines and policy-makers should recognize the substantial variation in treatment outcomes across trials and settings. Future research should evaluate the effects of treatments and treatment combinations on both falls but also more related outcomes including fractures, frailty, health-related quality of life, and participation.

REFERENCES

1. Lamb SE, Becker C, Gillespie LD et al. Reporting of complex interventions in clinical trials: development of a taxonomy to classify and describe fall-prevention interventions. *Trials.* 2011;12.
2. Lord SR, Menz HB, Tiedemann A. A physiological profile approach to falls risk assessment and prevention. *Phys Ther.* 2003;83:237–52.
3. Ambrose AF, Paul G, Hausdorff JM. Risk factors for falls among older adults: a review of the literature. *Maturitas.* 2013;75:51–61.
4. Koch M, Gottschalk M, Baker DI et al. An impairment and disability assessment and treatment protocol for community-living elderly persons. *Phys Ther.* 1994;74:286–94.
5. Bruce J, Ralhan S, Sheridan R et al. The design and development of a complex multifactorial falls assessment intervention for falls prevention: the Prevention of Falls Injury Trial (PreFIT). *BMC Geriatr.* 2017;17:116.
6. Tinetti ME, Baker DI, McAvay G et al. A multifactorial intervention to reduce the risk of falling among elderly people living in the community. *N Engl J Med.* 1994;331:821–7.
7. Close J, Ellis M, Hooper R et al. Prevention of falls in the elderly trial (PROFET): a randomised controlled trial. *Lancet.* 1999;353:93–7.
8. Davison J, Bond J, Dawson P et al. Patients with recurrent falls attending Accident & Emergency benefit from multifactorial intervention: a randomised controlled trial. *Age Ageing.* 2005;34:162–8.
9. Lamb SE, Fisher JD, Gates S et al. A national survey of services for the prevention and management of falls in the UK. *BMC Health Serv Res.* 2008;8:233.
10. Hopewell S, Adedire O, Copsey BJ et al. Multifactorial and multiple component interventions for preventing falls in older people living in the community. *Cochrane Database Syst Rev.* 2018;7:CD012221.

11. Hopewell S, Copsey B, Nicolson P et al. Multifactorial interventions for preventing falls in older people living in the community: a systematic review and meta-analysis of 41 trials and almost 20 000 participants. *Br J Sports Med.* 2010;54:1340–50.

12. Guirguis-Blake JM, Michael YL, Perdue LA et al. Interventions to prevent falls in older adults: updated evidence report and systematic review for the US Preventive Services Task Force. *J Am Med Assoc.* 2018;319:1705–16.

13. Tricco AC, Thomas SM, Veroniki AA et al. Comparisons of interventions for preventing falls in older adults: a systematic review and meta-analysis. *J Am Med Assoc.* 2017;318:1687–99.

14. Cameron ID, Dyer SM, Panagoda CE et al. Interventions for preventing falls in older people in care facilities and hospitals. *Cochrane Database Syst Rev.* 2018;9:CD005465.

15. Forstmeier W, Wagenmakers EJ, Parker TH. Detecting and avoiding likely false-positive findings: a practical guide. *Biol Rev Camb Philos Soc.* 2017;92:1941–68.

16. Copsey B, Hopewell S, Becker C et al. Appraising the uptake and use of recommendations for a common outcome data set for clinical trials: a case study in fall injury prevention. *Trials.* 2016;17:131.

17. Lamb SE, Jorstad-Stein EC, Hauer K et al. Development of a common outcome data set for fall injury prevention trials: the Prevention of Falls Network Europe consensus. *J Am Geriatr Soc.* 2005;53:1618–22.

18. Gates S, Fisher J, Cooke M et al. Multifactorial assessment and targeted intervention for preventing falls and injuries among older people in community and emergency care settings: systematic review and meta-analysis. *Br Med J.* 2008;336:130–3.

19. Bruce J, Hossain A, Lall R et al. Clinical and cost-effectiveness of alternative falls prevention interventions in primary care: the Prevention of Falls Injury Trial (PreFIT). *Health Technol Assess.* 2019.

20. Cremer A, Rousseau A-L, Boulestreau R et al. Screening for orthostatic hypotension using home blood pressure measurements. *J Hypertens.* 2019;37:923–7.

21. Mol A, Bui Hoang PTS, Sharmin S et al. Orthostatic hypotension and falls in older adults: a systematic review and meta-analysis. *J Am Med Dir Assoc.* 2019;20:589–97.e5.

22. Simonsick EM, Maffeo CE, Rogers SK et al. Methodology and feasibility of a home-based examination in disabled older women: the Women's Health and Aging Study. *J Gerontol A Biol Sci Med Sci.* 1997;52:M264–74.

23. Lee H, Lamb SE. Advancing physical therapist interventions by investigating causal mechanisms. *Phys Ther.* 2017;97:1119–21.

24. Lee H, Herbert RD, Lamb SE et al. Investigating causal mechanisms in randomised controlled trials. *Trials.* 2019;20:524.

25. Sherrington C, Fairhall NJ, Wallbank GK et al. Exercise for preventing falls in older people living in the community. *Cochrane Database Syst Rev.* 2019;1:CD012424.

26. Lamb SE, Bruce J, Hossain A et al. Screening and intervention to prevent falls and fractures in older people. *N Engl J Med.* 2020;383:1848–59.

27. Bhasin S, Gill TM, Reuben DB et al. A randomized trial of a multifactorial strategy to prevent serious fall injuries. *N Engl J Med.* 2020;383:129–40.

26

Fall Prevention in Hospitals

Anne-Marie Hill

Falls are one of the most frequent adverse events that occur in hospitals [1, 2]. Fall rates range from 3.4 to 11 falls per 1000 bed days in acute and rehabilitation wards [3–6]. These rates translate to significant numbers of patients falling during a hospital stay; for example, in England there were over 250,000 falls in hospitals 2015/2016 [1], and it is estimated that nearly one million patients fall in US hospitals each year [2]. For these patients, a hospital admission intended to improve health may result in serious injuries and even death.

While approximately 70% of falls result in no harm [1], studies in a broad range of hospital settings have found that between 20% and 40% of in-hospital falls result in physical injury [7–10]. Serious adverse outcomes such as fractures and head injuries occur in approximately 1% to 2% of falls [7, 8], and deaths occur in a small number of cases [8, 10]. Falls are known to also result in negative psycho-social consequences, such as admission to a nursing home, developing a fear of falls, and personal social and financial costs to the patient and their family [11, 12]. Falls result in increased costs to health care systems since fall injuries may cause increased lengths of stay, further treatment requirements, and possible litigation [1, 13].

How and Where Falls in Hospitals Occur

Patients over 65 years of age have a particularly high risk of falling. A national falls report in 2017 demonstrated that of 247,000 falls, 77% occurred in patients over 65 years old [1]. This is because older patients admitted to hospital because of acute illness often have gait and balance disorders, acute confusion, underlying cognitive impairment and are taking psychotropic medications [6, 14–16]. Older patients also are more likely to become acutely confused during their hospital stay because of their acute illness, their predisposition to become delirious due to pre-existing cognitive impairment, age-related changes to vision and hearing, and less ability to withstand insult to their homeostasis [17, 18]. Delirium is a medical emergency and an important contributing factor to falls [17, 18].

Fall rates are particularly high in medical, geriatric, and rehabilitation wards, as these wards contain large numbers of older patients [6]. One study found that fall rates in geriatric units were 10.7 per thousand patient days compared to 3.2 in surgical units [6]. Other groups at very high risk of falls include patients diagnosed with stroke [19], and patients in mental health units [1].

Falls occur most often in patients' bedrooms and when patients are alone [9, 20–22]. National and prospective studies have identified that over 80% of patient falls occur when patients are unobserved by staff [10, 22, 23]. Bedside transfers and attempts to go to the toilet comprise tasks associated with falls when patients are alone [6, 9, 22]. Epidemiological studies have also found that falls tend to occur early in the hospital stay [24, 25], most likely because patients are unfamiliar with the ward environment, they are more acutely unwell early in their hospital stay, their mobility is worse during this period, and staff are not familiar with caring for the newly admitted patient.

Is It Possible to Identify Patients at Risk of Falling?

Numerous studies have identified patient risk factors for falls, including older age, history of falls, impaired mobility, cognitive impairment, male gender, stroke, and psychoactive medication use [14–16]. Multiple screening tools have been developed to screen all patients and identify those at risk of falls [26, 27].

However, screening patients and rating their fall risk has been found to be an ineffective approach to reducing falls in the hospital setting. Studies have consistently identified that risk screening tools have only modest success in predicting which hospital patients are more likely to fall [12, 28, 29], or which patients are at risk of injurious falls [30]. Limitations in the predictive validity and practical used of screening tools means they are unlikely to have a meaningful effect on fall prevention [28]. Patients' fall risk is likely to alter during their admission according to their medical problems and importantly organizational policies regarding fall prevention, ward environment, and staff actions also impact on patient safety. National guidelines now recommend that a patient-centred approach be used to identify all modifiable risk factors for each patient, subsequently addressing each factor appropriately [2, 20, 31]. Guidelines also recommend that all patients over the age of 65 years be considered at high risk of falls when admitted to hospital [2, 20, 31].

Do Patients Have an Understanding About Their Risk of Falling in Hospital?

Qualitative studies have found that patients have low levels of awareness about their risk of falls and believe that they will not fall during their hospital admission [32–34]. These findings demonstrate why patients may attempt to initiate mobility tasks unassisted that are not safe for them to complete independently [9, 10, 22]. Previous qualitative studies have identified that communication failure between staff and patients, perceptions that staff are too busy, and desires to test physical boundaries influence older patients to take risks that could result in a fall [35]. Patients have also identified barriers to engaging in safe behaviour regarding fall prevention, including feeling overconfident or desiring to be independent, and thinking that staff would be delayed in providing assistance [36].

Implementing Best Practice for Fall Prevention in Hospitals

Falls in hospital can be conceptualized as events that occur due to a combination of patient, staff, and environmental factors [9, 21, 37]. The case study (Box 26.1) illustrates why a comprehensive approach to fall prevention in hospitals should address patient, staff, and environmental conditions.

Box 26.1 Case Study

John (80 years old) is admitted to a medical ward with a diagnosis of angina and shortness of breath. He has mild cognitive impairment, age-related visual impairment, and lower limb weakness. Alone in his room, John decides to go to the toilet. He has been told to seek assistance but is not sure whether he should ring the bell. His walking aid is not positioned by the bed and since he often walks inside at home with no aid he goes directly to the toilet without using his aid. He is unfamiliar with the bathroom and doesn't turn on the light. John reaches round to the toilet rail and overbalances, falling onto the hard tiles. He calls out and staff enter the room. John sustains bruises and skin tears.

Why has John fallen? John has NOT fallen only because he has medical problems of shortness of breath, reduced mobility, cognitive impairment, age-related visual impairment, and lower limb weakness. The environment is unfamiliar to him. His walking aid is not in reach. He does not have a clear understanding about using the bell. Staff are not present. If John has a toileting care plan in place, it has not been devised such that he seeks or receives assistance for toileting when needed. Staff have not communicated with John such that he has a clear understanding of what constitutes safe behaviour.

If John was receiving staff assistance or the environment was set up correctly with his aid and bell in reach, if he had his glasses on, and was familiar with the room environment he may not have fallen. John's fall is a combination of patient, environmental, and staff-related factors.

How can John's safety be addressed during admission? John, like every older patient, needs a tailored individualized plan that addresses not only his medical problems, but maintains his safety and promotes his functional recovery. A systematic hospital-wide approach that ensures the environment is safe, every patient receives an individualized fall prevention plan, and staff assistance for mobility is provided where required is key to preventing older patients like John from falling, thus facilitating their recovery. Protecting patients from preventable harm such as falls requires a system-wide approach to safety and quality.

Briefly, it is also critical that hospitals implement fall prevention policy and practice within the framework of national standards that health care regulators have developed to deliver high-quality health care [38, 39]. Safety and quality in all aspects of patient care is formulated around adopting these standards, including addressing a culture of safety and consistently high standards of clinical care [38, 39].

What Is the Best Available Evidence for Reducing Falls in Hospital?

A number of systematic reviews have synthesized the evidence for reducing falls in hospitals. These reviews have included different groups of studies, with differing trial design and settings [40–42].

A recent systematic review [40] that synthesized 24 randomized controlled trials (RCTs) concluded that multi-factorial interventions in hospitals may reduce the rate of falls in hospitals. Sub-group analysis suggested that reduction may be more likely in the sub-acute setting. A narrative review of five RCTs conducted in acute medical and surgical wards only, suggested that interventions that provided targeted fall interventions in addition to usual care, based on individualized patient fall risk assessment and management were effective in reducing falls, although not fall-related injuries, while multi-factorial interventions that were not tailored did not have a significant effect in these settings [41]. Another review which evaluated multiple systematic reviews and included evidence from another two RCTs also suggested that multi-component programmes reduce falls by approximately 30% [43].

However, since all multi-factorial trials implement different combinations of interventions with differing designs and results, synthesizing these trials has only resulted in low GRADE evidence [44] with high heterogeneity of the trials included [21, 40, 43]. Trials were conducted in a range of ward types and differing patient groups depending on hospital admission criteria. Different intervention designs are difficult to compare. There are differences between trials with regard to methods of collecting falls data. For example, falls are under-reported if hospital reporting systems alone are used [23, 45]. Multiple systematic reviews have emphasized that the optimal combination, targeting, and intensity of intervention components is not established and that further high-quality trials are required [40, 43, 46].

Regarding which components of multi-factorial interventions are effective, a systematic review of 21 studies suggested that components common to successful trials include risk assessments for patients, patient and staff education, bedside signs and wristband alerts, footwear advice, scheduled and supervised toileting, and medication reviews [42]. An earlier comprehensive clinical review on hospital fall prevention suggested that intervention components most commonly included in successful trials comprise a post fall review, patient education, staff education, footwear advice, and addressing issues related to toileting [21]. This review suggested that these interventions have a plausible mechanism of effect that aligns with the profile of patients who fall and the circumstances of falls, in that patients are unaware of their risk of falls and mobilize without staff being present to provide necessary assistance [10, 21–23, 33]

What Single Interventions Have Shown Evidence for Effectiveness to Be Included in Hospital Fall Prevention Programmes?

Trials which test single interventions can assist to determine which components of multi-factorial interventions contribute to reducing falls in hospital.

Environmental Conditions

Some multi-factorial interventions have delivered environmental strategies such as monitoring the bedside environment for safety [40]. Evaluating and modifying the hospital environment, including lighting, flooring, fittings, signage, and other environmental factors have not been undertaken as the main interventions specifically in hospital-based fall prevention randomized clinical trials. However, it is accepted that these factors contribute to fallsents [2, 9, 22]. Hence, they form an essential component of comprehensively addressing patient safety in hospital, including fall prevention. Further research is required to evaluate which types of environmental improvements could be most effective in reducing inpatient falls [20].

Equipment: Bed Alarms, Low Beds, and Patient Socks

There is strong evidence from RCTs that bed alarms do not reduce falls [47–49]. Bed alarms also have the potential to disturb patients and staff workflow [47–49]. Systematic implementation of low beds, which can be placed at floor level, for use on wards is also not effective in reducing falls [50]. An RCT conducted in acute medical and surgical wards included low beds and bed alarms in a multi-factorial intervention, alongside a toileting plan and risk alert sign at patients' bedsides was found to be ineffective in reducing falls [51]. These environmental interventions should only be used for an older patient if an individual assessment suggests a strong rationale. Socks which are described as non-slip have also been suggested as a fall reduction strategy, but there is inconclusive evidence that non-slip socks reduce falls [52]. These socks are less adequate than normal footwear and provide less slip resistance than bare feet [53].

Patient Sitters

Patient companions or 'sitters' provide supervision to patients considered at high risk of falls in range of hospital settings [54]. It seems plausible that such supervision, particularly for patients with cognitive impairment, could reduce falls, as around 80% of falls occur when patients are unobserved. However, sitters can only prevent falls if they provide an immediate verbal or physical response to patients attempting to move unsafely. This would imply that a patient would need the sitter to be in continuous close proximity and this may agitate confused older patients. Sitters themselves also report that there are numerous barriers to reducing falls in these patients at high risk [55], and at present the current evidence indicates providing sitters does not reduce patient falls [54, 56].

Patient Call Bells

It is critical to provide effective call bell systems. Effective call bell systems that can be modified for all patients and bed settings allow patients to immediately alert staff to their need for assistance. They are fundamental to comprehensive fall prevention programmes, as they reduce the likelihood of patients attempting to mobilize unassisted [2]. A national audit found that only 81% of patients could see and reach their call bell [57]. Qualitative studies clearly demonstrate that patients do not have a clear understanding about the rationale of seeking staff assistance, do not ring the bell for assistance and identify multiple barriers to using existing call bell systems to maintain their safety on hospital wards [35, 36, 58]. Therefore, providing patients with education about how and when to use the call bell is essential.

Patient Education

A cluster RCT demonstrated that patient education, provided in addition to usual care, significantly reduces falls and injurious falls in rehabilitation settings [4]. These findings are consistent with two other RCTs which also demonstrated that patient education effectively reduced falls in rehabilitation settings [5, 7]. This education was provided to patients with better levels of cognition and staff feedback was provided to assist staff to understand and respond to the patients who received the education [4]. While the education was provided only to patients with better cognition (approximately 50% of patients on the wards in the RCT), there was a trend indicating falls rates were also reduced in those with cognitive impairment. This education programme raised patients' awareness of their risk of falls and confidence to use their call bells to seek staff assistance [36, 37, 59]. Process evaluations conducted as part of this trial demonstrated that falls and fall-related injury were reduced through education stimulating a response which addressed the causes of falls at the patient, staff, and environment levels.

> **Box 26.2 Example of Plain Language Summary for Reducing Fall Risk for Older Patients (and Their Families) Who Are Admitted to a Hospital**
>
> - Be aware that ALL older people are at risk of falling while in hospital. This risk is even higher if you have fallen before, or have cognitive or mobility problems. Falls occur most frequently inside patient rooms, often near your bed.
> - Falls frequently occur because you have new medical problems that led to your admission. You may not have your usual level of strength. Therefore, follow staff guidance about moving out of your bed, especially when using the toilet. You may be instructed to seek staff assistance prior to getting out of bed or going to the toilet. Staff are experienced in assisting patients. Maintain your safety by asking and waiting for help at all times.
> - Always tell staff if you have had any prior falls, and if you have cognitive or mobility problems. If you transfer to another ward, repeat this information to new staff.
> - If you use a walking aid at home it is vital to also use it in hospital. If you have not brought your aid with you ask staff to immediately issue you with a walking aid when you are admitted.
> - If you care for an older person who is confused or unable to communicate effectively, speak to hospital staff about their history of falls and any mobility problems. Communicate regularly with staff about any concerns you have regarding their care and safety.

Therefore, providing patients with education can benefit those with impaired levels of cognition through ward and staff practice change [36, 37, 59]. Another RCT conducted in acute wards that included tailored patient education, with staff being provided with tailored information at the bedside to align with the patients' education also significantly reduced falls (but not injurious falls) [60].

Box 26.2 provides an example of a plain language summary for reducing fall risk that can be given to older patients (and their families) who are admitted to a hospital.

Reducing Falls by Managing Delirium

Providing tailored care for older patients with delirium is important to improve their medical outcomes and also their safety, including reducing falls [61]. Between 29% and 64% of older people become delirious while in hospital [17]. It is known that patients who are confused have increased rates of falls compared to those who are not confused or cognitively impaired [4], as well as increased mortality and functional decline [17]. A systematic review of four RCTs that evaluated multi-component non-pharmacologic delirium interventions found the interventions significantly reduced fall rates [18]. The elements of these interventions were based on the Hospital Elder Life Program [62]. This includes providing confused patients with orientation, early supported mobility, ensuring visual and hearing aids are worn, sleep–wake cycle preservation, ensuring adequate hydration, and reducing psychoactive medication use [62]. These interventions have a plausible mechanism for reducing falls, since they address care for older people with acute confusion such that these patients are more prepared to undertake safe mobility and receive adequate supervision and fall risk modification by staff.

Medication Reviews

Psychoactive medications are known to be associated with inpatient falls and delirium and have detrimental effects on mobility [15, 17, 21, 63]. There is limited evidence about the effect of medication reviews as a single intervention in hospitals and these reviews have not been routinely included in multi-factorial interventions [42, 43]. However, reducing these medications is recommended for decreasing the incidence of both falls and delirium [17, 20, 31]. A large time-series trial in hospital evaluated a computer algorithm to assist doctors reduce their prescriptions of psychoactive medications for older people. This trial demonstrated significant reductions in prescription of these medications and a significant reduction in fall rates [64].

Recommendations for Addressing Fall Prevention in Hospitals

Fall prevention guidelines have been developed by national health systems [2, 20, 31]. Health care organizations should use these guidelines to develop a systematic and comprehensive plan to address fall prevention. A national audit recently demonstrated that there are significant gaps in hospitals' clinical care and fall prevention policies and practice regarding actioning and translating evidence for reducing falls [57]. Organizations require leadership and policies that facilitate systematic translation of fall prevention evidence into sustained and effective clinical practice throughout the organization [38, 39]. This includes collecting and analysing fall incidence data, training staff, clinical leadership, systematic auditing, and feedback [2, 42, 43]. Key elements for a comprehensive hospital fall prevention programme are outlined below.

Recognize that All Older Patients Are at Risk of Falling

All patients over the age of 65 years are at risk of falls regardless of their location in a hospital. Also identify patients who are below the age of 65 years who may have increased risk of falls. This includes patients with acute confusion, other cognitive problems, stroke, and other neurological conditions [2, 20].

Institute Universal Precautions for All Older Patients in Hospital

There is strong evidence that over 80% of falls occur when patients are undertaking activities unassisted [9, 10, 22, 23]. Therefore fundamental safety precautions should underpin all fall prevention programmes. Universal precautions are:

- The hospital environment should be safely maintained, including suitable fittings such as wall and toilet rails and adequate lighting and flooring, and furniture stability and layout [20].

- Aspects of the environment directly adjusted for individual patients must be regularly monitored by staff. This includes bed height, working patient call bells within reach [57], mobility aids and drinks positioned in patients' reach, and optimal lighting.

- Provide individualized safety education for patients who have good levels of cognition, including the provision of clear guidance about call bell use and mobility [4, 20].

- Assess and monitor all older patients for confusion or delirium, using standardized assessment tools [17, 18]. Institute treatments promptly, including appropriately adjusting fall prevention care plans.

- Ensure all older patients with cognitive impairment receive tailored care from point of hospital admission that is specifically modified for this population. Specifically trained staff and providing a 'dementia friendly' environment are important for this group of patients to ensure that their safety and clinical care are optimized [61].

- Monitor all older patients daily, particularly patients with cognitive impairment, to ensure their vision and hearing is optimized, i.e. ensure they are wearing their glasses and hearing aids.

- Address continence problems with a tailored continence plan which includes monitoring hydration needs and ensure patients receive required assistance to complete toileting activities.

- Have mandated post-fall guidelines [2, 65]. A key means of preventing further falls and improving an older person's recovery in hospital is to treat each fall as an important event to be investigated and prevented from re-occurring. While post-fall assessment is essential to identify injuries such as fractures or head injury, even minor falls which cause no apparent injuries should be investigated by the multi-disciplinary team because an older patient falling is often an indication of infection or the onset of delirium. Additionally, a history of falling is one of the strongest predictors of having another fall [14, 21].

- Conduct post-fall analyses to review ward practice, identify gaps in clinical care and ensure that modified post-fall management is not only recorded in the clinical care plan, but is enacted by clinical staff.

Assess Every Older Patient's Individual Fall Risk

Every older patient requires an individualized assessment of their risk of falls, followed by appropriate management of modifiable and non-modifiable risks identified. All professions should be involved in systematically conducting this multi-factorial assessment and addressing risk factors during admission. Guidelines recommend this multi-factorial approach should assess and address medication use, poor mobility (including transfer ability and walking aid use), impaired cognition, unsafe footwear, health problems, continence problems, visual impairment, history of falls, and syncope, including the presence of postural drop in blood pressure [20, 31].

A systematic approach to providing patient-centred care for reducing a patient's risk of falls requires a purpose-designed fall risk assessment and management plan either separately completed or integrated with the patients' overall clinical care plan. Regardless of how this assessment is performed, the risk factors addressed should be clearly embedded into the patient's clinical care plan.

Embed Fall Prevention Programmes Within a Strong Quality Improvement System

All staff, regardless of discipline or work role, including students on clinical placement, should complete fall prevention training. This includes review of ward policies and practices whenever staff transfer between locations within the hospital. All staff should also be instructed to focus on preventing falls by immediately addressing environmental hazards and providing timely assistance to patients to mobilize safely.

Quality improvement departments must mandate individualized clinical assessment and management of fall risk. This includes providing staff training and support and a fall incident reporting system which provides timely analysis and feedback to clinical staff. A high-quality audit and feedback loop should also be regularly implemented as audits readily identify gaps in fall prevention practice [57, 66] to identify whether hospital policies regarding falls are being enacted effectively. This is critical for providing effective, safe clinical care. Additionally, a workplace culture that prioritizes patient safety is important as part of a whole-organization approach to fall prevention and other aspects of patient safety [67].

Conclusions

Falls are a serious adverse event that can hinder patients' recovery trajectory and may result in permanent disability or even death. Hospitals need to implement a system-wide culture of safety that addresses fall prevention at patient, ward, and organizational levels.

REFERENCES

1. NHS Improvement. The incidence and costs of inpatient falls in hospitals. 2017. https://improvement.nhs.uk/resources/incidence-and-costs-inpatient-falls-hospitals/ (accessed July 2019).

2. Ganz DA, Huang C, Saliba D et al. Preventing falls in hospitals. A Toolkit for improving quality of care. U.S. Department of Health and Human Services. Agency for Health Care Research and Quality (AHRQ). 2013. www.ahrq.gov/professionals/systems/hospital/fallpxtoolkit/index.html (accessed April 2021).

3. Bouldin EL, Andresen EM, Dunton NE et al. Falls among adult patients hospitalized in the United States: prevalence and trends. *J Patient Saf.* 2013;9:13–17.

4. Hill A-M, McPhail SM, Waldron N et al. Fall rates in hospital rehabilitation units after individualised patient and staff education programmes: a pragmatic, stepped-wedge, cluster-randomised controlled trial. *Lancet.* 2015;385:2592–9.

5. Haines TP, Bennell KL, Osborne RH et al. Effectiveness of targeted fall prevention programme in subacute hospital setting: randomised controlled trial. *Br Med J.* 2004;328:676.

6. Schwendimann R, Buhler H, De Geest S et al. Characteristics of hospital inpatient falls across clinical departments. *Gerontology.* 2008;54:342–8.

7. Haines TP, Hill A-M, Hill KD et al. Patient education to prevent falls among older hospital inpatients: a randomized controlled trial. *Arch Intern Med.* 2011;171:516–24.

8. Healey F, Scobie S, Oliver D et al. Falls in English and Welsh hospitals: a national observational study based on retrospective analysis of 12 months of patient safety incident reports. *Qual Saf Health Care.* 2008;17:424–30.

9. Hignett S, Sands G, Griffiths P. In-patient falls: what can we learn from incident reports? *Age Ageing.* 2013;42:527–31.

10. Staggs VS, Mion LC, Shorr RI. Assisted and unassisted falls: different events, different outcomes, different implications for quality of hospital care. *Jt Comm J Qual Patient Saf.* 2014;40:358–64.

11. Turner N, Jones D, Dawson P et al. The perceptions and rehabilitation experiences of older people after falling in the hospital. *Rehabil Nurs.* 2019;44:141–50.

12. Hill A-M, Jacques A, Chandler AM et al. In-hospital sequelae of injurious falls in 24 medical/surgical units in four hospitals in the United States. *Jt Comm J Qual Patient Saf.* 2019;45:91–7.

13. Morello RT, Barker AL, Watts JJ et al. The extra resource burden of in-hospital falls: a cost of falls study. *Med J Aust.* 2015;203:367.

14. Deandrea S, Bravi F, Turati F et al. Risk factors for falls in older people in nursing homes and hospitals. A systematic review and meta-analysis. *Arch Gerontol Geriatr.* 2013;56:407–15.

15. O'Neil CA, Krauss MJ, Bettale J et al. Medications and patient characteristics associated with falling in the hospital. *J Patient Saf.* 2018;14:27–33.

16. Oliver D, Daly F, Martin FC et al. Risk factors and risk assessment tools for falls in hospital in-patients: a systematic review. *Age Ageing.* 2004;33:122–30.

17. Inouye SK, Westendorp RG, Saczynski JS. Delirium in elderly people. *Lancet* 2014;383:911–22.

18. Hshieh TT, Yue J, Oh E et al. Effectiveness of multicomponent non-pharmacological delirium interventions. *JAMA Intern Med.* 2015;175:512–20.

19. Wong JS, Brooks D, Mansfield A. Do falls experienced during inpatient stroke rehabilitation affect length of stay, functional status, and discharge destination? *Arch Phys Med Rehabil.* 2016;97:561–6.

20. National Institute for Health and Care Excellence (NICE). Falls in Older People: Assessing Risk and Prevention. Clinical Guideline [CG161]. 2013. www.nice.org.uk/guidance/cg161 (accessed April 2021).

21. Oliver D, Healey F, Haines TP. Preventing falls and fall-related injuries in hospitals. *Clin Geriatr Med.* 2010;26:645–92.

22. de Jong LD, Francis-Coad J, Waldron N et al. Does free-text information in falls incident reports assist to explain how and why the falls occurred in a hospital setting? *J Patient Saf.* 2018;[e-pub ahead of print]. doi:10.1097/pts.0000000000000533.

23. Hill A-M, Hoffmann T, Hill K et al. Measuring falls events in acute hospitals: a comparison of three reporting methods to identify missing data in the hospital reporting system. *J Am Geriatr Soc.* 2010;58:1347–52.

24. Rapp K, Ravindren J, Becker C et al. Fall risk as a function of time after admission to sub-acute geriatric hospital units. *BMC Geriatr.* 2016;16:173.

25. Corsinovi L, Bo M, Ricauda Aimonino N et al. Predictors of falls and hospitalization outcomes in elderly patients admitted to an acute geriatric unit. *Arch Gerontol Geriatr.* 2009;49:142–5.

26. Coker E, Oliver D. Evaluation of the STRATIFY falls prediction tool on a geriatric unit. *Outcomes Manag.* 2003;7:8–14;quiz 15–16.

27. Morse JM, Black C, Oberle K et al. A prospective study to identify the fall-prone patient. *Soc Sci Med.* 1989;28:81–6.

28. Healey F, Haines TP. A pragmatic study of the predictive values of the Morse falls score. *Age Ageing.* 2013;42:462–8.

29. Oliver D, Papaioannou A, Giangregorio L et al. A systematic review and meta-analysis of studies using the STRATIFY tool for prediction of falls in hospital patients: how well does it work? *Age Ageing.* 2008;37:621–7.

30. Mion LC, Chandler AM, Waters TM et al. Is it possible to identify risks for injurious falls in hospitalized patients? *Jt Comm J Qual Patient Saf.* 2012;38:408–13.

31. Australian Commission on Safety and Quality in Healthcare. Preventing Falls and Harm from Falls in Older People: Best Practice Guidelines for Australian Hospitals. 2009. www.safetyandquality.gov.au/publications-and-resources/resource-library/preventing-falls-and-harm-falls-older-people-best-practice-guidelines-australian-hospitals (accessed April 2021).

32. Haines TP, McPhail SM. Threat appraisal for harm from falls: insights for development of education-based intervention. *Open Longev Sci.* 2011;5:9–15.

33. Lee DC, McDermott F, Hoffmann T et al. 'They will tell me if there is a problem': limited discussion between health professionals, older adults and their caregivers on fall prevention during and after hospitalization. *Health Educ Res.* 2013;28:1051–66.

34. Twibell RS, Siela D, Sproat T et al. Perceptions related to falls and fall prevention among hospitalized adults. *Am J Crit Care*. 2015;24:e78–85.

35. Haines TP, Lee DC, O'Connell B et al. Why do hospitalized older adults take risks that may lead to falls? *Health Expect*. 2012;18:233–49.

36. Hill A-M, Francis-Coad J, Haines TP et al. 'My independent streak may get in the way': how older adults respond to fall prevention education in hospital. *BMJ Open*. 2016;6:e012363.

37. Hill A-M, McPhail SM, Francis-Coad J et al. Educators' perspectives about how older hospital patients can engage in a fall prevention education programme: a qualitative process evaluation. *BMJ Open*. 2015;5:e009780.

38. Australian Commission on Safety and Quality in Health Care. National Safety and Quality Health Service (NSQHS) Standards. www.safetyandquality.gov.au/standards/nsqhs-standards (accessed April 2021).

39. National Health Service Improvement. Improvement Hub: Patient Safety. https://improvement.nhs.uk/improvement-hub/patient-safety/ (accessed April 2021).

40. Cameron ID, Dyer SM, Panagoda CE et al. Interventions for preventing falls in older people in care facilities and hospitals. *Cochrane Database Syst Rev*. 2018;2018:CD005465.

41. Avanecean D, Calliste D, Contreras T et al. Effectiveness of patient-centered interventions on falls in the acute care setting compared to usual care: a systematic review. *JBI Database System Rev Implement Rep*. 2017;15:3006–48.

42. Miake-Lye IM, Hempel S, Ganz DA et al. Inpatient fall prevention programs as a patient safety strategy: a systematic review. *Ann Intern Med*. 2013;158:390–6.

43. Hempel S, Newberry S, Wang Z et al. Hospital fall prevention: a systematic review of implementation, components, adherence, and effectiveness. *J Am Geriatr Soc*. 2013;61:483–94.

44. Guyatt G, Oxman AD, Akl EA et al. GRADE guidelines: 1. Introduction-GRADE evidence profiles and summary of findings tables. *J Clin Epidemiol*. 2011;64:383–94.

45. Shorr RI, Mion LC, Chandler AM et al. Improving the capture of fall events in hospitals: combining a service for evaluating inpatient falls with an incident report system. *J Am Geriatr Soc*. 2008;56:701–4.

46. LeLaurin JH, Shorr RI. Preventing falls in hospitalized patients: state of the science. *Clin Geriatr Med*. 2019;35:273–83.

47. Oliver D. Do bed and chair sensors really stop falls in hospital? *Br Med J*. 2018;360:k433.

48. Shorr RI, Chandler AM, Mion LC et al. Effects of an intervention to increase bed alarm use to prevent falls in hospitalized patients: a cluster randomized trial. *Ann Intern Med*. 2012;157:692–9.

49. Sahota O, Drummond A, Kendrick D et al. REFINE (REducing Falls in In-patieNt Elderly) using bed and bedside chair pressure sensors linked to radio-pagers in acute hospital care: a randomised controlled trial. *Age Ageing*. 2014;43:247–53.

50. Haines TP, Bell RA, Varghese PN. Pragmatic, cluster randomized trial of a policy to introduce low-low beds to hospital wards for the prevention of falls and fall injuries. *J Am Geriatr Soc*. 2010;58:435–41.

51. Barker AL, Morello RT, Wolfe R et al. 6-PACK programme to decrease fall injuries in acute hospitals: cluster randomised controlled trial. *Br Med J*. 2016;352:h6781.

52. Hartung B, Lalonde M. The use of non-slip socks to prevent falls among hospitalized older adults: a literature review. *Geriatr Nurs.* 2017;38:412–16.

53. Chari S, Haines T, Varghese P et al. Are non-slip socks really 'non-slip'? An analysis of slip resistance. *BMC Geriatr.* 2009;9:39.

54. Lang CE. Do sitters prevent falls? A review of the literature. *J Gerontol Nurs.* 2014;40:24–33; quiz 34–5.

55. de Jong LD, Weselman T, Kitchen S, Hill A-M. Exploring hospital patient sitters' fall prevention task readiness: a cross-sectional survey. *J Eval Clin Pract.* 2020;26:42–9.

56. Wood VJ, Vindrola-Padros C, Swart N et al. One to one specialling and sitters in acute care hospitals: a scoping review. *Int J Nurs Stud.* 2018;84:61–77.

57. Royal College of Physicians. National Audit of Inpatient Falls: Audit Report 2017. www .rcplondon.ac.uk/projects/outputs/naif-audit-report-2017 (accessed July 2019).

58. Carroll DL, Dykes PC, Hurley AC. Patients' perspectives of falling while in an acute care hospital and suggestions for prevention. *Appl Nurs Res.* 2010;23:238–41.

59. Hill A-M, Waldron N, Francis-Coad J et al. 'It promoted a positive culture around fall prevention'. Staff response to a patient education programme: a qualitative evaluation. *BMJ Open.* 2016;6:e013414.

60. Dykes C, Carroll DL, Hurley A et al. Fall prevention in acute care hospitals. *J Am Med Assoc.* 2010;304:1912–18.

61. Royal College of Psychiatrists' Centre for Quality Improvement. Healthcare Quality Improvement Partnership (HQIP). National Audit of Dementia. 2017. www.hqip.org.uk /a-z-of-nca/dementia-care-in-general-hospitals/ (accessed April 2021).

62. Inouye SK, Bogardus ST Jr., Baker DI et al. The Hospital Elder Life Program: a model of care to prevent cognitive and functional decline in older hospitalized patients. *J Am Geriatr Soc.* 2000;48:1697–706.

63. Diaz-Gutierrez MJ, Martinez-Cengotitabengoa M, Saez de Adana E et al. Relationship between the use of benzodiazepines and falls in older adults: a systematic review. *Maturitas.* 2017;101:17–22.

64. Peterson JF, Kuperman GJ, Shek C et al. Guided prescription of psychotropic medications for geriatric inpatients. *Arch Intern Med.* 2005;165:802–7.

65. National Institute for Health and Care Excellence (NICE). Falls in Older People. Quality Standard [QS86]. 2015. www.nice.org.uk/guidance/qs86 (accessed April 2021).

66. Francis-Coad J, Etherton-Beer C, Bulsara C et al. Using a community of practice to evaluate fall prevention activity in a residential aged care organisation: a clinical audit. *Aust Health Rev.* 2016;41:13–18.

67. Mardon RE, Khanna K, Sorra J et al. Exploring relationships between hospital patient safety culture and adverse events. *J Patient Saf.* 2010;6:226–32.

27

Fall Prevention in Residential Aged Care Facilities

Clemens Becker, Kilian Rapp, and Patrick Roigk

The chapter synthesizes the current knowledge about falls, fall-related injuries, and fall prevention among residents of nursing homes, residential care, and assisted living. These groups are from here on referred to as residents of long-term care (LTC) facilities. Evidence on the efficacy and effectiveness of fall prevention measures is cross-linked to the findings of systematic reviews, meta-analyses, and the most recent Cochrane review published in 2018 [1]. Evidence based on controlled studies is not available for all relevant questions. Therefore, scientific evidence is augmented by recommendations based on observational data and the authors' two decades of experience with large-scale implementation projects on fall prevention in German LTC facilities. The type of institutional care, and the qualification and cooperation of the staff differ significantly between countries and different care systems. In addition, resident case mix and care culture can differ considerably across countries. This should always be kept in mind. In order to update the knowledge, we performed a narrative literature search including study registries and databases. For the update, 46 registered or published studies from 2010 onwards were considered.

Relevance of Falls

Older people living in LTC facilities are at high risk for falls and injuries. Repeated falls and their consequences are key reasons why many older people are admitted to LTC. Falls threaten residents' remaining independence by reducing their ability to perform activities of daily living and participate in social activities, and this can be exacerbated by associated fear of falling. Furthermore, risk and history of falling can be considered 'justification' for the use of restrictive measures, including the use of physical restraints. Reducing the risk of falling, therefore, can improve residents' quality of life.

Epidemiology of Falls and Fall-Related Injuries

A summary of studies performed in LTC facilities calculated a mean fall rate of 1.7 falls per person-year (range: 0.6–3.6) [2]. These rates are considerably higher than the fall rate observed in older people living in the community (mean: 0.65, range: 0.3–1.6). In a facility with 100 beds, a fall can be expected every other day. The analysis of nearly 70,000 falls recorded in several hundred LTC facilities in Germany showed that more than 62% of falls occurred in residents' rooms, 13% in their bathrooms, 22% in common areas, and 3% outside [3]. More falls occurred during sit-to-stand or stand-to-sit transfers (41%) than when walking (36%), which differs from community dwellers where more falls are associated with walking activities. Nearly one-quarter of falls required the consultation of a physician or an accident and emergency department (A&E) or hospital visit, a higher proportion than is seen in community-living people. Falls in LTC facilities result in more serious complications with 10% to 25% of such falls resulting in fractures or traumatic brain injury [4].

The most common serious complications of falls in long-term care are hip fractures. The big difference in hip fracture rates between female residents in LTC facilities and females in the total population is even more marked than the above-mentioned difference in fall rates, possibly due to a higher prevalence of osteoporosis in residents of LTC facilities (see Figure 27.1) [5].

In Germany, residents of LTC facilities contribute about 20% to the overall burden of femoral fractures in older people, even though their corresponding person-years account only for 4% of the total (Figure 27.2) [6]. Women remain by far the largest group in absolute numbers of hip fractures. However, male residents should not be considered to be at low risk, as their hip fracture incidence is still considerably higher than the incidence of women of the same age living in the community [6,7].

While hip fractures are the most common form of fractures in LTC facilities, other fall-related injuries such as pelvic fractures, vertebral fractures, or traumatic brain injuries are also common.

Since 2013 the video-based analysis of falls experienced in LTC facilities in Vancouver has added new insights into fall mechanisms and possible preventive efforts [8]. One of the most relevant findings is the high rate of head impact during falls occurring in LTC facilities. More than 30% led to a visible head impact and thereby to a possible moderate or even severe traumatic brain injury. Another striking finding was the poor design of assistive devices with resultant non-use of walking aids and wheelchairs.

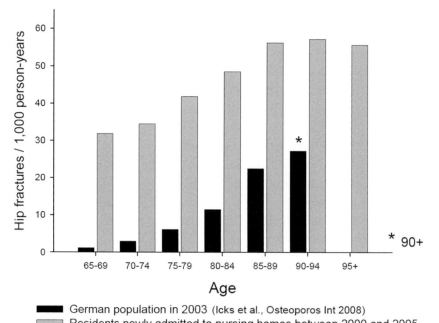

Figure 27.1   Comparison of hip fracture rates between older women living in the community and long-term care facilities. Adapted from Icks A, Haastert B, Wildner M et al. Trend of hip fracture incidence in Germany 1995–2004: a population-based study. Osteoporos Int 2008;19:1139–1145 [7], and Rapp K, Becker C, Lamb SE, Icks A, Klenk J. Hip fractures in institutionalized elderly people: incidence rates and excess mortality. *J Bone Miner Res.* 2008;23:1825–31 [74].

Risk Factors

Most LTC residents have numerous fall risk factors [9], with one study finding fall history (OR: 3.06), walking aid use (OR: 2.08), and moderate disability (OR: 2.08) as the strongest risk factors [10]. Poor vision, cognitive impairment, orthostatic hypotension, urinary incontinence [11], and nocturia are further common risk factors [9,12–15]. In addition, CNS co-morbidities such as dementia, depression, stroke, and Parkinson's disease lead to attention deficits, executive dysfunction, and visual field loss, and contribute to a higher propensity to fall. Drug side effects and interactions also increase the risk of falling [16–18]. The pathophysiologic mechanisms of psychotropic drugs, such as sedatives and antipsychotics, include impaired reactive balance control, and reduced attention and dual-task capacities. Risk factors may

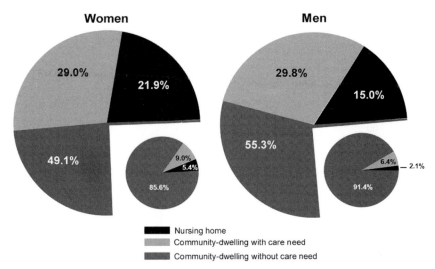

Figure 27.2   Percentage contribution of community-dwelling people with and without care needs and residents from nursing homes to the overall burden of femoral fractures (big diagrams) and their corresponding percentage of person-years under observation (small diagrams) in women and men aged 65 years or more. Adapted from Rapp K, Becker C, Cameron ID et al. Femoral fracture rates in people with and without disability. *Age Ageing* 2012;41:653–8 [6].

vary with different degrees of function and thereby exposure [19]. The risk of fall-related fractures, for example, is lowest in those residents with the most limited physical function [20]. A natural experimental design study demonstrated that the risk of fracture was greatest in the immediate time period after admission to LTC [21] (Figure 27.3). The most likely mechanism is an excess risk of falling due to an unfamiliar environment.

LTC facility design and environmental factors such as light and ergonomics contribute to falls and fall-related injuries. Building standards have been developed to minimize environmental hazards, but evidence for whether these measures are effective is not clear. Pragmatically, standards from age-friendly environments and dementia-sensitive architecture should be applied [22].

Fall Risk Assessment in Residents of Nursing Homes

Fall risk screening and assessment tools for LTC facilities have been developed based on the known risk factors. These instruments are often advocated and sometimes mandated, but their efficacy in relation to assisting fall prevention strategies has been questioned, as almost all residents of LTC facilities will score at moderate to high risk [23,24]. The comparison between

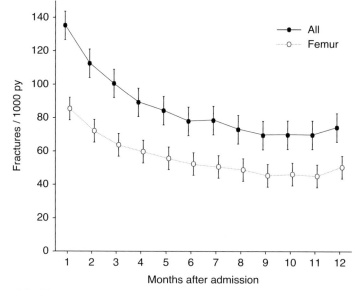

Figure 27.3   Risk of fracture in the time period following admission to a long-term care facility. Adapted from Rapp K, Lamb SE, Klenk J et al. Fractures after nursing home admission: incidence and potential consequences. Osteoporos Int 2009;20:1775–83 [21].

different fall risk assessment methods such as a single item screens using the resident's fall history, a nurse's global judgement, or a labour-intensive assessment tool did not demonstrate a clear superiority of one method [25] even if applied under the rigour of a research study. Standardized instruments administered at fixed intervals are time-consuming and do not adequately respond to a resident's dynamic health condition, possibly affecting fall risk over short periods. Therefore, the use of tools to predict falls in this high-risk population is not recommended [23,24]. We recommend a risk assessment focused on modifiable risk factors. A regular medication review is needed for every resident as part of best practice medical care. A mobility assessment is required for every person living in a LTC facility to identify their capacity to take part in an exercise programme. Vision, mood, and cognitive function should be addressed, and safe mobility is an implicit part of this process. An assessment based on these principles should be performed within the first days after admission to a LTC facility and repeated regularly.

LTC is a highly regulated and controlled environment. This allows a careful analytical approach of architectural and organizational measures for fall prevention using work safety approaches as part of a facility assessment. Lighting, flooring, walking aid maintenance, and room design are areas to improve environmental safety.

Managing Falls and Fall Prevention in Long-Term Care

The management of fall prevention should aim to be part of the routine care in LTC facilities as falls are so common and harmful. Routines should be regularly re-evaluated in a quality improvement process. One of the biggest challenges worldwide is the high proportion of inexperienced staff working in LTC facilities and high staff turnover [26,27]. This requires patience and sustainable management strategies. As it is in the community, the implementation of evidence from research studies to 'real world' practice in LTC facilities is a challenge.

Benchmarking and Documentation

Each LTC facility should have an IT-based system for documenting falls and fall-related injuries. Fall event reports should be brief, but precise, and include information about time and location of falls, activities associated with falls, and consequences of falls. Reports should be analysed on a three- to six-month basis with a timely feedback system to staff members. Each major event such as a fracture or an intra-cranial bleed should be discussed. Annually, the number of falls, fallers, and injuries should be analysed and compared in a benchmark process considering the case mix. A system should be in place so that the institution can be categorized as low/moderate/high risk and the quality of the documentation can be ascertained. The most frequent failures of documentation systems are the under-reporting of 'non-injurious' falls and the lack of timely feedback to staff [28].

Running or Starting a Fall Prevention Programme

This section presents suggestions for developing a fall prevention programme, bearing in mind that LTC facility care differs considerably across regions and countries. A quality improvement (QI) system and strong leadership are required to implement sustainable fall prevention within LTC facilities. The fall prevention programme needs to reflect the case mix and legally mandated tasks. Some changes will take months if not years to become routine. Furthermore, the identification and integration of staff champions in the QI initiatives can greatly assist in improving the quality of care and increase job satisfaction [29]. Initially, a baseline assessment of at least three months should be conducted before choosing the improvement modules to be implemented. The current Cochrane review remains unclear regarding whether multi-factorial programmes are effective in reducing the fall rate or the risk of falling in LTC facilities [1]. Negative studies are a reminder that programmes with low intensity might even be harmful [30]. Although it is difficult to prove in controlled trials, most experts agree that organizational commitment, leadership, and staff qualifications are essential components for implementing successful programmes. It has been demonstrated that structured process-of-care approaches can strengthen these initiatives [31]. Our state-wide implementation study of a non-randomized multi-factorial fall prevention programme showed a reduction of femoral fractures by 18% in the first year [32]. However, the reduction was only transient, which demonstrated that sustainability of fall prevention is an additional challenge [27,33].

Specific Fall Prevention Interventions

Most successful RCTs in LTC facilities have used complex interventions. None of the studies have used factorial designs to tease out which single components were most likely to reduce the number of falls. However, the shared components of most successful fall intervention programmes include knowledge improvement, attitudinal change, and the employment of staff with good qualifications [1]. As definitive RCT evidence is lacking, the following recommendations on the possible effects of single-component interventions relate to lower-level expert opinion based on discussion of the literature and insights gained from our programmes [34–36].

Staff Roles

LTC nursing staff have the most important role in implementation and sustainability. An ambivalent attitude and the lack of staff empowerment and self-efficacy will threaten the success of change [37]. The second most important component is inter-disciplinary communication. The interaction between nursing staff, physicians, administration, informal caregivers, and therapists is needed. As mentioned earlier in this chapter, many residents suffer a fall-related fracture soon after admission. In this early phase, timely responses are required with regard to assistance with toileting and transfers, and the provision of hip protectors for the first days or weeks. Staff must be made aware of the specific 'fall patterns' in their LTC facility and be cognizant that most falls occur in resident rooms and toilets, and are strongly associated with sit-to-stand transfers. Staff also need to be aware that in the early post-admission period, medication review and environmental adaptations are important [38,39].

For residents who have become familiar with the facility, the options for prevention change. In this period, exercise programmes and medication adjustments should be discussed. As the functional status of LTC residents can rapidly change, staff need the skills to identify 'hot' precipitating risk factors (e.g. an infection or reduced mobility following a fall) and should implement adaptive strategies immediately.

Environment and Clothing

The role and importance of extrinsic risk factors in LTC has been often debated [10], as there is a complex interaction between residents' functional status and their social and physical environment. A standardized chair height might be sufficient for many residents, but might be problematic for short or tall residents. An 'optimized' light design with increased luminance might be beneficial for residents with macular degeneration but create too much glare for residents with cataracts. Individual prescription is particularly important in the residents' rooms (walking patterns and navigation, adjusted transfer heights) with the aim of reducing person–environment mismatches in the individual's private space. This could be complemented by the provision of attractive pathways in public areas to encourage mobility in general.

Systematic review evidence indicates hip protectors probably reduce the risk of hip fractures in long-term care (see Chapter 24) [40,41]. However, there is concern that some models are insufficient to reduce the fall impact [42,43]. Shock-absorbing floor surfaces in resident rooms have also been suggested as a fall injury prevention strategy, but a recent definitive RCT found this strategy did not prevent serious fall injuries [44]. Other fall and fall injury prevention strategies being explored include footwear modifications, ergonomic improvement in furniture design [45], and intelligent assistive devices.

Training in assistive device use, maintenance, and design has been studied in other populations [46]. It seems reasonable to provide training in appropriate use with new devices and critically assess the capacity of residents with cognitive impairment to safely use them. Common user problems with assistive devices are sit-to-stand transfers and use during night-time walking.

Exercise

Although exercise has been found to be the most effective single intervention to prevent falls in the community, in LTC it has failed to reduce falls as a single intervention in most studies [1,47,48]. However, exercise as a single intervention reduced falls by 55% (incidence rate ratio: 0.45, 95% CI: 0.17, 0.74) in one recent randomized controlled trial conducted in LTC residents [49] and it would be unethical to withhold exercise to LTC residents, as regular exercise is beneficial for other health issues and can help general mobility. Most of the successful multifactorial programmes have included an exercise component within their suite of interventions. Often, the provision of exercise programmes is the best way to increase physical activity. Exercise has better uptake and adherence than other fall prevention strategies perceived to have negative connotations such as removal of hazards and hip protection.

The recommended duration, frequency, and intensity of exercise for frail old people are well established and the safety of such programmes demonstrated. Some examples of programmes that have been conducted in LTC include the HIFE [50], Otago [51], and Ulm [35] exercise programmes. It is recommended that the frequency of exercise sessions should be at least twice weekly and contain both challenging balance training and progressive strength training [52]. Secondary analysis has questioned the effectiveness of exercise in residents with severe dementia [53], but many studies have included participants with mild and moderate cognitive deficits with success [54–56]. Group programmes, however, are not feasible if several participants require too high a level of supervision. A recent evaluation of 40 exercise classes several years after implementation showed that adherence to the original programme was low. Therefore, ongoing trainer education seems to be crucial [57].

Vision

Vision impairment is a well-established risk factor for falls, but no single intervention trials to correct vision impairment have been conducted in LTC facilities. It should be noted that environmental approaches to improve contrast and light design appear difficult in LTC due to the co-existence of eye diseases (macular degeneration, glaucoma, cataract, and diabetic and hypertensive retinopathy) that require different lighting conditions.

Incontinence

More than 25% of falls occur when either walking to the bathroom or in the bathroom, and particularly during the night. Urinary incontinence (UI) and nocturia are well-established problems associated with falls, but very few trials have addressed this problem using a theory-based approach [58,59]. Efforts to improve incontinence such as assessment by a continence specialist nurse [60], scheduled nocturnal prompted voiding, or medical interventions to address urge incontinence appear under-used [61].

Medication Review and Pharmacological Interventions

The number of medical conditions and symptoms of LTC residents frequently leads to a high number of prescriptions. Psychoactive drugs are clearly associated with the risk for falls and deprescribing of inappropriate medication in LTC has been a research focus in recent years [62–64]. Although newer psychoactive medications (such as atypical neuroleptics and selective serotonin reuptake inhibitors) are generally better tolerated than the older agents, the most recent review concluded that most of these newer medications are not associated with fewer falls than the older agents [65]. Medication review to reduce orthostatic hypotension appears to be an important component [66]. The geriatric medicine-prescribing principles of prescribing the lowest effective dose, regularly reviewing medications and reducing or stopping medications whenever possible appear to be reasonable guidance to follow [67].

Finally, it is recommended that LTC residents should be prescribed Vitamin D in sufficient dosage (1000 IU per day) [1,64], as in addition to beneficial effect on bone health, Vitamin D is also effective in reducing falls and increasing muscle strength in people with severe Vitamin D deficiency [68,69].

Other Interventions

The evidence for fall prevention in disease-specific conditions is limited in general and particularly in LTC, and studies are required to determine whether people with Parkinson's disease, stroke, or epilepsy might benefit from specific interventions. Residents with dementia comprise the largest disease group of LTC facility residents. A secondary analysis of our first intervention trial showed that residents with cognitive impairment had a greater benefit than the residents without cognitive problems [54]. However, studies from Sweden and England have not found this to be the case [66,70]. Overall, the inclusion or exclusion from fall prevention programmes within LTC facilities based upon diagnosis appears not to be justified at this stage.

Physical Restraints and Falls

The use of restraints to avoid falls and fall-related injuries is still common in many countries [71]. This is a classical treatment paradox as the protective effect has never been demonstrated in controlled trials [72]. A short-term 'benefit' is seen as the justification to continue this questionable practice. Numerous studies have demonstrated that fall-related injuries and other side effects are increased if restraint effects are observed over longer time periods [73].

Conclusions

There is limited evidence that 20–30% of falls in long-term care are preventable [1]. There are marked differences between fall prevention in the community and in institutions. Whereas structured exercise is the key component in home-dwelling persons, exercise in LTC is only one component that has to be administered in combination with other interventions to be effective. Most successful programmes have used a combination of education, attitudinal change, and organizational efforts to ensure success. These comprehensive interventions are difficult to disentangle. Currently, there is no evidence to demonstrate that specific programmes (e.g. for stroke or demented patients) are superior to generic programmes including all residents with the capacity to stand or walk.

There are several options to further improve the effectiveness in translational efforts. LTC in many countries is a medically neglected area. One key component therefore is to develop and support good geriatric practice in LTC facilities. Another aspect is the improvement of uptake and adherence of fall prevention measures by staff members with knowledge and skills in aged care. The inclusion of expertise from organizational psychology may also strengthen the efforts. Another component is the inclusion of injury prevention models to better interpret location, time, and activities associated with falls. This could lead to the development of appropriate environmental adaptations. Lastly, it is essential to consider admission or return to an LTC facility as a time of high risk requiring different efforts to reduce falling.

LTC facilities have high rates for falls and fall-related injuries, so the prevention of fall-related injuries in mobile residents is a major goal. The prevention of hip fractures is crucial, as these fall-related injuries can drastically reduce the quality of life during a person's last phase of life. The implementation of the interventions outlined above should help to reduce falls in LTC facilities.

REFERENCES

1. Cameron ID, Dyer SM, Panagoda CE et al. Interventions for preventing falls in older people in care facilities and hospitals. *Cochrane Database Syst Rev.* 2018;2018:CD005465.
2. Rubenstein LZ. Falls in older people: epidemiology, risk factors and strategies for prevention. *Age Ageing.* 2006;35(2):ii37–41.
3. Rapp K, Becker C, Cameron ID et al. Epidemiology of falls in residential aged care: analysis of more than 70,000 falls from residents of Bavarian nursing homes. *J Am Med Dir Assoc.* 2012;13:187.e1–6.
4. Yang Y, Mackey DC, Liu-Ambrose T et al. Clinical risk factors for head impact during falls in older adults: a prospective cohort study in long-term care. *J Head Trauma Rehabil.* 2017;32:168–77.
5. Zimmerman SI, Girman CJ, Buie VC et al. The prevalence of osteoporosis in nursing home residents. *Osteoporos Int.* 1999;9:151–7.
6. Rapp K, Becker C, Cameron ID et al. Femoral fracture rates in people with and without disability. *Age Ageing.* 2012;41:653–8.
7. Icks A, Haastert B, Wildner M et al. Trend of hip fracture incidence in Germany 1995–2004: a population-based study. *Osteoporos Int.* 2008;19:1139–45.
8. Simon Fraser University. Technology for Injury Prevention in Seniors. 2019. www.sfu.ca /tips/ResearchProjects/videofalls.html (accessed April 2021).

9. Rubenstein LZ, Josephson KR, Robbins AS. Falls in the nursing home. *Ann Intern Med.* 1994;121:442–51.

10. Deandrea S, Bravi F, Turati F et al. Risk factors for falls in older people in nursing homes and hospitals. A systematic review and meta-analysis. *Arch Gerontol Geriatr.* 2013;56:407–15.

11. Chiarelli PE, Mackenzie LA, Osmotherly PG. Urinary incontinence is associated with an increase in falls: a systematic review. *Aust J Physiother.* 2009;55:89–95.

12. Luukinen H, Koski K, Laippala P et al. Risk factors for recurrent falls in the elderly in long-term institutional care. *Public Health.* 1995;109:57–65.

13. van Doorn C, Gruber-Baldini AL, Zimmerman S et al. Dementia as a risk factor for falls and fall injuries among nursing home residents. *J Am Geriatr Soc.* 2003;51:1213–18.

14. Thapa PB, Gideon P, Cost TW et al. Antidepressants and the risk of falls among nursing home residents. *N Engl J Med.* 1998;339:875–82.

15. Kron M, Loy S, Sturm E et al. Risk indicators for falls in institutionalized frail elderly. *Am J Epidemiol.* 2003;158:645–53.

16. Leipzig RM, Cumming RG, Tinetti ME. Drugs and falls in older people: a systematic review and meta-analysis. I. Psychotropic drugs. *J Am Geriatr Soc.* 1999;47:30–9.

17. Leipzig RM, Cumming RG, Tinetti ME. Drugs and falls in older people: a systematic review and meta-analysis. II. Cardiac and analgesic drugs. *J Am Geriatr Soc.* 1999;47:40–50.

18. Hartikainen S, Lonnroos E, Louhivuori K. Medication as a risk factor for falls: critical systematic review. *J Gerontol A Biol Sci Med Sci.* 2007;62:1172–81.

19. Lord SR, March LM, Cameron ID et al. Differing risk factors for falls in nursing home and intermediate-care residents who can and cannot stand unaided. *J Am Geriatr Soc.* 2003;51:1645–50.

20. Khatib R, Santesso N, Pickard L et al. Fracture risk in long term care: a systematic review and meta-analysis of prospective observational studies. *BMC Geriatr.* 2014;14:130.

21. Rapp K, Lamb SE, Klenk J et al. Fractures after nursing home admission: incidence and potential consequences. *Osteoporos Int.* 2009;20:1775–83.

22. Marquardt G, Bueter K, Motzek T. Impact of the design of the built environment on people with dementia: an evidence-based review. *HERD.* 2014;8:127–57.

23. Perell KL, Nelson A, Goldman RL et al. Fall risk assessment measures: an analytic review. *J Gerontol A Biol Sci Med Sci.* 2001;56:M761–6.

24. Scott V, Votova K, Scanlan A et al. Multifactorial and functional mobility assessment tools for fall risk among older adults in community, home-support, long-term and acute care settings. *Age Ageing.* 2007;36:130–9.

25. Lundin-Olsson L, Jensen J, Nyberg L et al. Predicting falls in residential care by a risk assessment tool, staff judgement, and history of falls. *Aging Clin Exp Res.* 2003;15:51–9.

26. Castle NG, Engberg J. Staff turnover and quality of care in nursing homes. *Med Care.* 2005;43:616–6.

27. Roigk P, Becker C, Schulz C et al. Long-term evaluation of the implementation of a large fall and fracture prevention program in long-term care facilities. *BMC Geriatr.* 2018;18:233.

28. Wagner LM, Capezuti E, Taylor JA et al. Impact of a falls menu-driven incident-reporting system on documentation and quality improvement in nursing homes. *Gerontologist.* 2005;45:835–42.

29. Woo K, Milworm G, Dowding D. Characteristics of quality improvement champions in nursing homes: a systematic review with implications for evidence-based practice. *Worldviews Evid Based Nurs.* 2017;14:440–6.

30. Kerse N, Butler M, Robinson E et al. Fall prevention in residential care: a cluster, randomized, controlled trial. *J Am Geriatr Soc.* 2004;52:524–31.

31. Rask K, Parmelee PA, Taylor JA et al. Implementation and evaluation of a nursing home fall management program. *J Am Geriatr Soc.* 2007;55:342–9.

32. Becker C, Cameron ID, Klenk J et al. Reduction of femoral fractures in long-term care facilities: the Bavarian fracture prevention study. *PLoS One.* 2011;6:e24311.

33. Schulz C, Lindlbauer I, Rapp K et al. Long-term effectiveness of a multifactorial fall and fracture prevention program in Bavarian nursing homes: an analysis based on health insurance claims data. *J Am Med Dir Assoc.* 2017;18:552.e7–17.

34. Jensen J, Lundin-Olsson L, Nyberg L et al. Fall and injury prevention in older people living in residential care facilities: a cluster randomized trial. *Ann Intern Med.* 2002;136:733–41.

35. Becker C, Kron M, Lindemann U et al. Effectiveness of a multifaceted intervention on falls in nursing home residents. *J Am Geriatr Soc.* 2003;51:306–13.

36. Rapp K, Lamb SE, Erhardt-Beer L et al. Effect of a statewide fall prevention program on incidence of femoral fractures in residents of long-term care facilities. *J Am Geriatr Soc.* 2010;58:70–5.

37. Vlaeyen E, Stas J, Leysens G et al. Implementation of fall prevention in residential care facilities: a systematic review of barriers and facilitators. *Int J Nurs Stud.* 2017;70:110–21.

38. Ray WA, Taylor JA, Meador KG et al. A randomized trial of a consultation service to reduce falls in nursing homes. *J Am Med Assoc.* 1997;278:557–62.

39. Rojas-Fernandez CH, Seymour N, Brown SG. Helping pharmacists to reduce fall risk in long-term care: a clinical tool to facilitate the medication review process. *Can Pharm J.* 2014;147:171–8.

40. Bentzen H, Forsen L, Becker C, et al. Uptake and adherence with soft- and hard-shelled hip protectors in Norwegian nursing homes: a cluster randomised trial. *Osteoporos Int.* 2008;19:101–11.

41. Santesso N, Carrasco-Labra A, Brignardello-Petersen R. Hip protectors for preventing hip fractures in older people. *Cochrane Database Syst Rev.* 2014:CD001255.

42. Minns RJ, Marsh AM, Chuck A et al. Are hip protectors correctly positioned in use? *Age Ageing.* 2007;36:140–4.

43. Laing AC, Feldman F, Jalili M et al. The effects of pad geometry and material properties on the biomechanical effectiveness of 26 commercially available hip protectors. *J Biomech.* 2011;44:2627–35.

44. Mackey DC, Lachance CC, Wang PT et al. The Flooring for Injury Prevention (FLIP) Study of compliant flooring for the prevention of fall-related injuries in long-term care: a randomized trial. *PLoS Med.* 2019;16:e1002843.

45. Lindemann U, Reicherz A, Nicolai S et al. Evaluation of an ergonomically modified bed to enhance mobilization in geriatric rehabilitation: a pilot study. *Z Gerontol Geriatr.* 2010;43:235–8.

46. Salminen AL, Brandt A, Samuelsson K et al. Mobility devices to promote activity and participation: a systematic review. *J Rehabil Med.* 2009;41:697–706.

47. McMurdo ME, Millar AM, Daly F. A randomized controlled trial of fall prevention strategies in old peoples' homes. *Gerontology.* 2000;46:83–7.

48. Mulrow CD, Gerety MB, Kanten D et al. A randomized trial of physical rehabilitation for very frail nursing home residents. *J Am Med Assoc.* 1994;271:519–24.

49. Hewitt J, Goodall S, Clemson L et al. Progressive resistance and balance training for falls prevention in long-term residential aged care: a cluster randomized trial of the sunbeam program. *J Am Med Dir Assoc.* 2018;19:361–9.

50. Toots A, Littbrand H, Lindelöf N et al. Effects of a high-intensity functional exercise program on dependence in activities of daily living and balance in older adults with dementia. *J Am Geriatr Soc.* 2016;64:55–64.

51. Gardner MM, Buchner DM, Robertson MC, et al. Implementation of an exercise-based falls prevention programme. *Age Ageing.* 2001;30:77–83.

52. Sherrington C, Michaleff ZA, Fairhall N et al. Exercise to prevent falls in older adults: an updated systematic review and meta-analysis. *Br J Sports Med.* 2017;51:1750–8.

53. Oliver D, Connelly JB, Victor CR et al. Strategies to prevent falls and fractures in hospitals and care homes and effect of cognitive impairment: systematic review and meta-analyses. *Br Med J.* 2007;334:82.

54. Rapp K, Lamb SE, Buchele G et al. Prevention of falls in nursing homes: subgroup analyses of a randomized fall prevention trial. *J Am Geriatr Soc.* 2008;56:1092–7.

55. Kovacs, E., Sztruhar Jonasne, I., Karoczi CK, et al. Effects of a multimodal exercise program on balance, functional mobility and fall risk in older adults with cognitive impairment: a randomized controlled single-blind study. *Eur J Phys Rehabil Med.* 2013;49:639–48.

56. Jansen CP, Diegelmann M, Schilling OK et al. Pushing the boundaries: a physical activity intervention extends sensor-assessed life-space in nursing home residents. *Gerontologist.* 2018;58:979–88.

57. Roigk P, Rupp K, Becker C et al. Long-term evaluation of the fidelity of a strength and balance training in long-term care facilities: the Bavarian Fall and Fracture Prevention Programme (BF2P2). *Physioscience.* 2018;14:5–12.

58. Schnelle JF, Alessi CA, Simmons SF et al. Translating clinical research into practice: a randomized controlled trial of exercise and incontinence care with nursing home residents. *J Am Geriatr Soc.* 2002;50:1476–83.

59. Brown JS, Vittinghoff E, Wyman JF et al. Urinary incontinence: does it increase risk for falls and fractures? Study of Osteoporotic Fractures Research Group. *J Am Geriatr Soc.* 2000;48:721–5.

60. Klay M, Marfyak K. Use of a continence nurse specialist in an extended care facility. *Urol Nurs.* 2005;25:101–2, 107–8.

61. Leung FW, Schnelle JF. Urinary and fecal incontinence in nursing home residents. *Gastroenterol Clin North Am.* 2008;37:697–707.

62. Kua CH, Yeo CYY, Char CWT et al. Nursing home team-care deprescribing study: a stepped-wedge randomised controlled trial protocol. *BMJ Open.* 2017;7:e015293.

63. Wouters H, Quick EH, Boersma F et al. Discontinuing inappropriate medication in nursing home residents (DIM-NHR Study): protocol of a cluster randomised controlled trial. *BMJ Open.* 2014;4:e006082.

64. Ailabouni N, Mangin D, Nishtala PS. Deprescribing anticholinergic and sedative medicines: protocol for a Feasibility Trial (DEFEAT-polypharmacy) in residential aged care facilities. *BMJ Open.* 2017;7:e013800.

65. Seppala L, Wermelink A, De Vries M et al. Falls-risk-increasing drugs: a systematic review and meta-analysis: II. Psychotrophics. *J Am Med Dir Assoc.* 2018;19:371.e11–17.

66. Shaw FE, Bond J, Richardson DA et al. Multifactorial intervention after a fall in older people with cognitive impairment and dementia presenting to the accident and emergency department: randomised controlled trial. *Br Med J.* 2003;326:73.

67. Zermansky AG, Alldred DP, Petty DR et al. Clinical medication review by a pharmacist of elderly people living in care homes: randomised controlled trial. *Age Ageing.* 2006;35:586–91.

68. Chapuy MC, Arlot ME, Duboeuf F et al. Vitamin D3 and calcium to prevent hip fractures in the elderly women. *N Engl J Med.* 1992;327:1637–42.

69. Beaudart C, Buckinx F, Rabenda V et al. The effects of vitamin D on skeletal muscle strength, muscle mass, and muscle power: a systematic review and meta-analysis of randomized controlled trials. *J Clin Endocrinol Metab.* 2014;99:4336–45.

70. Jensen J, Nyberg L, Gustafson Y et al. Fall and injury prevention in residential care – effects in residents with higher and lower levels of cognition. *J Am Geriatr Soc.* 2003;51:627–35.

71. Hofmann H, Hahn S. Characteristics of nursing home residents and physical restraint: a systematic literature review. *J Clin Nurs.* 2014;23:3012–24.

72. Sze TW, Leng CY, Lin SK. The effectiveness of physical restraints in reducing falls among adults in acute care hospitals and nursing homes: a systematic review. *JBI Libr Syst Rev.* 2012;10:307–51.

73. Castle NG, Engberg J. The health consequences of using physical restraints in nursing homes. *Med Care.* 2009;47:1164–73.

74. Rapp K, Becker C, Lamb SE et al. Hip fractures in institutionalized elderly people: incidence rates and excess mortality. *J Bone Miner Res.* 2008;23:1825–31.

Part III

Implications for Practice

28

Strategies to Promote Uptake and Adherence to Fall Prevention Programmes

Anne Tiedemann, Leanne Hassett, and Catherine Sherrington

Despite the strong evidence that many falls are preventable [1], there has been a failure to implement prevention evidence into routine clinical practice across the population of older people. Lack of uptake and adherence to effective fall prevention programmes is well documented. For example, reported participation rates are as low as 6% for balance-promoting activities among older people in Australia [2].

This low uptake may be in part explained by the way older people perceive the concept of fall prevention and how it relates to them personally, with research showing both a lack of recognition of the relevance of fall prevention [3] and a perception that falls are inevitable in older age. A deeper understanding of preferences and values is clearly needed. It has been suggested that fall prevention exercise programmes that are labelled with a positive health message, such as 'healthy ageing' or 'improving balance and mobility' are likely to be more acceptable to some older people than those which describe themselves as 'fall prevention' programmes or focus solely on risk reduction [4]. Understanding the influences on older people participating in fall prevention programmes and getting the messages right from the start is likely to result in greater interest from older people.

It is important to consider the programme-level factors that promote uptake and continued participation in health-promoting strategies by older people. In terms of fall prevention programmes, factors such as moderate duration activity, programme accessibility and convenience, emphasis on social aspects, strong leadership, and individual tailoring lead to greater uptake and adherence [5, 6].

Strategies for promoting health behaviour change among older people in relation to various health conditions have also been recommended. Some of these are relevant to fall prevention and are discussed below.

Older People's Perceptions of Falls

In order to understand the reasons for low uptake and adherence to fall prevention interventions it is firsty important to be aware of what is known about older people's perceptions of falls and the messages they receive about how to prevent them. A better understanding of the way older people view fall prevention messages is crucial since health-promotion messages that threaten personal independence and identity may lead to a reduction in the perceived immediate threat of falls and the need to take action to reduce the risk [7].

Qualitative research conducted by Yardley et al. [8] in the United Kingdom identified a lack of awareness about the role of exercise in preventing falls. This research highlighted a belief by some older people that falls can be prevented by reducing exposure to hazards, using walking aids, and restricting activity. Furthermore, the study participants regarded advice about fall prevention as useful in principle but not personally relevant or appropriate. They also perceived fall prevention advice as common sense that was more applicable to older or more disabled individuals and the suggestion that fall prevention was relevant to all older people could be perceived to be patronizing and cause distress. This highlights an element of stigma associated with falling in older age. Other research has identified a perception by some older people that they are to blame for falling, with common fall-related responses including anger, fear, and embarrassment [4].

Factors Associated with Adherence to Fall Prevention Programmes

When recommending a fall prevention programme to an individual, it is important that their preferences are considered and factors that may promote or restrict participation are considered. Barriers and enablers to participation vary from person to person and can be classified as individual-level or programme-level factors. Individual-level factors include socioeconomic status, health, motivation, and physical and psychological factors, whereas programme-level factors may include the location and delivery mode of the programme, the cost, and the attributes of the person delivering the programme [5, 6].

One study that explored older people's preferences with regard to fall prevention exercise programmes identified the attributes of exercise programmes with the highest utility values to be: home-based exercise and no need to use transport, an improvement of 60% in the ability to do daily tasks at home, no costs, and decreasing the chances of falling to 0%. The attributes with the lowest utility were a travel time of 30 minutes or more and out-of-pocket costs of AUD$50 per session [6]. These findings have significance for the development and implementation of fall prevention programmes and suggest a need to focus on improving programme accessibility and convenience rather than relying on the likely programme-related health benefits to entice people to participate.

A systematic review that investigated programme-level factors associated with adherence to group-based fall prevention exercise identified three key factors [9].

Firstly, the authors found that interventions that included a flexibility component, such as yoga or extended warm up/cool down, were associated with lower adherence, perhaps indicating low confidence in the efficacy of these exercise approaches. The study also found that programmes with a duration of 20 weeks or more elicited lower adherence, perhaps implying that participants feel overwhelmed by longer-term programmes, and the need for inter-term breaks. Lastly, programmes that were offered in two or fewer sessions per week were associated with lower adherence, which may be explained by low perceived effectiveness of programmes with fewer sessions each week, a slower rate of perceived progress when participating in these programmes or lower group cohesion as a result of less frequent group contact. These results indicate a need for careful planning of programme characteristics and flexibility in the way programmes are delivered and marketed.

Behaviour-Change Strategies

The behaviour-change wheel framework includes the COM-B 'behaviour system' at the hub that considers an individual's capability, opportunity, and motivation (Figure 28.1) as being key influencers on behaviour change [10]. This framework

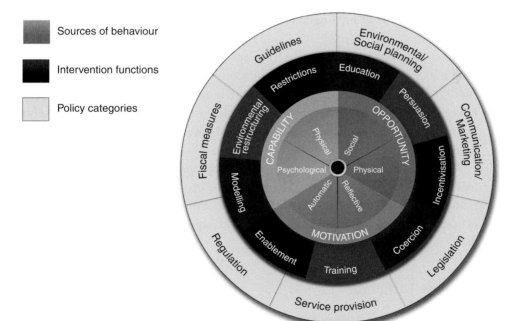

Figure 28.1   The behaviour-change wheel. Reproduced with permission from Michie S, van Stralen MM, West R. The behaviour change wheel: a new method for characterising and designing behaviour change interventions. Implement Sci. 2011;6:1–11 [10].

may assist with the implementation of fall prevention interventions by identifying effective behaviour-change techniques (BCTs).

Capability refers to the ability of the individual to engage in a behaviour, in terms of both their psychological and physical capacities. In the context of exercise for the prevention of falls, capability can be supported by instructor supervision, individualized tailoring of exercise, modification of exercises to suit individual abilities, embedding exercise into activities of daily living, and addressing the physical and psychological concerns of older people in relation to exercise capacity.

Opportunity encompasses the factors that are external to the individual that encourage and prompt the desired behaviour and incorporate both physical and social opportunity. In the context of exercise for fall prevention, physical opportunity may be improved by offering home exercise programmes for people unable to attend in a group setting, or transport to attend group programmes. Alternatively, offering community-based group exercise programmes may increase social opportunity by making it socially normal for older people to be exercising.

Opportunity could also be improved with the use of technology to provide remote supervision to support the uptake and ongoing participation in exercise programmes. Health professional support could also be provided by telephone and exercise could be integrated into activities of daily living to improve opportunity.

Other practical approaches that can improve opportunity include reduced cost or free access to group-based programmes, provision of programmes near place of residence, provision of transport to exercise venues, and offering programmes at times suitable for the target population. Health professional referral and support to participate in fall prevention programmes is another avenue for boosting opportunity.

Motivation is defined as both automatic and reflective brain processes that galvanize and guide behaviour. Motivation can be stimulated by various means, including goal-setting, habit formation, self-monitoring, social modelling, and action and coping planning strategies. These approaches are described in more detail below.

Behaviour-Change Techniques

BCTs are considered the active ingredients of an intervention to change behaviours [11]. Goal-setting and feedback on the behaviour are two examples of the 93 different BCTs included in the BCT taxonomy [12]. One study conducted in the Netherlands used a Delphi process to determine the most promising BCTs included in an effective nation-wide fall prevention intervention [13]. The three most promising BCTs identified were goal-setting (behaviour), graded tasks, and behavioural practice/rehearsal, whereas information about health consequences, salience of consequences, and information about emotional consequences were considered the least promising.

Goal-setting is a key BCT included in behaviour-change interventions [14] since it encourages people to create a sense of urgency and motivation to invest time and energy to reduce the difference between their current and desired states in terms of health-promoting behaviours [15]. As such it may be useful in increasing adherence to fall prevention programmes. Goal setting is often undertaken through a collaborative process between the client and the health professional, involving goal selection and action planning [16].

According to self-regulation theory [17], goal setting serves as an important motivational cue to change behaviour. In this theory it is proposed that behaviour is influenced by the interaction between the persons' immediate environment, their biological system and cues from the person's cognitions and goals [18]. To maximize goal effectiveness, it is recognized that goals should meet SMART criteria: Specific, Measurable, Attainable, Realistic, and Timely [15]. So rather than a general goal such as 'I want to improve my balance' or 'I want to reduce my risk of falling', using the SMART criteria to set a goal would result in a goal such as 'I will undertake balance exercises three times each week for the next six weeks, starting today'.

Research has identified the value that older people place on their ability to maintain independence in carrying out activities of daily living [4]. This highlights a key area that is likely to be an important focus of goal-setting for older people.

Social Support

Having appropriate social support within a fall prevention programme may be a strong motivator for an older person to initiate and sustain participation. Within self-determination theory of behaviour change [19], social contexts that promote competence (i.e. feeling competent at doing a task or behaviour), autonomy (i.e. feeling some choice or say in what to do), and relatedness (i.e. feeling related or connected to others) promote intrinsic motivation to participate in a behaviour in that context [18]. Health professionals, exercise leaders, and designers of fall prevention programmes can use these three needs to motivate older people to change their behaviour from not participating in fall prevention programmes to becoming regular participants. For example, a tailored approach can provide the correct level of exercise challenge to promote competence, and the provision of a range of exercise options enables people to choose what best suits them.

Relatedness or social support can be a strong driver for change. Social support can be provided through offering fall prevention programmes in group settings where people can engage with each other socially and support each other. Alternatively, social support from family, neighbours, or health professionals can also support engagement in fall prevention interventions where individual or home-based interventions are preferred.

Health Coaching

Some people require a more supported approach to reach their health goals. Health coaching has recently been gaining attention in the field of health behaviour change. Health coaching is a person-centred process that commonly involves motivational interviewing, participant-directed goal setting, and encourages self-discovery. Health coaches, also commonly known as activity counsellors or wellness coaches, support individuals to make changes to their behaviour by raising awareness of problems and possible solutions while also reducing the individual's uncertainty about change. Health coaching by physiotherapists experienced with exercise prescription for older adults appears to be particularly well received by those at risk of falls [20]. A case study of a health coaching intervention delivered by a physiotherapist is outlined in Box 28. 1.

A recently published systematic review with meta-analysis demonstrated that health coaching had a small, statistically significant effect on physical activity among people aged 60 years and over with a variety of medical conditions [21]. Health coaching can be delivered by health professionals with a range of professional backgrounds and can be delivered in a face-to-face format or via the telephone. This makes it a potentially cost-effective intervention strategy that has potential for delivery to people in remote locations.

Other Potential Approaches to Promoting Participation

The use of peers (i.e. other older people) to support and motivate older people to participate in fall prevention exercise programmes is a low cost and sustainable approach that has received some attention. Peers may take on the role of programme instructor/leader or co-participant/buddy attending the programme with the older person. Research into the use of peer leaders in the fall prevention field has demonstrated a positive impact on strength, balance, and falls, and importantly on sustained participation in group-based exercise in New Zealand [22].

The Active, Connected, Engaged (ACE) programme [23] is a theory-informed, pragmatic intervention developed in the United Kingdom. ACE involves peer volunteers (i.e. other older people) supporting socially

Box 28.1 Case Study of a Health Coaching Approach Delivered by a Physiotherapist

Case study: Ms X, 85 years old

Session 1
Six-month goals
1. Undertake 20 minutes of moderate intensity walking, three times/ week
2. Lose 3 kg

Two-week goals
1. Perform sit to stand ×10, heel raises 10, heel raises ×10, three times/week
2. Perform single leg stand 3×10 seconds each leg, five times/week
3. Five minutes of walking three times/week
4. Wear Fitbit daily to monitor progress
5. Synchronise Fitbit with iPad every two to three days
6. Call health coach in two weeks

Session 2
- Had flu last week so has not been as active as she would like. Feels much better now. Weather was bad in first week.
- Has been using stairs instead of lift at work. Feels she's climbing stairs more easily. Goes straight up stairs at train station – breathing is easier.
- Loves Fitbit.
- Has been to gym ×2/week but a bit expensive. Keen to find a cheaper option.

Barriers during six month review
Bronchitis, back pain, foot pain, dog died, another bad cold, wary of cold weather, worked 28 days straight, helped daughter move house, trigeminal neuralgia, brother very ill.

Change in status since beginning
Balance exercises embedded in day – tandem walking along corridor at work, etc. Joined gym. Given programme but does not get supervision while there. Different from last gym with exercise physiologists. Spends approximately 40 minutes at gym using bike, treadmill, weights. Does own balance exercises, sit to stand, etc.

Participant comments
'You can understand how running becomes addictive…I'm enjoying the feeling of being more fit.'

'I feel a remarkable improvement in my breathing and ability to do things. I walked to the Opera House and felt fine walking up the stairs!'

'I really feel the benefits…I can walk anywhere now!'

disengaged, inactive older adults to be more active. Peer volunteers and participants meet up to seven times over a six-month period to promote motivation, address participation barriers, and attend local activities together. A feasibility trial undertaken in Bristol, United Kingdom, found the intervention was acceptable, feasible, and had a positive impact on the health and well-being of both the older participants and the peer volunteers. This approach has potential to support participation in group-based fall prevention exercise programmes but is yet to be formally explored.

Conclusions

This chapter has outlined the importance of proactive, specifically tailored strategies to assist older people to achieve lasting behaviour change with respect to the uptake and continued adherence to participation in exercise for the prevention of falls. By considering the factors that influence behaviour generally and in the context of falls, in terms of older people's perceptions and preferences, fall prevention strategies are likely to be more acceptable and long-term adherence will be more achievable. The effectiveness of fall prevention interventions is influenced by the beliefs and attitudes of older people and other personal and practical barriers to uptake and ongoing participation. This is definitely an area where one size does not fit all.

REFERENCES

1. Sherrington C, Fairhall NJ, Wallbank GK et al. Exercise for preventing falls in older people living in the community. *Cochrane Database Syst Rev.* 2019;1:CD012424.
2. Merom D, Pye V, Macniven R et al. Prevalence and correlates of participation in fall prevention exercise/physical activity by older adults. *Prev Med.* 2012;55:613–17.
3. Haines TP, Day L, Hill KD et al. "Better for others than for me": a belief that should shape our efforts to promote participation in falls prevention strategies. *Arch Gerontol Geriatr.* 2014;59:136–44.
4. Calhoun R, Meischke H, Hammerback K et al. Older adults' perceptions of clinical fall prevention programs: a qualitative study. *J Aging Research.* 2011;2011:867341.
5. Bunn F, Dickinson A, Barnett-Page E et al. A systematic review of older people's perceptions of facilitators and barriers to participation in falls-prevention interventions. *Ageing Soc.* 2008;28:449–72.
6. Franco MR, Howard K, Sherrington C et al. Eliciting older people's preferences for exercise programs: a best-worst scaling choice experiment. *J Physiother.* 2015;61:34–41.
7. Woodhead G, Calnan M, Dieppe P et al. Dignity in old age: what do older people in the United Kingdom think? *Age Ageing.* 2004;33:165–70.
8. Yardley L, Donovan-Hall M, Francis K et al. Older people's views of advice about falls prevention: a qualitative study. *Health Educ Res.* 2006;21:508–17.

9. McPhate L, Simek EM, Haines TP. Program-related factors are associated with adherence to group exercise interventions for the prevention of falls: a systematic review. *J Physiother.* 2013;59:81–92.

10. Michie S, van Stralen MM, West R. The behaviour change wheel: a new method for characterising and designing behaviour change interventions. *Implement Sci.* 2011;6.1 11.

11. Michie S, Atkins L, West R. The behaviour change wheel. In: *A Guide to Designing Interventions.* London: Silverback Publishing; 2014.

12. Michie S, Abraham C, Whittington C et al. Effective techniques in healthy eating and physical activity interventions: a meta-regression. *Health Psychol.* 2009;28:690–701.

13. Vestjens L, Kempen G, Crutzen R et al. Promising behavior change techniques in a multicomponent intervention to reduce concerns about falls in old age: a Delphi study. *Health Educ Res.* 2015;30:309–22.

14. O'Hara BJ, Gale J, McGill B et al. Weight-related goal setting in a telephone-based preventive health-coaching program: demonstration of effectiveness. *Am J Health Promot.* 2016;31:491–501.

15. Mann T, de Ridder D, Fujita K. Self-regulation of health behavior: social psychological approaches to goal setting and goal striving. *Health Psych.* 2013;32:487–98.

16. Bodenheimer T, Handley MA. Goal-setting for behavior change in primary care: an exploration and status report. *Patient Educ Couns.* 2009;76:174–80.

17. Kanfer FH, Gaelick L. (Eds.) Self-management methods. In: *Helping People Change: A Textbook of Methods.* New York: Pergamon Press; 1991.

18. Michie S, West R, Campbell R et al. *ABC of Behaviour Change Theories.* London: Silverback Publishing; 2014.

19. Deci EL, Ryan RM. *Intrinsic Motivation and Self-Determination in Human Behaviour.* New York: Plenum Publishing Co; 1985.

20. Haynes A, Sherrington C, Wallbank G et al. "Someone's got my back": older people's experience of the Coaching for Healthy Ageing program for promoting physical activity and preventing falls. *J Aging Phys Act.* 2020;29:296–307.

21. Oliveira JS, Sherrington C, Amorim AB et al. What is the effect of health coaching on physical activity participation in people aged 60 years and over? A systematic review of randomised controlled trials. *Br J Sports Med.* 2017;51:1425–32.

22. Waters DL, Hale LA, Robertson L et al. Evaluation of a peer-led falls prevention program for older adults. *Arch Phys Med Rehabil.* 2011;92:1581–6.

23. Stathi A, Withall J, Thompson JL et al. Feasibility trial evaluation of a peer volunteering active aging intervention: ACE (Active, Connected, Engaged). *Gerontologist.* 2019;60:571–82.

29

Translating Fall Prevention Research into Practice

Kathryn M. Sibley, Alexandra M.B. Korall, and Alexie J. Touchette

Moving Fall Prevention Evidence into Action: Easier Said Than Done

Generating a comprehensive body of high-quality evidence that demonstrates the problem of falls, identifies causal mechanisms and risk factors, and determines effective interventions for reducing falls is critical for establishing a strong foundation on which to reduce the global burden of falls. While the establishment of such an evidence base is absolutely necessary, this alone will not have an impact on incidence of falls. Assumptions should not be made about the diffusion of fall prevention evidence into clinical practices and health systems [1]. There is growing recognition that most efforts to date attempting to incorporate health research into health care practices and policies are grossly ineffective, and thereby, inefficient [2, 3]. The challenges of moving health evidence into care practices and decision-making are not unique to fall prevention. In fact, published reports have estimated that there is a 17-year time lag between established health evidence reaching clinical practice [3].

There is consistent and persistent evidence of gaps in fall prevention care around the world (including the United States [4, 5], Canada [6], United Kingdom [7], Netherlands [8], Australia [9, 10], and Denmark [11]). Most recently, a 2014 Danish study demonstrated that just 2% of 1100 health records from people aged 50 and over treated in an emergency department for a fall in two regions included evidence of fall-risk screening according to national recommendations [11]. Furthermore, in a Canadian study published in 2006, only two of 54 older adults who presented to an emergency department with a fall-related complaint received care consistent with international guidelines [6]. The impacts of poor uptake may be profound, as this study also determined that six months following discharge, physiological fall risk profiles deteriorated by almost 30%, functional ability, balance confidence, and depression all significantly worsened, and 10% of patients experienced fall-related fractures [6].

Knowledge Translation and Implementation Science: Emergence of a New Discipline in Health

Growing recognition of the inherent challenges associated with moving research into action has led to the emergence of a new disciplinary focus dedicated to understanding, improving, and accelerating research and practice for using health evidence in real-world settings. In the context of health, this explicit shift has evolved largely subsequent to the evidence-based medicine paradigm [12]. However, this emerging discipline has long-standing multi-disciplinary roots in the social sciences stemming from Diffusion of Innovations Theory [13].

There is no globally recognized term used to identify and describe this type of work. One terminology system that originated in Canada known as knowledge translation has been adopted by several international agencies including the World Health Organization [2]. *Knowledge translation* (KT) is defined as a dynamic and iterative process that includes the synthesis, dissemination, exchange, and ethically sound application of knowledge to improve health, the health care system, and health service delivery (Table 29.1). KT takes place within a complex system of interactions between researchers and knowledge users which may vary in intensity, complexity, and level of engagement depending on the nature of the research, the findings, and the needs of the particular knowledge user [14]. Within each domain of KT there are active networks growing a scholarly and practical foundation. This chapter focuses on one dimension of KT application: implementation science pertaining to the prevention of falls and/or fall-related injuries in older adults. *Implementation science* refers to the theoretical approaches and scientific study of methods to promote the systematic uptake of clinical research findings and other evidence-based practices into routine practice,

Table 29.1 Components of knowledge translation

Component	Definition	Synonyms or examples
Synthesis	The process of synthesizing results from individual research studies and interpreting in the context of global evidence	Examples: systematic, scoping, and realist reviews
Exchange	Partnerships between research producers and users *in* the research process to generate more usable and solutions-focused research	Synonym: integrated knowledge translation
Dissemination	Sharing and communicating research findings to increase knowledge, awareness, and enhance attitudes with target audiences, with an emphasis beyond traditional academic users	Examples: presentations, social media, mass media
Application	Use of knowledge in practice and decision-making settings	Synonym: implementation

and hence to improve the quality of health care, health systems, and health service delivery [15].

It is important to acknowledge that, despite the critical importance of improving health care systems and health service delivery, implementation must be supplemented with complementary efforts to ensure optimal improvements in health outcomes. For example, adherence to evidence-based strategies by older adults, families, and/or caregivers is often necessary to achieve improvements in health outcomes.

Theoretical approaches: guiding roadmaps for implementation

There is a strong interest in the theoretical underpinnings of implementation [15, 16]. The use of theoretical approaches is advocated in implementation science to provide better understanding of how and why implementation succeeds or fails in various settings and populations [16], to develop implementation interventions, and to allow for an incremental accumulation of knowledge [15]. However, explicit use of theoretical approaches in rehabilitation KT and implementation research has historically been low [17, 18].

Theoretical approaches used in implementation science include: (i) *process models* that describe and/or guide the process of moving knowledge into action, (ii) *determinant frameworks and theories* that identify and explain the many factors influencing implementation, and (iii) *evaluation frameworks* that identify implementation outcomes that need to be considered [16]. One challenge facing those wishing to use theoretical approaches is the sheer volume of available options and the absence of universally accepted gold standards [19]. As it is beyond the scope of this chapter to review all theoretical approaches in implementation, it focuses on one highly cited process model that has been adopted by health research agencies worldwide: The *Knowledge-to-Action (KTA) Framework* [2, 20] (Figure 29.1).

The KTA Framework combines the critical features of over 30 planned-action theories [20]. The KTA Framework describes two key phases to move from knowledge production to implementation: the *knowledge creation phase*, which encompasses knowledge inquiry, synthesis, and the development of knowledge products or tools, and the *action cycle*. The action cycle involves identifying the problem and knowledge-to-practice gaps, adapting knowledge to local context, identifying barriers and facilitators to knowledge use, selecting, tailoring and implementing interventions, monitoring knowledge use, evaluating outcomes, and sustaining knowledge use. Each component of the KTA Framework has an important role, along with unique features, approaches, and methodologies for addressing each component. Some components are typically addressed as distinct

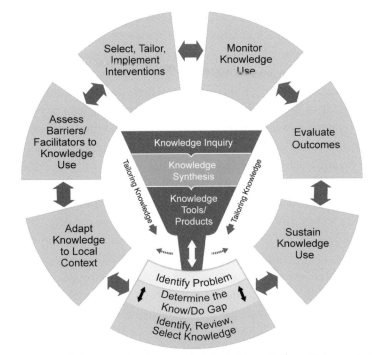

Figure 29.1   The Knowledge-to-Action Framework. Adapted from Graham ID, Logan J, Harrison MB et al. Lost in knowledge translation: Time for a map? J Contin Educ Health Prof. 2006;26:13–24 [20].

projects, while others are commonly grouped together within a single project. The remainder of this chapter describes each KTA component and highlights relevant fall prevention examples for each. Sibley et al.'s study is an example of a fall prevention research programme focusing on balance measurements that was designed using the KTA Framework and can be reviewed at [21–23].

The KTA Framework and Its Application in Fall Prevention

Knowledge Creation Phase

The knowledge creation phase is represented as a funnel. At the top is *knowledge inquiry*: the large body of primary research that includes basic and clinical science. This is particularly true in the fall prevention literature, where a PubMed database search of the medical subject heading (MeSH) terms 'accidental falls' and 'aged' returns 17,645 items (searched December 1, 2020). Most content in this book is based on this type of primary evidence. It is noteworthy that the knowledge inquiry component of KTA represents most academic research activities but is in reality only one step required for moving knowledge into action.

The next component is *knowledge synthesis*. Syntheses are widely regarded as the cornerstone of implementation [24]. Syntheses are emphasized as a 'key ingredient' for implementation because a critical examination of whether there is sufficient evidence to support changing behaviour on a broad scale is essential for maximizing impact and reducing research waste. If the body of evidence is small, mixed, or of low quality, the knowledge (in most cases, a particular treatment or intervention) may not be ready for widespread implementation [25]. The large body of primary evidence in fall prevention facilitates knowledge synthesis. The most recent Cochrane Reviews on fall prevention, widely regarded for their rigorous methodological approach, highlight strong evidence for the effects of balance and functional exercise in community-dwelling older adults but persisting uncertainties about the effects of interventions in residential care homes or hospital settings [26, 27]. Novel synthesis methods can be applied to fall prevention evidence. For example, network meta-analysis, a statistical technique that compares multiple treatments and facilitates interpretation of complex evidence, compared 25 fall prevention intervention components for older adults and concluded that exercise was likely the most effective intervention for reducing falls, injurious falls, fractures, and hip fractures [28].

This second-generation knowledge is refined in the next component which develops *knowledge tools and products* to disseminate evidence and facilitate knowledge uptake. Examples of these tools and products include practice guidelines, logic models, infographics, and online resources. There are multiple examples in fall prevention, including the United Kingdom's National Institute for Health and Care Excellence (NICE) guidelines for assessing risk and prevention of falls in older people [29], as well as specific guidelines for evidence-based interventions such as exercise [30]. The goal of this component is that knowledge becomes more useful to the end user. As methods used to develop knowledge tools and products can vary widely in quality [31], rigorous guidance for developing, reporting, and evaluating guidelines [32] and online resources [33] are emerging.

Action Cycle

The action cycle identifies the steps required for a unit of knowledge (usually a treatment or intervention) to reach widespread use. Table 29.2 describes examples of studies that used the action cycle. This table provides details of studies that addressed fall prevention treatments or interventions supported by evidence from systematic reviews and meta-analyses [26–28] and/or used a theoretical approach or implementation evidence to inform study aims and objectives, implementation strategies, outcome selection, and/or the interpretation of results. Although it is possible to enter the action cycle at any component, typically the first step involves *identifying the problem*, which establishes a 'know–do' gap.

Table 29.2 Description of some fall prevention studies that used the Knowledge-to-Action Framework action cycle

Action cycle components[a]	First author	Year published	Country	Year data collected	Setting	Fall prevention focus	Theoretical approach(es) used	How theoretical approach(es) was/were used[b]
Identify gap/problem	Lillevang-Johannsen [11]	2017	Denmark	2014	Hospital	Fall risk assessment	None reported	N/A
Identify gap/problem	Rubenstein [5]	2004	United States	1998	Community	Fall risk assessment and management	None reported	N/A
Identify gap/problem	Said [9]	2016	Australia	2012	Community	Fall risk identification, assessment, and management	None reported	N/A
Identify gap/problem	Tirrell [4]	2015	United States	2012	Hospital	Fall risk assessment	None reported	N/A
Identify gap/problem	Day [10]	2014	Australia	2012	Community	Fall risk assessment, planning, management, and monitoring	None reported	N/A
Identify gap/problem	Askari [8]	2016	Netherlands	2010	Community	Fall detection and management	None reported	N/A
Identify gap/problem	Banerjee [7]	2012	United Kingdom	2005	Hospital	Fall risk assessment and bone health	None reported	N/A
Identify gap/problem	Salter [6]	2006	Canada	2003	Hospital	Fall risk assessment and management	None reported	N/A
Adapt to local context	Hendriks [49]	2008	Netherlands	Not specified	Community	Multi-faceted assessment programme	None reported	N/A
Identify gap/problem; **Barriers and facilitators;**	Zachary [39]	2012	United States	Not specified	Residential/ long-term care/nursing	Multi-component fall prevention education, medication management, and home safety information	Theory of Organizational Change [69], Diffusion of Innovations Theory [13]	Informed instrument development and guided outcomes measurement
Barriers and facilitators	Meyer [38]	2016	Australia	Not specified	Community	Home-based exercise programme	Knowledge-to-Action Framework [20]	Overarching guide/ framework for study
Barriers and facilitators	Shaw [42]	2013	Canada	Not specified	Community	Fall risk assessment and education	Consolidated Framework for Implementation Research [40]	Discussed in background and used to support/ explain results
Barriers and facilitators; **Intervene;**	Thomas [53]	2014	Australia	2012	Hospital	Fall risk assessment and management		Discussed in background and

Table 29.2 (cont.)

Action cycle components[a]	First author	Year published	Country	Year data collected	Setting	Fall prevention focus	Theoretical approach(es) used	How theoretical approach(es) was/were used[b]
Monitor and evaluate								
Barriers and facilitators; Adapt to local context; **Intervene;** Monitor and Evaluate; Sustain	Sibley [23]	2016	Canada	Not specified	Rehabilitation Hospital	Assessment of reactive balance	Theoretical Domains Framework [43, 44]	Discussed in background and informed intervention
Intervene; **Monitor and Evaluate;** Sustain	Li [58]	2016	United States	2012	Community	Community exercise programme	RE-AIM Framework [54]	Guided outcomes measurement/ develop evaluation strategy
Intervene; **Monitor and Evaluate; Sustain**	Li [56]	2013	United States	2010	Community	Community exercise programme	RE-AIM Framework [54]	Guided outcomes measurement/ develop evaluation strategy
Intervene; **Monitor and Evaluate;** Sustain	Roigk [55]	2018	Germany	2005	Residential/ Long term care/ Nursing	Prevention of hip fracture	RE-AIM Framework [54]	Guided outcomes measurement/ develop evaluation strategy
Adapt; **Monitor and Evaluate**	Day [58]	2016	Australia	2011	Community	Community exercise programme	RE-AIM Framework [54] Diffusion of Innovations Theory [13]	Discussed in background, test influence of variables predicted to be relevant by theory, guided outcomes measurement/ develop evaluation strategy, used to support or explain the results

a. The primary KTA stage is bolded.

b. References for theories taken from the article.

Formal, data-driven assessments of gaps are recommended [34]. A number of methods have been used to identify gaps, including examination of administrative data [4–7, 9, 11] and self-report surveys to document current practice [8, 10]. Table 29.3 provides some examples of fall prevention studies that were designed to identify 'know–do' gaps.

A critical subsequent step is to *assess barriers and facilitators to knowledge use* in a particular setting. The factors influencing knowledge use are numerous and complex, often operating simultaneously at individual patient and health professional, organizational, and/or system levels [35–37]. For example, a systematic review of 19 qualitative studies explored factors influencing the implementation of fall prevention programmes from the perspectives of older adults and health professionals. They identified three overarching concepts: practical considerations (including economic factors, access to the intervention, and time), social and cultural adaptations across communities, and psychosocial considerations (including the role of fall risk in shaping an individual's identity and defining expertise related to power differentials between older adults, caregivers, and health professionals) [35]. Methodologically, identification of barriers and facilitators may be determined through quantitative approaches such as surveys [38] or using qualitative approaches such as interviews [38, 39]. An example of each of these approaches is shown in Table 29.4. There is no evidence establishing superiority of either approach.

Although use of theoretical approaches is minimal in existing studies of factors influencing fall prevention implementation, there are several determinant frameworks that can help guide this work. For example, the Consolidated Framework for Implementation Research (CFIR) [40] is a highly cited [41] framework that prompts users to consider five domains that influence the complex nature of implementation (see Table 29.5). A user guide can be found at cfirguide.org. Although existing application of CFIR in fall prevention is limited [42], its comprehensive nature is highly relevant. Additionally, the COM-B System and Theoretical Domains Framework (TDF) are two commonly used determinant frameworks. The COM-B system purports that behaviour is influenced by physical and psychological capability, physical, and social opportunity, and reflective and automatic processes (i.e. motivation). The TDF is more granular than the COM-B system, identifying 14 domains influencing the behaviour of health professionals (see Table 29.5) [43, 44]. Each domain of the TDF has been mapped to a corresponding component of the COM-B system, for which each component has been mapped to relevant behaviour-change strategies [45, 46]. Published guidance on using the TDF is also available [47].

Adapting knowledge to the local context is an important component as it is recognized that users may already be adopting some aspects of the evidence, and/

Table 29.3 Description of some of fall prevention studies that evaluated gaps in practice

First author	Year published	Gap assessment	Comparator	Methods
Lillevang-Johannsen [11]	2017	Compliance to national guideline recommendations that fall risk assessment should be completed in all patients 65 years or older admitted to the emergency department due to a fall	National guideline: Danish Health Authority recommendations [70]	Record audit
Rubenstein [5]	2004	Examination of fall risk assessment and management strategies for at risk community-dwelling older adults	Quality indicators: six process of care quality indicators for falls and gait instability developed through literature review and expert panel consideration	Medical record abstraction of administrative data, patient quality-of-care interviews
Said [9]	2016	Compliance of clinical practice to national guidelines for high fall risk patients discharged home after rehabilitation	Audit tool: development guided by the *Best Practice Guidelines for Australian Hospitals* and the *Best Practice Guidelines for Australian Community Care* [71, 72]	Retrospective medical record audit
Tirrell [4]	2015	Compliance to international guidelines in emergency department evaluations of older adult fallers	International Guideline: *American Geriatrics Society, British Geriatrics Society Clinical Practice Guideline for Prevention of Falls in Older Persons* [73] and the *Geriatric Emergency Department Guidelines* [74]	Chart review

Study	Year	Objective	Comparator / Guideline	Method
Askari [8]	2016	Examination of quality of fall detection and management in older adults by general practitioners	National Guideline: The Assessing Care Of Vulnerable Elders (ACOVE) quality indicators [75]	Patient questionnaire
Banerjee [7]	2012	Examine integrated falls services against national standards	Audit tool: indicators of the structure and process of high-quality care developed by multidisciplinary steering group representing professional and patient organizations relevant to falls and bone health	Two rounds of national organizational audit, one patient-level national clinical audit
Salter [6]	2006	Compliance to international guidelines in older adults admitted to the emergency department due to a fall	International guideline: The *American Geriatrics Society, British Geriatrics Society, American Academy of Orthopaedic Surgeons* [76]	Medical chart examination, daily patient diary of falls submitted monthly, patient interview, physician reconciliation where needed
Day [10]	2014	Examination of current fall prevention practices among Hospital Admission Risk Programmes for people at high risk of hospitalization	No comparator	Cross-sectional survey

Table 29.4 Description of two fall prevention studies that assessed barriers to knowledge use

First author	Year published	Barriers/facilitators assessments	Methods
Zachary [39]	2012	Barriers to implementing multicomponent fall prevention education in senior centres	Telephone interview with centre directors
Meyer [38]	2016	Barriers and facilitators to delivering home exercise programme based on the OTAGO exercise programme	Older adult and physiotherapist focus groups, physiotherapist surveys & data recording sheets

or may have feasibility considerations for their setting. A challenge in implementation lies in that there may be tensions in navigating feasibility considerations and the essential components of the knowledge. Guidelines for the adaptation process are emerging in the literature [48]. Many are specifically focused on adapting clinical practice guidelines, although the principles of adaptation can be applied more broadly. For example, Hendriks et al. [49] reported on the adaptation of a British multi-disciplinary fall prevention programme with established effects on falls and functioning to a Dutch context through a structured consensus process using a nominal group to achieve consensus on protocol adaptations.

The preceding action cycle components are considered key ingredients in implementation science that are essential to conduct prior to launching implementation [25]. They are necessary for both appropriately justifying the need for and developing an implementation intervention. The implementation intervention refers to the activities and strategies intended to enhance uptake of the primary evidence or knowledge itself, and its role in the action cycle is highlighted in the *select, tailor and implement intervention* component. Implementation science has been building an evidence foundation on which to inform how to implement [24]. For example, audit and feedback, a technique which summarizes clinical performance over a period of time, has been studied in over 140 trials and consistently demonstrates small positive effect sizes that may be meaningful at a population level [50]. The implementation evidence base is also clearly demonstrating what is not effective. For example, systematic reviews have well established that didactic educational interventions are not effective at changing clinician behaviour, particularly for complex behaviours [51]. For example, syntheses of rehabilitation implementation research have revealed that most studies adopted primarily passive education strategies and found no clear effect of such strategies [17]. A 2010 systematic review of fall prevention implementation

Table 29.5 Description of three Implementation framework domains

Consolidated Framework for Implementation Research (CFIR)	Theoretical Domains Framework (TDF)	RE-AIM Framework
1. Characteristics of the intervention under consideration	1. Knowledge: awareness of the existence of something	1. Reach: proportion of the target population that participated in the intervention
2. Economic, social, and political environment in which an organization using the intervention exists (the 'outer setting')	2. Skills: ability or proficiency acquired through practice	2. Effectiveness: impact of an intervention on important outcomes
3. Structural, cultural, and political conditions of the organization itself (the 'inner setting')	3. Social/professional role and identity: a coherent set of behaviours and displayed personal qualities of an individual in a social or work setting	3. Adoption: proportion and representativeness of settings that adopt a given policy or programme
4. Characteristics of the individuals adopting an intervention	4. Beliefs about capabilities: acceptance of the truth, reality, or validity about an ability, talent, or facility that a person can put to constructive use	4. Implementation: the extent to which the intervention is implemented as intended in the real word
5. Features of the implementation process	5. Optimism: confidence that things will happen for the best or desired goals will be attained	5. Maintenance: the extent to which a programme or policy becomes institutionalized or part of the routine organizational practices and policies
	6. Beliefs about consequences: acceptance of the truth, reality, or validity about outcomes of a behaviour in a given situation	
	7. Reinforcement: increasing the probability of a response by arranging a dependent relationship or contingency between the response and a given stimulus	
	8. Intentions: a conscious decision to perform a behaviour or a resolve to act in a certain way	
	9. Goals: mental representations of outcome or end states that an individual wants to achieve	

Table 29.5 (*cont.*)

Consolidated Framework for Implementation Research (CFIR)	Theoretical Domains Framework (TDF)	RE-AIM Framework
	10. Memory, attention and decision processes: ability to retain information, focus selectively on aspects of the environment and choose between alternatives	
	11. Environmental context and resources: any circumstance of a person's situation or environment that discourages or encourages the development of skills and abilities, independence, social competence and adaptive behaviour	
	12. Social influences: interpersonal processes that can cause individuals to change their thoughts, feelings or behaviours	
	13. Emotion: a complex reaction pattern involving experiential, behavioural and physiological elements, by which the individual attempts to deal with a personally significant matter or event	
	14. Behavioural regulation: anything aimed at managing or changing objectively observed or measured actions	

interventions also found that most used training of health care professionals [52]. Although the absence of theoretical approaches to intervention development compounds our limited understanding about effective implementation interventions, there is emerging use of the TDF to inform the selection of implementation intervention components and link them to identified barriers to specific fall prevention and rehabilitation practices [23, 53]. Table 29.6 provides the details of two examples of this

Monitoring knowledge use and *evaluating outcomes* are two critical action cycle components that are often operationalized into a single project or study in tandem with the delivery of an implementation intervention. Knowledge use refers to the specific effects of an intervention on the implementation target, and can occur at a conceptual level (reflected by changes in understanding or attitudes), an instrumental level (reflected by changes in behaviour), and/or at a strategic level (to gain power, profit, or influence a decision) [20]. These may also be referred to as process variables, reflecting the importance of evaluating the effectiveness of implementation distinct from the evidence-based treatment/intervention itself. Outcomes refer to individual- and/or system-level variables that reflect the target outcome of the evidence-based treatment or intervention (in fall prevention: fewer falls, fractures, hospitalizations, etc.). RE-AIM is a commonly used evaluation framework incorporating knowledge use variables and outcomes that recommends measurement of five key constructs (see Table 29.5) [54]. The RE-AIM framework has been used in multiple fall prevention implementation studies and applied in a number of ways, ranging from prospective, quantitative, and comprehensive approaches [55–57] to retrospective, qualitative and/or selective use of framework components [58]. Some of these studies are described in Table 29.7. With regard to research and evaluation designs for monitoring knowledge use and evaluating outcomes, much of implementation research to date is limited to quasi-experimental designs, as a whole and in fall prevention [56, 58]. While there are practical advantages to such approaches when implementing complex interventions in complex settings, there are recognized limitations in establishing causality. Moving forward, there are calls and increased work to encourage use of more rigorous designs that also account for the practical realities of implementation research in complex environments. These include stepped wedge designs where all groups receive the intervention but have a variable control phase and random allocation to timing of intervention commencement [59], which are beginning to be applied in fall prevention [60].

The final component in the action cycle is *sustain knowledge use*. Sustainability may be defined by five constructs, including following a defined period of time, the programme, clinical intervention, or implementation strategies continue to be delivered, and/or individual behaviour is maintained, activities may evolve or be adapted while continuing to produce benefits [61]. Sustainability is historically under-studied in implementation science [62]. A 2013 review exploring sustainability of community-based fall prevention programmes included 19 studies [63], and a few additional studies have rigorously evaluated sustainability since then

Table 29.6 Examples of methods to develop implementation interventions and description of components of implementation interventions in two fall prevention studies

First author	Year published	Methods to develop implementation intervention	Target population	Components of implementation intervention
Thomas [53]	2014	Guide for using TDF [77] was used to identify barriers and facilitators of practice change and identify behaviour-change strategies most likely to improve the identification and treatment of patients at risk of falls after discharge from the hospital; project governance committee was established and met monthly for 18 months to review and provide feedback on proposed interventions; the chosen behaviour change strategies were pilot tested with key stakeholders (physiotherapists, community fall prevention team, and consumers) and modified based on feedback	Health care professionals and organizations	Education sessions for physiotherapists on guideline recommendations and consequences of not meeting recommendations; development of a 'pathway' to assist physiotherapists to meet recommendations for identifying and managing fall risk; modification of an existing initial assessment form to include prompts for identifying and managing fall risk; development of standardized processes for high-quality handover at discharge; dissemination of patient education package [78]; 'Snapshot audits' of the intervention strategies over three months; outcome feedback provided to staff; establishment of physiotherapy department 'fall committee' responsible for ongoing sustainability of practice change; intervention processes incorporated into standardized operating procedures and made widely available; allocation of staff time to oversee identification and referral processes on an ongoing basis

| Sibley [23] | 2016 | Health professionals | Twelve-month multi-component behaviour-change intervention comprised of the nine behaviour-change techniques: (i) group meetings: seven interactive 60-minute group meetings including didactic education, hands-on practice, ongoing review of experiences concerns, troubleshooting, (ii) local champions: physiotherapist research team members who work to engage participants and foster through feedback, maintaining regular communication with participants, serving as a resource, providing reminders, and encouraging use of the test, (iii) health record modifications: reactive balance measure administration form added to health record to act as a reminder/prompt for test use and instructions | Guide for using TDF [77] was used to develop the intervention; 6 barriers & the the layout of this page should be improved facilitators to reactive balance assessment identified by physiotherapists were mapped by the research team to 8 TDF domains; relevant TDF domains mapped to 9 behaviour change strategies and informed selection of reactive balance measure to implement |

Table 29.7 Description of four fall prevention studies that monitor knowledge use and evaluate outcomes

First author	Year published	Study design	Outcomes
Li [58]	2016	Prospective cohort study within 48-week, single-group, pre-post design, and exit survey	Adoption: proportion of centres that agreed to participate by the total number of centres approached in the dissemination geographic area; Reach: proportion and representativeness of older adults who participated in programme; Implementation: project implementation costs and extent to which instructors successfully implemented three pre-specified programme protocol components (60-min sessions delivered twice weekly for 48 weeks, adherence to teaching and training protocols, class participation rate ≥75%; Effectiveness: degree to which fall incidence reduced and physical performance measures improved, and cost effectiveness; perceived improvements in balance, leg strength, mobility, intention to continue with exercises
Li [56]	2013	Monitor: Prospective cohort study within pre- post design	Adoption: proportion of providers approached who agreed to participate and proportion of participating providers who made referrals; Reach: proportion of individuals enrolled relative to total number of all referrals during study period; Implementation: extent to which instructors successfully implemented pre-specified programme protocol components: delivered twice-weekly 60-min sessions for 24 weeks, adhered to teaching and training protocols, participation and retention rates ≥75%
Roigk [55]	2018	Prospective cohort study, non-randomized trial	Adoption: percentage of eligible sites that adopted programme; Reach: percentage of eligible residents reached by programme; Implementation: percentage of participating sites offering fall and fracture prevention classes, percentage of residents attending fall and fracture prevention classes, percentage of residents owning hip protectors, percentage of residents using hip protectors, percentage of eligible sites that provided regular individual environmental adaptation advice, costs caused by programme implementation in first 18 months; Effectiveness: reduction in monthly falls frequency during 24-week programme implementation, change in limits of stability, stride length, walking velocity, functional reach, Timed Up and Go Test, Sit-to-Stand Test, and balance efficacy from baseline to 24 weeks
Day [58]	2016	Qualitative, semi-structured individual and group interviews	Compatibility, relative advantage, complexity, trialability, observability

Table 29.8 Description of some of fall prevention studies that that evaluated sustainability

First author	Year published	Study design	Outcomes
Li i [58]	2016	Six month post-intervention cross-sectional, observational follow-up and six-month post-intervention cross-sectional follow-up survey	Maintenance: proportion of centres that continued offering programme during six months following implementation period, and sustained participation by participating older adults
Li [56]	2013	A post-programme survey conducted with providers, follow-up survey for programme participants conducted three months post-intervention	Maintenance: clinician willingness to continue to make referrals after 24-week study completed and percentage of participants who continued exercises 12 weeks after programme
Roigk [55]	2018	Cross-sectional survey to examine availability of the programme, cross-sectional structured observations of programmes for fidelity, time-series design for incident femoral fractures	Maintenance: availability of programme in participating sites during follow-up, fidelity of exercise components in the fall and fracture prevention classes according to the initial protocol, and incident femoral fractures three to nine years after implementation

[55, 56, 58] (see Table 29.8). The factors most commonly identified as influencing sustainability of fall prevention programmes included financial support and participation, though it was recognized that many types and combinations of factors were described. While often considered as the last component in the action cycle, its cyclical nature prompts readers to consider and plan for sustainability issues during implementation planning. For example, in a 2016 study developing an implementation intervention for measuring reactive balance in rehabilitation settings, the authors explicitly considered potential for sustainability in selecting a measure to implement [23].

Advancing Implementation of Fall Prevention Evidence: Future Directions

As the fall prevention evidence foundation matures, research and practice efforts can turn to understanding, developing, and applying implementation processes for moving knowledge into action. It was beyond the scope of this chapter to systematically map and comprehensively appraise the nature of all fall prevention implementation research activity. The exemplars identified highlight burgeoning recognition of the need to explicitly focus on implementation of evidence-based fall prevention practice. Literature searching identified some gaps in the state of fall prevention implementation science which warrant discussion. First, multiple implementation studies that included fall prevention treatments or interventions that are not supported by systematic review evidence were identified [64–66]. This has important implications as implementation theory suggests that some fall prevention strategies currently being scaled up might not be ready for widespread implementation. Implementation efforts and resources should be directed at implementing interventions with a strong evidence base to optimize potential impact. Second, the lack of details provided in some reports surrounding the content of the implementation intervention [56, 67] limits advancement of implementation science. Finally, the absence of theoretical approaches or empirical evidence to select and tailor components of fall prevention implementation interventions may also contribute to sub-optimal impact and research waste. Although few studies met all inclusion criteria, this should not be interpreted as meaning that fall prevention implementation studies have been performed poorly. On the contrary, studies were encountered that implemented fall prevention treatments and interventions based on the results of rigorous knowledge syntheses [58] and used theoretical approaches [53], as well as those that provided explicit rationales for their selection of implementation strategies based on theoretical and/or empirical evidence [68]. A great opportunity for future research lies in merging the evidence base of implementation science with the evidence base of fall prevention. Doing so will offer the greatest potential for effectively moving fall prevention efforts into action while also rigorously advancing the growing field of Implementation Science.

REFERENCES

1. Fixsen D, Scott V, Blase K et al. When evidence is not enough: the challenge of implementing fall prevention strategies. *J Safety Res.* 2011;42:419–22.
2. *Knowledge Translation in Health Care: Moving from Evidence to Practice. 2nd Edn.* Straus SE, Tetroe J, Graham ID. (Eds.) UK: John Wiley & Sons; 2013.
3. Balas E, Boren S. Managing clinical knowledge for health care improvement. In: Bemmel J, McCray AT. (Eds.) *Yearbook of Medical Informatics: Patient Centered Systems.* Stuttgart, Germany: Schattauer Verlagsgesellschaft; 2000:65–70.
4. Tirrell G, Sri-On J, Lipsitz LA et al. Evaluation of older adult patients with falls in the emergency department: discordance with national guidelines. *Acad Emerg Med.* 2015;22:461–7.

5. Rubenstein LZ, Solomon DH, Roth CP et al. Detection and management of falls and instability in vulnerable elders by community physicians. *J Am Geriatr Soc.* 2004;52:1527–31.

6. Salter AE, Khan K, Donaldson MG et al. Community-dwelling seniors who present to the emergency department with a fall do not receive guideline care and their fall risk profile worsens significantly: a 6-month prospective study. *Osteoporos Int.* 2006;17.672–83.

7. Banerjee J, Benger J, Treml J et al. The National Falls and Bone Health Audit: Implications for UK emergency care. *Emerg Med J.* 2012;29:830.

8. Askari M, Eslami S, Rijn M et al. Assessment of the quality of fall detection and management in primary care in the Netherlands based on the ACOVE quality indicators. *Osteoporos Int.* 2016;27:569–76.

9. Said CM, Batchelor F, Shaw K et al. Preparing patients at high risk of falls for discharge home after rehabilitation: do we meet the guidelines? *Geriatr Gerontol Int.* 2016;16:570–6.

10. Day L, Trotter MJ, Hill KD et al. Implementation of evidence-based falls prevention in clinical services for high-risk clients. *J Eval Clin Pract.* 2014;20:255–9.

11. Lillevang-Johannsen M, Grand J, Lembeck M et al. Falls in elderly patients are not treated according to national recommendations. *Dan Med J.* 2017;64:A5418.

12. Estabrooks C, Derksen L, Winther C et al. The intellectual structure and substance of the knowledge utilization field: a longitudinal author co-citation analysis, 1945 to 2004. *Implement Sci.* 2008;3:49.

13. Rogers EM. *Diffusion of Innovations.* New York: Free Press; 2003.

14. Canadian Institutes of Health Research. About Knowledge Translation. www.cihr-irsc.gc.ca/e/29418.html (accessed April 2021).

15. Eccles MP, Armstrong D, Baker R et al. An implementation research agenda. *Implement Sci.* 2009;4:18.

16. Nilsen P. Making sense of implementation theories, models and frameworks. *Implement Sci.* 2015;10:53.

17. Jones CA, Roop SC, Pohar SL et al. Translating knowledge in rehabilitation: systematic review. *Phys Ther.* 2015;95:663–77.

18. Colquhoun HL, Letts LJ, Law MC et al. A scoping review of the use of theory in studies of knowledge translation. *Can J Occup Ther.* 2010;77:270–9.

19. Strifler L, Cardoso R, McGowan J et al. Scoping review identifies significant number of knowledge translation theories, models, and frameworks with limited use. *J Clin Epidemiol.* 2018;100:92–102.

20. Graham ID, Logan J, Harrison MB et al. Lost in knowledge translation: time for a map? *J Contin Educ Health Prof.* 2006;26:13–24.

21. Sibley KM, Bentley DC, Salbach NM et al. A theory-based multi-component intervention to increase reactive balance measurement by physiotherapists in three rehabilitation hospitals: an uncontrolled single group study. *BMC Health Serv Res.* 2018;18:724.

22. Sibley KM, Salbach NM. Applying knowledge translation theory to physical therapy research and practice in balance and gait assessment: case report. *Phys Ther.* 2015;95:579–87.

23. Sibley KM, Brooks D, Gardner P et al. Development of a theory-based intervention to increase clinical measurement of reactive balance in adults at risk of falls. *J Neurol Phys Ther.* 2016;40:100–6.

24. Grimshaw JM, Eccles MP, Lavis JN et al. Knowledge translation of research findings. *Implement Sci.* 2012;7:50.

25. Proctor E, Powell B, Baumann A et al. Writing implementation research grant proposals: ten key ingredients. *Implement Sci.* 2012;7:96.

26. Cameron ID, Dyer SM, Panagoda CE et al. Interventions for preventing falls in older people in care facilities and hospitals. *Cochrane Database Syst Rev.* 2018;2018:CD005465.

27. Sherrington C, Fairhall NJ, Wallbank GK et al. Exercise for preventing falls in older people living in the community. *Cochrane Database Syst Rev.* 2019;1:CD012424.

28. Tricco AC, Thomas SM, Veroniki AA et al. Comparisons of interventions for preventing falls in older adults: a systematic review and meta-analysis. *J Am Med Assoc.* 2017;318:1687–99.

29. National Institute for Health and Care Excellence. *Falls: Assessment and Prevention of Falls in Older People*. London, England: NICE; 2013.

30. Sherrington C, Michaleff ZA, Fairhall N et al. Exercise to prevent falls in older adults: an updated systematic review and meta-analysis. *Br J Sports Med.* 2017;51:1750–8.

31. Brouwers MC, Kho ME, Browman GP et al. AGREE II: advancing guideline development, reporting and evaluation in health care. *Can Med Assoc J.* 2010;182:E839–42.

32. Burgers JS, Fervers B, Haugh M et al. International assessment of the quality of clinical practice guidelines in oncology using the Appraisal of Guidelines and Research and Evaluation Instrument. *J Clin Oncol.* 2004;22:2000–7.

33. Levac D, Glegg SM, Camden C et al. Best practice recommendations for the development, implementation, and evaluation of online knowledge translation resources in rehabilitation. *Phys Ther.* 2015;95:648–62.

34. Sibley KM, Straus SE, Webster F et al. Moving balance and mobility evidence in to action: a primer in knowledge translation. *Gait Posture.* 2011;33:527–31.

35. Child S, Goodwin V, Garside R et al. Factors influencing the implementation of fall-prevention programmes: a systematic review and synthesis of qualitative studies. *Implement Sci.* 2012;7:91.

36. McInnes E, Askie L. Evidence review on older people's views and experiences of falls prevention strategies. *Worldviews Evid Based Nurs.* 2004;1:20–37.

37. McPhate L, Simek EM, Haines TP. Program-related factors are associated with adherence to group exercise interventions for the prevention of falls: a systematic review. *J Physiother.* 2013;59:81–92.

38. Meyer C, Williams S, Batchelor F et al. Enhancing adoption of a home-based exercise program for mild balance dysfunction: a qualitative study. *J Aging Phys Act.* 2016;24:53–60.

39. Zachary C, Casteel C, Nocera M et al. Barriers to senior centre implementation of falls prevention programmes. *Inj Prev.* 2012;18:272–6.

40. Damschroder LJ, Aron DC, Keith RE et al. Fostering implementation of health services research findings into practice: a consolidated framework for advancing implementation science. *Implement Sci.* 2009;4:50.

41. Kirk MA, Kelley C, Yankey N et al. A systematic review of the use of the Consolidated Framework for Implementation Research. *Implement Sci.* 2016;11:72.

42. Shaw J, Sidhu K, Kearney C et al. Engaging home health care providers in a fall prevention best practice initiative. *Home Health Care Serv Q.* 2013;32:1–16.

43. Michie S, Johnston M, Abraham C et al. Making psychological theory useful for implementing evidence based practice: a consensus approach. *Qual Saf Health Care.* 2005;14:26–33.

44. Cane J, O'Connor D, Michie S. Validation of the theoretical domains framework for use in behaviour change and implementation research. *Implement Sci.* 2012;7:37.

45. Michie S, Johnston M, Francis J et al. From theory to intervention: mapping theoretically derived behavioural determinants to behaviour change techniques. *Appl Psychol.* 2008;57:660–80.

46. Michie S, van Stralen MM, West R. The behaviour change wheel: a new method for characterising and designing behaviour change interventions. *Implement Sci.* 2011;6:42.

47. Atkins L, Francis J, Islam R et al. A guide to using the Theoretical Domains Framework of behaviour change to investigate implementation problems. *Implement Sci.* 2017;12:77.

48. Fervers B, Burgers JS, Voellinger R et al. Guideline adaptation: an approach to enhance efficiency in guideline development and improve utilisation. *BMJ Qual Saf.* 2011;20:228–36.

49. Hendriks MRC, Bleijlevens MHC, van Haastregt JCM et al. A multidisciplinary fall prevention program for elderly persons: a feasibility study. *Geriatr Nurs.* 2008;29:186–96.

50. Ivers NM, Grimshaw JM, Jamtvedt G et al. Growing literature, stagnant science? Systematic review, meta-regression and cumulative analysis of audit and feedback interventions in health care. *J Gen Intern Med.* 2014;29:1534–41.

51. Forsetlund L, Bjørndal A, Rashidian A et al. Continuing education meetings and workshops: effects on professional practice and health care outcomes. *Cochrane Database Syst Rev.* 2009;2009:CD003030.

52. Goodwin V, Jones-Hughes T, Thompson-Coon J et al. Implementing the evidence for preventing falls among community-dwelling older people: a systematic review. *J Safety Res.* 2011;42:443–51.

53. Thomas S, Mackintosh S. Use of the theoretical domains framework to develop an intervention to improve physical therapist management of the risk of falls after discharge. *Phys Ther.* 2014;94:1660–75.

54. Glasgow RE, Vogt TM, Boles SM. Evaluating the public health impact of health promotion interventions: the RE-AIM framework. *Am J Public Health.* 1999;89:1322–7.

55. Roigk P, Becker C, Schulz C et al. Long-term evaluation of the implementation of a large fall and fracture prevention program in long-term care facilities. *BMC Geriatr.* 2018;18:233.

56. Li F, Harmer P, Stock R et al. Implementing an evidence-based fall prevention program in an outpatient clinical setting. *J Am Geriatr Soc.* 2013;61:2142–9.

57. Li F, Harmer P, Fitzgerald K. Implementing an evidence-based fall prevention intervention in community senior centers. *Am J Public Health.* 2016;106:2026.

58. Day L, Trotter MJ, Donaldson A et al. Key factors influencing implementation of falls prevention exercise programs in the community. *J Aging Phys Act.* 2016;24:45–52.

59. Hemming K, Haines TP, Chilton PJ et al. The stepped wedge cluster randomised trial: rationale, design, analysis, and reporting. *Br Med J.* 2015;350:h391.

60. Hill A-M, McPhail SM, Waldron N et al. Fall rates in hospital rehabilitation units after individualised patient and staff education programmes: a pragmatic, stepped-wedge, cluster-randomised controlled trial. *Lancet.* 2015;385:2592–9.

61. Moore JE, Mascarenhas A, Bain J et al. Developing a comprehensive definition of sustainability. *Implement Sci.* 2017;12:110.

62. Greenhalgh T, Robert G, Macfarlane F et al. Diffusion of innovations in service organizations: systematic review and recommendations. *Milbank Q.* 2004;82:581–629.

63. Lovarini M, Clemson L, Dean C. Sustainability of community-based fall prevention programs: a systematic review. *J Safety Res.* 2013;47:9–17.

64. Fortinsky RH, Baker D, Gottschalk M et al. Extent of implementation of evidence-based fall prevention practices for older patients in home health care. *J Am Geriatr Soc.* 2008;56:737–43.

65. Sze PC, Lam PS, Chan J et al. A primary falls prevention programme for older people in Hong Kong. *Br J Community Nurs.* 2005;10:166–71.

66. Lohse GR, Leopold SS, Theiler S et al. Systems-based safety intervention: reducing falls with injury and total falls on an orthopaedic ward. *J Bone Joint Surg Am.* 2012;94:1217–22.

67. Gawler S, Skelton DA, Dinan-Young S et al. Reducing falls among older people in general practice: the ProAct65+ exercise intervention trial. *Arch Gerontol Geriatr.* 2016;67:46–54.

68. Waldron N, Dey I, Nagree Y et al. A multi-faceted intervention to implement guideline care and improve quality of care for older people who present to the emergency department with falls. *BMC Geriatr.* 2011:11.

69. Steckler A, Goodman RM, Kegler MC. Mobilizing organisations for health enhancement: theories of organisational change. In: Glanz K, Rimer BK, Lewis FM. (Eds.) *Health Behavior and Health Education: Theory, Research, and Practice. 3rd Edn.* San Francisco: Jossey-Bass; 2002:335–60.

70. Brot C, Skjøth T, Nielsen K. Faldpatienter i den kliniske hverdag – rådgiv-ning fra Sundhedsstyrelsen. 2006. https://www.sst.dk/~/media/1E493E28DB284605A110EEAF1 EAE0503.ashx

71. Australian Commission on Safety and Quality in Health Care. Preventing falls and harm from falls in older people: best practice guidelines for Australian hospitals. 2009. www .safetyandquality.gov.au/wp-content/uploads/2012/01/Guidelines-HOSP1.pdf (accessed April 2021).

72. Australian Commission on Safety and Quality in Health Care. Preventing falls and harm from falls in older people: best practice guidelines for Australian hospitals. 2009. www .safetyandquality.gov.au/wp-content/uploads/2012/01/Guidelines-COMM.pdf (accessed April 2021).

73. American Geriatrics Society, British Geriatrics Society. Panel on prevention of falls in older persons. Summary of the updated American Geriatrics Society/British Geriatrics Society clinical practice guideline for prevention of falls in older persons. *J Am Geriatr Soc.* 2011;59:148–57.

74. American College of Emergency Physicians, American Geriatrics Society, Emergency Nurses Association et al. Geriatric emergency department guidelines. *Ann Emerg Med.* 2014;63:e7–25.

75. van Der Ploeg E, Depla MFIA, Shekelle P et al. Developing quality indicators for general practice care for vulnerable elders; transfer from US to The Netherlands. *Qual Saf Health Care*. 2008;17:291.

76. Guideline for the prevention of falls in older persons. American Geriatrics Society, British Geriatrics Society, and American Academy of Orthopaedic Surgeons Panel on Falls Prevention. *J Am Geriatr Soc*. 2001;49:664–72.

77. French S, Green S, O'Connor D et al. Developing theory-informed behaviour change interventions to implement evidence into practice: a systematic approach using the Theoretical Domains Framework. *Implement Sci*. 2012;7:38.

78. Australian Government Department of Health. Don't Fall For It. Falls Can Be Prevented! www.health.gov.au/internet/main/publishing.nsf/Content/phd-pub-injury-dontfall-cnt.htm (accessed April 2021).

30

Interventions Reduce Falls, but What Is the Cost for Better Health Outcomes?

Jennifer C. Davis, Teresa Liu-Ambrose, and Chun-Liang Hsu

Cost of Falls

Falls and fall-related injuries among older adults represent a substantial health burden. Approximately 30% of older adults experience at least one fall each year, and half of these individuals fall recurrently [1, 2]. Fall-related non-fatal injuries are associated with increased morbidity, decreased functioning, and increased health care resource utilization [3, 4]. Fall-related injuries such as fracture account for 10-15% of emergency department presentations of those aged 65 years and older [5, 6]. With the number of adults aged 65 and older expected to increase to 1 in 5 by 2050, the economic burden imposed by falls is expected to increase proportionally [7].

Two systematic reviews [8, 9] have examined the cost of falls among older adults. One demonstrated that mean cost of falls ranged from USD$3,476 per faller to USD$10,749 per injurious fall and USD$26,483 per fall requiring hospitalization, with the total cost incurred by falls approximated to USD$9 billion annually (2008 US prices) [8]. The other systematic review found that fall-related costs of prevalence-based studies accounted for 0.85% and 1.5% of the total health care expenditures, and 0.07% to 0.20% of the GDP [9]. Higher direct costs were noted for women in higher age groups, fractures, and those living in residential care. Mean costs per fall, per fall-related hospitalization, and per faller ranged from USD$1,059 to USD$10,913, USD$5,654 to USD$42,840 and USD$2,044 to USD$25,955 (2006 US prices), respectively, with costs dependent on fall severity [9].

Since publication of these reviews [8, 9], a US study documented the economic burdens of fatal and non-fatal falls [10]. Between 2012 and 2015, the cost of fatal falls rose from USD$616.5 to USD$637.5 million while the cost of non-fatal falls rose from USD$30 to USD$31.3 billion [10]. The average cost of a non-fatal fall was USD$9,780 and the average cost of a fatal fall was USD$26,340 [10]. Costs of falls differed significantly by sex, age, and treatment setting (i.e. hospitalized falls were more expensive than other settings). Women aged 85 years and older accounted for 9% of the population but incurred approximately one-third of the total hospital-related costs [10]. This study provides additional economic evidence that the greatest potential to save money within our health care system is to prevent falls by targeting effective fall prevention interventions to high-risk groups [10, 11].

Effective Interventions Exist, but at What Cost?

Fall prevention strategies are commonly classified into three categories: (i) individually customized multi-factorial interventions [12], (ii) multi-component regimens targeting the same multiple factors to all participants [13], and (iii) single-factor interventions.

Two systematic reviews have examined studies conducting economic evaluations of fall prevention programmes among older adults [11, 14]. The more recent review included 31 studies that conducted economic evaluations of various fall prevention programmes [14]. Of these, 11 studies included a multi-factorial intervention, while the remaining 20 studies included a variety of single-factor interventions [14]. This review concluded fall prevention programmes are cost-effective for adults aged 60 years and older with home assessment/modifications (incremental cost-effectiveness ratio (ICER) <$40,000/quality adjusted life year (QALY)) and medication adjustments (ICER <$13,000/QALY) being the most cost-effective types of intervention [14]. Nineteen studies performed a cost–utility analysis (CUA) with QALYs as the measure of effectiveness. QALYs were generally derived indirectly using the SF-36 and the EQ-5D [15, 16]. Health care system and societal perspectives were applied with the same frequency (n = 13) [14].

The following criteria were adopted by the review to ensure comparability of the ICERs as well as the results of the CUAs and QALYs: (i) conversion of the ICERs to 2016 US dollars; (ii) a lower bound willingness to pay (WTP) threshold of $50,000 per QALY and an inflation-adjusted threshold of USD$100,000 per QALY, and (iii) no comparison for ICERs of CEAs were conducted with a threshold due to CEAs lacking a common denominator to permit comparisons [14]. Studies were categorized based on intervention type (9 exercise, 6 home assessment, 4 medication adjustment, 11 multi-factorial approach such as general education on fall prevention with exercise programme and environmental modifications, and 13 were based on other types of programme such as vitamin D, cataract surgery, cardiac pacing, and cognitive behavioural therapy). Briefly, for exercise-based programmes, the ICERs of CEAs fell within the range of USD$186 to USD$4,446 per fall prevented (injurious or not) and ICERs of CUAs fell within the range of USD$30,013 to USD$80,860 per QALY (six studies were cost effective above the USD$50,000 per QALY threshold); for home-assessment-based programmes, the ICERs of CEAs fell within the range of USD$548 to USD$5,313 per fall prevented and ICERs of CUAs fell within the range of USD$2,158 to USD$39,281 per QALY; the evaluation for medication-adjustment-based programme suggested it is generally cost-effective for older adults; for multi-factorial programmes, the ICERs of CEAs fell within the range of $1,666 to $125,909 and ICERs of CUAs fell within the range of USD$20,427 to USD$112,598 per QALY (seven studies were above the USD$50,000 per QALY threshold); for other programmes, seven studies were deemed cost-effective with nine studies above the inflation-adjusted threshold of USD$100,000 per QALY [14].

One reason that exercise was not deemed most cost-effective in this systematic review may be related to compliance [17]. Despite the efficacy of exercise interventions in preventing falls, adherence rates to such programmes are low. Most studies reported adherence rates of around 50% or lower [18-21]. In a prospective cohort study in a fall prevention clinic, adherence to a multi-factorial geriatrician-based fall prevention programme was found to be lowest for recommendations involving behavioural change such as exercise (58%) and lifestyle modifications (35%), and highest for factors requiring less behavioural change such as medication reductions, referral to a health care professional, and laboratory tests/investigations [17]. Hence, it is important to interpret the results of the economic evaluations with caution and with consideration of adherence rates to the various intervention strategies. Future research should evaluate factors driving adherence to provide targets for future intervention strategies.

The original systematic review of economic evaluations of fall prevention programmes among older adults living in the community demonstrated targeting high-risk groups provided the best value for money (i.e. prevented the *greatest number of falls* for the lowest incremental costs) [11]. Three programmes were cost saving in sub-groups of seniors: (i) a multi-factorial programme targeted at eight fall risk factors, (ii) the home-based Otago Exercise Programme delivered to people aged ≥80 years, and (iii) a home safety programme for those recently discharged from hospital, if delivered to participants with a previous fall. Of these three programmes, the home-based exercise programme in people aged ≥80 years may have the broadest applicability in that it is able to target the greatest number of individuals and thus provide the best value for money [11].

Trial-Based versus Model-Based Economic Evaluations

Trial-based economic evaluations (TBEEs) are embedded in the design of a clinical trial [22, 23]. Generally, measures to ascertain costs prospectively are used along with a prospectively collected quality-of-life instrument data, using instruments such as the Euro-Qol EQ-5D questionnaire [15] or the Short Form 12 or 36 [16]. A number of strengths are embedded into TBEEs. First, economic data are collected prospectively alongside an existing trial, making the addition of an economic evaluation feasible with minimal addition of resources needed for the trial [23]. Secondly, the roots of economic evaluation are embedded within the epidemiological tradition that regards randomized clinical trials (RCT) as a gold standard for trial design [23]. The RCT design that TBEEs generally accompany also enables the direct comparison of costs and outcomes simultaneously in the same target population [23].

Nevertheless, TBEEs are subject to bias, often secondary to the decisions researchers make when designing the concurrent TBEE. A number of factors make ICERs determined from CEAs alongside RCTs different from real-world ICERs. These choices include: comparator, types of cost items, outcomes measures, clinical relevance of outcomes measures, valuation methods for estimating QALYs, and perspective of the economic evaluation [23]. Some of these choices subsequently predispose the study to the following limitations: (i) the comparator used in the trial may not represent a real-world comparator affecting study generalizability, (ii) a non-representative participant sample that does not reflect the target population, and (iii) insufficient collection of data on health services.

One study examined the sources of systematic error (i.e. bias) that are specific to TBEEs as pre-trial bias, bias during the trial, and bias post-trial [23]. Pre-trial bias included: (i) overly narrow cost and outcome perspective, (ii) inefficient comparator bias, (iii) cost measurement omission bias, and (iv) intermittent data collection bias. During trial bias included: (i) invalid cost-valuation bias, (ii) ordinal ICER bias, (iii) double counting of cost and outcome bias, (iv) inappropriate discounting bias, and (v) limited sensitivity analysis bias. Post-trial bias included: sponsor/funder bias and reporting and dissemination bias (i.e. under-reporting null or negative findings). These biases underscore the importance of following guidelines for conducting and reporting economic evaluations described below.

Model-based economic evaluations (MBEEs) utilize existing literature to model cost-effectiveness of different fall prevention intervention strategies [22]. MBEEs include a number of strengths. MBEEs allow for population-level questions relating to the efficiency of implementing fall prevention strategies to be explored [24]. Within models, elements of both costs and consequences can be tested to ascertain which parameters are exerting the strongest influence on whether or not a fall prevention intervention will be cost-effective [25]. MBEEs provide researchers with greater flexibility in varying parameters such as time or age of the population models which provides answers to more questions [26]. For example, MBEEs allow for estimation of the costs and consequences such as health outcomes over a longer time horizon such as a lifetime horizon (i.e. 25+ years). Another benefit of MBEEs is that they can utilize published evidence for efficacy and effectiveness. In the systematic review conducted by Olij et al. [14], 12 of the 31 included studies utilized MBEEs, with half of these using a lifetime horizon.

A limitation of MBEEs is the heterogeneity of the study methodology in terms of cost item collections, perspective of the economic evaluation, the time horizon in which the original study was conducted, study sample, method of assessing health outcomes and QALYs, and analytic methods [22]. Given the variation introduced from this heterogeneity, modelling variation around key cost and health outcome parameters is critical. Lastly, it is important to be aware that MBEEs are often populated in part by data from TBEEs; therefore, risk of bias present in TBEEs transfers to MBEEs in these cases.

Of the two systemic reviews conducted on MBEEs of fall prevention interventions, the most recent one did not separate the results of MBEEs from trial-based economic evaluations [11, 14]. One economic modelling study examined the efficiency, using a Markov model, of a public health programme for fall prevention and found that the ICER was $AUD28,931 per QALY gained and the programme cost AUD$700 per person [24]. The cost-effectiveness of this programme was primarily driven by the cost of residential aged care and older adults' probability of falls [24]. Importantly, the parameters that drive efficiency for one study should be interpreted with caution, as these parameters are likely to vary by intervention type, demographics of the population studied, and the health care system providing the care. A decision analytic model was used to assess the cost effectiveness of a hypothetical home assessment and modification programme to prevent falls [27]. The ICER was GBP1,052 per fall prevented over a one-year period [27]. The assumed probability of a fall and assumed effectiveness of the intervention were key variables that affected the magnitude of the incremental cost effectiveness ratio. From these two studies, it is clear that intervention effectiveness is an important parameter to accurately estimate MBEEs.

Of the nine economic evaluations of fall prevention strategies, only two conducted a cost–benefit [28] or cost–utility [29] study. Beard et al. [28] conducted a cost–benefit analysis using people in two different geographic areas as the controls. Although the programme required a large budget, both comparisons yielded a net monetary benefit-to-cost ratio for the intervention of 20.6 to 1. Sach et al. [29] conducted a cost–utility analysis that provided estimates for QALYs using the EQ-5D. For this study evaluating expedited cataract surgery, incremental cost per QALY gained over the participants' lifetime after surgery was estimated at USD$23,273; this is within range of the maximum WTP threshold of the cost per QALY. To provide a basis for comparison with other chronic conditions, the ICER reported for aspirin in primary prevention of age-related cardiovascular disease was USD$14,355 [30]. Thus, providing surgery requires only an addition of USD$9,000 per QALY. Further, fall prevention studies that report QALYs are needed for comparison across health care interventions and health services.

Of the 31 economic evaluations (trial-based and model-based) included in the systematic review by Olij et al., approximately 33% of the ICERs with QALYs as outcomes were above the WTP threshold of USD$50,000 and just 14% were above the threshold of USD$100,000 per QALY [14]. With regard to the various fall prevention programme types, approximately 50% from exercise interventions, 50% from multi-factorial interventions, and 66% from other interventions were deemed cost-effective with ICERs greater than the threshold of USD$50,000 per QALY, for which an average of less than USD$2,000 per fall prevented (exercise and medication-adjustment programmes) and greater than USD$2,000 per fall prevented (multi-factorial programmes) were estimated.

Importantly, whether using TBEEs or MBEEs, all economic evaluations should follow the published guidelines for conducting and reporting of economic evaluations. There are several generalized checklists for economic evaluations for all conditions [22, 31]. In addition, one guideline addresses the challenges unique to economic evaluations of fall prevention strategies[32].

Methodological Limitations of Economic Evaluations of Fall Prevention Interventions

Measuring outcomes in economic evaluations of fall prevention interventions poses distinct challenges for cost-effectiveness and cost–utility studies. For CEAs, how health outcomes are valued matters. For example, the health outcomes should contain clinically meaningful units that can be translated into clinically usable and tangible information. For CUAs, there are challenges in valuing health outcomes using common metrics to assess health gains or losses more broadly. A commonly used metric for CUAs is the QALY. The QALY is a metric that attempts to account for both quality of life and time spent in specific quality states.

Some limitations for using QALYs as a measure of benefit in older people and in conditions such as falls have been noted [33] – preference-based utility instruments such as the EQ-5D and SF-6D may lack sensitivity in older adults who fall. The inherent problem with using QALYs as an outcome for a complex intervention may be due to the potential of such an intervention to produce multiple benefits for older people. This makes it difficult to determine the component of the intervention that proved most useful. Robertson et al. [34] have also shown quality-of-life measures are insensitive to change because trial participants' health state utility values were too high to see a change in published fall prevention studies, despite the beneficial outcomes of the trials. For example, the instruments used to estimate health state utility values that are used to calculate QALYs may have a ceiling effect among high-functioning people. Data indicate that participants who participate in RCTs are higher functioning than those who do not [35].

Future Directions: Methods Considerations and Evidence for Health Policy

Ultimately, the goal of clinical research is to inform policy decisions. Economic evaluation provides the missing evidence to link clinical research with health policy decisions, whether this be through maintaining the status quo, investment, or disinvestment [36, 37]. Economic evaluations provide a framework to guide health care decision-makers in how to most efficiently use resources allocated to health care. To adequately promote effective fall prevention strategies and lessen the burden of fall-related injury, it is essential to engage policy-makers by providing information on the value of population-specific interventions [36]. Although there is an increasing application of evidence-informed policy-making based on efficacy and effectiveness data, this trend needs to be broadened to a global scale for effective fall prevention [38, 39].

REFERENCES

1. Campbell AJ, Borrie MJ, Spears GF. Risk factors for falls in a community-based prospective study of people 70 years and older. *J Gerontol*. 1989;44:M112–17.
2. Tinetti ME, Speechley M, Ginter SF. Risk factors for falls among elderly persons living in the community. *N Engl J Med*. 1988;319:1701–7.
3. Davis JC, Dian L, Khan KM et al. Cognitive status is a determinant of health resource utilization among individuals with a history of falls: a 12-month prospective cohort study. *Osteoporos Int*. 2016;27:943–51.
4. Laurence BD, Michel L. The fall in older adults: physical and cognitive problems. *Curr Aging Sci*. 2017;10:185–200.
5. National Center for Injury Prevention and Control: statistics and activities. *Int J Trauma Nurs*. 1998;4:18–22.
6. Sattin RW, Lambert Huber DA, DeVito CA et al. The incidence of fall injury events among the elderly in a defined population. *Am J Epidemiol*. 1990;131:1028–37.
7. Wiener JM, Tilly J. Population ageing in the United States of America: implications for public programmes. *Int J Epidemiol*. 2002;31:776–81.
8. Davis JC, Robertson MC, Ashe MC et al. International comparison of cost of falls in older adults living in the community: a systematic review. *Osteoporos Int*. 2010;21:1295–306.
9. Heinrich S, Rapp K, Rissmann U et al. Cost of falls in old age: a systematic review. *Osteoporos Int*. 2010;21:891–902.
10. Burns ER, Stevens JA, Lee R. The direct costs of fatal and non-fatal falls among older adults: United States. *J Safety Res*. 2016;58:99–103.

11. Davis JC, Robertson MC, Ashe MC et al. Does a home-based strength and balance programme in people aged > or =80 years provide the best value for money to prevent falls? A systematic review of economic evaluations of falls prevention interventions. *Br J Sports Med*. 2010;44:80–9.

12. Gates S, Fisher JD, Cooke MW et al. Multifactorial assessment and targeted intervention for preventing falls and injuries among older people in community and emergency care settings: systematic review and meta-analysis. *Br Med J*. 2008;336:130–3.

13. Kempton A, Van Beruden E, Sladden T et al. Older people can stay on their feet: final results of a community-based falls prevention programme. *Health Promot Int*. 2000;15:27–33.

14. Olij BF, Ophuis RH, Polinder S et al. Economic evaluations of falls prevention programs for older adults: a systematic review. *J Am Geriatr Soc*. 2018;66:2197–204.

15. Dolan P, Roberts J. Modelling valuations for Eq-5d health states: an alternative model using differences in valuations. *Med Care*. 2002;40:442–6.

16. Brazier JE, Roberts J. The estimation of a preference-based measure of health from the SF-12. *Med Care*. 2004;42:851–9.

17. Davis JC, Dian L, Parmar N et al. Geriatrician-led evidence-based Falls Prevention Clinic: a prospective 12-month feasibility and acceptability cohort study among older adults. *BMJ Open*. 2018;8:e020576.

18. Arkkukangas M, Soderlund A, Eriksson S et al. One-year adherence to the Otago Exercise Program with or without motivational interviewing in community-dwelling older adults. *J Aging Phys Act*. 2018;26:390–5.

19. Findorff MJ, Wyman JF, Gross CR. Predictors of long-term exercise adherence in a community-based sample of older women. *J Women's Health*. 2009;18:1769–76.

20. Picorelli AM, Pereira DS, Felicio DC et al. Adherence of older women with strength training and aerobic exercise. *Clin Interv Aging*. 2014;9:323–31.

21. Picorelli AM, Pereira LS, Pereira DS et al. Adherence to exercise programs for older people is influenced by program characteristics and personal factors: a systematic review. *J Physiother*. 2014;60:151–6.

22. Drummond M, Sculpher M, Claxton K et al. *Methods for Economic Evaluation. 4th Edn.* New York: Oxford University Press; 2015.

23. Evers SM, Hiligsmann M, Adarkwah CC. Risk of bias in trial-based economic evaluations: identification of sources and bias-reducing strategies. *Psychol Health*. 2015;30:52–71.

24. Farag I, Howard K, Ferreira ML et al. Economic modelling of a public health programme for fall prevention. *Age Ageing*. 2015;44:409–14.

25. Eldridge S, Spencer A, Cryer C et al. Why modelling a complex intervention is an important precursor to trial design: lessons from studying an intervention to reduce falls-related injuries in older people. *J Health Serv Res Policy*. 2005;10:133–42.

26. Bradley F, Wiles R, Kinmonth AL et al. Development and evaluation of complex interventions in health services research: case study of the Southampton heart integrated care project (SHIP). The SHIP Collaborative Group. *Br Med J*. 1999;318:711–15.

27. Smith RD, Widiatmoko D. The cost-effectiveness of home assessment and modification to reduce falls in the elderly. *Aust NZ J Public Health*. 1998;22:436–40.

28. Beard J, Rowell D, Scott D et al. Economic analysis of a community-based falls prevention program. *Public Health.* 2006;120:742–51.

29. Sach TH, Foss AJ, Gregson RM et al. Falls and health status in elderly women following first eye cataract surgery: an economic evaluation conducted alongside a randomised controlled trial. *Br J Ophthalmol.* 2007;91:1675–9.

30. Pignone M, Earnshaw S, Pletcher MJ et al. Aspirin for the primary prevention of cardio-vascular disease in women: a cost-utility analysis. *Arch Intern Med.* 2007;167:290–5.

31. Husereau D, Drummond M, Petrou S et al. Consolidated Health Economic Evaluation Reporting Standards (CHEERS): explanation and elaboration. A report of the ISPOR Health Economic Evaluation Publication Guidelines Good Reporting Practices Task Force. *Value Health.* 2013;16:231–50.

32. Davis JC, Robertson MC, Comans T et al. Guidelines for conducting and reporting economic evaluation of fall prevention strategies. *Osteoporos Int.* 2011;22:2449–59.

33. Harwood RH. Economic evaluations of complex services for older people. *Age Ageing.* 2008;37:491–3.

34. Robertson MC, Campbell AJ, Gardner MM et al. Preventing injuries in older people by preventing falls: a meta-analysis of individual-level data. *J Am Geriatr Soc.* 2002;50:905–11.

35. Vind AB, Andersen HE, Pedersen KD et al. Baseline and follow-up characteristics of participants and nonparticipants in a randomized clinical trial of multifactorial fall pre-vention in Denmark. *J Am Geriatr Soc.* 2009;57:1844–9.

36. Bryant T. Role of knowledge in public health and health promotion policy change. *Health Promot Int.* 2002;17:89–98.

37. Mitton C, Donaldson C. Priority Setting Toolkit: A Guide to the Use of Economics in Healthcare Decision Making. London: BMJ Publishing Group; 2004.

38. Bowen S, Zwi AB. Pathways to "evidence-informed" policy and practice: a framework for action. *PLoS Med.* 2005;2:e166.

39. Buse K, Dickinson C, Gilson L et al. How can the analysis of power and process in policy-making improve health outcomes? *World Hosp Health Serv.* 2009;45:4–8.

31

Bringing It All Together

Stephen R. Lord, Catherine Sherrington, and Vasi Naganathan

The vast amount of literature on the many risk factors for falls and the various intervention options can make interpretation and implementation of the evidence difficult. This chapter overviews the research findings presented in previous chapters to assist the reader to integrate this information and use it to guide their own research and/or practice. It concludes with a brief review of select research issues that need to be addressed in the future.

Understanding and Predicting Falls

Falls occur due to a mismatch between an individual's physiological function, environmental requirements, psychological function, and behaviour. Falls become more common with increased age (Chapter 1). This is due to a combination of physiological ageing and deconditioning, as well as the increased prevalence of heath conditions and medication use. As with other aspects of ageing, the key issue is loss of intrinsic capacity and functional ability rather than chronological age [1]. A life-course population-based approach to understanding and maintaining intrinsic capacity and functional ability would probably prevent many falls but is difficult to evaluate in research studies.

Physiological Function

A range of body structures and functions are involved in maintaining the body in an upright position to undertake daily tasks without falling. The appropriate coordination of these structures and functions is crucial for safe balance and mobility (Chapters 2–3). To avoid falling, a sighted ambulant person needs adequate vision to observe environmental challenges such as uneven or slippery surfaces, adequate proprioception (awareness of where body parts are in space), adequate reaction time to respond to unexpected perturbations, and adequate muscle strength to extend the legs against gravity with spare capacity to enable a stronger activation to regain an upright position in case of a trip. Adequate coordination of these functions enables the correct muscles to be activated at the correct times with the correct amount of force to successfully undertake tasks such as walking and stair climbing (Chapters 2–4). Postural control (balance) reflects the successful coordination of these functions, so the role of the brain is crucial (Chapter 7).

Understanding and avoiding injuries from falling (Chapter 5) as well as avoiding falling per se is an important area of research due to the burden of fall-related injuries on individuals and health systems (Chapter 1).

Adequate cardiovascular and respiratory function also ensures oxygen transport to the muscles and the brain to enable these functions to occur. Diseases and medications may also have this impact. Balance control can also be adversely affected by acute medical problems such as infections, chronic conditions such as diabetes, and progressive conditions such as Parkinson's disease (Chapter 10). The impact of medications on successful balance control and falls varies according to dose, interactions, and metabolism but it is known that psychoactive medications are particularly associated with falls (Chapter 11). New technologies hold great promise for fall risk assessment and detection (Chapter 13) but added value compared to simpler approaches needs to be demonstrated.

Environmental Context

It is important to consider the interaction between the environment in which an individual is undertaking tasks and his or her physiological functioning (Chapter 12). An individual with a high level of function in the physiological systems crucial to fall avoidance is still likely to fall in very challenging environments. For example, sportspeople often fall during competitions and young fit people may fall while hiking or walking on icy surfaces. The key distinction is that an older person with impaired physiology may fall in an unchallenging environment such as walking across a room or have a fall precipitated by a seemingly minor environmental challenge. Health professionals should therefore seek to understand the context of falls reported by their clients.

Footwear (Chapter 6), aids, and appliances (Chapter 22) can change the person's interaction with the environment. Inappropriate footwear can increase the risk of falls. People with impairments in one or more body systems can also learn to compensate for these with other strategies such as the use of a cane for those with visual impairments or walking aids for those with insufficient leg muscle strength or poor postural control.

Behavioural Context

A person's cognition (Chapter 8), psychological state (Chapter 9), and behaviour are also crucial contributors to their risk of falling. People choose which tasks they undertake and how they undertake them. Behaviour is likely to be influenced by cognitive ability, insight, and level of support available. Some individuals with a high physiological risk of falling may be able to avoid falling by increased awareness and use of assistance when required. Individual variations in attitudes and behaviour may explain differences between measured fall risk and actual falls experienced [2].

Fall-Risk Assessment

As falls are not inevitable, fall-risk screening and assessment tools (Chapter 14) can help predict who will fall, understand the likely causes for an individual's falls, and guide the implementation of evidence-based interventions. It is important to note that many fall prevention trials have been targeted at the general population and do not involve fall-risk assessment so this assessment may not be essential in all contexts.

Preventing Falls

Interpreting Effect Sizes in Fall Prevention Trials

Randomized controlled trials with falls as an outcome typically compare the number of falls experienced by people randomized to the intervention group with the number of falls experienced by people randomized to the control group using a rate ratio. If there were the same number of falls in both groups, the rate ratio would be 1. A rate ratio of 0.7 means there were 30% fewer falls in the intervention group compared to the control group. Rate ratios are reported with 95% confidence intervals reflecting the certainty of the effect estimate, with a smaller confidence interval indicating more certainty. Trials also often compare the proportion of people experiencing one or more falls in each group (i.e. 'fallers') using a risk ratio. Similarly, if there were the same proportion of fallers in both groups the risk ratio would be 1. A risk ratio of 0.7 means there were 30% fewer fallers in the intervention group compared to the control group.

Single Fall Prevention Interventions in Community Dwellers

Exercise is the most commonly studied single fall prevention intervention. The 2019 Cochrane review of exercise for fall prevention included 108 trials and confirmed that exercise can prevent falls in the community in terms of the rate of falls (number of falls experienced per person) and the number of people experiencing one or more falls per year (proportion of fallers in each group) [3]. This review categorized exercise programmes as primarily involving different types of exercise according to criteria established by the European Union-funded ProFaNE group [4]. As not all exercise modalities were equally effective in preventing falls, the impact of different types of exercise was explored independently. This led to the conclusion that: (i) exercise that primarily targeted functional abilities or balance, (ii) exercise with multiple components (most commonly function/balance and strength), and (iii) Tai Chi were effective forms of exercise to prevent falls. Conversely, there was no evidence that strength training alone, walking alone, or dance prevents falls. These findings remain unchanged in the update of this review reported in Chapter 16.

Training of voluntary stepping to avoid a fall shows promise as a fall prevention strategy (Chapter 17) as do exergames, cognitive-motor interventions (Chapter 18) and behavioural approaches to address fear of falling (Chapter 19). These approaches can also be incorporated into multi-component exercise interventions recommended for all older adults by WHO Physical Activity Guidelines [5].

Several single non-exercise interventions targeted to people with particular risk factors have now been found to prevent falls in trials. There is evidence to support: (i) a multi-faceted podiatry intervention in people with disabling foot pain (Chapters 6 and 22), (ii) insertion of a cardiac pacemaker in people with cardioinhibitory carotid sinus hypersensitivity (Chapter 20), (iii) cataract removal in those with operable cataracts (Chapter 21), and (iv) gradual reduction in psychoactive medications (Chapter 20). There is also evidence that daily or weekly doses of vitamin D can prevent falls in those with low vitamin D (but not in an unselected population), that a GP-based medication review can prevent falls (Chapter 20) [6], and that replacement of multi-focal glasses with single-lens glasses can prevent falls in those who regularly walk outdoors (Chapter 21). Environmental fall prevention interventions can prevent falls in high-risk people (Chapter 23) and hip protectors can prevent hip fractures if worn at the time of falls (Chapter 24).

Multi-Factorial Fall Prevention Interventions in Community Dwellers

As a range of risk factors can cause falls, another common approach is to assess for the presence of risk factors and target interventions to the risk factors identified. It is difficult to draw conclusions about the optimal approach from meta-analyses of multi-factorial interventions as the many trials in this area have included a range of approaches and some studies have methodological issues (Chapter 25). Two examples of particularly successful multi-factorial interventions are from earlier trials [7, 8]. Tinetti et al. [7] found that targeting fall risk factors in a systematic way with medication adjustment, behavioural instructions, and/or exercise led to a 30% lower fall rate in the intervention compared to the control group. Close et al. [8] tested a detailed medical and occupational-therapy assessment for community dwellers who presented to an accident and emergency department with a fall, and found marked reductions in the risk of falling and of recurrent falls as well as significantly lower risks of hospitalization and functional decline. Other multi-factorial interventions have been less successful. Elley et al. [9] found a general-practice-based programme that involved a home-based fall-risk assessment by a nurse and referral to community services, and exercise where indicated, did not prevent falls (IRR: 0.96, 95% CI: 0.70, 1.34). There is some evidence that interventions provided as part of studies have greater impacts than referral-based programmes [10], presumably due to better adherence to interventions. It may be that intervention effects have become diluted over time as fall prevention interventions are more commonly applied to control groups.

Building on Exercise as an Intervention Approach in the Community?

It has been suggested that single interventions are as effective as multiple interventions at a population level and are cheaper to deliver [11]., and that tailoring to individually assessed risk factors may not be essential for multiple component interventions, i.e. the provision of more than one intervention to groups of people without screening and targeting can also be successful [12]. Given the importance of physical function as a risk factor for falls, an approach worthy of investigation is to provide exercise for everyone and add additional interventions to address risk factors not amenable to exercise intervention as required.

Preventing Falls in Hospitals and Care Facilities

Optimal approaches to the prevention of falls in hospitals and residential care facilities are less clear than in the community. In hospitals, multi-faceted programmes have been found to prevent falls in longer-stay settings but risk-factor screening interventions have not been found to work in large trials in acute hospital settings [13]. The most promising interventions focus on communication between patients and staff about the risk of falls and safe mobility on the ward, particularly when using the bathroom, where many hospital falls occur (Chapter 26).

There is evidence that vitamin D can prevent falls in residential care (Chapter 27), probably because vitamin D levels are low among residents. A well-supported multi-faceted programme from Germany that included exercise prevented falls [14] but this programme was not effective in other settings when rolled out with fewer resources (Chapter 27). A promising recent trial of an exercise intervention in residential care needs replication (Chapter 16) [15].

Making Changes and Justifying Them

Less is known about how best to prevent falls within complex health and community systems without providing additional resources. Advances in this area will be helped by understanding of behaviour-change principles as they apply to older adults and to health professionals (Chapter 28), as well as implementation science (Chapter 29). Trial-based and modelled cost-effectiveness analyses of fall prevention interventions (Chapter 30) can guide the choice of interventions as well as funding decisions by health policy-makers.

Future Research Directions

There is a considerable body of knowledge about the various fall risk factors and the effectiveness of a range of intervention strategies for the prevention of falls. Indeed, since the second edition of this book was published in 2007, advances have been made in many of the research areas suggested as priorities. However, as in every area of scientific study, the findings of one study often pose questions for another. In this final section, we present a brief review of select research issues that need to be addressed in the future.

Remote Fall-Risk Assessments and Fall Detection

Several studies have demonstrated it is feasible to monitor activity in older people living at home with wearable sensors. Applications developed for smart phones can accurately perform long-term activity monitoring [16], offering scope for automated fall detection and incorporation of remote fall assessments into clinical care. However, wearable fall detection devices are still not sufficiently reliable, primarily due to their inability to distinguish falls from other activities. The research into remote fall-risk assessments has likely reported overoptimistic results due to the considerable number of variables entered as putative risk factors, small sample sizes, questionable modelling decisions, and lack of external validation. In consequence, the derived models are unlikely to work well in everyday use and provide useful prognostic tools [17]. Future prospective studies are needed with designs that permit external validation.

Primary Prevention of Falls for Middle-Aged People

There is strong evidence that sub-clinical vision, sensation, strength, reaction time, and balance declines occur in middle age [18, 19]. Further, reduced strength in the middle years predicts greater declines in balance over time [20, 21], and an increased incidence of falls has been reported in women from the age of 40 years [22]. Except for trials aimed at preventing falls in people with neurological conditions, all fall prevention trials to date have been conducted in older people. Studies undertaken in younger groups could involve a 'postural stress test' that would allow the safe evaluation of an individual's ability to withstand a perturbation while walking. This could be supplemented with profiling of sensorimotor, balance, and gait performances and targeted interventions aimed at addressing identified impairments for the primary prevention of falls.

Reactive Step Training

As outlined in Chapter 17, reactive step training involves exposure to repeated slips or trips to generate rapid balance responses. Systematic review evidence from four trials indicates reactive stepping can improve balance recovery after slips and reduce falls longer-term by 48% in older people [23]. These interventions have required individual supervision and special treadmills or walkways with participants walking in a body harness. They have also been short term in nature, with the notion that such interventions have lasting protection against falls [24]. Reactive step training may enhance fall prevention programmes by addressing aspects of balance control (i.e. reactive responses), often not included in exercise programmes. However, further trials are required to ensure the benefits of reactive step training is an effective fall prevention intervention.

Psychoactive Medication Withdrawal

Psychoactive medications have been consistently shown to be significant and independent risk factors for falls, and in an early study, Campbell et al. found that it is possible to reduce falls by withdrawing these medications [25]. Subsequent studies, however, have not demonstrated success in preventing falls by reducing fall-risk-inducing drugs, with a recent systematic review involving 1309 participants showing that fall-risk-inducing drugs withdrawal strategies (mostly targeting centrally acting medications) does not significantly reduce fall rates (RaR: 0.98, 95% CI: 0.63, 1.51) in older people over a 6- to 12-month follow-up period [26]. Further work is required to identify alternatives to pharmacological treatment of sleep disorders and anxiety in older people. As benzodiazepine withdrawal has been shown to be difficult, strategies for preventing initial use of these medications would be important to identify. To be successful, such strategies would need to be an acceptable alternative to medication use by older people, their doctors, and other health professionals.

Medications for Fall Prevention

Only limited research has addressed fall-related risk factors such muscle weakness and poor functional mobility. Recently, the role of myostatin inhibitors has received attention. Animal and human Phase 1 studies have shown myostatin inhibition stimulates protein synthesis in muscle fibres, resulting in muscle hypertrophy, increased bone density, and decreased fat tissue – a combination considered to be truly a holy grail [27]. Further, a proof-of-concept randomized controlled trial in 201 people aged ≥75 years with muscle weakness and a history of falls has demonstrated that a humanized myostatin antibody can increase appendicular lean body mass over six months [28]. The myostatin inhibitor also reduced fat mass and brought about improvements in power-intensive performance-based measures (fast walking, stair climbing, and chair stands). However, the beneficial effects of myostatin inhibition need to be determined using primary outcomes such as falls and fractures.

Methylphenidate (used since the 1950s as a treatment for attention deficit hyperactivity disorder) has recently received attention with respect to its role in cognitive performance and control of gait. These studies have shown methylphenidate can improve executive function and gait velocity, and reduce gait variability [29, 30]. However, the short half-life of this medication and unfavourable side effects limits its utility. Nonetheless, similar agents with a longer half-life and more favourable side-effect profiles may emerge over time.

Acetylcholinesterase inhibition has also been considered to have a role in fall prevention. Donepezil, galantamine, and rivastigmine have all been investigated, with the largest and most recent trial examining the use of rivastigmine in 130 participants with mild PD [31]. Participants assigned to rivastigmine had a 45% fall rate reduction over the 32-week trial period, and at the end of the trial had improved step time variability for normal and dual-task walking compared with participants assigned to placebo. A Phase 3 study is currently underway to determine if these promising findings can be confirmed.

Cognitive-Motor Interventions

Cognitive-motor training involves a combination of physical and cognitive tasks, often reflecting the multi-task nature of daily activities. Interactive, exercise-based videogames (exergames) combine player movement, enjoyment, and performance feedback, and, as outlined in Chapter 18, may comprise an effective means for delivering cognitive-motor exercise. A systematic review of 37 trials investigating the efficacy of exergames for addressing fall risk in older people found most trials were of a pilot nature with many containing methodological limitations [32]. Nonetheless, most reported that exergame training improved physical (e.g. balance and strength) and cognitive (e.g. attention, executive function) measures and were of equal efficacy in reducing fall risk as traditional training programmes. Adequately powered studies are now required, comparing cognitive-motor training to appropriate controls to establish definitive evidence for the effects of cognitive-motor interventions for preventing falls in older people.

Fall Prevention in People at High Risk of Falls

Further research is needed to establish optimal approaches to fall prevention in clinical groups with balance impairments (e.g. stroke, frailty, dementia), and older people after hospital discharge, and while in hospital and residential care settings. The effectiveness and cost-effectiveness of the delivery of fall prevention interventions in the context of usual health services also requires more investigation.

Behaviour Change

Behaviour of individual older adults, their caregivers, and health professionals are crucial for fall avoidance and adoption of fall prevention interventions. It is now understood that there is more to behaviour change than giving information or instructions. Behaviours are influenced by many individual and systems factors. This understanding now needs to be more systematically applied to the development and evaluation of fall prevention interventions.

Fall Prevention in Low- and Middle-Income Settings

There is an urgent need to explore fall prevention interventions in low- and middle-income settings, as the majority of the studies to date have been undertaken in higher-income countries [33]. It is likely that the main principles behind fall prevention strategies such as exercise will apply across countries, but the design and delivery of programmes will need refinement to ensure the programmes are acceptable in different settings. Health service interventions designed in high-income countries are unlikely to be broadly relevant to low- and middle-income settings.

Implementation of Effective Fall Prevention Intervention

More work needs to be undertaken to maximize the uptake of interventions that have been shown to be successful. Research now needs to establish the most effective approaches to implementation. For example, participation by community-living older people in the types of exercise found to prevent falls is limited. Strategies to address this important evidence-to-implementation gap, may include health professionals encouraging their clients to be more active, systems to support health professionals to refer patients to suitable community exercise opportunities, and support of community organizations to deliver suitable exercise opportunities. These approaches require investigation in research studies.

Fall Injury Prevention in the Community

Much more is known about the prevention of falls than the prevention of fall-related injuries. There is an urgent need to explore the impact of fall prevention interventions on falls requiring medical attention, fractures, and brain injuries. Cochrane reviews [3] highlight the importance of attention to the design of studies, as many included studies had design features that increased the risk of bias. Two recent large trials of implementation of fall prevention interventions into community health systems found no significant effect on primary fall injury outcomes [34, 35]. In both trials intervention adoption appears to have been sub-optimal. This highlights the challenge of delivering interventions in large trials (and in 'real-world' practice) and the need to distinguish between more controlled efficacy/explanatory trials and more pragmatic effectiveness trials [36].

Fall Injury Prevention with Compliant Flooring

Compliant flooring for fall injury prevention in residential aged care is attractive in theory, but evidence from a recent high-quality randomized trial found that the provision of compliant flooring in this setting did not reduce serious fall-related injuries [37]. Further studies are required to identify a flooring type that can effectively reduce injury while not causing problems with manual handling and meeting occupational health and safety requirements (as compliant flooring can make pushing furniture and people in wheelchairs more difficult).

Conclusions

Falls and fall-related injuries are likely to be major health care problems for older people for the foreseeable future. Consequently, the identification and implementation of effective fall prevention strategies will remain an important public health priority. Much has been learned about risk factors for falls and fractures in recent years, but further work remains to be done to fully understand the role of certain medical, physiological, psychological, and environmental factors in predisposing older people to falls. Currently, known effective interventions include exercise, expedited cataract surgery, podiatric interventions, occupational therapy interventions, and targeted multi-factorial interventions. Greater understanding is required regarding optimal approaches to multi-factorial interventions, fall prevention in hospital and residential care, behaviour-change strategies, cost-effectiveness of fall prevention interventions and fall-injury prevention. Further progress will be made if advances from new technologies can be successfully incorporated into fall prevention initiatives and if implementation strategies can be put in place to apply the findings from research studies to the broad community of older people.

REFERENCES

1. WHO. *World Report on Ageing and Health*. Switzerland: World Health Organisation; 2015.
2. Delbaere K, Close JCT, Brodaty H et al. Determinants of disparities between perceived and physiological risk of falling among elderly people: cohort study. *Br Med J*. 2010;341:c4165.

3. Sherrington C, Fairhall NJ, Wallbank GK et al. Exercise for preventing falls in older people living in the community. *Cochrane Database Syst Rev.* 2019;1:CD012424.

4. Lamb SE, Jørstad EC, Hauer K et al. Development of a common outcome data set for fall injury prevention trials: the Prevention of Falls Network Europe consensus. *J Am Geriatr Soc.* 2005;53:1618–22.

5. Bull FC, Al-Ansari SS, Biddle S et al. World Health Organization 2020 guidelines on physical activity and sedentary behaviour. *Br J Sports Med.* 2020;54:1451–62.

6. Gillespie LD, Robertson MC, Gillespie WJ et al. Interventions for preventing falls in older people living in the community. *Cochrane Database Syst Rev.* 2012:CD007146.

7. Tinetti ME, Baker DI, McAvay G et al. A multifactorial intervention to reduce the risk of falling among elderly people living in the community. *N Engl J Med.* 1994;331:821–7.

8. Close J, Ellis M, Hooper R et al. Prevention of falls in the elderly trial (PROFET): a randomised controlled trial. *Lancet.* 1999;353:93–7.

9. Elley CR, Robertson MC, Garrett S et al. Effectiveness of a falls-and-fracture nurse coordinator to reduce falls: a randomized, controlled trial of at-risk older adults. *J Am Geriatr Soc.* 2008;56:1383–9.

10. Gates S, Fisher JD, Cooke MW et al. Multifactorial assessment and targeted intervention for preventing falls and injuries among older people in community and emergency care settings: systematic review and meta-analysis. *Br Med J.* 2008;336:130–3.

11. Campbell AJ, Robertson MC. Rethinking individual and community fall prevention strategies: a meta-regression comparing single and multifactorial interventions. *Age Ageing.* 2007;36:656–62.

12. Hopewell S, Adedire O, Copsey BJ et al. Multifactorial and multiple component interventions for preventing falls in older people living in the community. *Cochrane Database Syst Rev.* 2018;7:CD012221.

13. Barker AL, Morello RT, Wolfe R et al. 6-PACK programme to decrease fall injuries in acute hospitals: cluster randomised controlled trial. *Br Med J.* 2016:h6781.

14. Becker C, Kron M, Lindemann U et al. Effectiveness of a multifaceted intervention on falls in nursing home residents. *J Am Geriatr Soc.* 2003;51:306–13.

15. Hewitt J, Goodall S, Clemson L, Henwood T, Refshauge K. Progressive resistance and balance training for falls prevention in long-term residential aged care: a cluster randomized trial of the Sunbeam Program. *J Am Medical Dir Assoc.* 2018;19:361–9.

16. Del Rosario MB, Wang K, Wang J et al. A comparison of activity classification in younger and older cohorts using a smartphone. *Physiol Meas.* 2014;35:2269–86.

17. Shany T, Wang K, Liu Y et al. Review: are we stumbling in our quest to find the best predictor? Over-optimism in sensor-based models for predicting falls in older adults. *Healthc Technol Lett.* 2015;2:79–88.

18. Low Choy NL, Brauer SG, Nitz JC. Age-related changes in strength and somatosensation during midlife: rationale for targeted preventive intervention programs. *Ann NY Acad Sci.* 2007;1114:180–93.

19. Choy NL, Brauer S, Nitz J. Linking stability to demographics, strength and sensory system function in women over 40 to support pre-emptive preventive intervention. *Climacteric.* 2008;11:144–54.

20. Wu F, Callisaya M, Wills K et al. Both baseline and change in lower limb muscle strength in younger women are independent predictors of balance in middle age: a 12-year population-based prospective study. *J Bone Miner Res*. 2017;32:1201–8.

21. Wu F, Callisaya M, Laslett LL et al. Lower limb muscle strength is associated with poor balance in middle-aged women: linear and nonlinear analyses. *Osteoporos Int*. 2016;27:2241–8.

22. Nitz JC, Choy NL. Falling is not just for older women: support for pre-emptive prevention intervention before 60. *Climacteric*. 2008;11:461–6.

23. Okubo Y, Schoene D, Lord SR. Step training improves reaction time, gait and balance and reduces falls in older people: a systematic review and meta-analysis. *Br J Sports Med*. 2017;51:586–93.

24. Bhatt T, Yang F, Pai YC. Learning to resist gait-slip falls: long-term retention in community-dwelling older adults. *Arch Phys Med Rehab*. 2012;93:557–64.

25. Campbell AJ, Robertson MC, Gardner MM et al. Psychotropic medication withdrawal and a home-based exercise program to prevent falls: a randomized, controlled trial. *J Am Geriatr Soc*. 1999;47:850–3.

26. Lee J, Negm A, Wong E, Holbrook A. Does deprescribing fall-associated drugs reduce falls and its complications? A systematic review. *Innov Aging*. 2017;1:268.

27. Buehring B, Binkley N. Myostatin: the holy grail for muscle, bone, and fat? *Curr Osteoporos Rep*. 2013;11:407–14.

28. Becker C, Lord SR, Studenski SA et al. Myostatin antibody (LY2495655) in older weak fallers: a proof-of-concept, randomised, phase 2 trial. *Lancet Diabetes Endocrinol*. 2015;3:948–57.

29. Shorer Z, Bachner Y, Guy T et al. Effect of single dose methylphenidate on walking and postural stability under single- and dual-task conditions in older adults: a double-blind randomized control trial. *J Gerontol A Biol Sci Med Sci*. 2013;68:1271–80.

30. Ben-Itzhak R, Giladi N, Gruendlinger L et al. Can methylphenidate reduce fall risk in community-living older adults? A double-blind, single-dose cross-over study. *J Am Geriatr Soc*. 2008;56:695–700.

31. Henderson EJ, Lord SR, Close JC et al. The ReSPonD trial: rivastigmine to stabilise gait in Parkinson's disease a phase II, randomised, double blind, placebo controlled trial to evaluate the effect of rivastigmine on gait in patients with Parkinson's disease who have fallen. *BMC Neurol*. 2013;13:188.

32. Schoene D, Valenzuela T, Lord SR et al. The effect of interactive cognitive-motor training in reducing fall risk in older people: a systematic review. *BMC Geriatr*. 2014;14:107.

33. Ng C, Fairhall N, Wallbank G et al. Exercise for falls prevention in community-dwelling older adults: trial and participant characteristics, interventions and bias in clinical trials from a systematic review. *BMJ Open Sport Exerc Med*. 2019;5:e000663.

34. Bhasin S, Gill TM, Reuben DB et al. A randomized trial of a multifactorial strategy to prevent serious fall injuries. *New Engl J Med*. 2020;383:129–40.

35. Lamb SE, Bruce J, Hossain A et al. Screening and intervention to prevent falls and fractures in older people. *New Engl J Med*. 2020;383:1848–59.

36. Sedgwick P. Explanatory trials versus pragmatic trials. *Br Med J*. 2014;349:g6694.

37. Mackey DC, Lachance CC, Wang PT et al. The Flooring for Injury Prevention (FLIP) Study of compliant flooring for the prevention of fall-related injuries in long-term care: a randomized trial. *PLoS Med*. 2019;16:e1002843.

Index